AF510763

Perspective Press

THE PHARMACY TECHNICIAN

FIFTH EDITION

MORTON PUBLISHING COMPANY
www.morton-pub.com

Morton Publishing

Fifth Edition

Printed in the United States of America.

Morton Publishing Company
925 West Kenyon Avenue, Unit 12
Englewood, CO 80110
phone: 1-303-761-4805
fax: 1-303-762-9923
www.morton-pub.com

International Standard Book Number

ISBN 13: 978-1-61731-070-6

10 9 8 7 6 5 4 3

Library of Congress Control Number: 2012952073

Cover design by Hannah Hogan; cover photo courtesy Elisanth_/iStockphoto®

NOTICE

To the best of the Publisher's knowledge, the information presented in this book follows general practice as well as federal and state regulations and guidelines. However, please note that you are responsible for following your employer's and your state's policies and guidelines.

The job description for pharmacy technicians varies by institution and state. Your employer and state can provide you with the most recent regulations, guidelines, and practices that apply to your work.

The Publisher of this book disclaims any responsibility whatsoever for any injuries, damages, or other conditions that result from your practice of the skills described in this book for any reason whatsoever.

Contents

Contents

Preface

The Pharmacy Technician and ***The Pharmacy Technician Workbook & Certification Review*** have successfully trained thousands of practicing pharmacy technicians and are officially endorsed by the American Pharmacists Association (APhA).

Features

This book has been specially designed and developed to make learning easier and more productive. It provides clear, concise, current, and practical coverage of a broad range of topics.

Each chapter begins with a **new Thinking it Through case scenario** and questions for students to think about as they read the chapter.

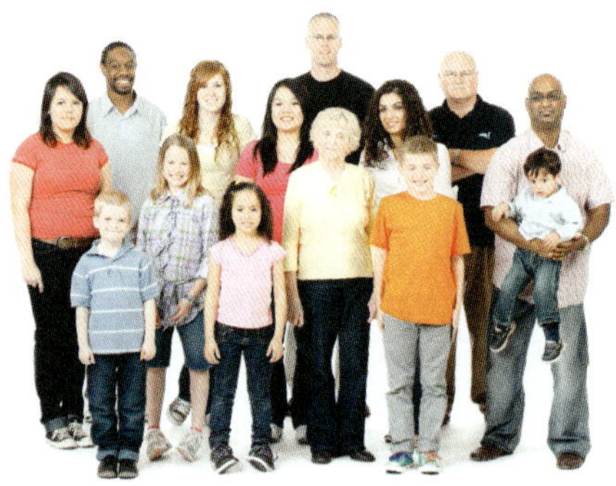

11

FACTORS AFFECTING DRUG ACTIVITY

LEARNING OBJECTIVES

At the completion of study, the student will:

- ✔ enumerate physiological factors that influence drug disposition and lead to variation in drug response.
- ✔ describe how common disease states can lead to altered drug response.
- ✔ understand common adverse drug reactions and that such reactions can occur in one patient but not another.
- ✔ describe the mechanisms of drug–drug interactions that affect the disposition of one or both drugs and result in either increases or decreases in therapeutic or side effects.
- ✔ explain the types of drug–drug interactions that do not alter the drugs' disposition but interact at the site of action.
- ✔ describe drug–diet interactions that alter drug disposition.

THINKING IT THROUGH

You decide to ask your family members how they react to a single 325 mg dose of aspirin when they get a headache. You know you don't have any problems taking aspirin, but it doesn't always get rid of your headache, and you end up taking some other drug like ibuprofen.

Your mom says aspirin gives her terrible nausea so she just doesn't take it. Your older uncle says he "almost died" when he took a dose of aspirin—he couldn't breathe and it felt like his chest was going to explode. Your dad says three aspirins seem to be the best dose for him, and that it works better with a cup of coffee. Your aunt is on warfarin therapy; her doctor told her to take only the 81 mg size of aspirin, but not for headaches—he said to take Tylenol® for headache.

As you read this chapter, identify which factors might be affecting each family member's experience with aspirin.

312 313

A distinctive **facing-page design** makes it easier to identify important points and make connections between concepts.

Illustrations are always on the same spread as corresponding text discussions.

The **topic sentence** for each paragraph in the major columns is in bold to emphasize the main points.

THE FILL PROCESS

Once prescription information is finalized in the computerized prescription system, a label and receipt are printed out.

At this point, the correct medication must be selected from pharmacy stock and the prescribed amount measured or counted and packaged. If the prescription calls for a compounded product, the technician must follow pharmacy policy in its preparation.

The pharmacy technician completes the fill process by placing the correct amount of medication into an appropriate container and labeling it correctly.

This includes placing the computer-generated label on the container so it sticks firmly, is straight, and is easy to read and placing the appropriate auxiliary labels on the container (see page 107). In addition, some medications such as oral contraceptives require Patient Package Inserts (PPI). Medication Guides (MedGuides) may also be provided voluntarily by some manufacturers. Both PPIs and MedGuides provide information on how to safely use medications and are part of FDA-approved labeling.

A pharmacist must check the final product and its label.

When finished with preparation, the technician initials the pharmacy copy of the label and organizes the finished product, prescription order, and the stock bottle that the medication was taken from for the pharmacist to check. The pharmacist signs off on the prescription via computer or by initialing the pharmacy copy of the label information, indicating the prescription was correctly filled. At this point the prescription may be released to the patient.

Rx safety you should know: common errors

Being aware that serious medication errors can happen is the first step in preventing them. Medication errors include, but are not limited to, dispensing:

- ✔ the wrong medication
- ✔ the wrong strength, dosage form, or quantity
- ✔ the wrong directions
- ✔ the medication to the wrong patient
- ✔ a medication on a forged or altered prescription

ISMP, The Institute for Safe Medication Practices, is an excellent resource for drug safety information. Visit www.ismp.org for a list of commonly confused drug names and more.

SAFETY CONSIDERATIONS

The technician should consider these factors when filling prescriptions:

Is the prescription for a high-alert medication?
High-alert medications are medications that are known to cause significant harm to the patient if an error is made. Examples of high-alert medications can be found online at http://www.ismp.org/tools/highalertmedications.pdf.

Are the instructions logical?
Are the directions, quantity, and strength typical for this medication? For example, is the dosing schedule q pm or prn? Does the Sig. read: 4 ml or .4 ml?

Are the directions clear?
Are the directions clearly translated in an unambiguously, avoiding any misinterpretation by the patient? For example, does "Take two tablets daily" mean "Take one tablet twice daily" or "Take two tablets once daily"?

Are there look-alike names?
Are there any look-alike drug names that could be confused with the intended medication? For example, did the prescriber write Janumet® or Sinemet®; Zovirax® or Zyvox®?

Pay attention to warnings!
When a DUR warning screen appears, such as a high-alert medication, a high-dose alert, or a drug interaction, the pharmacist must be notified as per pharmacy's rules—some pharmacies allow warnings to be printed for review with the final check, while others require immediate pharmacist review.

Check against the original!
During the fill process, always refer to the original prescription first and then refer to the label.

Don't add information!
Never add information based on what you assume the prescriber meant.

PRESCRIPTIONS 5

Rx tip

A number of drugs have moved from prescription-only to over-the-counter status. Many insurance companies have responded by agreeing to pay for select OTC medications with a valid prescription. Examples of over-the-counter medications that were previously available by prescription only are: Allegra®, Prevacid OTC®, and Zaditor® eye drops.

THE PHARMACY TECHNICIAN'S ROLE

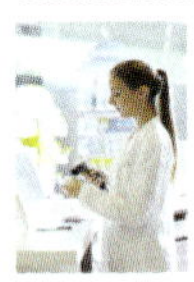

The pharmacy technician's responsibilities include:

- ✔ assisting the pharmacist in routine, technical aspects of prescription filling
- ✔ treating each patient, their personal information, and their medications with respect
- ✔ accepting new prescriptions from patients, obtaining all necessary information, and keying it into the computer in an efficient, and accurate manner
- ✔ alerting the pharmacist whenever a DUR warning screen appears while filling a prescription
- ✔ faxing or telephoning refill and clarification requests to prescribers
- ✔ consulting formularies and responding appropriately to third-party adjudication messaging such as: non-preferred drug, prior authorization or step-edit required
- ✔ quickly locating the correct medication for dispensing, calculating quantities, repackaging medication, and locating the corresponding patient medication guide
- ✔ compounding a prescription under supervision
- ✔ recording the dispensing of controlled drugs
- ✔ checking the work of other technicians, as instructed by a pharmacist
- ✔ referring patients to a pharmacist for counseling on the use of prescription and over-the-counter medications, or any other question requiring judgement
- ✔ ALWAYS ensuring the accuracy and safety of the prescription by incorporating quality control checks into every step in the process

THE PHARMACIST'S ROLE

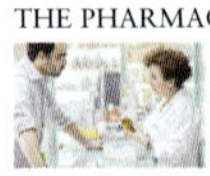

Photo courtesy catalina mas sebastian/E+/Getty Images

The pharmacist uses his/her expertise to ensure physicians' orders are carried out accurately and safely by checking that:

- ✔ the correct medication, strength, and dosage form is dispensed to the correct patient
- ✔ the directions for the patient are clear, accurate, and unambiguous
- ✔ the patient knows how to take the medication and how and when to refill it
- ✔ there are no potential problems with drug allergies, drug-drug, or drug-disease interactions. Information from DUR warnings are essential to this process.
- ✔ the patient understands the expected beneficial effects of the medication and any potential side effects the patient should be aware of
- ✔ the prescriber has been contacted regarding the prescription if appropriate
- ✔ the prescription has been accurately billed to the patient and/or the appropriate third party

In addition:

- ✔ only a pharmacist may counsel patients on the use of OTC medications
- ✔ only a pharmacist may receive telephone requests for new prescriptions

104 105

Rx Safety You Should Know notes and **Rx Tips** highlight safety information, indicate points of emphasis, and offer useful tips.

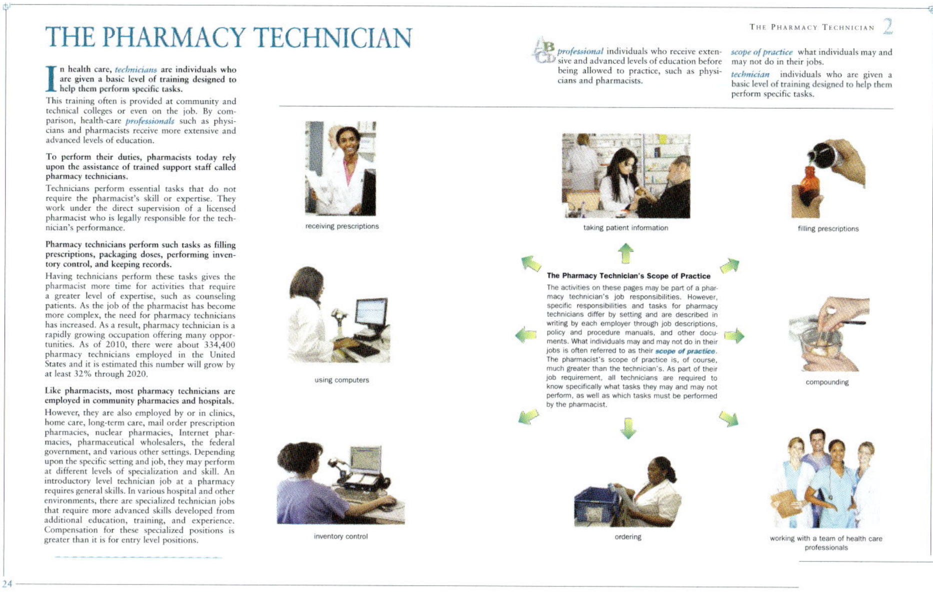

24

THE PHARMACY TECHNICIAN

In health care, *technicians* are individuals who are given a basic level of training designed to help them perform specific tasks.

This training often is provided at community and technical colleges or even on the job. By comparison, health-care *professionals* such as physicians and pharmacists receive more extensive and advanced levels of education.

To perform their duties, pharmacists today rely upon the assistance of trained support staff called pharmacy technicians.

Technicians perform essential tasks that do not require the pharmacist's skill or expertise. They work under the direct supervision of a licensed pharmacist who is legally responsible for the technician's performance.

Pharmacy technicians perform such tasks as filling prescriptions, packaging doses, performing inventory control, and keeping records.

Having technicians perform these tasks gives the pharmacist more time for activities that require a greater level of expertise, such as counseling patients. As the job of the pharmacist has become more complex, the need for pharmacy technicians has increased. As a result, pharmacy technician is a rapidly growing occupation offering many opportunities. As of 2010, there were about 334,400 pharmacy technicians employed in the United States and it is estimated this number will grow by at least 32% through 2020.

Like pharmacists, most pharmacy technicians are employed in community pharmacies and hospitals.

However, they are also employed by or in clinics, home care, long-term care, mail order prescription pharmacies, nuclear pharmacies, Internet pharmacies, pharmaceutical wholesalers, the federal government, and various other settings. Depending upon the specific setting and job, they may perform at different levels of specialization and skill. An introductory level technician job at a pharmacy requires general skills. In various hospital and other environments, there are specialized technician jobs that require more advanced skills developed from additional education, training, and experience. Compensation for these specialized positions is greater than it is for entry level positions.

THE PHARMACY TECHNICIAN 2

professional individuals who receive extensive and advanced levels of education before being allowed to practice, such as physicians and pharmacists.

scope of practice what individuals may and may not do in their jobs.

technician individuals who are given a basic level of training designed to help them perform specific tasks.

receiving prescriptions

taking patient information

filling prescriptions

The Pharmacy Technician's Scope of Practice

The activities on these pages may be part of a pharmacy technician's job responsibilities. However, specific responsibilities and tasks for pharmacy technicians differ by setting and are described in writing by each employer through job descriptions, policy and procedure manuals, and other documents. What individuals may and may not do in their jobs is often referred to as their ***scope of practice***. The pharmacist's scope of practice is, of course, much greater than the technician's. As part of their job requirement, all technicians are required to know specifically what tasks they may and may not perform, as well as which tasks must be performed by the pharmacist.

using computers

compounding

inventory control

ordering

working with a team of health care professionals

The fifth edition retains its highly visual presentation and offers **an updated art program** with many new real-world photos.

Illustrations are used extensively to provide information, reinforce text discussions, and show step-by-step procedures.

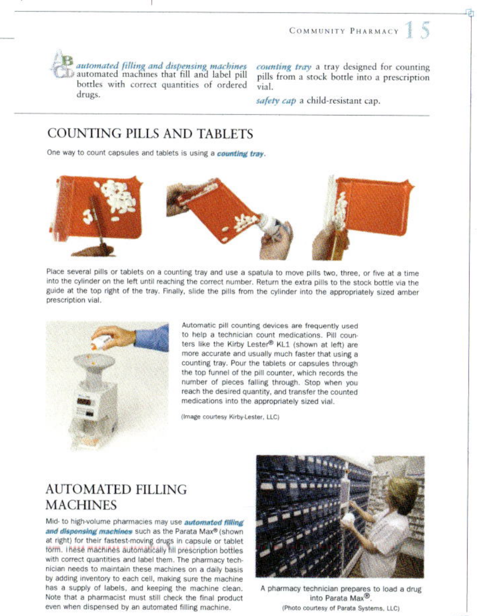

COMMUNITY PHARMACY 15

automated filling and dispensing machines automated machines that fill and label pill bottles with correct quantities of ordered drugs.

counting tray a tray designed for counting pills from a stock bottle into a prescription vial.

safety cap a child-resistant cap.

COUNTING PILLS AND TABLETS

One way to count capsules and tablets is using a ***counting tray***.

Place several pills or tablets on a counting tray and use a spatula to move pills two, three, or five at a time into the cylinder on the left until reaching the correct number. Return the extra pills to the stock bottle via the guide at the top right of the tray. Finally, slide the pills from the cylinder into the appropriately sized amber prescription vial.

Automatic pill counting devices are frequently used to help a technician count medications. Pill counters like the Kirby Lester® KL1 (shown at left) are more accurate and usually much faster that using a counting tray. Pour the tablets or capsules through the top funnel of the pill counter, which records the number of pieces falling through. Stop when you reach the desired quantity, and transfer the counted medications into the appropriately sized vial.

(Image courtesy Kirby-Lester, LLC)

AUTOMATED FILLING MACHINES

Mid- to high-volume pharmacies may use ***automated filling and dispensing machines*** such as the Parata Max® (shown at right) for their fastest-moving drugs in capsule or tablet form. These machines automatically fill prescription bottles with correct quantities and label them. The pharmacy technician needs to maintain these machines on a daily basis by adding inventory to each cell, making sure the machine has a supply of labels, and keeping the machine clean. Note that a pharmacist must still check the final product even when dispensed by an automated filling machine.

A pharmacy technician prepares to load a drug into Parata Max®.

(Photo courtesy of Parata Systems, LLC)

407

A **running glossary** defines all the key terms on each spread. **New** to this edition, **corresponding key terms are highlighted in *bold green italics*** where they appear in the text discussion to make them easier to locate.

Example—Flow Rate Calculation

Calculating flow rates can help prevent errors, decrease pharmacy waste, and help keep IV drips from running out before a new one arrives.

A medication order reads: Milrinone 0.75 mcg/kg/min; patient wt = 154 lbs. Milrinone is available as a premade IVPB with a concentration of 200 mcg/ml. Remember: 1 kg = 2.2 lbs. (wt = 154 lbs = 70 kg).

Question: How long will a 100 ml vs. a 200 ml ready-to-use (RTU) IVPB last?

Step 1: Calculate rate in ml/hr:

$$\frac{0.75 \text{ mcg}}{\text{kg x min}} \times 70 \text{ kg} \times \frac{60 \text{ min}}{1 \text{ hr}} \times \frac{1 \text{ ml}}{200 \text{ mcg}} = 15.75 \text{ ml/hr}$$

Step 2: Calculate how long the 100 ml vs. 200 ml bag will last:

100 ml IVPB	200 ml IVPB
$\frac{100 \text{ ml}}{15.75 \text{ ml/hr}} = 6.3 \text{ hrs}$	$\frac{200 \text{ ml}}{15.75 \text{ ml/hr}} = 12.6 \text{ hrs}$

Answer: In this case it may be more advantageous to use a 200 ml bag since it will need to be replaced only every 12 hours instead of every 6 hours.

A new design and step-by-step format for the calculation examples makes them easier to locate and follow.

FACTORS AFFECTING DRUG ACTIVITY 11

CRITICAL THINKING QUESTIONS

1. Why is it important to know something about the physical characteristics of a patient?
2. How can you easily distinguish between an adverse drug reaction and a drug–drug interaction?
3. Not all drug–drug interactions occur immediately. Some require days or weeks to develop. Why?

THINKING IT THROUGH WRAP-UP

Your mom says she doesn't take aspirin because of the nausea. Nausea when taking aspirin is a very common adverse effect. For almost all drugs that cause gastrointestinal adverse effects, nausea, vomiting, and diarrhea are the three most common reactions.

Since your uncle said he "almost died," either literally or figuratively, he might have been describing an anaphylactic reaction to the aspirin. If you wanted to confirm your suspicion, you could ask him how quickly the reaction came on and how long it lasted.

Your dad says coffee makes the aspirin work better. The most likely explanation is that the caffeine is adding to the pain relieving effect of aspirin through a potentiation drug–drug interaction. But the caffeine may also provide either an additive or synergistic effect. Coffee has been shown to decrease the absorption of alendronate, so a complexation interaction may also be occurring, which would explain why your dad takes three aspirins, instead of the normal two tablet dose.

Your aunt's doctor is advising her to take only small doses of aspirin because it has a synergistic effect with warfarin's effect of thinning blood. Tylenol® does not contain aspirin and so does not have that effect.

A **Thinking it Through Wrap-Up** section at the end of the chapter discusses answers to the questions in the opening scenario. In addition, an extensive Review provides a Key Concepts summary, Match the Terms exercises, Choose the Best Answer multiple choice questions, and **new Critical Thinking questions** with discussion-based answers in the back of the book.

Key Chapter-by-Chapter Changes in the Fifth Edition

This text has been extensively revised and updated throughout. Some of the more significant individual chapter changes are:

The beginning of Chapter 1 on *Pharmacy & Health Care* has been revised and reorganized to provide a two-spread narrative of the history of medicine prior to the "Medicine through the Ages" time line. A revised and updated spread on Pharmacy Today follows the time line, with a new discussion of Medication Therapy Management services.

In Chapter 2 on *The Pharmacy Technician,* the discussion of the PTCE is revised to reflect its new "blueprint" and nine Knowledge Domains.

The Regulation time line in Chapter 3 on *Drug Regulation & Control* is updated through 2012 to include the 2003 Medicare Modernization Act, the 2005 Combat Methamphetamine Act, the 2010 Patient Protection and Affordable Care Act, and the 2012 FDA Safety and Innovation Act. The chapter has new discussions of Patient Package Inserts (PPI), Medication Guides (MedGuides), and tall man lettering. In addition, an expanded discussion of Law & The Technician has a new section on Compounding: Federal and State Regulations and USP Guidelines that includes a discussion of the NECC tragedy. A new spread on Ethics and Compliance provides the AAPT Code of Ethics and discussions of basic values in ethical considerations, federal guidelines for compliance, and ethical/institutional review boards.

Chapter 4 on *Terminology* has expanded tables on root words and their meanings, expanded tables on common terminology, and new "Fill in the Meaning" end-of-chapter exercises.

Chapter 5, *Prescriptions*, has been updated to reflect non-paper transmission of prescriptions. It also emphasizes safety throughout, adding information on the The Joint Commission's Do Not Use List of abbreviations, Patient Package Inserts (PPI), MedGuides, high-alert medications, and tall man lettering.

A new design for Examples in Chapter 6 on *Calculations* makes them much easier to locate and follow. The chapter also has a clarified section on Alligations and revised discussions of Calculation of Children's Doses and Calculations for Business.

Chapter 7 on *Routes & Formulations* has, among its many revisions, a clearer discussion of aqueous and nonaqueous solutions, a new discussion of rapidly dissolving tablets, a clearer discussion of injectable administration routes, and a new discussion of Smart Pumps.

Chapter 8, *Compounding*, now comes before the more specialized chapter on *Parenterals: Compounding Sterile Formulations* (Chapter 9). It has a revised discussion of USP–NF compounding regulations and Compounding vs. Manufacturing. The section on Stability and Beyond-Use Dates now directly follows the section on Regulations. A reorganized and revised section on Equipment moves the material on Mortars and Pestles and on Spatulas to the later discussion on Mixing Solids and Semisolids, which is now two spreads and includes information on Electric Mortars and Pestles and Ointment Mills. The chapter also includes a new spread on compounding tablets.

Chapter 9, *Parenterals: Compounding Sterile Formulations,* has a reorganized discussion of Administration Devices which now comes earlier in the chapter since they are referred to throughout the rest of the chapter. The chapter also has a revised discussion of plastic bags v. glass bottles for LVP solutions, a reorganized discussion of SVPs, revised discussions of Clean Rooms and ISO Class 5 and Class 7 environments, and a reorganized spread on Working with Vials that includes a new section on Multiple Dose Vials and Overflow Volumes. The discussion of Quality Assurance & Infection Control now precedes the spread on Parenteral Incompatibilities.

Chapter 10, *Basic Biopharmaceutics*, has a clarified discussion of dose-response curve and revised, reorganized, and expanded discussions of Bioavailability and Bioequivalence.

Chapter 11, *Factors Affecting Drug Activity*, has a reorganized spread on Adverse Drug Reactions, providing more drug examples.

Chapter 12, *Information*, has thoroughly updated references, including web addresses.

Chapter 13, *Inventory*, has a revised and updated discussion of Automated Dispensing Systems, reorganized info on ordering, receiving, and storing controlled substances, and new information on 340B Drug Pricing Program.

Chapter 14, *Financial Issues*, has a new section on Coordination of Benefits, and new information on online platforms for Medication Therapy Management (MTM) and MTM-billable services.

Chapter 15, *Community Pharmacy*, has been heavily revised and reorganized throughout. Among its many revisions is an expanded discussion of disease state management and clinic services, along with a new discussion of MTM services, which is now in the opening spread on Community Pharmacy. A new spread on Regulations includes additional discussion of MTM under MMA, an extensive discussion of CMEA, and a new discussion of the Red Flag Rule. The Customer Service spread has a new section on Customer Satisfaction, Productivity, and Efficiency. The sections on Processing Prescriptions and Preparing the Prescription are greatly expanded with many new real-wold images and practical information for such tasks as using counting trays, automatic counting machines (Kirby Lester®), automated filling machines (Parata Max®), and Fillmaster®.

In Chapter 16 on *Hospital Pharmacy,* the sections on Organization of Medications and on Unit Dose System now precede the section on Sterile Products. An expanded section on Technician Roles now has two spreads, with many new photographs. The chapter also has new coverage of REMS (Risk Evaluation and Mitigation Strategy). As in Chapter 6, a new design for the worked examples make them much easier to follow.

Chapter 17, *Other Environments,* has a new spread on Nuclear Pharmacy.

Chapter 18, *Common Drugs & Their Uses,* updates the drugs in text and tables throughout and provides 10 new sets of drill exercises for matching brand and generic drugs.

Companion Workbook

The Pharmacy Technician Workbook and Certification Review, Fifth Edition offers hundreds of carefully explained key terms and concepts, over 1,000 exercises and problems for self-testing, *In the Workplace* sample documents and job-related information, and lists of the top 200 brand name drugs cross-referenced with corresponding generic names and classifications, the top 200 brand name drugs by classification, the top generic drugs by classification, the top 50 Canadian drugs, and commonly refrigerated drugs. New to the fifth edition are 15 labs with exercises to provide hands-on activities to enhance learning. This workbook can be used in preparation for national certification exams such as the Pharmacy Technician Certification Exam (PTCE) and the Exam for Certification of Pharmacy Technicians (ExCPT). It provides two certification practice exams, one in the format of the PTCE and one in the format of the ExCPT, both of which have been revised as per their respective new exam "blueprints." In addition, the *Workbook* contains a Calculations Practice Exam for practice in solving quantitative problems on the certification exams. ISBN 13: 978-1-61731-072-0.

ACKNOWLEDGMENTS

CONTRIBUTORS

We would like to thank the following people for their contributions to this book. Aside from developing and/or revising their specific chapter(s), they have been a great help with the whole book from making suggestions to providing general, and often frequent, assistance.

Mary F. Powers, Ph.D., R.Ph., Professor, University of Toledo College of Pharmacy & Pharmaceutical Sciences

Mary developed the Financial Issues and Calculations chapters, revised Chapter 18 on Common Drugs and Their Uses, revised and updated Chapters 1–3 and 17, and prepared most of the lists of drugs in Appendices. In addition, Mary is the author of the Workbook accompanying this text. Once again, Mary has provided help and feedback throughout the development of the entire project, for which we are very grateful.

Robert P. Shrewsbury, Ph.D., R.Ph., Associate Professor of Pharmaceutics, University of North Carolina-Chapel Hill; member of the USP Expert Committee on Compounding

Bob developed Chapters 4, 7, 8, 9, 10, and 11, as well as the Appendix on Commonly Refrigerated Drugs.

Brenda Vonderau, B.Sc. (Pharm.), Director, Clinical Product Development, Catamaran

Brenda developed the chapter on Prescriptions.

Cindy B. Johnson, R.Ph., L.C.S.W., RxMentor Pharmacist, Humana

Cindy developed the Information chapter.

Steve Johnson, B.S., R.Ph., Meditech Lead Analyst, Catholic Health Initiatives

Steve revised the Inventory chapter.

Ruth Gilman-Duke, Pharm.D., Pharmacist, CVS Pharmacy

Ruth developed the Community Pharmacy chapter and helped provide many photographs used throughout the book.

Pamela Nicoski-Lenaghan, Pharm.D., BCPS, Clinical Pharmacist, Loyola University Medical Center, and Britta Young, Pharm.D., Clinical Pharmacist, Ann & Robert H. Lurie Children's Hospital of Chicago

Pamela and Britta developed the Hospital Pharmacy chapter, including providing extensive photography.

Melanie V. Duhaine, R.N., B.S.N., M.Ed., Director of Nursing, Fairchild Manor, Senior-Associates of Western New York

Melanie developed what was the Classifications Appendix for the first three editions.

REVIEWERS

In addition we would like to thank the following reviewers who provided feedback on the previous editions, which we used to help prepare the fifth edition: James Austin, R.N., B.S.N., CPhT, Program Chair, Pharmacy Technology Program, Weatherford College; Ashley Bures, CVS; CVS Pharmacy; Marisa Fetzer, Institute of Technology; Claudia Johnson, M.S.N., R.N.C., A.P.N., Allied Health Instructor, Pharmacy Technician Program, Polytech Adult Education; Mary Anna Marshall, CPhT, Instructor for PTCB Examination Review, CVS/Pharmacy Regional Intern Coordinator, and Teacher in the Pharmacy Technician Program, Hanover High School; Russell C. McGuire, Ph.D., Vice President of Allied Health Programs, Education Corporation of America; Tony David Ornelas, CPhT; Alexandria Zarrina Ostowari, Course Developer, Allied Business School; Becky Schonscheck, Director of Curriculum Development, Anthem Education Group; Jacqueline T.

Smith R.N., CPhT, Department Chair–Pharmacy Technician, National College; Peter E. Vonderau, Sr., R.Ph., Pharmacy Manager, Scolari's Food & Drug, Inc.; Walgreen Co.; and Deborah Zenzal R.N., M.S., CPC CCS-P RMA, Department Chair, Allied Health, Penn Foster Schools.

Image Credits

We gratefully acknowledge permission to use the following images:

Chapter One: Page 2 and page 15, top middle, Stuart Rayner Photography/iStockphoto®; page 7, Alex Raths/iStockphoto®; page 12, Steve Cole/Christie & Cole Studio, Inc./iStockpoto®; page 13, Mark Bowden/bowdenimages/iStockphoto®; page 14, Christopher Futcher/Kaspi - Kilikpela's Aperture Studio Photography, Inc./iStockphoto®; page 15, top left, Kali Nine, LLC/iStockphoto®; page 15, middle, photo courtesy Dell, Inc.; page 15, lower, Christian Martínez Kempin/iStockphoto®.

Chapter Two: Pages 22 and 27, stokkete/iStockphoto®; page 24, top, Sean Locke/Digital Planet Design/iStockphoto®; page 25, top left, Mustafa Arican/iStockphoto®; page 25, lower right, Kali Nine, LLC/iStockphoto®; page 26, Christopher Futcher/Kaspi - Kilikpela's Aperture Studio Photography, Inc./iStockphoto®; page 28, Hanson Ng/Design Pics/Getty Images.

Chapter Three: Page 38, Jeremy Edwards/iStockphoto®; page 42, Christopher Futcher/Kaspi - Kilikpela's Aperture Studio Photography, Inc./iStockphoto®; page 48, Endocet® label and stock bottle courtesy Endo Pharmaceuticals, Inc.; page 51, Diazepam label reprinted with permission of Mylan Pharmaceuticals, Inc. All rights reserved.; page 51, Endocet® stock bottle courtesy Endo Pharmaceuticals, Inc.; page 58, Christian Martínez Kempin/iStockphoto®; page 60, Mustafa Arican/iStockphoto®.

Chapter Five: Page 96 and page 99, lower middle, Sean Locke/Digital Planet Design/iStockphoto®; page 98, middle, and page 105, lower, Catalina Mas Sebastian/E+/Getty Images; page 98, lower, Steve Debenport Imagery/iStockphoto®; page 99, middle top, Steve Cole/Christie & Cole Studio, Inc./iStockpoto®; page 99, lower left, VisualPhotos.com; page 100, clock courtesy the Florida Center for Instructional Technology; page 105, top, stokkete/iStockphoto®; page 106, lower, Mustafa Arican/iStockphoto®; page 107, Sean Locke/Digital Planet Design/iStockphoto®.

Chapter Six: Page 118, Keith Brofsky/Photodisc/Getty Images; page 158, Christopher Futcher/Kaspi - Kilikpela's Aperture Studio Photography, Inc./iStockphoto®.

Chapter Seven: Page 197, lower middle, ADVAIR DISKUS® 250/50 inhalation device copyright GlaxoSmithKline. Used with permission.; page 199, CLEAN & CLEAR® and PERSA-GEL® are registered trademarks of Johnson & Johnson. Used with permission.; page 201, lower right, NuvaRing® image reproduced with permission of MSD Oss B.V., a subsidiary of Merck & Co., Inc., Whitehouse Station, New Jersey, USA. All rights reserved.

Chapter Eight: Pages 208 and 212, BSIP/Universal Images Group/Getty Images; page 210, left, Christopher Futcher/Kaspi - Kilikpela's Aperture Studio Photography, Inc./iStockphoto®; page 210, right, McIninch/iStockphoto®; page 211, savaskeskiner, www.istavrit.biz/iStockphoto®; page 229, right column, middle, Unguator® image courtesy Unguator® Technologies; page 229, right column, lower, EXAKT 50 image courtesy EXAKT Technologies, Inc.

Chapter Nine: Page 261, Administration set and volume control chamber illustrations adapted from Figure 2.4 and 2.9 respectively in Hunt, *Training Manual for Intravenous Admixture Personnel, Fifth Edition.* ®Copyright 1995 Baxter Healthcare Corporation.

Chapter Ten: Page 290 and page 304, Floortje/iStockphoto®.

Chapter Eleven: Page 312, Christopher Futcher/Kaspi - Kilikpela's Aperture Studio Photography, Inc./iStockphoto®; page 314, left column, above, Cameron Whitman/Cameron Whitman Photography/iStockphoto®; page 314, left column, below, Christopher Futcher/Kaspi - Kilikpela's Aperture Studio Photography, Inc./iStockphoto®; page 314 right column, above, Johnny Greig/iStockphoto®; page 314, right column, below, McIninch/iStockphoto®; page 324, image courtesy the Florida Center for Instructional Technology.

Chapter Twelve: Page 332 and page 340, Hanson Ng/Design Pics/Getty Images; page 342, photo courtesy Dell, Inc.

Chapter Thirteen: Page 350, Adie Bush/Cultura/Getty Images; page 353, right column, above, savaskeskiner, www.istavrit.biz/iStockphoto®; page 354, 355, and 362, Endocet® stock bottle courtesy Endo Pharmaceuticals, Inc.; page 355, top left, stokkete/iStockphoto®; page 357, top, Parata Max® photo courtesy of Parata Systems, LLC; page 357, lower, Talyst AutoCarousel photo courtesy of Talyst; page 358, right, photo courtesy Dell, Inc.

Chapter Fourteen: Page 378, middle, photos courtesy Dell, Inc.

Chapter Fifteen: Page 392 and page 402, Francis Twitty, Pinmyst Studios/iStockphoto®; page 394 Mark Bowden/bowdenimages/iStockphoto®; page 395, top, Mustafa Arican/iStockphoto®; page 395, lower, Gene Chutka/iStockphoto®; page 399, top, Sean Locke/Digital Planet Design/iStockphoto®; page 400, Steve Debenport Imagery/iStockphoto®; page 407, middle, Kirby Lester® KL1 image courtesy Kirby-Lester, LLC; page 407, lower, Parata Max® photo courtesy Parata Systems, LLC; page 408, upper right, Fillmaster® photo used with permission of Fillmaster Systems LLC; page 408, lower left, QVAR® image courtesy of Teva Respiratory, LLC; page 408, lower middle, Lotemax® Ophthalmic Gel photo courtesy Bausch & Lomb, Incorporated; page 408, lower right, Clindamycin Phosphate Topical Gel photo used with permission of Pfizer, Inc.; page 409, lower left, VisualPhotos.com; page 410, lower, Steve Debenport Imagery/iStockphoto®; page 411, upper, Andrey Popov/iStockphoto®; page 411, lower, Steve Debenport Imagery/iStockphoto®.

Chapter Sixteen: Page 424, lower right, Mustafa Arican/iStockphoto®; page 427, lower right, Hanson Ng/Design Pics/Getty Images; page 435 and page 436, middle, images courtesy Epic Systems Corporation. Used with permission.

Chapter Seventeen: Page 460 and page 463, upper, Bruce Kluckhohn/TIME & LIFE Images/Getty Images; page 463, middle, Erich Spieldiener/iStockphoto®; page 463, lower, Mark Bowden/bowdenimages/iStockphoto®; page 464, McIninch/iStockphoto®; page 467, lower, Kali Nine, LLC/iStockphoto®.

Chapter Eighteen: Page 474, Nicola Bilic/iStockphoto®.

We would also like to thank the following people for helping produce original photography for the text: Kristi L. Bernal, Mary Dean, Sohrab Forouhar, Iris Johnson, Ryan Mignagaray, Nina Urbina, and Shannon Wetzel.

Finally, we would like to thank Ned Richardson for preparing all the new and revised in-text art, Hannah Hogan for designing and preparing the cover for the *Fifth Edition*, and Tamara Newnam for preparing art in the previous editions. At Morton Publishing Company, Rayna Bailey did a very thorough and helpful job proofreading the text and workbook, Joanne Saliger answered InDesign® riddles, Jes Haggerty took on the role of marketing manager, and Dona Mendoza and Chrissy Morton were, as always, very helpful.

Perspective Press

APhA

American Pharmacists Association

Basic Pharmacy and Pharmacology Series

Dear Student or Instructor,

The American Pharmacists Association (APhA), the national professional society of pharmacists in the United States, and Morton Publishing Company, a publisher of educational texts and training materials in health care, are pleased to present this outstanding textbook, *The Pharmacy Technician, Fifth Edition*. It is one of a series of distinctive texts and training materials for basic pharmacy and pharmacology training published under this banner: *American Pharmacists Association Basic Pharmacy and Pharmacology Series*.

Each book in the series is oriented toward developing an understanding of fundamental concepts. In addition, each text presents applied and practical information on the skills necessary to function effectively in positions such as technicians and medical assistants who work with medications and whose role in health care is increasingly important. Each of the books in the series uses a visual design to enhance understanding and ease of use and is accompanied by various instructional support materials. We think you will find them valuable training tools.

The American Pharmacists Association and Morton Publishing thank you for using this book and invite you to look at other titles in this series, which are listed below.

Thomas E. Menighan, BSPharm, MBA
Executive Vice President
Chief Executive Officer
American Pharmacists Association

Douglas N. Morton
President
Morton Publishing Company

Titles in this series:

The Pharmacy Technician, Fifth Edition
The Pharmacy Technician Workbook and Certification Review, Fifth Edition
Medication Workbook for Pharmacy Technicians: A Pharmacology Primer

THE
PHARMACY TECHNICIAN
Fifth Edition

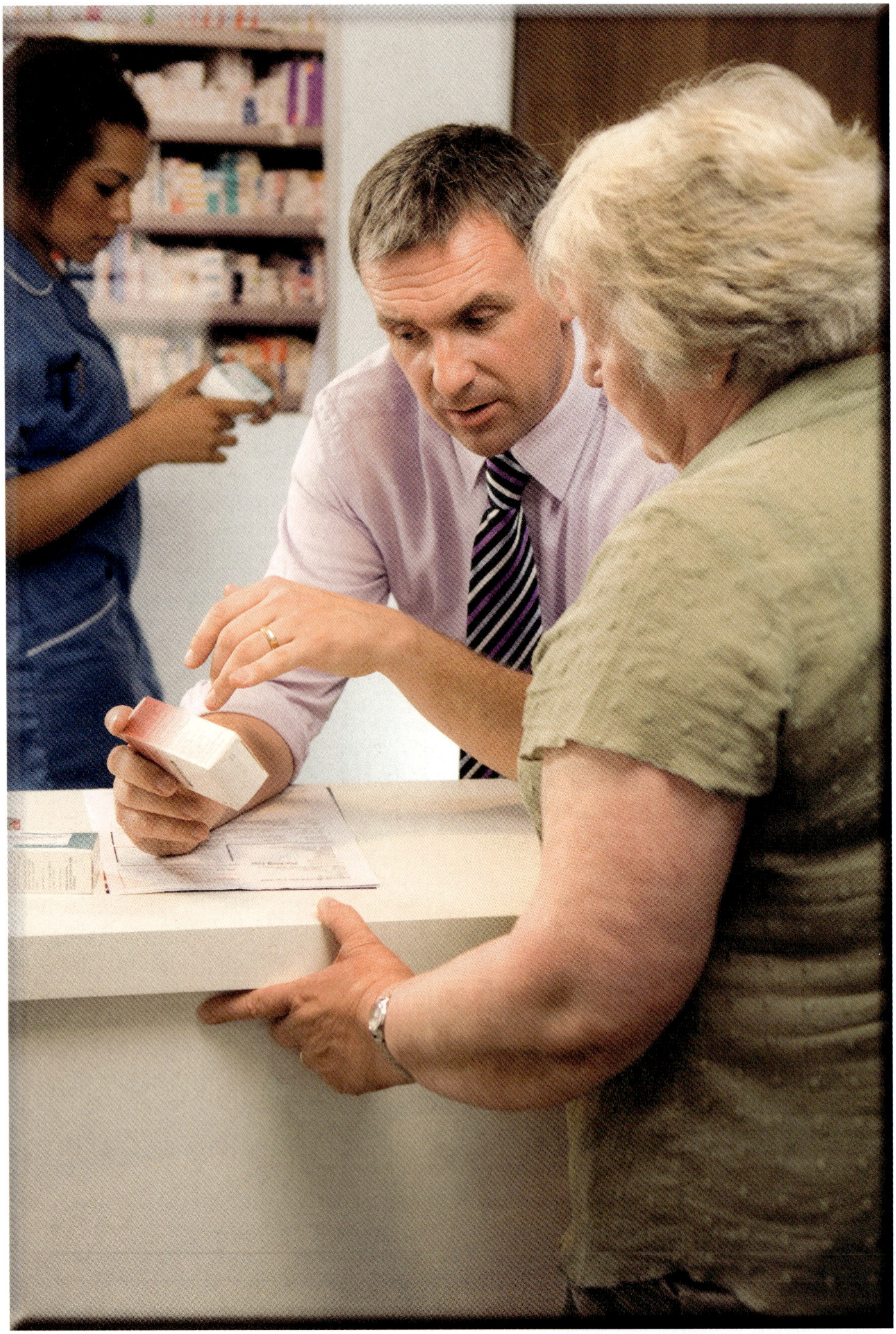

1

PHARMACY & HEALTH CARE

LEARNING OBJECTIVES

At the completion of study, the student will:

- ✔ be familiar with the history of pharmacy from ancient times through today.
- ✔ have an overall understanding of the pharmacy profession as well as the settings and economic environment in which it operates.
- ✔ have a general understanding of how computers are used in pharmacy.

THINKING IT THROUGH

Sarah and fifteen of her coworkers were recently laid off from a local tire company where Sarah had worked for 10 years. The company has shifted much of its operations oversees and it is not likely she will be called back to work. The employees who were laid off were given a severance package as well as payment to train for a new career at the local community college. After meeting with a career counselor to help find the type of training she would find most rewarding, Sarah decided she would like to pursue a career in health care, possibly as a pharmacy technician.

As you read this chapter, keep in mind the following questions:

1. What are some reasons for pursuing a career in health care, and in particular as a pharmacy technician?
2. What are some of the primary environments today for employment as a pharmacy technician?

FROM MEDICINE'S ORIGINS ...

Our knowledge of medicine through the ages goes back thousands of years.

Like many ancient peoples, Sumerians living between the Tigris and Euphrates rivers around 4000 B.C. believed that demons were the cause of illness. They studied the stars and the intestines of animals for clues to the supernatural causes of man's condition and fate. In many cultures, physicians were priests, and sometimes considered gods or demigods. The Egyptian Imhotep, for example, born around 3000 B.C., was a priest, an adviser to pharaohs, and the first physician known by name. After his death, he was named a demigod and eventually a god: the Egyptian god of medicine.

The supernatural approach to treating illness gradually gave way to a more scientific approach, based on observation and experimentation.

Around 400 B.C., the Greek physician Hippocrates developed a more scientific approach, which has guided Western medicine for much of the time since. He promoted the idea of diagnosing illness based on careful observation of the patient's condition, not supernatural or other external elements. He also wrote the oath that physicians recited for centuries and still honor today: the Hippocratic oath. From Hippocrates and others following in his footsteps, an approach to medicine in which natural causes were examined scientifically gradually grew to become the dominant approach to treating human illness.

panacea a cure-all (from the Greek *panakeia,* same meaning).

pharmacology the study of drugs—their properties, uses, application, and effects (from the Greek *pharmakon*: drug, and *logos*: word or thought).

MEDICAL MYTH

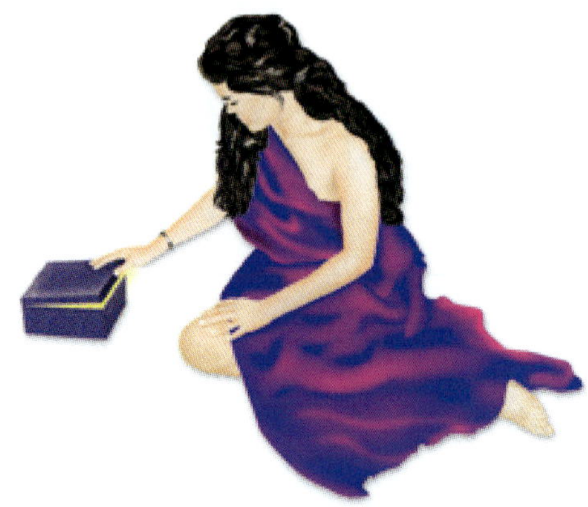

Pandora's Box

As punishment for Prometheus's theft of fire for mankind, the Greek god Zeus created Pandora and had her collect gifts for man from the gods. These gifts were really punishments that included disease and pestilence. They were released upon the world when Pandora opened her box.

The Greek god of Medicine

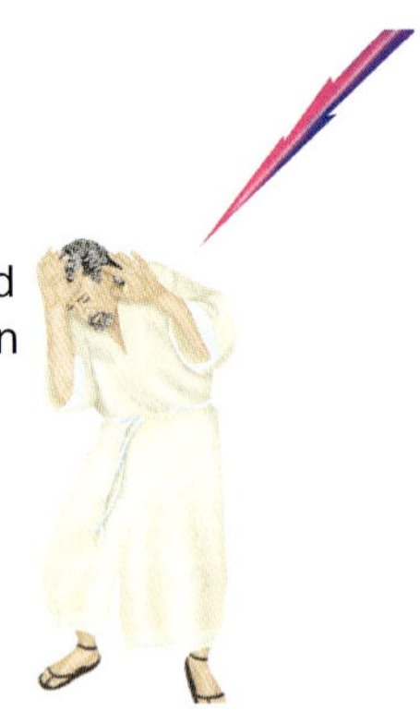

The ancient Greek Aesculapius was said to have been such an extraordinary physician that he could keep his patients from dying and even raise the dead. This skill angered Pluto, the god of the underworld, because it reduced the number of his subjects. At Pluto's request, Zeus killed Aesculapius with a lightning bolt, then named him the god of medicine. Aesculapius' daughter, ***Panacea***, became the goddess of medicinal herbs.

NATURE'S MEDICINE

Nature's Aspirin

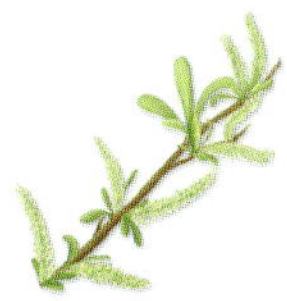

The ancient Greek physicians Hippocrates and Dioscorides both wrote about the pain relieving ability of the bark of a white willow tree that grew in the Mediterranean. In the 1800's, more than 2,000 years after Hippocrates' time, the active ingredient in the willow bark, salicylic acid, was derived by chemists. However, because of difficulties in taking salicylic acid internally, acetylsalicylic acid, popularly known as aspirin, was developed and it eventually became the most widely used drug in the world.

A Treatment for Malaria

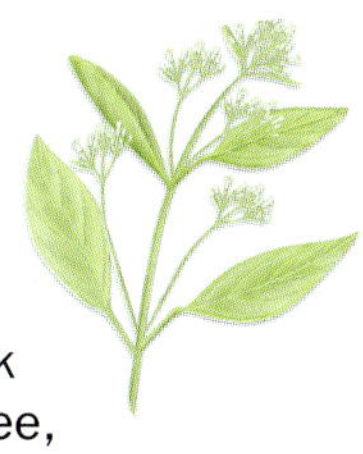

Malaria had long been one of the most deadly diseases in world history, until quinine, made from the bark of the Peruvian Cinchona tree, was discovered. Popularly called *Jesuit's powder* for the Spanish priests that sent it to Europe from the New World, its use, along with preventive measures aimed at eradicating the cause of malaria, finally brought this deadly disease under control.

The First Anesthetic

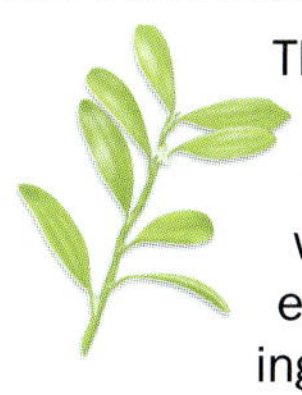

The Indians of the Andes chewed coca leaves for their medicinal effects, which included increased endurance. The active ingredient in the leaves was cocaine, which in 1884 was shown to be the first effective local anesthetic by Carl Koller, a Viennese surgeon. This discovery revolutionized surgery and dentistry, since previously anesthesia was administered on a general basis—that is, to the whole body. Eventually, because of its harmful properties when abused, a man-made substitute was developed, called procaine or Novocain®.

Besides looking to the supernatural, several ancient cultures also looked to the natural world for medical remedies, many of which are still used today.

Early man understood that plants and other natural materials had the power to treat or relieve illness. The ancient Sumerians used about 250 natural medicines derived from plants, many of which are still used today. Around 3000 B.C., the Chinese Emperor Shen Nung is said to have begun eating plants and other natural materials to determine which were poisonous and which were beneficial. One of the first known practitioners of trial and error drug testing, he is believed to have established 365 herbs that could be used in health treatments, and herbal medicine remains a major component of Chinese medicine today.

In 100 A.D. the Indian physician Charaka wrote the Charaka Samhita, which among other things described over 500 herbal drugs that had been known and used in India for many centuries.

About the same time, Avicenna, who was perhaps the greatest Islamic physician, wrote a five volume encyclopedia, one volume of which was devoted to natural medications and another to compounding drugs from individual medications; his writings dominated medical thinking in Europe for centuries. By 1500, the Indians of Mexico had a well-established ***pharmacology*** that included more than 1,200 drugs and was clearly the result of many hundreds of years of medical practice. One plant, the sarsaparilla, became very popular in Europe for kidney and bladder ailments and can be found to this day in many medicinal teas.

Western man also has used nature as a source for many of the drugs still in use today.

In 1785, the British physician William Withering published his study of the foxglove plant and the drug it contained, digitalis, which became widely used in treating heart disease. Foxglove had been used since ancient times in various remedies but Withering described a process for creating the drug from the dried leaves of the plant and established a dosage approach. And in 1943 Russell Marker created the hormone progesterone, the first reliable birth control drug, from a species of Mexican yam.

... TO MODERN MEDICINE

Today, while we still rely on many drugs derived from natural sources, we use more than twice as many *synthetic* drugs as naturally derived ones.

Synthetic drugs, and the ability to mass-produce them, often have advantages in cost, effect, and availability over natural drugs.

Some of these man-made drugs have replaced natural drugs and others are for entirely new uses.

The creation in 1899 of the easier-to-take acetylsalicylic acid, or aspirin, from salicylic acid was one of the first discoveries to prompt more pharmaceutical research and development. Then in Britain in 1928 Alexander Fleming discovered a fungus that produces a chemical that kills bacteria. He named the chemical penicillin and it was the first ***antibiotic*** drug. Its discovery was followed shortly by World War II in which the ability to mass produce penicillin was critical to Allied success.

This and other war-related drug needs stimulated the U.S. pharmaceutical industry to dramatically boost its capacity and production.

Ever since, pharmaceutical research and development in the United States has grown substantially, making it the world's leading producer of pharmaceuticals.

Due in part to the dramatic growth in pharmaceutical medicine, the average life span in the United States has increased by over 30 years since 1900.

In 1900 the average American lived only into their late 40s. By 2012 the average life expectancy at birth in the United States had risen to 78.7 years. Similar changes were seen throughout the industrialized world and to a lesser extent in developing countries. The growth of hospitals, advances in the treatment of disease, improved medical technology, better understanding of nutrition and health, and the rapid increase in the number of effective drugs and vaccines have all contributed to this profound change in improved life experience.

antibiotic a substance that harms or kills microorganisms like bacteria and fungi.

synthetic combining simpler chemicals into more complex compounds, creating a new chemical not found in nature.

The Age of Antibiotics

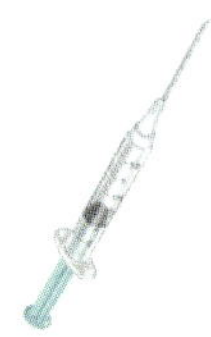

In World War I, more soldiers died from infections than the wounds themselves. Although penicillin was discovered as an antibiotic in 1928, it was difficult to produce and for years not much was made of the discovery. With the start of World War II, however, British scientists looked again at penicillin and established that it was effective in fighting infections. Already under attack from Germany and unable to develop mass production methods for penicillin, the British sought help in the United States. In 1942 the Pfizer pharmaceutical company was able to develop a method for mass production of the drug, and by D-Day the Allied army was well stocked with it. Its use saved many thousands of lives during the war and revolutionized the pharmaceutical industry. A period of intense research and discovery in the field of antibiotics began, and many new antibiotics were developed that have dramatically contributed to improved health and increased life expectancy.

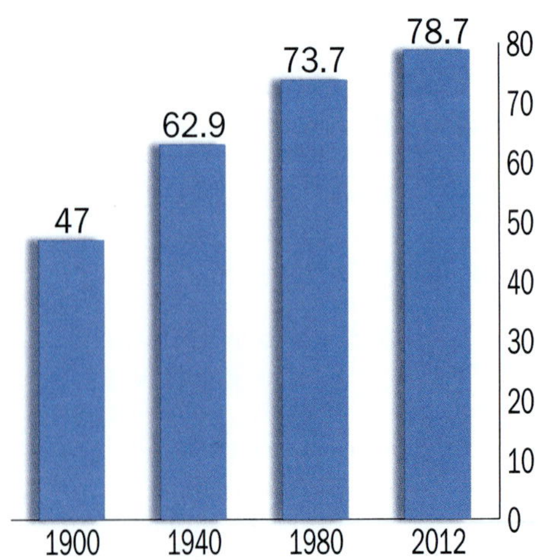

Source: www.data360.org

average life expectancy in the United States

THE DRUG INDUSTRY

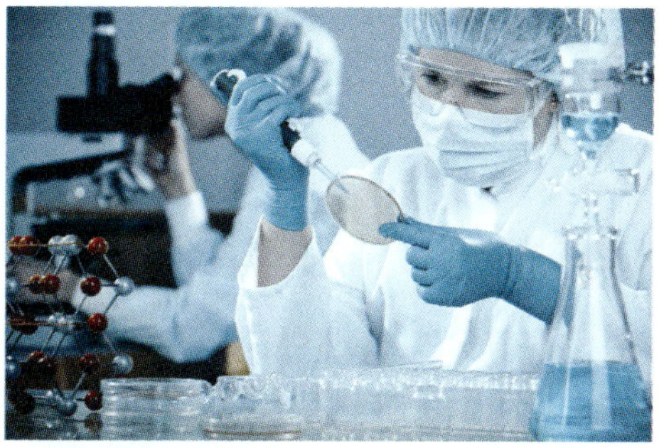

Patenting Discoveries

Patenting new discoveries is an important part of the pharmaceutical development process because it protects against illegal copying of the discovery. The company holding the patent is able to control the marketing of the product and use this as a way to recover their original investment. Since patenting generally occurs long before a drug is approved, however, a company usually has only about 10 years of patent protection left in which to market their product without competition from direct copies called generic versions. For more information, see the section on New Drug Approval and Marketed Drugs in Chapter 3.

With the increasing availability of powerful drugs, their regulation became more important than ever.

Leaders and governments have long sought to regulate the use of medicinal drugs because of their effect on the population's health. The explosive growth of pharmaceuticals made governments throughout the world keenly aware of the importance of setting and maintaining standards for their distribution and use.

In the United States, drug regulation is performed by the Food and Drug Administration.

FDA activity is a major factor in the nation's public health and safety. Before a drug can be marketed, it must be shown through testing that it is safe and effective for its intended use. Once marketed, the FDA monitors drugs to make sure they work as intended, and that there are no serious negative (adverse) effects from their use. If drugs that are marketed are found to have significant adverse effects, the FDA can recall them (take them off the market).

The discovery of new drugs requires a major investment of time, research, and development.

The pharmaceutical industry employs thousands of scientists and devotes about one-sixth of its income to research and development. Bringing a new drug to market is a long and difficult process in which the vast majority of research does not produce a successful drug. Thousands of chemical combinations must be tried in order to find one that might work as hoped. Once a potentially useful drug is created, it must undergo an extensive testing and approval process before it can be made available to the public. In the United States, the length of time from the beginning of development through testing and to ultimate FDA approval is often more than 10 years.

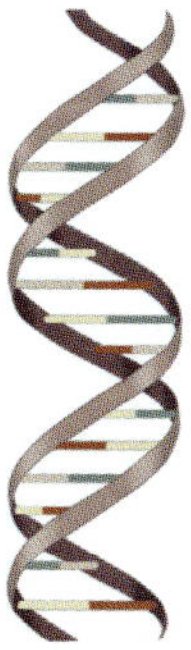

It's in the Genes

One of the most exciting areas of pharmaceutical research is performed by molecular biologists studying human genes. While antibiotics are the answer for many infectious diseases, many other diseases that seemed based on heredity are effectively untreatable. The study of the human genome has shown that many diseases are related to genetic defects. This has led to the creation of new drugs that can successfully treat many diseases previously considered untreatable. As a result, the field of biotechnology has become the most dynamic area of pharmaceutical research and development.

MEDICINE THROUGH THE AGES — A TIME LINE —

4000 B.C.

Ancient Sumerians studied the stars and animal intestines to divine man's fate and physical condition.

3000 B.C.

The **Egyptian Imhotep,** born in 3000 B.C., was a priest, adviser to pharaohs, and the first physician known by name. After his death he was eventually named the Egyptian god of medicine.

1500 B.C.

The most complete record of ancient Egyptian medicine and pharmacology, called the **Papyrus Ebers,** dates back to 1500 B.C. This 1,100 page scroll document includes about 800 prescriptions using 700 drugs, mostly derived from plants.

500 B.C.

The **Greek Alcmaeon,** a student of Pythagorus, saw diseases as a result of a loss of the body's natural equilibrium, rather than the work of the gods.

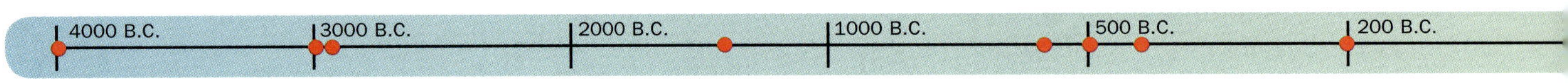

3000 B.C.

The **Chinese Emperor Shen Nung** is said to have begun tasting plants and other natural materials to determine which were poisonous and which were beneficial. One of the first known practitioners of trial and error drug testing, he is credited with establishing hundreds of herbal medicines.

600 B.C.

A cult following **Aesculapius, the Greek god of Medicine**, established centers where medicine was practiced. These early clinics became training grounds for the great Greek physicians of later years.

400 B.C.

A number of medical documents were written by different Greek physicians under the name **Hippocrates.** These works avoided the supernatural and religious approaches to medicine and instead were grounded in scientific reasoning based on close observation of the patient. They also contained writings about the conduct of physicians, including the famous Hippocratic oath.

200 B.C.

The first official Chinese pharmacopeia, the **Shen Nung Pen Tsao**, listing 365 herbs for use in health treatments, is believed to have been published. This can be considered an early Chinese forerunner to the FDA approved drug list.

tip

Since the use of drugs goes so far back in history, we use many terms based on Greek or Latin words.

100 B.C.

King Mithridates of Pontos practiced an early form of immunization by taking small amounts of poisons so that he could build up his tolerance of them. It is said that he was so successful that when he eventually decided to kill himself through poisoning, he was unable to do so, and had to be killed by someone else. The potion Mithridates developed, Mithridaticum, was believed to be good at promoting health and was used for 1500 years.

77 B.C.

Dioscorides, a Greek physician, wrote the **De *Materia Medica***, five books that described over 600 plants and their healing properties. His work was the main influence for Western ***pharmaceutics*** for over 1600 years. One of the remedies he described was made from the bark of a type of willow tree, the active ingredient of which was salicylic acid, the natural drug on which acetylsalicylic acid (aspirin) is based. He also described how to get opium from poppies.

100 A.D.

The **Indian physician Charaka** wrote the **Charaka Samhita**, the first great book of Indian medicine, which among other things described over 500 herbal drugs that had been known and used in India for many centuries.

162 A.D.

The Greek physician **Galen** went to Rome and became the greatest name in Western medicine since Hippocrates, both through his practice and extensive writings, nearly 100 of which survive. He believed there were four humours in man that needed to be in balance for good health, and he advocated bleeding to assist that balance. He also believed in the vigorous application of a scientific approach to medicine and his emphasis on education, observation, and logic formed the cornerstone for Western medicine.

900 A.D.

The **Persian Rhazes** wrote one of the most popular textbooks of medicine in the Middle Ages, the **Book of Medicine Dedicated to Mansur**. A man of science, Rhazes was also an alchemist who believed he could turn lesser metal into gold. When he failed to do this, he was ordered to be beaten over the head with his own chemistry book until either his head or the book broke. Apparently, it was a tie. Rhazes lost sight in one eye but lived to continue his work.

1000 A.D.

Perhaps the greatest Islamic physician was **Avicenna**. His writings dominated medical thinking in Europe for centuries. He wrote a five volume encyclopedia, one volume of which was devoted to natural medications and another to compounding drugs from individual medications.

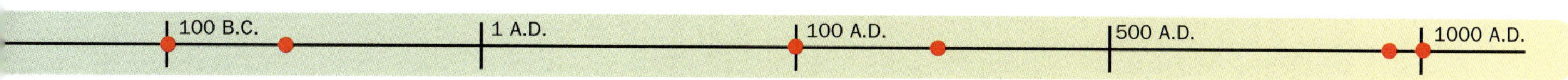

materia medica generally pharmacology, but also refers to the drugs in use (from the Latin *materia*, matter; and *medica*, medical).

pharmaceutics of or about drugs; also, a drug product.

MEDICINE THROUGH THE AGES — A TIME LINE —

1500 A.D.

In the early 1500s, a Swiss alchemist who went by the name of **Paracelsus** rejected the humoural philosophy of Galen and all previous medical teaching other than Hippocrates. Though he had many critics, he is generally credited with firmly establishing the use of chemistry to create medicinal drugs. Included in his work is the first published recipe for the addictive drug laudanum, which became a popular though tragically abused drug for the next 300 years.

1630 A.D.

Jesuits sent **quinine** back to Europe in the early 1600s. Also called Jesuit's powder, it was the first drug to be used successfully in the treatment of malaria.

1785 A.D.

The **British Physician, William Withering**, published his study of the **foxglove** plant and the drug it contained, **digitalis**, which became widely used in treating heart disease. Foxglove had been used since ancient times in various remedies but Withering described a process for creating the drug from the dried leaves of the plant and established a dosage approach.

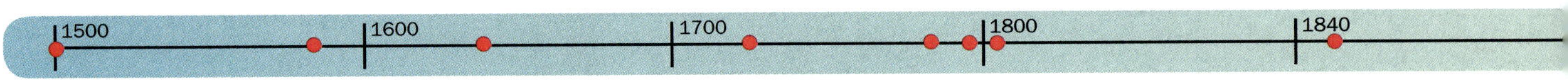

1500 A.D.

When the Spanish found them, the **Indians of Mexico** had a well established pharmacology that included more than 1,200 drugs and was clearly the result of many hundreds of years of medical practice. One plant, the sarsaparilla, became very popular in Europe for its use on kidney and bladder ailments and can be found to this day in many medicinal teas.

1580 A.D.

In China, **Li Shi Zhen** completed the **Pen Tsao Kang Mu**, a compilation of nearly 2,000 drugs for use in treating illness and other conditions.

1721 A.D.

Dr. Zabdiel Boylston in Boston became the first person to administer a **smallpox vaccine** in what is now the United States. Boylston had already contracted the disease in an earlier epidemic. The first people he inoculated were his six-year-old son and two slaves, all of whom developed only a mild case of smallpox and then recovered. While much of the population was initially extremely suspicious, 249 people were eventually inoculated, six of whom died, compared to 844 deaths among the 5,980 people who contracted the disease naturally.

1796

Edward Jenner successfully developed a vaccine from the cowpox disease to inoculate against smallpox.

1803

The German pharmacist **Frederich Serturner** extracted morphine from opium.

1846

In Boston, the first publicized operation using **general anesthesia** was performed. Ether was the anesthetic.

antitoxin a substance that acts against a toxin in the body; also, a vaccine containing antitoxins, used to fight disease.

hormones chemicals produced by the body that regulate body functions and processes.

human genome the complete set of genetic material contained in a human cell.

1864

Louis Pasteur's experiments showed that microorganisms cause food spoilage, and that heat can be used to kill them and preserve the food. Though others had proposed principles of **germ theory** previously, Pasteur's work was instrumental in it becoming widely accepted.

1884

In 1884 **Carl Koller,** a Viennese surgeon, discovered that cocaine, the active ingredient in coca leaves, was useful as a local anesthetic in eye surgery, and cocaine became established as the **first local anesthetic**.

1928

In Britain, **Alexander Fleming** discovered a fungus that produces a chemical that kills bacteria. He named the chemical **penicillin**. It is the first antibiotic drug.

1943

Russell Marker created the hormone **progesterone**, the first reliable birth control drug, from a species of Mexican yam.

1951

James Watson and **Francis Crick** identified the structure of **DNA**, the basic component within the cell that contains the organism's genetic code.

1987

AZT became the first drug approved by the FDA for AIDS treatment.

1988

The **Human Genome Project** was started with the goal of mapping the entire DNA sequence in the ***human genome***. This information will provide a better understanding of hereditary diseases and allow the development of new treatments for them.

1989

Amgen, a **biotechnology** company that develops products based on advances in cellular and molecular biology, introduced its first product, Epogen, an anemia treatment for dialysis patients.

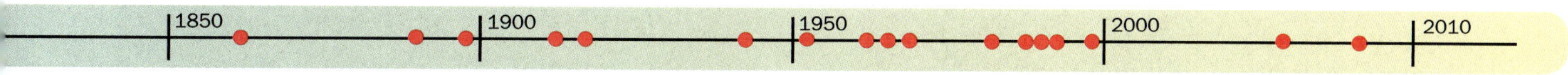

1890

Effective ***antitoxins*** were developed for diphtheria and tetanus, giving a major boost to the development of medicines that fight infectious disease.

1899

Acetylsalicylic acid, popularly known as **aspirin**, was developed because of difficulties in using salicylic acid, a drug contained in certain willow trees that had long been used in the external treatment of various conditions.

1921

In Toronto, Canada, **Frederick Banting** and **Charles Best** showed that an extract of the ***hormone*** **insulin** lowers blood sugar in dogs and so might be useful in treating the terrible disease diabetes. Then biochemist **James B. Collip** developed an extract of insulin pure enough to test on humans. The first human trial in January, 1922, proved successful and dramatically changed the prospects for all diabetics.

1955

Dr. Jonas Salk succeeded in developing a refined **injectable polio vaccine** from killed polio virus. (In 1954 polio had killed more than 13,000 and crippled more than 18,000 Americans.)

1957

Albert Sabin developed an **oral polio vaccine** using a weakened live virus that could be taken orally rather than by injection. However, because of risk of an associated disease from the live virus, only the injectable form of the vaccine was used to inoculate children after January 2000.

1960

The **birth control pill** was introduced.

1981

First documented cases of **AIDS.**

1996

HAART (Highly Active Anti-Retroviral Therapy) was introduced for AIDS treatment. Made up of a combination of one protease inhibitor and usually two antiretroviral drugs, it proves extremely effective in slowing HIV progress and was partially responsible for a 47% decrease in the AIDS death rate in 1997.

1996

Dolly the sheep was cloned as the first mammal to be **cloned** from an adult cell. She lived for almost seven years.

2006

Gardasil was marketed as the first preventative **HPV vaccine** and thereby the first vaccine to target a cause of cancer.

2008

Scientists in Japan created an **artificial DNA molecule** using four new artificial bases.

PHARMACY TODAY

A prescription drug is one that has been ordered or prescribed by a physician or other licensed prescriber to treat a patient.
Though physicians occasionally give patients the actual medication, in most cases the individual who dispenses the prescribed medication to the patient is a pharmacist. Pharmacists at the more than 50,000 community pharmacies account for approximately half of the distribution of prescription drugs in the United States. The rest reach consumers primarily through hospitals, mass merchandisers, food stores, mail order pharmacies, clinics, and nursing homes—all of which employ pharmacists for the dispensing of medications.

The sheer number of available drugs, their different names and costs, having multiple prescriptions from different physicians, and the involvement of third-party insurers are among the many factors that make using prescription drugs a complex area for consumers.
As a result, consumers rely on pharmacists to provide information and advice on prescription and over-the-counter medications in easy to understand language. They also routinely ask the pharmacist to make recommendations about less expensive generic substitutes for a prescribed drug.

Since the late twentieth century, the pharmacist's role has been expanding greatly to meet the need for greater pharmacist-patient consultation and even direct medication administration services.
In 1990 the United States Congress required pharmacists to provide counseling services to Medicaid patients in the Omnibus Budget Reconciliation Act (OBRA); a number of states require this for all patients, and it is generally considered a fundamental service for pharmacists to provide. Since 1990, state laws have gradually changed so that pharmacists can now administer immunizations in all 50 states. And in 2003 the Medicare Modernization Act (MMA) expanded the role of the pharmacist to provide Medication Therapy Management (MTM) services to some Medicare patients.

THE PHARMACIST

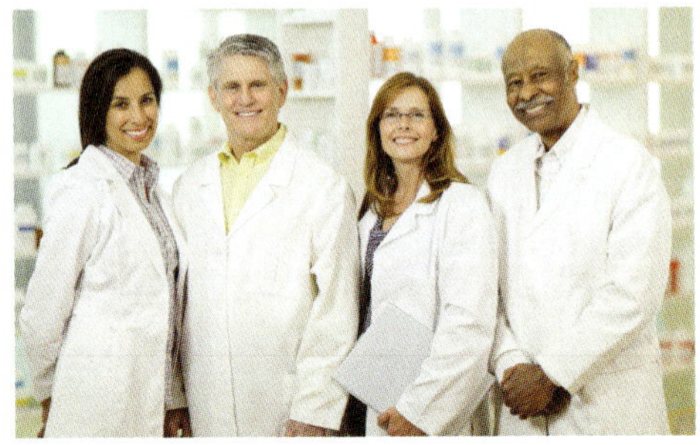

A Trusted Profession

Pharmacists consistently rank as one of the mostly highly trusted and ethical professions in the United States, according to Gallup Polls. In 2012, the top five professions were:

1. Nurses
2. Pharmacists
3. Medical Doctors
4. Engineers
5. Dentists

Education

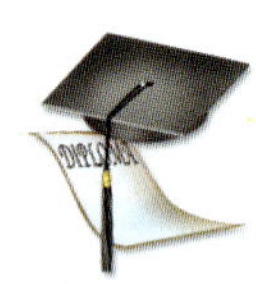

To become a pharmacist, an individual must have earned a Doctor of Pharmacy degree from an accredited college of pharmacy (of which there are about 119 in the United States), pass a state licensing exam (in some states), and perform experiential training under a licensed pharmacist. Once licensed, pharmacists must receive continuing education to maintain their license. Pharmacists seeking to teach, do research, or work in hospitals often must have postdoctoral training in the form of residency and fellowship training. Three out of five pharmacists work in community pharmacies; one out of four in hospitals.

Medication Therapy Management services provide patients with a comprehensive look at all of the medications they are taking rather than consultation on only the prescriptions dispensed on a given day.

Pharmacists work with the patients to look for ways to improve health outcomes such as better adherence to the drug therapy plan. In some cases, the pharmacist makes recommendations to the physician for changes in drug therapy. In an initial MTM encounter, the pharmacist could spend 30 or more minutes to gain information about the patient's total medication profile as well as other health information. Follow-up MTM encounters take less time. While pharmacists are not paid for routine counseling, they are paid for MTM services at approximately $1 to $3 per minute.

All of these developments have expanded the pharmacist's role in health care.

Even the traditional role of dispensing medications is has grown enormously: From 1999 to 2010, the number of prescriptions increased 50% (from 2.8 billion to 4.2 billion), and the number of pharmacists increased 49% (from 185,000 to 274,900). To help with both the volume of prescriptions and the increasingly complex environment, pharmacists use powerful computerized tools to manage customer profiles, inventory, pricing, and other key aspects of pharmacy. And, pharmacy technicians perform many tasks that pharmacists once performed.

PHARMACY SETTINGS

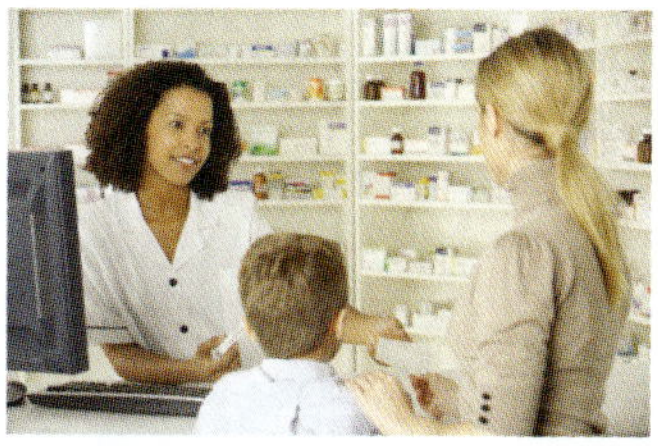

The primary environments for pharmacist and technician employment are:

- **community pharmacies:** independent and chain retail pharmacies.
- **hospitals:** in-patient and out-patient pharmacies.
- **mail order operations:** pharmacy businesses that provide drugs by mail to patients, a fast growing area.
- **long-term care:** residence facilities that provide care on a long-term rather than acute or short-term basis.
- **managed care:** care that is managed by an insurer, such as Kaiser Permanente.
- **home care:** care provided to patients in their home, often by a a home-care agency working with a home-care pharmacy.
- **compounding pharmacies**: specialized pharmacies that prepare compounded medications.

ECONOMIC TRENDS

Between 1970 and 2000, total health-care costs in the United States increased by over 1,500 percent to $1.3 trillion dollars. By 2010 the costs doubled to surpass $2.5 trillion dollars.

As a result of these escalating costs, there have been increasing efforts by government, industry, and consumers to find ways to control the costs of care. Though drugs represent only a small fraction of overall health-care expenses, they have also been included in these efforts.

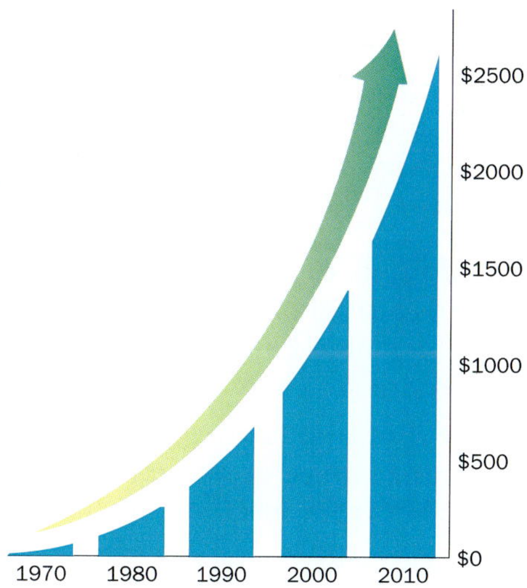

Source for illustration and data: U.S. Statistical Abstract

COMPUTERS IN PHARMACY

Pharmacies use powerful computerized tools that help productivity.

Computerized pharmacy management systems put customer profiles, product, inventory, pricing, and other essential information within easy access. They also automate elements like label printing, inventory management, stock reordering, and billing. As a result, pharmacies and pharmacists dispense more prescriptions and information than ever before.

Pharmacy computer systems may be developed by the user to meet specific needs, purchased ready-made, or provided by a drug wholesaler.

Wholesalers provide inventory management systems to their customers as part of their service. The wholesaler actually owns the system. It is primarily designed for placing orders with the wholesaler, though it may also contain various other elements. Large pharmacy chains have the business volume to justify the expense of developing comprehensive systems that are tailored to their needs. Smaller operations usually buy a commercially available system. Whatever the operation, a computerized pharmacy management system is an indispensable productivity tool.

Although each pharmacy computer system has its own specific features, many general principles of computer usage apply to all systems.

The most important element is stated in the classic computer axiom: garbage in, garbage out. That is, the information produced by the computer is only as good as the information that is entered into it. This means special care has to be taken when entering information (generally called *data*) to make sure it is correct. A simple mistake in data entry can result in the wrong medication being given to the wrong patient or any number of other serious problems.

In addition to traditional computers, pharmacies are increasingly using tablet computers such as the iPad, portable handheld electronic devices such as the iPod, iTouch, and smartphones.

These portable devices are especially useful for accessing drug information from online references as well as from specific software programs, applications, and apps.

A SAMPLE COMPUTER SYSTEM

Pharmacy computer systems generally offer most or all of these features, and may offer others as well.

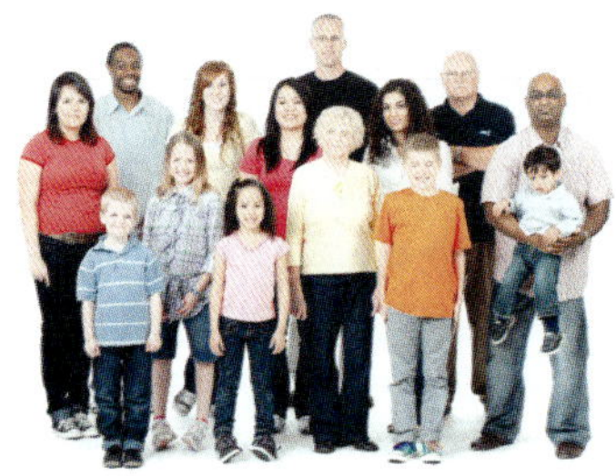

Patient Profile

Provides complete information about patients, including prescribers, insurer, medication history, and medical history, including allergies; identifies drug interactions for patients taking multiple medications.

Billing

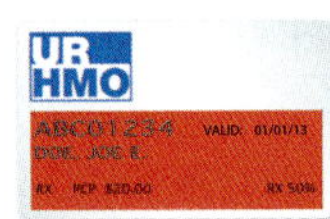

Checks policies of third parties such as HMOs and insurers; authorizes third-party transactions and credit cards electronically.

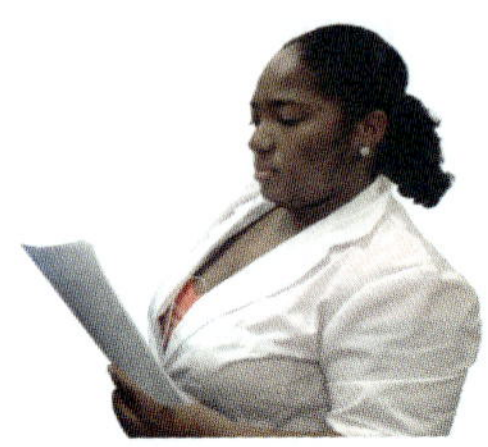

Management Reporting

Forecasting, financial analysis

data information that is entered into and stored in a computer system.

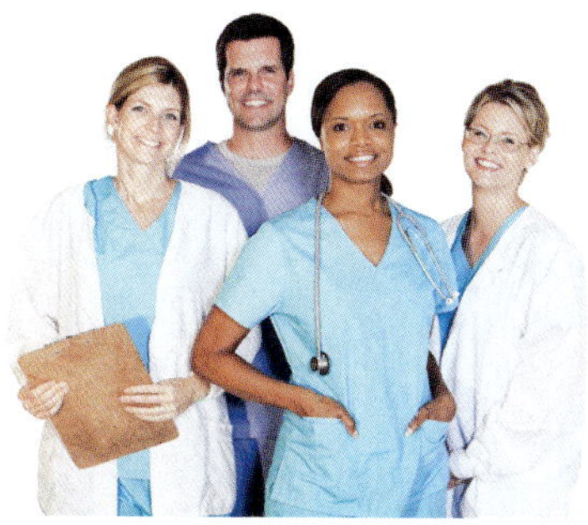

Prescriber Profile

Includes state identification numbers and affiliations with facilities and insurers.

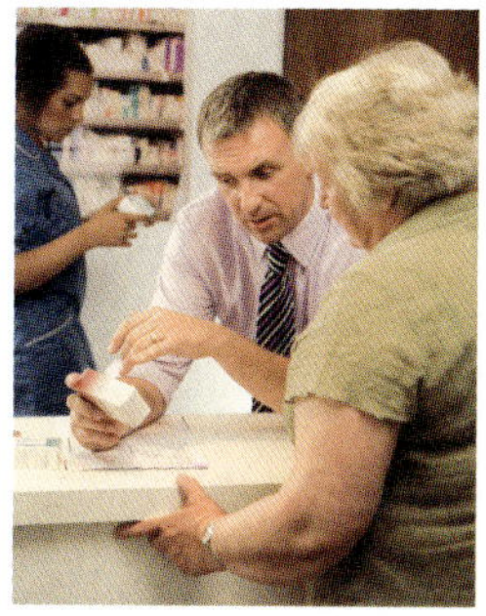

Education

Provides information for the patient about drugs, usage, interactions, allergies, etc.

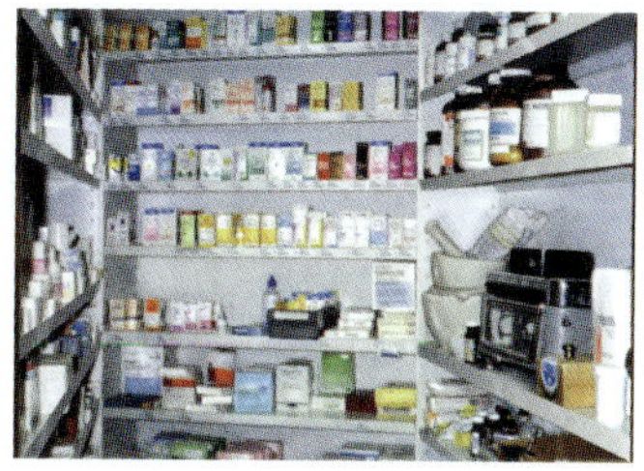

Product Selection

Locates items by various means (brand name, generic name, product code, category, supplier, etc.). Gives updates of prices and other product information.

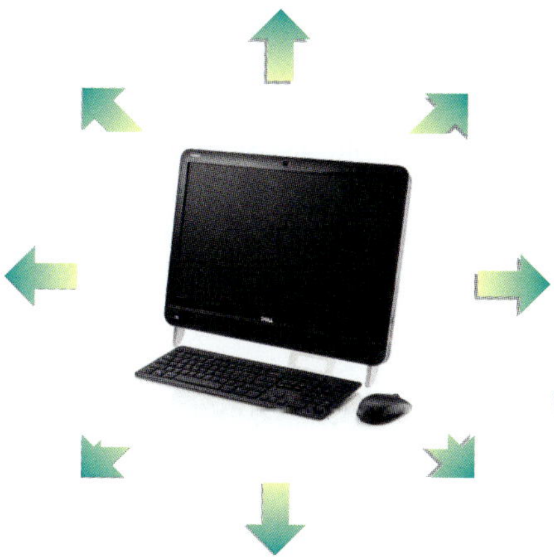

Photo courtesy Dell, Inc.

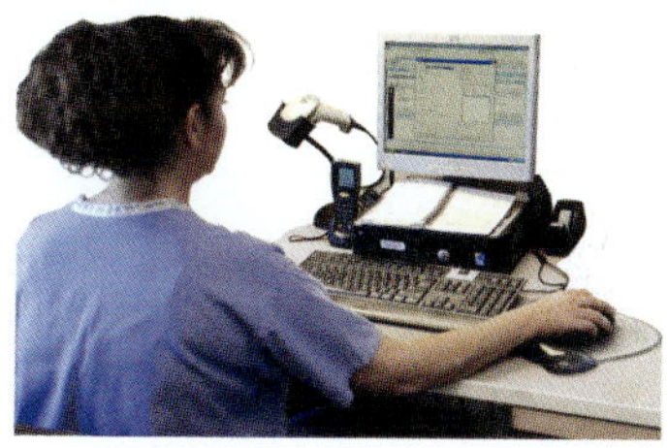

Inventory

Adjusts inventory as prescriptions are filled; analyzes turnover; produces status reports; automatically reorders based on inventory levels, generates purchase orders.

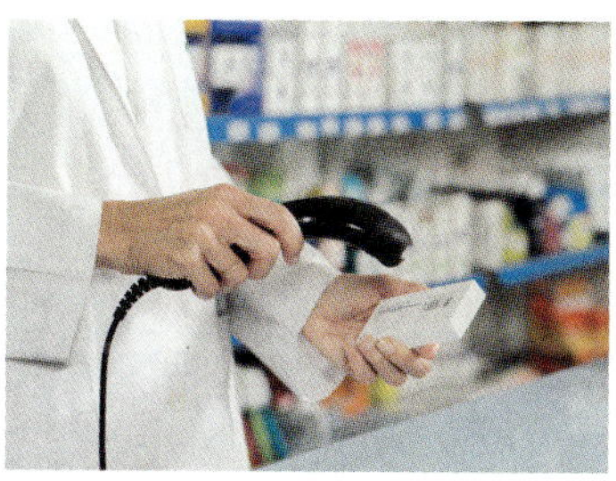

Pricing

Provides prices for medications and possible substitutes; automatically updates prices; scans prices from bar codes.

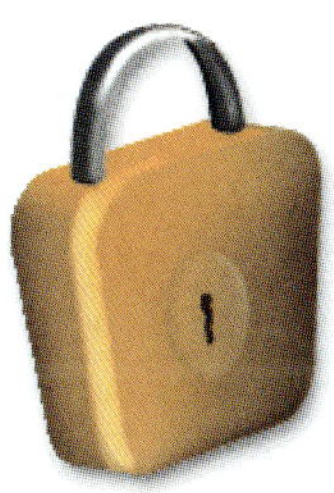

Security

Password protection restricts access to authorized users for different features.

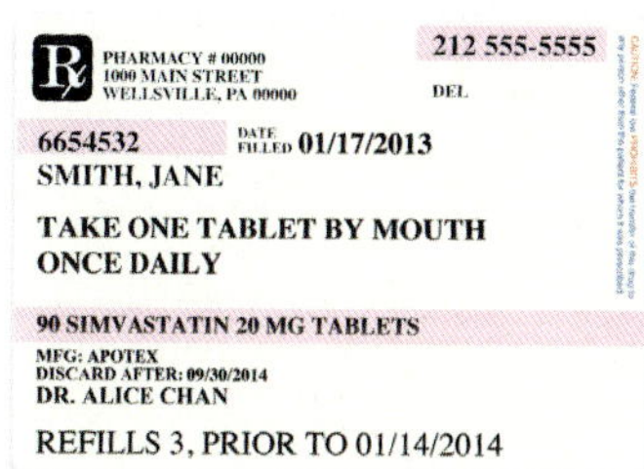

Labeling

Creates label, receipt, customer information, and usage instructions.

REVIEW

KEY CONCEPTS

FROM MEDICINE'S ORIGINS ...

- ✔ People have used drugs derived from plants to treat illnesses and other physical conditions for thousands of years.
- ✔ The ancient Greeks used the bark of a white willow tree to relieve pain. The bark contained salicylic acid, the natural forerunner of the active ingredient in aspirin.
- ✔ Cocaine was the first effective local anesthetic.

... TO MODERN MEDICINE

- ✔ The average life span in the United States increased by over 30 years since 1900.
- ✔ In World War I, more soldiers died from infections than the wounds themselves; in World War II, the mass production of the antibiotic penicillin saved thousands of lives and was seen as a critical factor in the success of the Allied forces.

MEDICINE THROUGH THE AGES—A TIME LINE

- ✔ The foxglove plant contains digitalis, which has been widely used in treating heart disease.
- ✔ Louis Pasteur's experiments showed that microorganisms cause food spoilage, and that heat can be used to kill them and preserve the food.
- ✔ Frederick Banting and Charles Best showed that an extract of the hormone insulin lowered blood sugar in dogs and might be useful in the treatment of diabetes.
- ✔ Alexander Fleming discovered the antibiotic chemical, penicillin.
- ✔ The Human Genome Project is an attempt to map the entire DNA sequence in the human genome. This information will provide a better understanding of hereditary diseases and how to treat them.

PHARMACY TODAY

- ✔ To become a pharmacist in the United States, an individual must graduate from an accredited college of pharmacy, pass a state licensing exam, and perform an internship working under a licensed pharmacist.
- ✔ Once licensed, pharmacists must receive continuing education to maintain their license.
- ✔ The cost of health care in the United States from 1970 to 2000 rose by over 1,500 percent.
- ✔ Medication Therapy Management services provide patients with a comprehensive look at all of the medications they are taking rather than consultation on only the prescriptions dispensed on a given day.

COMPUTERS IN PHARMACY

- ✔ Computerized pharmacy management systems put customer profiles, product, inventory, pricing, and other essential information within easy access. One result has been that pharmacies and pharmacists dispense more prescriptions and information than ever before.

SELF TEST

the answer key begins on page 569

MATCH THE TERMS

1. antibiotic ____
2. antitoxin ____
3. data ____
4. hormones ____
5. human genome ____
6. materia medica ____
7. panacea ____
8. pharmaceutical ____
9. pharmacognosi ____
10. synthetic ____

a. combining simpler chemicals into more complex ones, creating a new chemical not found in nature.
b. a cure-all.
c. a substance that acts against a toxin in the body.
d. a substance that harms or kills microorganisms like bacteria and fungi.
e. chemicals produced by the body that regulate body functions and processes.
f. the complete set of genetic material contained in a human cell.
g. the study of physical, chemical, biochemical, and biological properties of drugs as well as the search for new drugs from natural sources.
h. information that is entered into and stored in a computer system.
i. generally pharmacology, but also refers to the drugs in use.
j. of or about drugs; also, a drug product.

CHOOSE THE BEST ANSWER

1. The first physician known by name was
   a. Prometheus.
   b. Hippocrates.
   c. Imhotep.
   d. Aesculapius.

2. Hippocrates' approach to medicine was based on
   a. superstition.
   b. careful observation.
   c. astrology.
   d. animal behavior.

3. The ancient Greek goddess of Medicinal Herbs was
   a. Pandora.
   b. Panacea.
   c. Hippocrates.
   d. Euphrates.

4. Derived from the bark of a Peruvian tree, Jesuit's powder, used with other preventive measures, helps keep this disease under control.
   a. smallpox
   b. malaria
   c. polio
   d. tuberculosis

REVIEW

5. Aspirin is made from salicylic acid from the bark of the ________________ tree.
   a. white willow
   b. cinchona
   c. tea
   d. fig

6. __________________ was the first effective local anesthetic.
   a. Quinine
   b. Cocaine
   c. Heroin
   d. Morphine

7. From 200 B.C., an early forerunner to the FDA approved drug list
   a. De Materia Medica
   b. Papyrus Ebers
   c. Pen Tsao Kang Mu
   d. Shen Nung Pen Tsao

8. The ________ from _____ is an 1,100-page scroll document containing about 800 prescriptions using 700 drugs mostly derived from plants.
   a. Pen Tsao, 200 B.C.
   b. herbal, 200 B.C.
   c. Papyrus Ebers, 1500 B.C.
   d. De Materia Medica, 77 B.C.

9. The first great book of Indian medicine describing over 500 herbal drugs that had been used for centuries was written in
   a. 500 B.C.
   b. 500 A.D.
   c. 100 A.D.
   d. 1000 A.D.

10. The Persian Rhazes who wrote one of the most popular textbooks of medicine in the middle ages was a man of science and
    a. an alchemist.
    b. a sorcerer.
    c. a politician.
    d. a god.

11. _________ was a(n) _____ physician who wrote a five volume encyclopedia in _____, one of which was devoted to natural medicines and another compounding drugs from individual medications.
    a. Li Shi Zen, Chinese, 1580 A.D.
    b. Zabdiel Boylston, colonial, 1721 A.D.
    c. William Withering, British, 1785 A.D.
    d. Avicenna, Islamic, 1000 A.D.

12. The first operation with general anesthesia used
    a. digitalis.
    b. morphine.
    c. ether.
    d. cocaine.

13. ________________________ showed that heat can be used to kill microorganisms associated with food spoilage.
    a. Pasteur
    b. Banting and Best
    c. Watson and Crick
    d. Fleming

14. ____________________ discovered penicillin could kill some bacteria.
    a. Banting and Best
    b. Watson and Crick
    c. Fleming
    d. Marker

15. ______________________ are substances produced by the body to regulate body functions and processes.
    a. Hormones
    b. Antitoxins
    c. Antibiotics
    d. Genomes

16. ______________________ identified the structure of DNA.
    a. Watson and Crick
    b. Banting and Best
    c. Serturner
    d. Koller

17. The pharmaceutical manufacturing industry devotes about ____________ of its income to research and development.
    a. 1/10
    b. 1/6
    c. 1/3
    d. 1/2

18. __________________ protect(s) against illegal copying of new discoveries.
    a. Generics
    b. Brand names
    c. Patenting
    d. The FDA

19. The FDA is required to
    a. ensure that a drug is safe and effective for its intended use.
    b. to monitor a drug after it is marketed to ensure it works as intended.
    c. to monitor a drug for any adverse effects.
    d. all of the above.

20. The length of time from the beginning of development of a new drug to FDA approval is often more than __________ years.
    a. two
    b. five
    c. ten
    d. twenty

21. The first vaccine to target a cause of cancer:
    a. smallpox
    b. cowpox
    c. diphtheria
    d. Gardasil

22. The Omnibus Budget Reconciliation Act (OBRA) requires pharmacists to provide
    a. counseling services to all patients.
    b. mail-order medication to Medicaid patients.
    c. counseling services to Medicaid patients.
    d. HMO coverage to all patients.

23. To become a pharmacist in the United States,
    a. an individual must graduate from an accredited college of pharmacy, pass a state licensing exam, and perform experiential training working under a licensed pharmacist.
    b. an individual must graduate from a nonaccredited college of pharmacy and pass a state licensing exam.
    c. no internship experience is required unless the pharmacist intends to practice in community pharmacy.
    d. an individual must graduate from an accredited college of pharmacy, and perform an internship working under a licensed pharmacist, however, no examination is required.

REVIEW

24. The area of greatest employment for pharmacists is
    a. hospitals.
    b. mail order operations.
    c. community pharmacies.
    d. managed care.

25. Medicare Modernization Act (MMA) expanded the role of the pharmacist to include
    a. counseling.
    b. MTM services.
    c. home delivery.
    d. dispensing.

26. In managed care, care is managed by a(an)
    a. patient.
    b. physician.
    c. pharmacist.
    d. insurer.

27. Pharmacy computer systems generally offer
    a. labeling.
    b. pricing.
    c. prescriber profile.
    d. all of the above.

28. Information that is entered and stored into a computer, such as a patient's name, is called
    a. product.
    b. inventory.
    c. data.
    d. billing.

CRITICAL THINKING QUESTIONS

1. The first mammal to be cloned from an adult cell was Dolly the sheep. Why was this controversial?
2. Scientists have created an artificial DNA molecule. How might this be beneficial. Why might this be controversial?
3. Brian is thinking of pursuing a career as a pharmacy technician in a hospital. What are some reasons this career path could be a good choice?

THINKING IT THROUGH WRAP-UP

1. Economic trends show that health care costs escalated in the past half-century, and this trend is continuing. This trend is indicative of job opportunities in health care. The number of available drugs, the number or prescriptions written, and the complex nature of health insurance have led to expanded job opportunities in pharmacy. Federal regulation associated with OBRA and MMA have expanded the role of the pharmacist and also led to an expansion of job opportunities for pharmacy technicians.
2. Community pharmacies account for about half of the prescriptions dispensed and most job opportunities for pharmacy technicians are in the community pharmacy setting. Some other environments include hospitals, mail order operations, long-term care, and compounding pharmacies

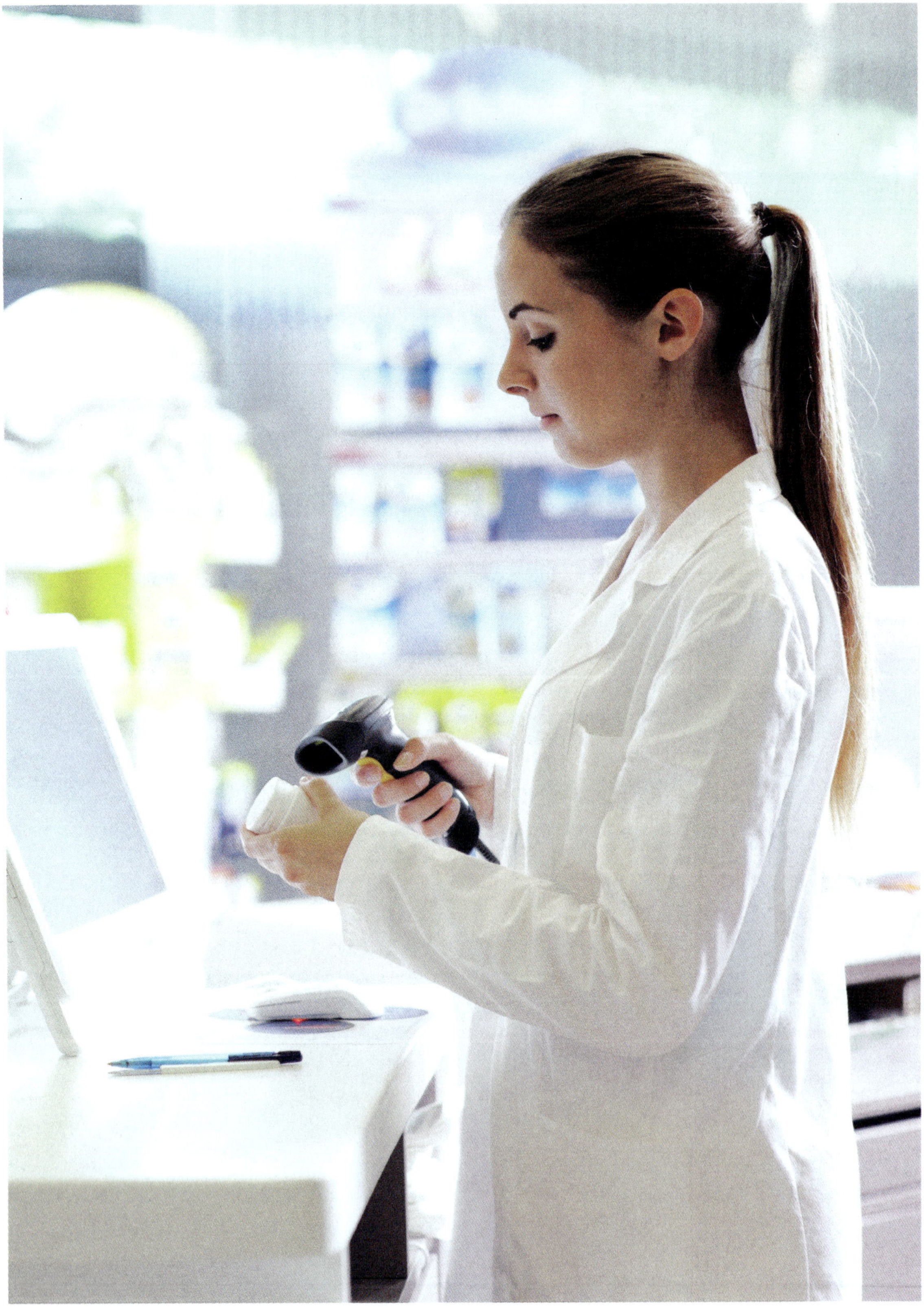

2

THE PHARMACY TECHNICIAN

LEARNING OBJECTIVES

At the completion of study, the student will:

- ✔ be familiar with the overall aspects of the pharmacy technician job and the general role of the pharmacy technician in relation to the pharmacist.
- ✔ know what personal standards are expected of the pharmacy technician.
- ✔ understand the overall scope of HIPAA regulations concerning interactions between health-care providers and patients as well as regarding the patient's health information.
- ✔ understand the range of training programs and what agencies establish training and certification regulations, and what organization accredits training programs.
- ✔ know what technicians must do in order to receive certification and how often it must be renewed.

THINKING IT THROUGH

Stacey works in a community pharmacy as a technician and wants to gain the CPhT credential. As you read this chapter, consider the following questions:

1. How can Stacey earn the CPhT credential?
2. What are some similarities and differences between the PTCE and ExCPT?
3. Once certified, how can Stacey maintain certification?

THE PHARMACY TECHNICIAN

In health care, *technicians* are individuals who are given a basic level of training designed to help them perform specific tasks.

This training often is provided at community and technical colleges or even on the job. By comparison, health-care ***professionals*** such as physicians and pharmacists receive more extensive and advanced levels of education.

To perform their duties, pharmacists today rely upon the assistance of trained support staff called pharmacy technicians.

Technicians perform essential tasks that do not require the pharmacist's skill or expertise. They work under the direct supervision of a licensed pharmacist who is legally responsible for the technician's performance.

Pharmacy technicians perform such tasks as filling prescriptions, packaging doses, performing inventory control, and keeping records.

Having technicians perform these tasks gives the pharmacist more time for activities that require a greater level of expertise, such as counseling patients. As the job of the pharmacist has become more complex, the need for pharmacy technicians has increased. As a result, pharmacy technician is a rapidly growing occupation offering many opportunities. As of 2010, there were about 334,400 pharmacy technicians employed in the United States and it is estimated this number will grow by at least 32% through 2020.

Like pharmacists, most pharmacy technicians are employed in community pharmacies and hospitals.

However, they are also employed by or in clinics, home care, long-term care, mail order prescription pharmacies, nuclear pharmacies, Internet pharmacies, pharmaceutical wholesalers, the federal government, and various other settings. Depending upon the specific setting and job, they may perform at different levels of specialization and skill. An introductory level technician job at a pharmacy requires general skills. In various hospital and other environments, there are specialized technician jobs that require more advanced skills developed from additional education, training, and experience. Compensation for these specialized positions is greater than it is for entry level positions.

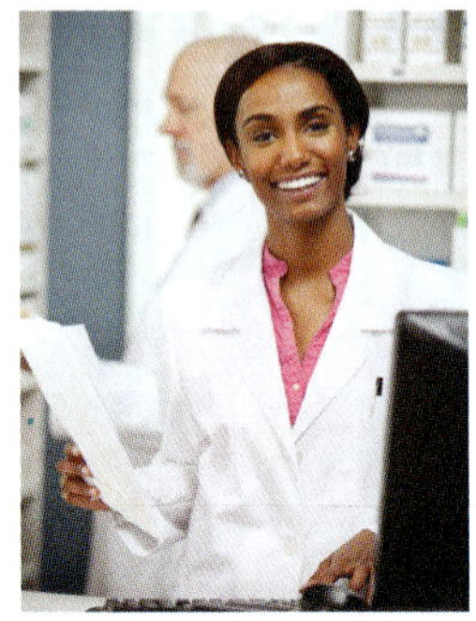

receiving prescriptions

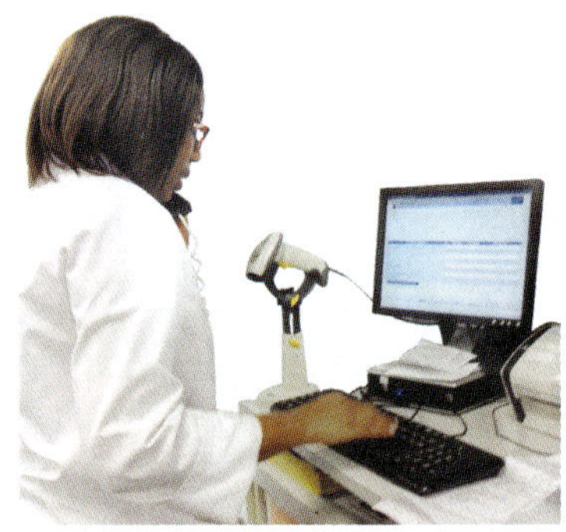

using computers

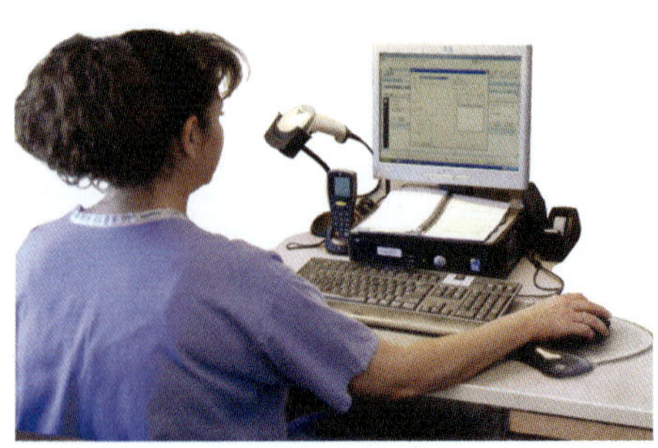

inventory control

professional individuals who receive extensive and advanced levels of education before being allowed to practice, such as physicians and pharmacists.

scope of practice what individuals may and may not do in their jobs.

technician individuals who are given a basic level of training designed to help them perform specific tasks.

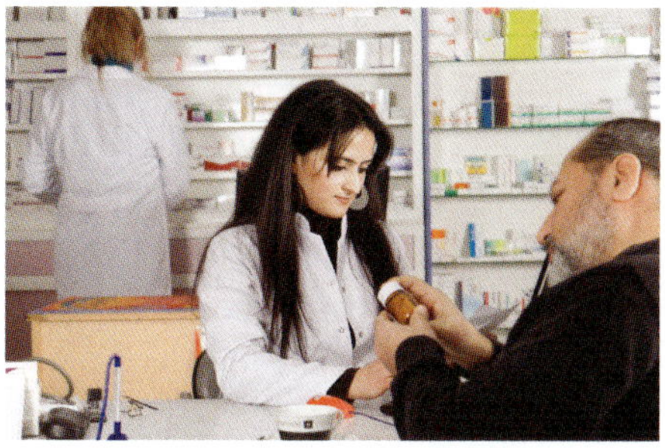

taking patient information

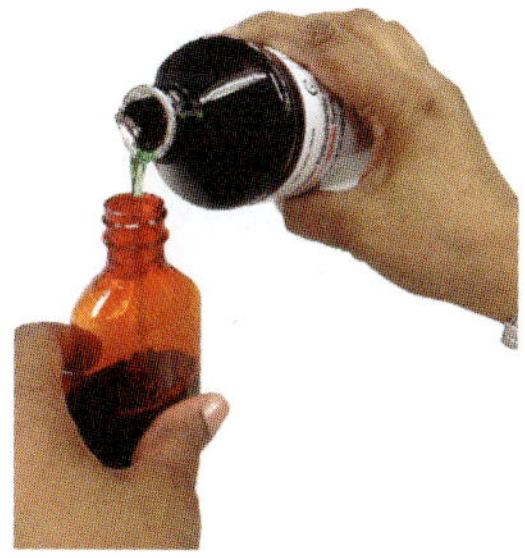

filling prescriptions

The Pharmacy Technician's Scope of Practice

The activities on these pages may be part of a pharmacy technician's job responsibilities. However, specific responsibilities and tasks for pharmacy technicians differ by setting and are described in writing by each employer through job descriptions, policy and procedure manuals, and other documents. What individuals may and may not do in their jobs is often referred to as their ***scope of practice***. The pharmacist's scope of practice is, of course, much greater than the technician's. As part of their job requirement, all technicians are required to know specifically what tasks they may and may not perform, as well as which tasks must be performed by the pharmacist.

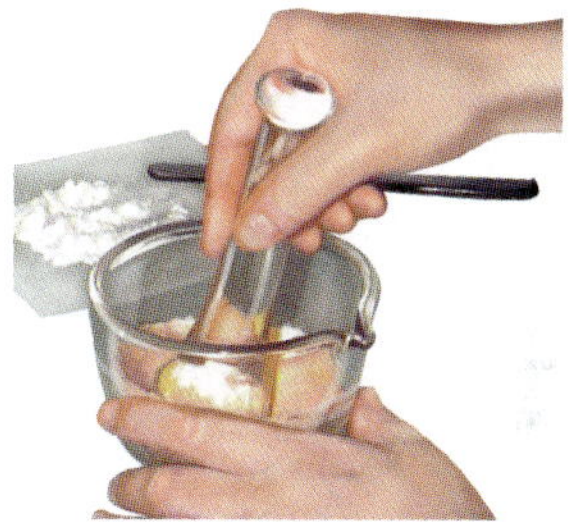

compounding

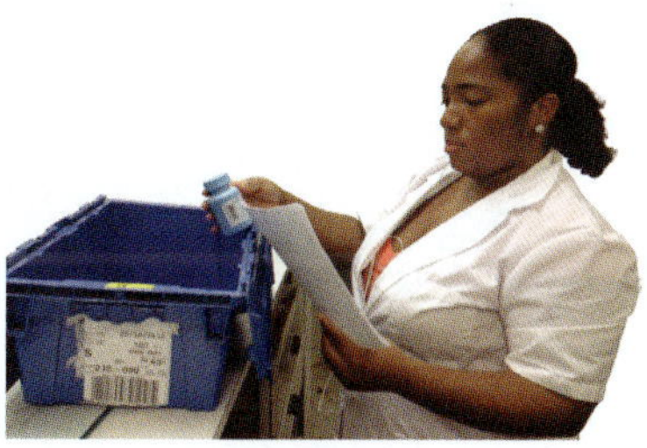

ordering

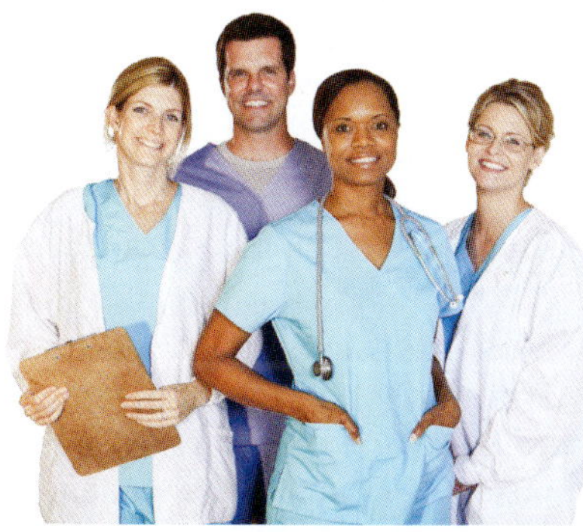

working with a team of health care professionals

PERSONAL STANDARDS

There are personal standards for pharmacy technicians.

Employers may specify these standards as part of the job requirement. Many, though not all, are outlined on these pages. There are standards for behavior, skill, health, hygiene, and appearance. Anyone seeking to become a pharmacy technician should take a ***personal inventory*** in each of these areas and what they must do to excel in them.

The pharmacy technician is a member of a team, the patient's health-care team.

For this team to succeed, all members, including the technician, must work together for the patient's welfare. If any member of the team fails to perform as required, there can be serious consequences for the patient. Anyone wishing to become a pharmacy technician must be able to work cooperatively with others, communicate effectively, perform as expected, and act responsibly. The patient's welfare depends upon it.

Respect for the Patient

The patient's welfare is the most important consideration in health care. To ensure this, various government laws and professional standards guarantee basic patient rights and require health-care providers to explain these rights to their patients.

The 1996 *Health Insurance Portability and Accountability Act (HIPAA)* made health-care providers responsible for the privacy and security of all identifiable patient health information (also called Protected Health Information or PHI), in any form, whether it is electronic, on paper or orally communicated. Among other things, this means that computer files must be protected; any electronic transmission of health information, including claims and billing, must be done via HIPAA–compliant electronic data interchange (EDI); there can be no discussion of patient information within earshot of others; no casual discussion with anyone, including a patient's family members or friends, of a patient or patient information; directing patients to a private area when discussing medications or other personal health issues; making sure files and documents are securely stored where no unauthorized person can access them.

THE TECHNICIAN: A PERSONAL INVENTORY

Technicians should possess the following personal qualities:

✔ **Dependable**

The patient, the pharmacist, and the patient's health-care team will depend upon you performing your job as required, including showing up on time for scheduled work hours. You must do what you are required to do, whether anyone is observing you or not.

✔ **Detail Oriented**

Patients must receive medications exactly as they have been prescribed. Drugs, whether prescription or over the counter, can be dangerous if misused, and mistakes by pharmacy technicians can be life threatening.

✔ **Trustworthy**

You will be entrusted with ***confidential*** patient information, dangerous substances, and perishable products. In addition, many drugs are very expensive and you will be trusted to handle them appropriately.

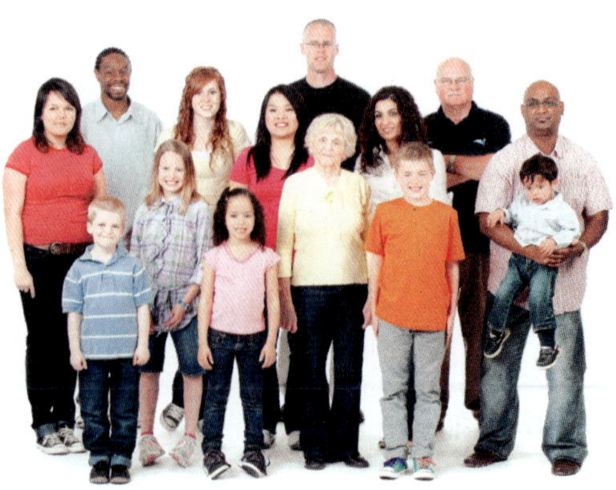

confidentiality the requirement of health-care providers to keep all patient information private among the patient, the patient's insurer, and the providers directly involved in the patient's care.

personal inventory an assessment of one's characteristics, skills, qualities, etc.

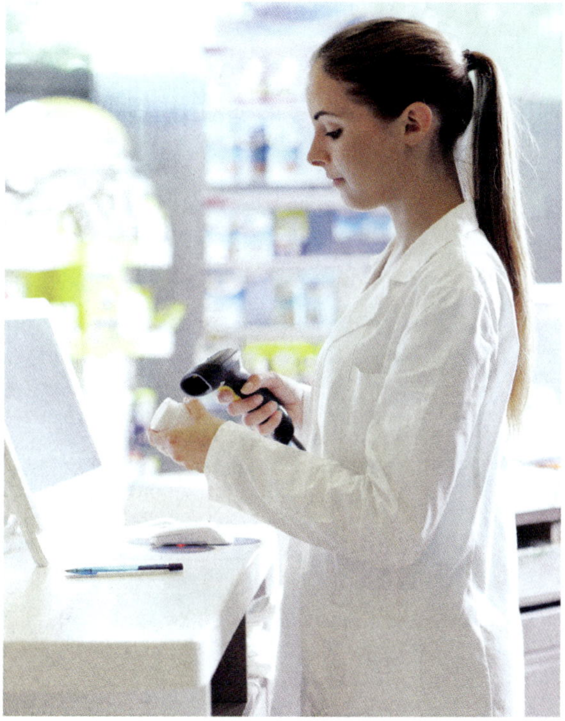

Technicians must follow these personal guidelines:

✔ **Health**

You must maintain good physical and mental health. If you become physically or mentally run-down, you will increase the chance of making serious mistakes.

✔ **Hygiene**

Practice good hygiene. You will interact closely with others. Poor hygiene may hurt your ability to be effective. You will also be expected to perform in infection free conditions and poor hygiene can violate this requirement.

✔ **Appearance**

Your uniform and personal clothing should be neat, clean, and functional. Shoes should be comfortable. Clothes should allow the freedom of movement necessary to perform your duties. Hair should be well-groomed and pulled back if long. Fingernails should be neat and trim.

Technicians must be capable and competent in the following skill areas:

✔ **Mathematics and Problem Solving**

You will routinely perform mathematical calculations in filling prescriptions and other activities.

✔ **Language and Terminology**

You must learn the specific pharmaceutical terminology and medical abbreviations (e.g., QID, QS) that will be used on your job.

✔ **Computer Skills**

You will regularly use computers for entering patient information, maintaining inventory, filling prescriptions, and so on.

✔ **Interpersonal Skills**

You will interact with patients/customers, your supervisor, coworkers, physicians, and others. You must be able to communicate, cooperate, and work effectively.

℞ **tip**

There are legal aspects to many of these standards. Failing to follow them can hurt your job performance and result in legal violations.

TRAINING & COMPETENCY

Training and competency requirements for pharmacy technicians differ from setting to setting.

Technician training is generally based on job requirements for the specific workplace, particular skills involved, any applicable professional standards, and state regulations. Specific training and certification requirements are set by each state's board of pharmacy. Regulations vary considerably but almost all states require some form of technician training.

An example of a model curriculum for technician training is that of the American Society of Health-System Pharmacists (ASHP).

The ASHP is the leading association for pharmacists practicing in hospitals and other health-care systems. Their curriculum provides a national standard for developing technician competency. It can be adapted to different pharmacy settings and the specific needs of an individual training program.

Training programs that meet ASHP standards receive ASHP accreditation.

Accreditation is a peer-review process to determine if a training program meets the standards of the accrediting body. The accreditation process is voluntary, but can provide evidence of commitment to quality. The ASHP has been accrediting pharmacy technician training programs in the United States since 1983 and its curriculum is endorsed by the Pharmacy Technician Educator's Council (PTEC).

The ASHP maintains a directory of over 250 schools and training institutions that offer technician training programs.

Most of these have been accredited by the ASHP and the remainder have applied for accreditation. They are found in community and technical colleges as well in community pharmacies, hospitals, and other institutions offering on-the-job training.

Your employer will monitor and document your competency.

Your employer is legally responsible for your performance and therefore your competency. In addition to daily monitoring, you will receive regularly scheduled performance reviews. Through these reviews and other means, your employer will document your competency to perform your job.

TRAINING

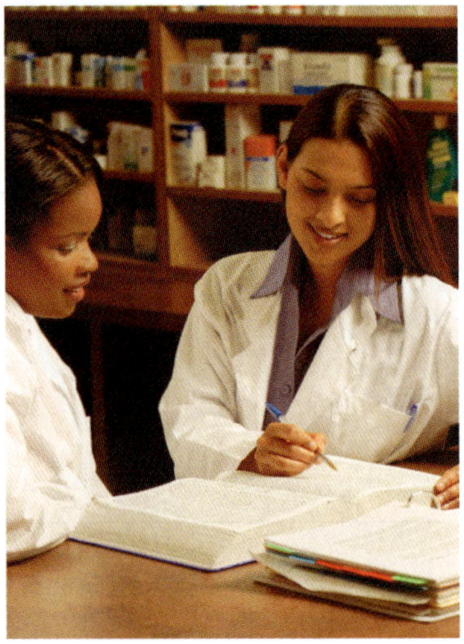

Photo courtesy Hanson Ng/Design Pics/Getty Images

Depending upon your setting, you will receive training in some or all of the following areas:

- drug laws
- terminology
- prescriptions
- calculations
- drug routes and forms
- drug dosage and activity
- infection control
- compounding
- preparing IV admixtures
- biopharmaceutics
- drug classifications
- inventory management
- pharmacy literature

An important part of training is exposure to actual workplace settings. Many technicians receive this in the form of on-the-job training from their employer or as internships through community colleges or other training programs.

competent being qualified and capable.

COMPETENCY

Testing

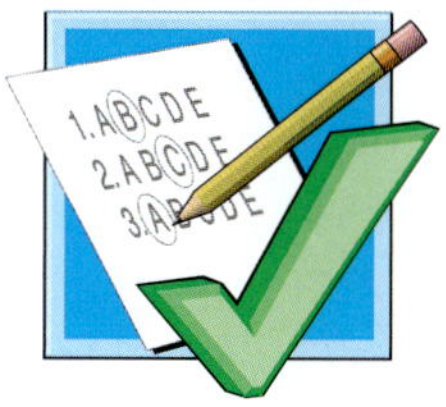

Demonstration of competency during training will generally be through written tests and practical demonstrations. In on-the-job training or internships, your performance will be directly judged by the supervising pharmacist.

Continuing Education

Pharmacy is a dynamic field that changes constantly. There are always new drugs, treatments, methods, and other developments. As a result, continuing education is a critical element in maintaining competency for pharmacy technicians. In order to perform your job as required, you must continually learn new information. Ultimately, this will make your job more interesting and make you more effective at your job.

Performance

After you have qualified as ***competent***, your employer will continue to monitor and document your performance throughout your employment. Documentation kept in files may include:

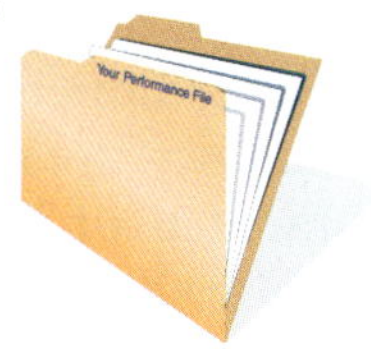

- performance reviews,
- complaints,
- and comments by your supervisor and and other appropriate personnel.

Most jobs also have a probation period during which time the pharmacy technician is expected to learn certain skill sets. If competency is not met, the technician may receive an extended probation period or be dismissed from the job.

Rx tip

For information regarding ASHP accredited programs, contact the American Society of Health-System Pharmacists, 7272 Wisconsin Ave., Bethesda, MD 20814, 301-657-3000 or visit www.ashp.org

State Training Requirements for Pharmacy Technicians

More and more states are requiring technicians to complete a formal training program and/or certification. Each state has different requirements. Information for the requirements for your state can be found on the website for your board of pharmacy. The National Association of Boards of Pharmacy® (NABP) website at www.nabp.net/boards-of-pharmacy/all.php provides links to the websites for all state boards of pharmacy in the U.S.

CERTIFICATION

Since there is no federal standard for training or competency, obtaining *certification* is a valuable career step for pharmacy technicians.

To receive certification in most states, technicians must pass a standardized national examination, such as the Pharmacy Technician Certification Exam (PTCE) offered by the Pharmacy Technician Certification Board (PTCB), the Exam for the Certification of Pharmacy Technicians (ExCPT) given by the National Healthcareer Association (NHA), or another exam approved by their state board. These exams test the technician's knowledge and competency in basic pharmacy functions and activity areas. While certification is mainly voluntary, as of June, 2012 the PTCB had certified over 450,000 pharmacy technicians.

Certification is a mark of achievement that employers, colleagues, and others will recognize.

If you pass a national certification examination, you will become a Certified Pharmacy Technician (CPhT). Beyond verifying your competence as a technician, this designation indicates you have a high level of knowledge and skill and can be given greater responsibilities. This in turn means that you may earn more and will probably cost your employer less time and money in training. Studies have also shown that certified technicians have lower turnover, higher morale, greater productivity, and make fewer errors. Some employers may pay for the cost of a certification exam (if successfully completed) and/or provide training assistance for a certification exam.

Certification must be renewed every two years.

Because pharmacy is a constantly changing field, maintaining skills and competence requires continuing education. In order to renew their certification every two years, CPhTs must meet requirements of 20 contact hours of pharmacy-related continuing education, including at least one hour in pharmacy law. Up to 10 contact hours of continuing education can occur at the CPhT's practice site under the supervision of a registered pharmacist, and these hours can be customized to fit the specific needs of the CPhT.

certification a legal document certifying that an individual meets certain objective standards, usually provided by a neutral professional organization.

PTCE AND ExCPT

Both PTCE and ExCPT are certified by the National Commission for Certifying Agencies (NCCA), last two hours, and are administered in a computerized testing environment. Candidates must have completed high school or have a GED and have no felony conviction.

Beginning in 2013, the PTCE will cover the following nine Knowledge Domains:

1. Pharmacology for Technicians (13.75%)
2. Pharmacy Law and Regulations (12.5%)
3. Sterile and Non-Sterile Compounding (8.75%)
4. Medication Safety (12.5%)
5. Pharmacy Quality Assurance (7.5%)
6. Medication Order Entry and Fill Process (17.5%)
7. Pharmacy Inventory Management (8.75%)
8. Pharmacy Billing and Reimbursement (8.75%)
9. Pharmacy Information Systems Usage and Application (10%)

In addition, PTCE candidates must have never been convicted of a pharmacy or drug-related misdemeanor. To pass, candidates must score at least 650 out of a possible 900.

ExCPT contains 110 multiple choice questions on these areas:

- regulations and technician duties (~25% of the exam);
- drugs and drug products (~23% of the exam);
- dispensing process (~52% of the exam).

In addition ExCPT candidates must be at least 18 years old and have completed a training program or have one year experience in the field. To pass, candidates must have a scaled score of 390 out of a possible 500.

tip
In accordance with the Americans with Disabilities Act (ADA), special accommodations will be provided for persons with documented disabilities taking a national certification exam.

Sample PTCE Questions

The sample questions below reflect the "choose the best answer" format of the PTCE. This type of question requires careful reading and judgment. In some cases, there may be more than one answer that is at least partially correct. However, there will only be one correct answer that is the best and most complete answer.

answers:
1. 4
2. 1
3. 1
4. 2
5. 4
6. 4

1. Pharmacies located in hospitals are required to follow regulations of this organization:

1. ASHP
2. USP
3. ASCP
4. TJC

2. Of the following schedules of drugs, which is for drugs with no accepted medical use in the United States?

1. Schedule I
2. Schedule II
3. Schedule III
4. Schedule IV

3. Of the following needles, which size is the most likely to cause coring?

1. 13G
2. 16G
3. 20G
4. 23G

4. A solution of Halperidol (Haldol®) contains 2 mg/ml of active ingredient. How many grams would be in 473 ml of this solution?

1. 9.46 g
2. 0.946 g
3. 0.0946 g
4. 0.00946 g

5. You have a 70% solution of Dextrose 1,000 ml. How many Kg of Dextrose is in 400 ml of this solution?

1. 280 kg
2. 28 kg
3. 2.8 kg
4. 0.28 kg

6. Which is the largest capsule size?

1. size 5
2. size 3
3. size 1
4. size 0

More sample exam questions and practice exams can be found in the workbook accompanying this text, *The Pharmacy Technician Workbook and Certification Review, Fifth Edition.*

tip
For information regarding the PTCE contact the Pharmacy Technician Certification Board at 2215 Constitution Avenue, NW, Washington, DC 20037-2985; ph. (800) 363-8012; fax (202) 429-7596; or e-mail contact@ptcb.org.

For information regarding ExCPT, contact the Exam for the Certification of Pharmacy Technicians, National Healthcareer Association, 11161 Overbrook Rd., Leawood, KS 66211; ph (800) 499-9092; fax (913) 661-6291; e-mail info@nhanow.com

REVIEW

KEY CONCEPTS

THE PHARMACY TECHNICIAN

- ✔ Pharmacy technicians perform essential tasks that do not require the pharmacist's expertise.
- ✔ Pharmacy technicians work under the direct supervision of a licensed pharmacist who is legally responsible for their performance.
- ✔ Specific responsibilities and tasks for pharmacy technicians differ by setting and are described by each employer through job descriptions, policy and procedure manuals, and other documents.
- ✔ Having technicians perform these tasks gives the pharmacist more time for activities that require a greater level of expertise, such as consulting with patients.
- ✔ What individuals may and may not do in their jobs is often referred to as their *scope of practice*.
- ✔ Most pharmacy technicians are employed in community pharmacies and hospitals but they are also employed in clinics, home care, long-term care, mail order prescription pharmacies, and various other settings.
- ✔ Hospitals and other environments have specialized technician jobs that require more advanced training and skills.

PERSONAL STANDARDS

- ✔ Pharmacy technicians are entrusted with confidential patient information, dangerous substances, and perishable products.
- ✔ Drugs, whether prescription or over the counter, can be dangerous if misused, and mistakes by pharmacy technicians can be life threatening.
- ✔ Pharmacy technicians routinely perform mathematical calculations in filling prescriptions and other activities.
- ✔ Pharmacy technicians must learn the specific pharmaceutical terminology that will be used on the job.
- ✔ Pharmacy technicians must be able to communicate, cooperate, and work effectively with others.

TRAINING AND COMPETENCY

- ✔ Standards for pharmacy technician training and/or competency are established by the state boards of pharmacy; regulations vary considerably but most states require some form of technician training.

CERTIFICATION

- ✔ Although certification is mainly voluntary, many states recognize national certification and some require pharmacy technicians to take the PTCE, ExCPT, or other exam approved by their state board.
- ✔ The CPhT designation, Certified Pharmacy Technician, is good for two years. It verifies an individual's competence as a technician, and indicates a high level of knowledge and skill.

SELF TEST

the answer key begins on page 569

MATCH THE TERMS

1. certification ____
2. competent ____
3. confidentiality ___
4. personal inventory ____
5. professionals ____
6. scope of practice ____
7. technicians ____

a. what individuals may and may not do in their jobs.

b. an assessment of one's personal characteristics, skills, qualities, etc.

c. the requirement of health-care providers to keep all patient information private among the patient, the patient's insurer, and the providers directly involved in the patient's care.

d. being qualified and capable to perform a task or job.

e. a legal proof or document that an individual meets certain objective standards, usually provided by a neutral professional organization.

f. individuals who are given a basic level of training designed to help them perform specific tasks.

g. individuals who receive extensive and advanced levels of education before being allowed to practice, such as physicians and pharmacists.

CHOOSE THE BEST ANSWER

1. ______________ are individuals who are given a basic level of training designed to help them perform specific tasks.
   a. LPNs
   b. DOs
   c. Professionals
   d. Technicians

2. In pharmacy, technicians perform essential tasks that do not require ______________ skill or expertise.
   a. the clerk's
   b. the pharmacist's
   c. scientific
   d. mathematical

3. Specialized technician jobs in hospitals have ______________ compensation than entry level positions.
   a. less
   b. about the same
   c. greater

4. Specific responsibilities and tasks for pharmacy technicians differ by setting and are described in writing by each
   a. technician.
   b. local police department.
   c. employer.
   d. state board of pharmacy.

5. The pharmacy technician can do the following functions except
   a. take patient information.
   b. fill prescription orders.
   c. compound prescription orders.
   d. advise patients on medications.

6. What individuals may and may not do on their jobs is referred to as their
   a. job responsibilities.
   b. scope of practice.
   c. opinion.
   d. employee guidelines.

REVIEW

7. The term that describes making an accounting of items on hand is a/an
   a. policy.
   b. inventory.
   c. ordering.
   d. reordering.

8. The Health Insurance Portability and Accountability Act of 1996
   a. governs how often insurance companies can merge with each other.
   b. makes insurers accountable to patients for reimbursement of approved medical costs.
   c. is a set of general rather than legal guidelines regarding the privacy of patient health information.
   d. requires health-care providers to be responsible for the privacy and security of a patient's protected health information.

9. Under HIPAA, PHI stands for
   a. Personal Health Information.
   b. Protected Health Information.
   c. Professional Health Information.
   d. Programmed Health Information.

10. Pharmacy technicians should be detail oriented. This means
    a. patients must receive medications exactly as they have been prescribed.
    b. an incorrect strength will always be detected by the pharmacist.
    c. technicians do not need to be careful because the pharmacist is supposed to find and correct all technician errors.
    d. it is unusual for a technician to pay attention to details.

11. Good hygiene is important for pharmacy technicians because of the interactions with other persons and the expectation of performing in ______________ conditions.
    a. warm
    b. cold
    c. infection free
    d. sunny

12. Pharmacy technicians must be capable and competent in mathematics and problem solving because
    a. all medications that are available on prescription cannot lead to overdose death.
    b. pharmacists always check their work.
    c. all medications come premixed and prepackaged.
    d. mathematical calculations are routinely used.

13. Pharmacy technicians must be capable and competent with computer skills because
    a. pharmacists will check their data entry.
    b. pharmacists do all of the computer work.
    c. pharmacists should operate the computer.
    d. technicians regularly use computers.

14. Pharmacy technicians must be capable and competent in the area of interpersonal skills. This means
    a. they must be able to communicate, cooperate, and work effectively.
    b. they must socialize with their coworkers.
    c. the pharmacist should obtain all confidential information from the patient.
    d. they must make friends with every patient.

15. Training and certification requirements for pharmacy technicians are set by
    a. each state's board of pharmacy.
    b. the ASHP
    c. the PTCB.
    d. the federal government.

16. The _____ is the leading association for pharmacists practicing in hospitals and other health-care systems.
    a. ASHP
    b. PTCB
    c. PTEC
    d. APhA

17. ________________ typically monitor and document competency of pharmacy technicians.
    a. Employers
    b. Technicians
    c. Pharmacists
    d. PTCB

18. Any complaints received regarding an employee's employment
    a. are discarded after two weeks.
    b. are discarded after one year.
    c. are discarded within one week after the complaint was received.
    d. may be kept in the employee's performance/personnel file.

19. Training that occurs in actual workplace settings is called
    a. performance-based training.
    b. on-the-job training.
    c. community college training.
    d. certified training.

20. ________________ is another term for being qualified and capable.
    a. Realistic
    b. Competent
    c. Professional
    d. Technical

21. In the United States, two organizations that performs pharmacy technician certification are the
    a. APhA and ASHP.
    b. PTCB and NHA.
    c. ASHP and PTEC.
    d. PTEC and APhA.

22. The ExCPT exam contains _______ multiple choice questions.
    a. 90
    b. 100
    c. 110
    d. 120

23. To take the PTCE exam, candidates
    a. need only submit an application form.
    b. must be working at a pharmacy.
    c. need to have completed an ASHP accredited training program.
    d. must have a high school diploma or GED by the application deadline and have never been convicted of a felony or a pharmacy or drug-related misdemeanor.

24. Certification must be renewed every
    a. three years.
    b. year.
    c. two years.
    d. four years.

REVIEW

25. After passing a pharmacy technician national certification exam, pharmacy technicians may use the following designation after their name:
    a. PT
    b. RPhT
    c. CPhT
    d. none of the above

26. CPhTs need ____________ of continuing education every ______________ years to renew certification.
    a. 30 hours, 2
    b. 10 hours, 1
    c. 30 hours, 3
    d. 20 hours, 2

27. Continuing education for CPhTs must contain __________ in pharmacy law every _________ years.
    a. one hour, one
    b. two hours, one
    c. one hour, two
    d. two hours, two

CRITICAL THINKING QUESTIONS

1. Why is attention to detail an important quality for a pharmacy technician?
2. What different types of computer skills are important for a pharmacy technician?
3. What are the benefits of certification for a pharmacy technician?

THINKING IT THROUGH WRAP-UP

1. Stacey can earn the CPhT credential by passing the PTCE exam or the ExCPT exam. Both exams assess the knowledge of technicians in areas of pharmacy technician work.
2. Both exams are national exams. The PTCE has 90 multiple choice questions while the ExCPT exam has 110 questions. Both exams are accredited by the National Commission for Certifying Agencies. The PTCE has more questions geared toward institutional pharmacy and the ExCPT has more questions geared toward community pharmacy.
3. Certification must be renewed every two years and certified technicians must meet continuing education requirements.

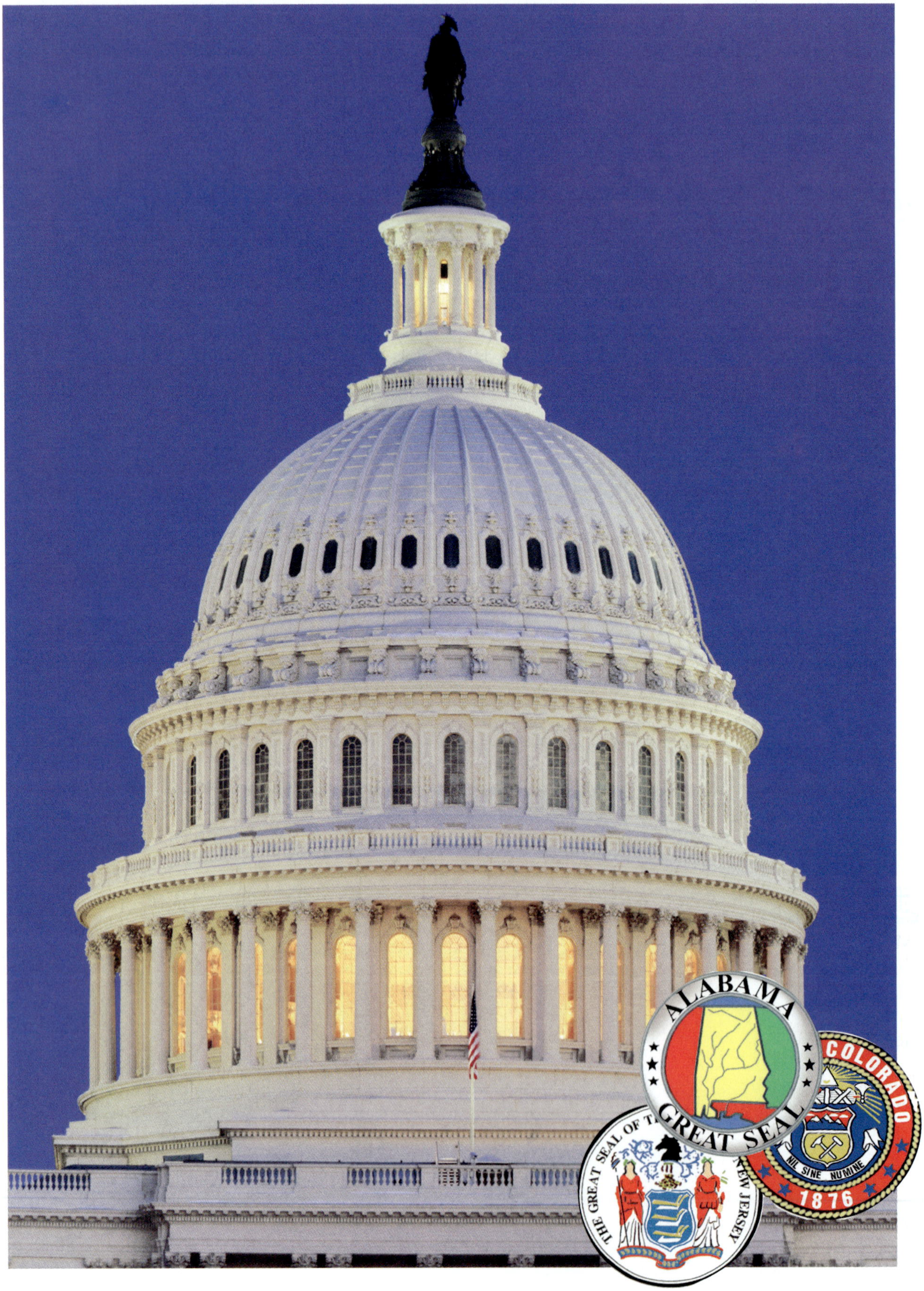
ALABAMA
GREAT SEAL
COLORADO
NIL SINE NUMINE
1876

3

DRUG REGULATION & CONTROL

LEARNING OBJECTIVES

At the completion of study, the student will:

- ✔ know the key legislative acts governing pharmacy practice.
- ✔ understand the FDA process for new drug approval.
- ✔ understand the process by which patents expire, making a drug eligible for release under a pharmaceutical or generic name, and what approval procedures manufacturers must go through.
- ✔ know the different requirements for labels and product labeling for stock medications, prescription containers, controlled substances, and over-the-counter drugs.
- ✔ know the restrictions for the different categories of over-the-counter drugs.
- ✔ know the five groups of controlled substances and restrictions for each.
- ✔ know when a DEA number is required and how to check it.
- ✔ know when and how to fill out and process DEA Form 222.
- ✔ be aware of other key DEA forms and when they are required.
- ✔ know the process for FDA drug recalls.

THINKING IT THROUGH

Mike works as a pharmacy technician at a local community pharmacy. Some OTC drugs are behind the counter, including pseudoephedrine 30 mg tablets, Sudafed® 30 mg tablets, Claritin–D 12 Hour®, Claritin–D 24 Hour®, and Alavert–D 12 Hour®. The pharmacist has told Mike he can sell these products to patients, but he has to follow federal rules governing their sale.

Susan, a 54-year-old regular customer, comes in and asks Mike if she can purchase two 100-count bottles of pseudoephedrine 30 mg tablets.

As you read this chapter, keep in mind the following questions:

1. What is the maximum number of tablets Susan can purchase today?
2. What is the maximum number of bottles of 100 tablets Susan can purchase within a month?

DRUG REGULATION

— A TIME LINE —

There are many laws in the United States concerning the safety and effectiveness of food, drugs, medical devices, and cosmetics. Regardless of whether a product is produced in the United States or is imported, it must meet the requirements of these laws. The leading enforcement agency at the federal level for these regulations is the Food and Drug Administration. On these pages are brief descriptions of U.S. federal laws and their significance.

Food and Drug Act of 1906

Prohibits interstate commerce in adulterated or misbranded food, drinks, and drugs. Government preapproval of drugs is required.

1927 Food, Drug and Insecticide Administration

The law enforcement agency is formed; would be renamed in 1930 as the Food and Drug Administration.

1950 Alberty Food Products v. U.S.

The U.S. Court of Appeals rules that the purpose for which a drug is to be used must be included on the label.

1951 Durham–Humphrey Amendment

Defines which drugs require a prescription by a licensed practitioner and requires them to include this ***legend*** on the label: "Caution: Federal Law prohibits dispensing without a prescription" or "Rx Only."

1962 Kefauver–Harris Amendment

Requires drug manufacturers to provide proof of safety and effectiveness before marketing a drug.

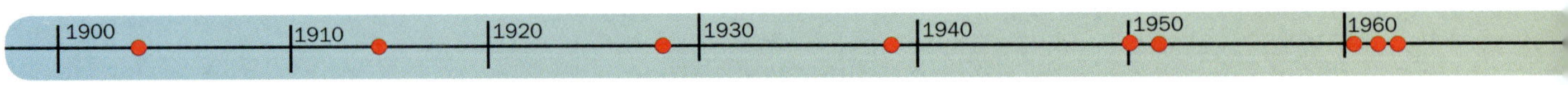

1914 Harrison Tax Act

In response to growing addiction to opiates and cocaine-containing medicines, the Harrison Tax Act establishes that manufacturers, pharmacists, importers, and physicians prescribing narcotics should be licensed and required to pay a tax.

1938 Food, Drug and Cosmetic (FDC) Act

In response to the fatal poisoning of 107 people, primarily children, by an untested sulfanilamide concoction, this comprehensive law requires new drugs be shown to be safe before marketing.

1965 Social Security Act

Establishes the Medicare program.

1966 Fair Packaging and Labeling Act

Requires all consumer products in interstate commerce to be honestly and informatively labeled.

The Thalidomide Lesson

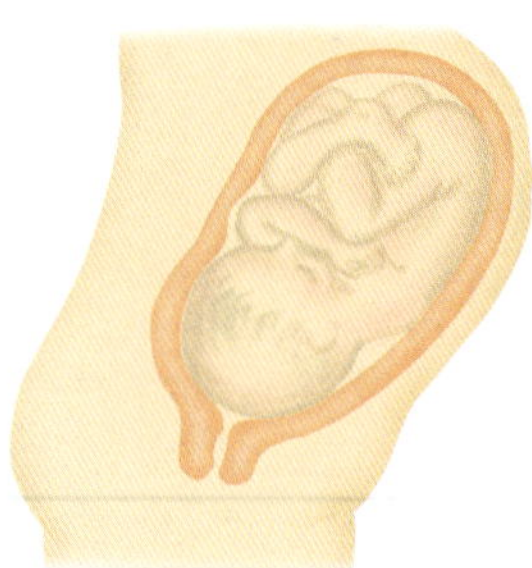

In 1962 the Kefauver-Harris Amendment was signed into law in part because a new sleeping pill containing the drug thalidomide was found to cause severe birth defects when used by pregnant women. This included lost limbs and other major deformities that affected thousands of children in Europe, where the drug had been widely used. After passage of the Kefauver-Harris Amendment, drugs had to be shown to be both safe and effective before they could be marketed in the United States.

Later studies found thalidomide to be safe and effective in treating multiple myeloma and leprosy and it is now approved for those uses. However, an FDA Alert remains on the drug stating that both men and women must agree in writing to their understanding of the risks of thalidomide and actions they must take while being treated with it.

legend drug any drug that requires a prescription and either of these *legends* on the label: "Caution: Federal law prohibits dispensing without a prescription," or "Rx only."

1970 Poison Prevention Packaging Act

Requires childproof packaging on all controlled and most prescription drugs dispensed by pharmacies. Non-childproof containers may only be used if the prescriber or patient requests one.

1970 Controlled Substances Act (CSA)

Classifies five levels of controlled substances that have potential for abuse and therefore restricts their distribution; establishes the Drug Enforcement Administration (DEA) as a division of the Justice Department.

1983 Orphan Drug Act

Provides incentives to promote research, approval, and marketing of drugs needed for the treatment of rare diseases.

1984 Drug Price Competition and Patent Term Restoration Act (Hatch–Waxman)

Allows for both the extension of drug patent terms and quicker introduction of lower-cost generic drugs.

1987 Prescription Drug Marketing Act

Restricts distribution of prescription drugs to legitimate commercial channels; requires drug wholesalers to be licensed by the states.

1996 Health Insurance Portability and Accountability Act

Among other things, this act defined the scope of health information that may and may not be shared among health-care providers without patient consent and provided for broad and stringent regulations to protect patients' right to privacy. These regulations govern the transfer of patient health information whether it is communicated electronically, on paper, or orally.

2003 Medicare Modernization Act

Establishes optional Medicare Part D to provide coverage for prescription drugs and Medication Therapy Management (MTM).

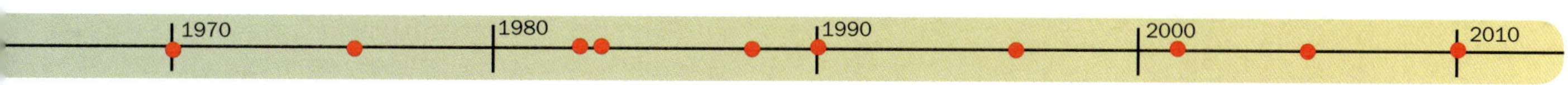

1976 Medical Device Amendment

Requires premarket approval for safety and effectiveness of life-sustaining and life-supporting medical devices.

1990 Omnibus Budget Reconciliation Act (OBRA)

Among other things, this act requires pharmacists to offer counseling to Medicaid patients regarding medications.

1990 Anabolic Steroid Control Act

Passed to "address the abuse of steroids by athletes, and, especially, youngsters and teenagers."

2005 Combat Methamphetamine Epidemic Act

Establishes strict controls on OTC sales of pseudoephedrine, ephedrine, and phenylpropanolamine.

2010 Patient Protection and Affordable Care Act

Health-care reform legislation of the 111th United States Congress intended to expand health insurance access for uninsured Americans.

2012 FDA Safety and Innovation Act

Establishes user fees to enhance access to medications and medical devices and made provisions for addressing drug product shortages in the United States.

safety you should know

The FDA's Center for Drug Evaluation and Research provides an Index to Drug-Specific Information (www.fda.gov/cder/drug/DrugSafety/DrugIndex.htm) with patient, consumer, and health-care professional information sheets, including FDA alerts. The center also works with drug manufacturers to develop risk management programs for drugs with FDA alerts, such as the iPLEDGE program for Accutane. Health care professionals, wholesalers, pharmacies, and patients must register in the iPLEDGE program to prescribe, distribute, fill prescriptions for, or use Accutane.

NEW DRUG APPROVAL

All new drugs, whether made domestically or imported, require FDA approval before they can be marketed in the United States.

A new drug is any drug proposed for marketing after 1938 that was not already recognized as safe and effective. This represents the vast majority of drugs on the market.

Before it is approved, a new drug must be shown to be both safe and effective and that its benefits substantially outweigh its risks.

It is the responsibility of the drug manufacturer (not the FDA) to provide proof of this to the FDA's Center for Drug Evaluation and Research (CDER). The proof is based on extensive testing, which begins in the laboratory, where chemical analysis is performed, and moves on to animal testing and then clinical trials with people. The FDA estimates that the testing process currently takes 8.5 years.

Clinical trials involve testing the drug on people.

Clinical tests begin with small numbers of participants over a short period of time and eventually expand into large groups of participants over long periods. Trial participants must give their informed consent. Among other things, it means the person must be told of the risks of the treatment along with other treatment options in language they can understand. Participants are also free to leave the trial at any time they wish.

pediatric having to do with the treatment of children.

placebo an inactive substance given in place of a medication.

TESTING

Animal Testing

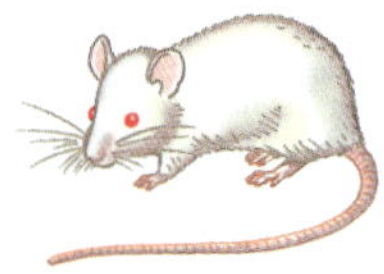

Once laboratory testing of a proposed new drug is finished, the drug is tested on animals before it will be tested on humans. Drug companies try to use as few animals and to treat them as humanely as possible. Since different species often react differently, more than one species is usually tested. Drug absorption into the bloodstream is monitored carefully. Only a fraction of a percent of drugs tested on animals are ever tested on humans.

Placebos

Placebos are inactive substances, not real medications, that are administered to give the patient the impression he or she is receiving a potentially effective medication. This provides a valuable comparison against patients who receive a test drug. Patients in trials must freely agree to the possibility that they may be given a placebo. They must also be informed of an effective treatment if one is available.

Testing Children

Children are not included in trials until a drug has been fully tested on adults. Drugs that have not been tested on children generally state on the label that their safety and effectiveness has not been established for children. Some drugs, however, may carry label information for ***pediatric*** use that is based on studies of adults and other pediatric treatment information. The Pediatric Labeling Rule mandates that all drugs have pediatric dosing and safety information on their labels if the drug has potential use for pediatric patients. The Pediatric Research Equity Act (PREA) was passed in 2003 requiring pharmaceutical companies to test on children any new drugs likely to be used to treat children.

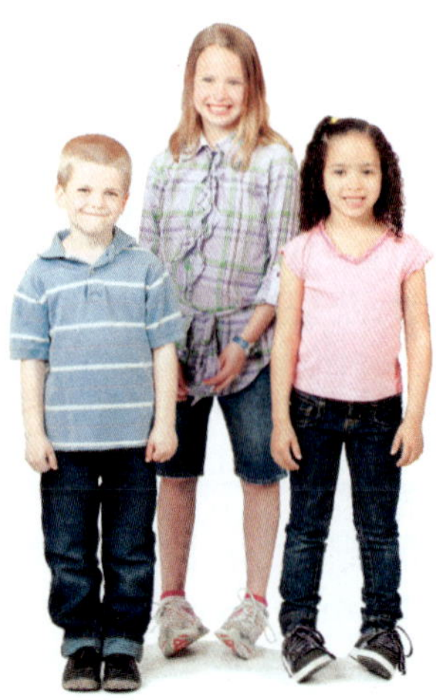

Testing Phases in Humans

There are three phases of testing a new drug in humans. Phase 1 begins with a small number of participants for a short time, increasing to a large number of participants for a longer period of time in phases 2 and 3. The goals of each phase also progress from indicating a minimal level of safety to ultimately verifying the safety, effectiveness and dosage for widespread use. Only about 25% of drugs tested in phase 1 successfully complete phase 3 and are approved for marketing. Once a drug becomes available to the public, additional information is collected about safety, efficacy, and uses, and this additional post-marketing surveillance is sometimes called phase 4.

phase 1

- 20–100 patients
- time: several months
- purpose: mainly safety

phase 2

- up to several hundred patients
- time: several months to two years
- purpose: short-term safety but mainly effectiveness

phase 3

- several hundred to several thousand patients
- time: one to four years
- purpose: safety, dosage, and effectiveness

Source: U.S. Food and Drug Administration

During the trial phase, a proposed new drug is called an investigational new drug (IND).

It is available for use only within the trial groups unless granted a special "treatment" status, which is sometimes given to provide relief to critically ill patients outside of clinical trials. An example of this is AZT, which was used on thousands of AIDS patients who were not part of a clinical trial prior to the drug receiving FDA approval. It is worth noting, however, that such drugs are extremely expensive and are excluded from coverage by most insurers and HMOs.

Tests are controlled by comparing the effect of a proposed drug on one group of patients with the effect of a different treatment on other patients.

Patients have the same condition and similar characteristics and are placed in either treatment groups or control groups at random to make sure the groups have essentially the same characteristics. The control group may receive no drug at all, a placebo, a drug known to be effective, or a different dose of the same drug.

The patients in a trial are always blind to the treatment, meaning they do not know if they are receiving the drug being tested or a placebo.

In a double-blind test, neither the patients nor the physicians know whether the patient is receiving the active drug or a placebo. This prevents patients and/or their physicians from imagining effects one way or the other. Medical results alone determine the drug's effectiveness and its safety.

℞ safety you should know

Medical devices and biological products such as insulin and vaccines must also meet FDA testing and approval requirements. The Center for Devices and Radiological Health (CDRH) is responsible for devices. The Center for Biologics Evaluation and Research (CBER) is responsible for biological products made from living organisms.

MARKETED DRUGS

A patent for a new drug gives its manufacturer an exclusive right to market the drug for a specific period of time under a brand name.

During this time, the manufacturer attempts to recover the costs of the drug's research and development. Many factors can affect the duration of a patent but they typically expire 20 years from the date of filing. Since the testing and approval process takes years to complete, for many years drugs reached the market with only half their patent time left. To compensate for this, the Hatch–Waxman Act of 1984 provided for up to five-year extensions of patent protection to the patent holders to make up for time lost while products went through the FDA approval process.

Once a patent for a brand drug expires, other manufacturers may copy the drug and release it under its pharmaceutical or generic name.

Manufacturers of generic drugs do not need to perform the safety and effectiveness testing required of new drugs. However, they need to demonstrate that the drug is ***pharmaceutically equivalent*** to the proprietary (patented brand) drug—that it has the same active ingredients, same dosage form, same route of administration, and same strength; and that it is ***therapeutically equivalent***—that the body's use of the drug is the same. This is measured by the rate and extent to which the active ingredients are absorbed into the bloodstream. Evaluations of generic drug products can be found in the FDA "Orange Book."

Over-the-counter (OTC) drugs are drugs that do not require a prescription.

They can be used upon the judgment of the consumer. There are over 100,000 OTC drugs in 80 therapeutic categories marketed. The FDA publishes acceptable ingredients for OTC drugs in *Drug Monographs*. The manufacturer of an OTC drug must follow monograph requirements to be able to market their drug without undergoing the FDA new drug approval process. Though some OTC drugs were available before FDA approval was required, the FDA has been reviewing them under the OTC Drug Review Program, and all new OTC drugs require FDA approval.

LABELS AND PRODUCT LABELING

While all drugs are required to have clear and accurate information for all labels, inserts, packaging, and so on, there are different information requirements for various categories of drugs. Information requirements for OTC drugs are designed to enable consumers to use them without medical advice. Manufacturers of prescription drugs do not include directions for use on their labels since such directions must be supplied by the prescriber and dispenser. In many cases, important associated information may not fit on the label itself, and it will be provided in the form of an insert, brochure, or other document that is referred to as ***product labeling***.

Patient Package Inserts (PPI) are required by the FDA for some potentially dangerous drugs and have information for patients on how to safely use the medication. Oral contraceptives are one type of medication with PPIs; PPIs must be provided to patients with the first dispensing and also with refills if 30 days has passed since the patient received a PPI. PPIs are part of the FDA-approved labeling.

Medication Guides (MedGuides) can be provided voluntarily by drug manufacturers for some drugs. MedGuides also contain information for patients on how to safely use a drug product. When provided by manufacturers, MedGuides are also part of the FDA-approved labeling.

pharmaceutical equivalent drug products that contain identical amounts of the same active ingredients in the same dosage form.

product labeling important associated information that is not on the label of a drug product itself, but is provided with the product in the form of an insert, brochure, or other document.

therapeutic equivalent pharmaceutical equivalents that produce the same effects in patients.

OTC LABELS

Over-the-counter medications do not require a prescription but sometimes prescriptions are written for them for insurance or other reasons. As a result, the pharmacy technician will deal with OTC medications regularly and should be familiar both with their label information and how to handle inquiries about them.

Many over-the-counter products have labels that are difficult to read, understand, or both. To the right is a label format adopted by the FDA to make it easier to read and understand the information currently contained on over-the-counter medication labels.

The following information should be contained on the labels of over-the-counter medications.

- product name
- name and address of manufacturer or distributor
- list of all active and other ingredients
- amount of contents
- adequate warnings
- adequate directions for use

Since OTC medications are not without risks, all patients requesting information on them should be referred to the pharmacist. OTC medications may have significant drug interactions with prescription drugs the patient may be taking, which could lead to serious adverse effects, including death.

Active Ingredient (In Each Tablet) **Purpose**

Chlorpheniramine Maleate 4 mg..Antihistamine

Uses: for the temporary relief of these symptoms of hay fever

- sneezing
- runny nose
- itchy,watery eyes

Warnings

Ask a Doctor Before Use

If You Have:

- glaucoma
- a breathing problem such as emphysema or chronic bronchitis
- difficulty in urination due to enlargement of the prostate gland

If You Are:

- taking sedatives or tranquilizers

When Using This Product:

- marked drowsiness may occur
- alcohol, sedatives, and tranquilizers may increase the drowsiness effect
- avoid alcoholic beverages
- use caution when driving a motor vehicle or operating machinery
- excitability may occur, especially in children

If pregnant or breast-feeding, ask a health professional before use.
Keep out of reach of children. In case of overdose, get medical help right away.

Directions:

Adults and children over 12 years:	Take 1 tablet every 4 to 6 hours as needed. Do not take more than 6 tablets in 24 hours.
Children 6 to under 12 years:	Take 1/2 tablet every 4 to 6 hours as needed. Do not take more than 3 tablets in 24 hours.
Children under 6 years:	Ask a doctor.

FDA label format for over-the-counter medications

safety you should know

- Federal laws require that a drug and/or its container not be imitative of another drug so that the consumer will be misled. Nevertheless, there are many drugs with similar sounding names in similar looking packages. It is therefore essential for pharmacy technicians to pay close attention to the details of drug names and packaging. Using the wrong drug can have very serious consequences. A list of some Look-alike and Soundalike drugs is in Appendix A.
- Manufacturers of drugs are encouraged to use tall man lettering on drugs that are prone to be confused with other look-alike or soundalike drugs. The distinguishing part of the drug's name is printed in upper case letters (e.g., predniSONE vs. prednisoLONE). The FDA and ISMP list of drug names with recommended tall man letters is online at http://www.ismp.org/tools/tallmanletters.pdf.

BEHIND-THE-COUNTER MEDICATIONS

While most OTC medications are not kept behind the pharmacy counter, some are, even if a prescription is not required. These medications may at times be sold without a prescription, but with restrictions on their sale. Three categories of behind-the-counter medications are OTC medications containing ephedrine and pseudoephedrine, exempt narcotics, and emergency contraceptives.

The ***Combat Methamphetamine Epidemic Act (CMEA)*** requires pharmacies to keep all OTC cold and allergy medications containing ephedrine, pseudoephedrine or phenylpropanolamine behind the counter (although phenylpropanolamine is no longer available in OTC medications).

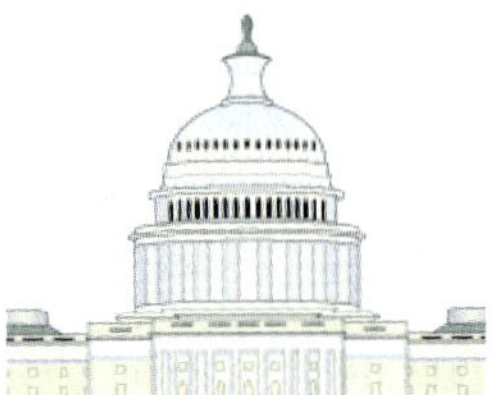

CMEA also sets daily and monthly restrictions on the amount of ephedrine or pseudoephedrine that can be sold to an individual (3.6 grams per day and 9 grams per month, of which not more than 7.5 grams may be imported by means of a common or contract carrier or the U.S. Postal Service). The law also requires purchasers to present photo identification and retailers to keep personal information about the purchasers for at least two years after each purchase. It is important to note that some state or local laws may call for additional restrictions on the sale of OTCs containing ephedrine and pseudoephedrine.

As part of CMEA, appropriately trained pharmacy technicians may be allowed to sell OTC medications containing ephedrine or pseudoephedrine. The following rules must be followed:

- ✔ The pharmacy or store cannot exceed the established daily and monthly limits per customer for the OTC sale of ephedrine or pseudoephedrine.
- ✔ The pharmacy or store must maintain written or electronic records for a period of two years that contain the following elements:
    - product name
    - quantity sold
    - name and address of purchaser
    - date and time of the sale
    - proof of identification
    - signature of the purchaser

OTC MEDICATIONS CONTAINING EPHEDRINE AND PSEUDOEPHEDRINE

The daily sales limit of pseudoephedrine base is 3.6 grams per purchaser, regardless of the number of transactions. The tables below show commonly available strengths of pseudoephedrine and the amounts of products that can be purchased in a day.

Note: The molecular weight of pseudoephedrine base is 165.23 while the molecular weight of pseudoephedrine HCl is 201.70. The quantities in the tables below are calculated for the commonly found HCl form of pseudoephedrine.

mg/ml of Pseudoephedrine HCl	Number of Milliliters (ml)
15 mg/1.6 ml	468
7.5 mg/5 ml	2,929
15 mg/5 ml	1,464
30 mg/5 ml	732
60 mg/5 ml	366

mg of Pseudoephedrine HCl	Number of Tablets
30 mg	146
60 mg	73
120 mg	36
240 mg	18

EXEMPT NARCOTICS

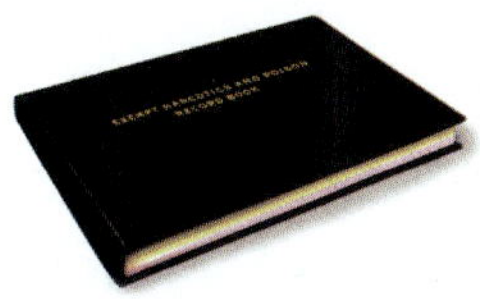

Exempt narcotics are medications that contain habit-forming ingredients but can be sold by a pharmacist without a prescription to persons at least 18 years of age. For example, there are some cough syrups that contain a small amount of codeine and do not require a prescription according to federal, state, or local law.

Certain rules apply to the sale of exempt narcotics:

- ✔ Dispensing of exempt narcotics is made only by a pharmacist, although the actual cash register transaction may be completed by a pharmacy technician after a pharmacist has approved and documented the dispensing.
- ✔ Limits for how many dosage units can be sold in any given 48-hour period are followed.
- ✔ Purchasers of exempt narcotics are at least 18 years old, and purchasers not known by the pharmacist must provide suitable identification.
- ✔ A bound record book containing the name and address of the purchaser, the name and quantity of exempt narcotic purchased, the date of each purchase, and the name or initials of the pharmacist who dispensed the substance to the purchaser is maintained.

EMERGENCY CONTRACEPTIVES

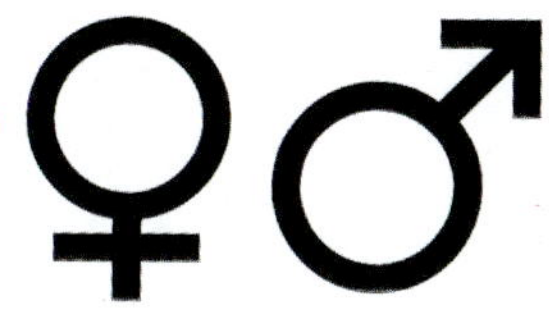

Plan B® is a drug indicated for emergency contraception (EC). It has ***dual marketing*** status, which means it has prescription drug status and OTC drug status.

While a prescription is required to dispense EC to patients under 17 years old, pharmacists may sell Plan B® without a prescription to individuals 17 years and older. A special program called CARE, which stands for Convenient Access, Responsible Education, provides that Plan B® is available only through pharmacies and other health care facilities licensed to dispense prescription drugs. Packages of Plan B® that can be sold OTC must bear the statement "Rx only for women younger than age 17." Pharmacies that stock Plan B® as an OTC must keep the product behind the counter and confirm the patient's age by requesting to see government-issued identification.

Additionally, pharmacists in some states have authority to prescribe and dispense EC under protocol to patients under 17 years old. Alaska, California, Hawaii, Maine, Massachusetts, New Hampshire, New Mexico, Vermont, and Washington law provides pharmacists with authority to prescribe and dispense EC under protocol.

Combat Methamphetamine Epidemic Act (CMEA) federal law that sets daily and monthly limits on OTC sale of pseudoephedrine and ephedrine.

Dual marketing status of medications like Plan B® that are classified as both prescription drugs and OTC drugs.

Exempt narcotics medications with habit-forming ingredients that could be dispensed by a pharmacist without a prescription to persons at least 18 years of age.

SAMPLE LABELS

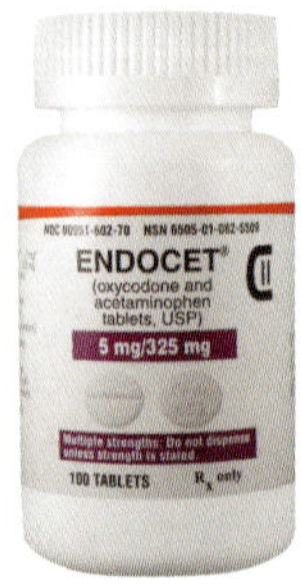

MANUFACTURER STOCK LABEL

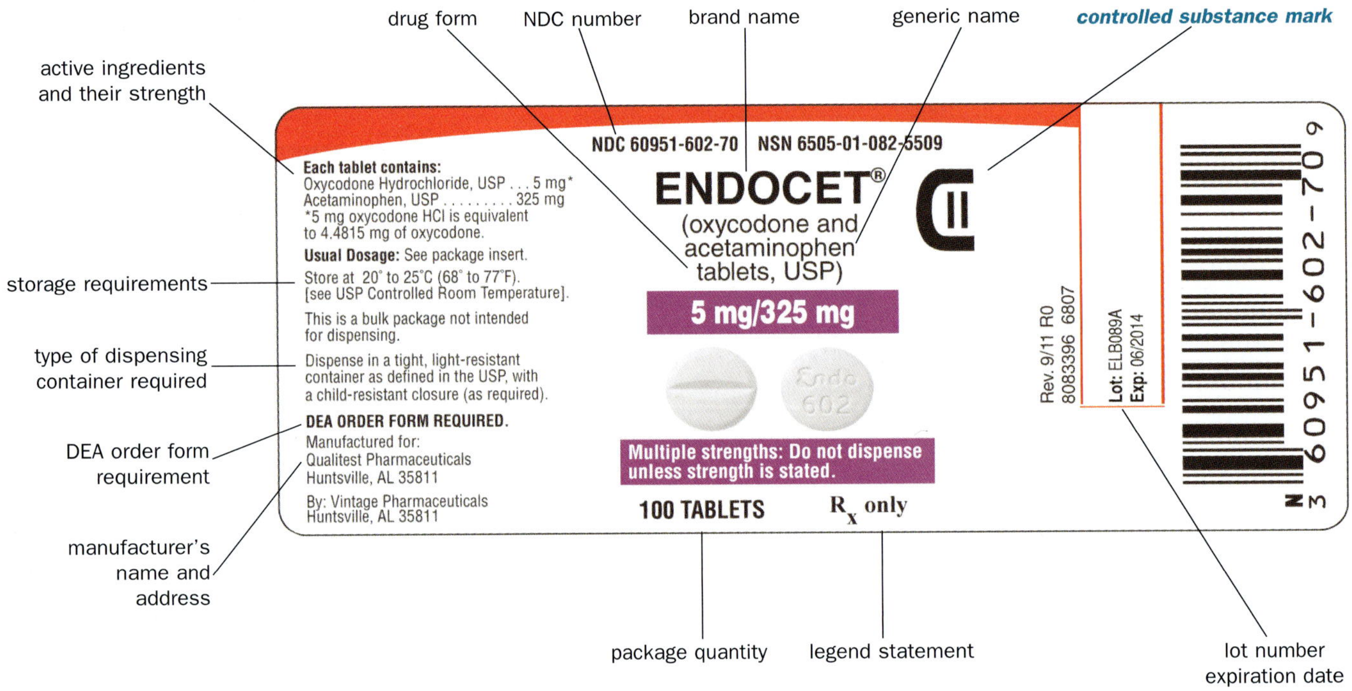

Product Labeling

In addition to a container label, manufacturer prescription drugs must also be accompanied by product labeling, sometimes called the "package insert" or "prescribing information," which includes information on the following: clinical pharmacology, indications and usage, contraindications, warnings, precautions, adverse reactions, drug abuse and dependence, dosage, and packaging. This information is designed to inform both the prescriber and the dispenser regarding the drug.

NDC (National Drug Code) Numbers

An NDC number is an identification number assigned by the manufacturer to a drug product. Each NDC number has three sets of numbers: the first set indicates the manufacturer; the second set indicates the medication, its strength, and dosage form; and the third set indicates the package size. Note that depending on whether it is an older or newer drug product, the first set of numbers could have four or five digits and the second set of numbers could have three or four digits. The last set of numbers always has two digits.

controlled substance mark the mark (CII–CV) that indicates the control category of a drug with a potential for abuse.

DISPENSED PRESCRIPTION DRUG LABELS

Minimum requirements on prescription labels for most drugs generally are as follows:

- ✔ name and address of dispenser
- ✔ prescription serial number
- ✔ date of prescription or filling
- ✔ expiration date
- ✔ name of prescriber

And any of the following that are stated in the prescription:

- ✔ name of patient
- ✔ directions for use
- ✔ cautionary statements

Certain drugs have greater requirements, and many states impose greater requirements.

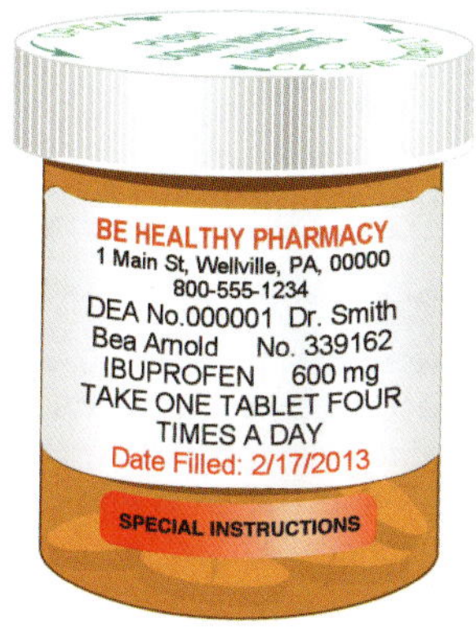

Typical elements on a prescription label:

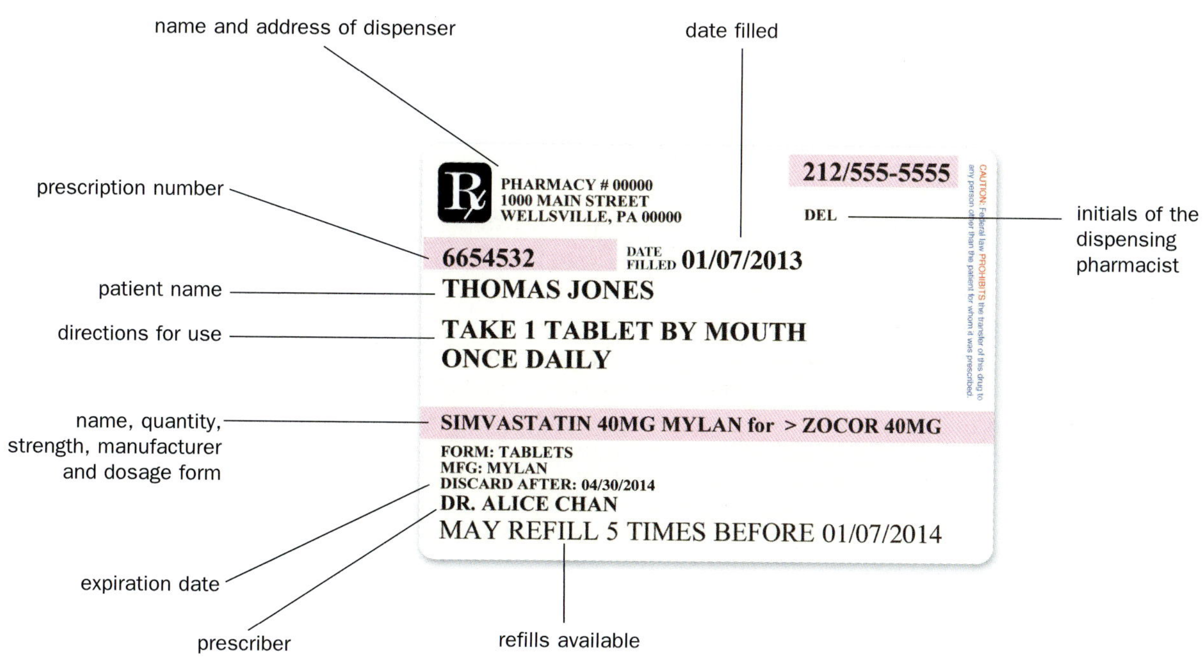

CONTROLLED SUBSTANCES

The government tightly controls the use of drugs that can be easily abused.

The Controlled Substances Act of 1970 (CSA) identified five groups, or schedules, of drugs as controlled substances and established strict distribution guidelines for them. This act also requires manufacturers, distributors, or dispensers of controlled substances to register with the Drug Enforcement Administration (DEA) of the Justice Department. This created a closed system in which only registered parties can distribute these drugs.

Controlled Substances Schedules

- **Schedule I:** Drugs with a high potential for abuse and no accepted medical use in the United States. They may not be prescribed. Heroin, various opium derivatives, and hallucinogenic substances are included on this schedule.
- **Schedule II:** Drugs that have a high potential for abuse which may lead to physical or psychological dependence but that also have currently accepted medical uses in the United States. Amphetamines, opium, cocaine, methadone, and various opiates are included on this schedule.
- **Schedule III:** Drugs with a potential for abuse less than those in Schedules I and II. These drugs have currently accepted medical uses in the United States, but their abuse may lead to moderate or low physical dependence or high psychological dependence. Anabolic steroids and various compounds containing limited quantities of narcotic substances such as codeine are included on this schedule.
- **Schedule IV:** Drugs with low potential for abuse relative to Schedule III drugs. These drugs have currently accepted medical uses in the United States, but their abuse may lead to limited physical dependence or psychological dependence. Phenobarbital, the sedative chloral hydrate, and the anesthetic methohexital are included in this group.
- **Schedule V:** Drugs with a low potential for abuse relative to Schedule IV drugs. These drugs have currently accepted medical uses in the United States, but their abuse may lead to limited physical dependence or psychological dependence. Compounds containing limited amounts of a narcotic such as codeine are included in this group.

Source: 21 USC (United States Code) Sec. 812 as of 1/2012. Note: these schedules are revised periodically. It is important to refer to the most current schedule.

REGULATIONS

Labels

Manufacturers must clearly label controlled drugs with their control classification.

Record Keeping

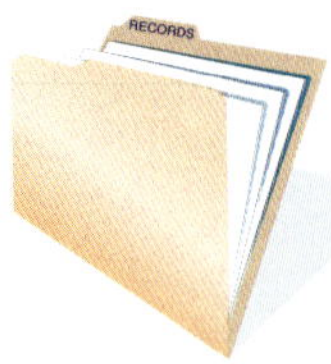

Distributors are required to maintain accurate records of all controlled substance activity, including accurate records of inventory and drugs dispensed. Schedule II records must be kept for seven years and all other records for two years, unless the state requirement is different. Schedule II prescription records must also be kept separate from noncontrolled drug records, though in some cases they may be kept with other controlled drug records.

Security for Controlled Drugs

Schedule II drugs are generally stored in a locked, tamper-proof narcotics cabinet that is usually secured to the floor or wall. Schedule III, IV, and V drugs may be kept openly on storage shelves in retail and hospital settings.

Joint Responsibility

By law, both the prescriber and the dispenser of the prescription have joint responsibility for the legitimate medical purpose of the prescription. This is primarily intended to ensure that controlled substances not be prescribed for inappropriate reasons.

DEA Number

All prescribers of controlled substances must be authorized by the DEA. Prescribers are assigned a DEA number, which must be used on all controlled drug prescriptions.

controlled substances five groups of drugs identified by the 1970 Controlled Substances Act (CSA) as having the potential for abuse and whose distribution is therefore strictly controlled by five control schedules set forth in the CSA.

SAMPLE LABELS

At right are two manufacturer labels, one for a C-IV product (Diazepam) and one for a C-II product (Endocet®). Note the prominent controlled substance marks.

C-I and C-II labels must also have "DEA Order Form Required" printed on them.

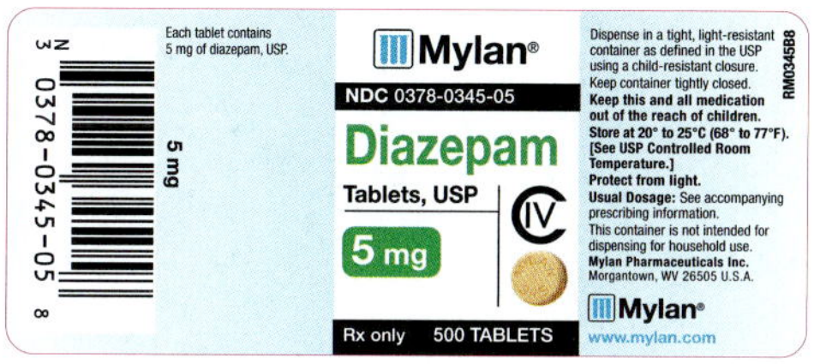

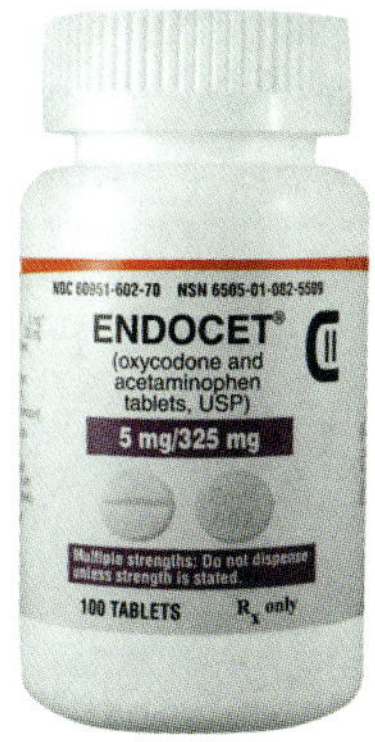

DEA 222 ORDER FORM

DEA Form 222 is used to order C-I and C-II substances. It must be filled out in pen, typewriter, or indelible pencil and be signed by an authorized person, in triplicate. Copy 1 is retained by the supplier, Copy 2 is forwarded to the DEA, and Copy 3 is retained by the purchaser (for example, the pharmacy). The purchaser must record on Copy 3 the number of containers received and the dates the drugs were received. Each form has its own unique serial number issued when the form is requested and all forms must be kept on-hand for two years, even if they are filled out incorrectly. This form can be requested online from www.deadiversion. usdoj.gov/drugreg/index.html. Note that C-III–C-V don't require federal order forms because of their lower potential for abuse.

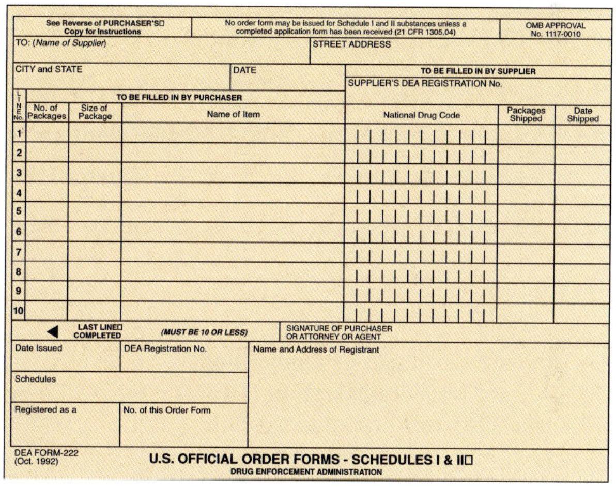
See Reverse of PURCHASER'S Copy for Instructions | No order form may be issued for Schedule I and II substances unless a completed application form has been received (21 CFR 1305.04) | OMB APPROVAL No. 1117-0010

TO: (*Name of Supplier*) | STREET ADDRESS

CITY and STATE | DATE | TO BE FILLED IN BY SUPPLIER | SUPPLIER'S DEA REGISTRATION No.

LINE No.	No. of Packages	Size of Package	Name of Item	National Drug Code	Packages Shipped	Date Shipped
1						
2						
3						
4						
5						
6						
7						
8						
9						
10						

(TO BE FILLED IN BY PURCHASER)

LAST LINE COMPLETED (*MUST BE 10 OR LESS*) | SIGNATURE OF PURCHASER OR ATTORNEY OR AGENT

Date Issued | DEA Registration No. | Name and Address of Registrant

Schedules

Registered as a | No. of this Order Form

DEA FORM-222 (Oct. 1992)

U.S. OFFICIAL ORDER FORMS - SCHEDULES I & II

DRUG ENFORCEMENT ADMINISTRATION

CONTROLLED SUBSTANCES PRESCRIPTIONS

Controlled substances prescriptions, particularly for Schedule II drugs, have greater requirements than other prescriptions, at both the federal and state levels. The DEA number must appear on the form and the patient's full street address must be entered for all controlled substances prescriptions.

On Schedule II prescriptions, the form must be signed by the prescriber. In many states, there are specific time limits that require Schedule II prescriptions be promptly filled. Quantities are limited and generally refills are not allowed.

Federal requirements for Schedules III–V are less stringent than for Schedule II. For example, faxed prescriptions are allowed and they may be refilled up to five times within a six-month period. However, state and other regulations may be stricter than federal requirements, so it is necessary to know the requirements for your specific job setting.

Working the DEA Formula: An Example

DEA numbers are required by federal law. They have two letters followed by seven single-digit numbers, e.g., AB1234563. To check a DEA number on a prescription, use the following formula: Add the sum of the first, third, and fifth digits to twice the sum of the second, fourth, and sixth digits; the total should be a number whose last digit is the same as the last digit of the DEA number on the prescription. For example, using the number AB1234563, since (1 + 3 + 5) + 2 X (2 + 4 + 6) = 33, the DEA number is consistent with the formula.

ADDITIONAL DEA FORMS

In addition to DEA Form 222, manufacturers, distributors, and dispensers of controlled substances are required to use other DEA forms to register with the DEA and monitor inventory.

Below is a list of all DEA forms and some samples of more commonly used forms. They are available online at www.deadiversion.usdoj.gov/drugreg/index.html.

DEA Forms

- DEA Form-224 (Application for New Registration)
- DEA Form-224a (Renewal Application for Registration)
- DEA Form-224b (Retail Pharmacy Registration Affidavit for Chain Renewal)
- DEA Form-222 (U.S. Official Order Forms—Schedule I & II)
- DEA Form-41 (Registrants Inventory of Drugs Surrendered)
- DEA Form-106 (Report of Theft or Loss of Controlled Substances)
- DEA Form-363 (New Application Registration)—Narcotic Treatment Program
- DEA Form-363a (Application for DEA Registration)—NTP renewal registration
- DEA Form-510 (Application for Registration)—for Chemical Registration

This is an example of **Application for New Registration (DEA Form-224)** for retail pharmacies, hospitals/clinics, practitioners, teaching institutions, and mid-level practitioners. The form requests information such as the business activity, drug schedules, state license number, and state controlled substance number (if required).

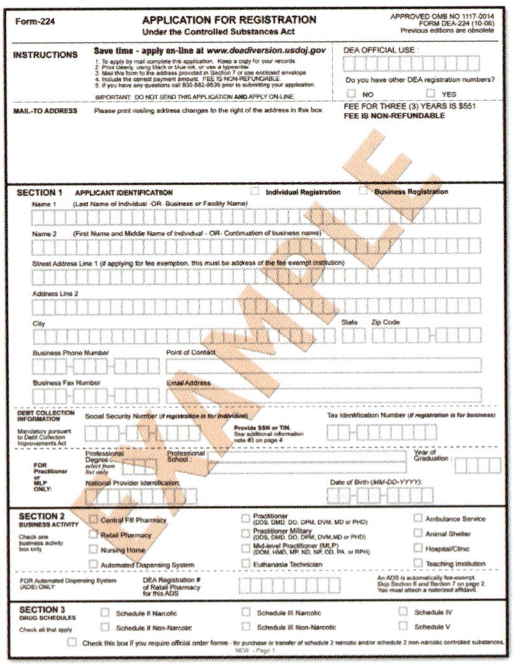

Form-224

APPLICATION FOR REGISTRATION
Under the Controlled Substances Act

APPROVED OMB NO 1117-0014
FORM DEA-224 (10-06)
Previous editions are obsolete

INSTRUCTIONS

Save time - apply on-line at *www.deadiversion.usdoj.gov*

1. To apply by mail complete this application. Keep a copy for your records.
2. Print clearly, using black or blue ink, or use a typewriter.
3. Mail this form to the address provided in Section 7 or use enclosed envelope.
4. Include the correct payment amount. FEE IS NON-REFUNDABLE.
5. If you have any questions call 800-882-9539 prior to submitting your application.

IMPORTANT: DO NOT SEND THIS APPLICATION AND APPLY ON-LINE.

DEA OFFICIAL USE :

Do you have other DEA registration numbers? ☐ NO ☐ YES

MAIL-TO ADDRESS — Please print mailing address changes to the right of the address in this box

FEE FOR THREE (3) YEARS IS $551
FEE IS NON-REFUNDABLE

SECTION 1 APPLICANT IDENTIFICATION ☐ Individual Registration ☐ Business Registration

Name 1 (Last Name of individual -OR- Business or Facility Name)

Name 2 (First Name and Middle Name of individual - OR- Continuation of business name)

Street Address Line 1 (if applying for fee exemption, this must be address of the fee exempt institution)

Address Line 2

City — State — Zip Code

Business Phone Number — Point of Contact

Business Fax Number — Email Address

DEBT COLLECTION INFORMATION — Mandatory pursuant to Debt Collection Improvements Act

Social Security Number (*if registration is for individual*)

Provide SSN or TIN. See additional information note #3 on page 4

Tax Identification Number (*if registration is for business*)

FOR Practitioner or MLP ONLY:

Professional Degree: *select from list only* — Professional School : — Year of Graduation :

National Provider Identification: — Date of Birth (*MM-DD-YYYY*):

SECTION 2 BUSINESS ACTIVITY — Check one business activity box only

☐ Central Fill Pharmacy
☐ Retail Pharmacy
☐ Nursing Home
☐ Automated Dispensing System
☐ Practitioner (DDS, DMD, DO, DPM, DVM, MD or PHD)
☐ Practitioner Military (DDS, DMD, DO, DPM, DVM,MD or PHD)
☐ Mid-level Practitioner (MLP) (DOM, HMD, MP, ND, NP, OD, PA, or RPH)
☐ Euthanasia Technician
☐ Ambulance Service
☐ Animal Shelter
☐ Hospital/Clinic
☐ Teaching Institution

FOR Automated Dispensing System (ADS) ONLY: DEA Registration # of Retail Pharmacy for this ADS

An ADS is automatically fee-exempt. Skip Section 6 and Section 7 on page 2. You must attach a notarized affidavit.

SECTION 3 DRUG SCHEDULES — Check all that apply

☐ Schedule II Narcotic
☐ Schedule II Non-Narcotic
☐ Schedule III Narcotic
☐ Schedule III Non-Narcotic
☐ Schedule IV
☐ Schedule V

☐ Check this box if you require official order forms - for purchase or transfer of schedule 2 narcotic and/or schedule 2 non-narcotic controlled substances.

NEW - Page 1

Source: www.deadiversion.usdoj.gov/drugreg/index.html and *Pharmacist's Manual*, U.S. Department of Justice, Drug Enforcement Administration, Office of Diversion Control.

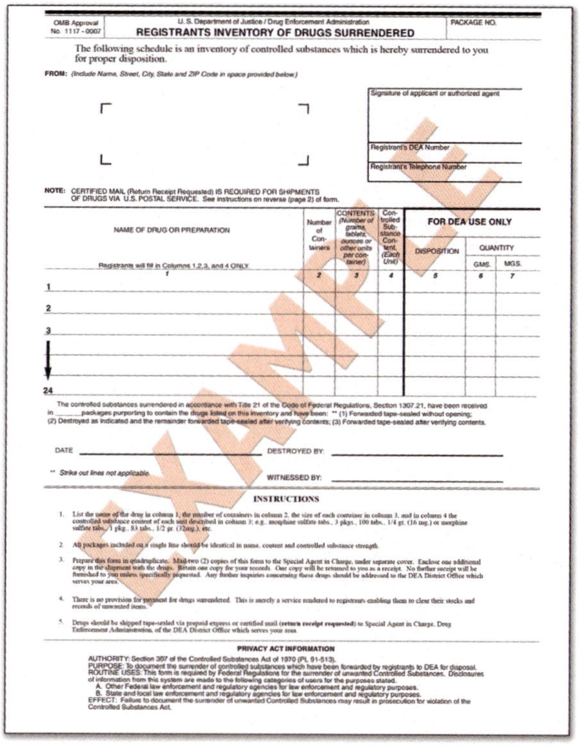

OMB Approval No. 1117 - 0007

U. S. Department of Justice / Drug Enforcement Administration

REGISTRANTS INVENTORY OF DRUGS SURRENDERED

PACKAGE NO.

The following schedule is an inventory of controlled substances which is hereby surrendered to you for proper disposition.

FROM: *(Include Name, Street, City, State and ZIP Code in space provided below.)*

Signature of applicant or authorized agent

Registrant's DEA Number

Registrant's Telephone Number

NOTE: CERTIFIED MAIL (Return Receipt Requested) IS REQUIRED FOR SHIPMENTS OF DRUGS VIA U.S. POSTAL SERVICE. See instructions on reverse (page 2) of form.

	NAME OF DRUG OR PREPARATION Registrants will fill in Columns 1,2,3, and 4 ONLY	Number of Containers	CONTENTS (Number of grams, tablets, ounces or other units per container)	Controlled Substance Content, (Each Unit)	FOR DEA USE ONLY DISPOSITION	QUANTITY GMS.	MGS.
	1	2	3	4	5	6	7
1							
2							
3							
24							

The controlled substances surrendered in accordance with Title 21 of the Code of Federal Regulations, Section 1307.21, have been received in ______ packages purporting to contain the drugs listed on this inventory and have been: ** (1) Forwarded tape-sealed without opening; (2) Destroyed as indicated and the remainder forwarded tape-sealed after verifying contents; (3) Forwarded tape-sealed after verifying contents.

DATE ______ DESTROYED BY: ______

** *Strike out lines not applicable.* WITNESSED BY: ______

INSTRUCTIONS

1. List the name of the drug in column 1, the number of containers in column 2, the size of each container in column 3, and in column 4 the controlled substance content of each unit described in column 3; e.g., morphine sulfate tabs., 3 pkgs., 100 tabs., 1/4 gr. (16 mg.) or morphine sulfate tabs., 1 pkg., 83 tabs., 1/2 gr. (32mg.), etc.
2. All packages included on a single line should be identical in name, content and controlled substance strength.
3. Prepare this form in quadruplicate. Mail two (2) copies of this form to the Special Agent in Charge, under separate cover. Enclose one additional copy in the shipment with the drugs. Retain one copy for your records. One copy will be returned to you as a receipt. No further receipt will be furnished to you unless specifically requested. Any further inquiries concerning these drugs should be addressed to the DEA District Office which serves your area.
4. There is no provision for payment for drugs surrendered. This is merely a service rendered to registrants enabling them to clear their stocks and records of unwanted items.
5. Drugs should be shipped tape-sealed via prepaid express or certified mail (**return receipt requested**) to Special Agent in Charge, Drug Enforcement Administration, of the DEA District Office which serves your area.

PRIVACY ACT INFORMATION

AUTHORITY: Section 307 of the Controlled Substances Act of 1970 (PL 91-513).
PURPOSE: To document the surrender of controlled substances which have been forwarded by registrants to DEA for disposal.
ROUTINE USES: This form is required by Federal Regulations for the surrender of unwanted Controlled Substances. Disclosures of information from this system are made to the following categories of users for the purposes stated.
A. Other Federal law enforcement and regulatory agencies for law enforcement and regulatory purposes.
B. State and local law enforcement and regulatory agencies for law enforcement and regulatory purposes.
EFFECT: Failure to document the surrender of unwanted Controlled Substances may result in prosecution for violation of the Controlled Substances Act.

EXAMPLE

This is an example of a **Registrants Inventory of Drugs Surrendered (DEA Form-41).** The form requests information such as the mailing address, DEA number, name of drug or preparation, number of containers, contents (number of grams, tablets, ounces, or other units per container), and controlled substance content in each unit.

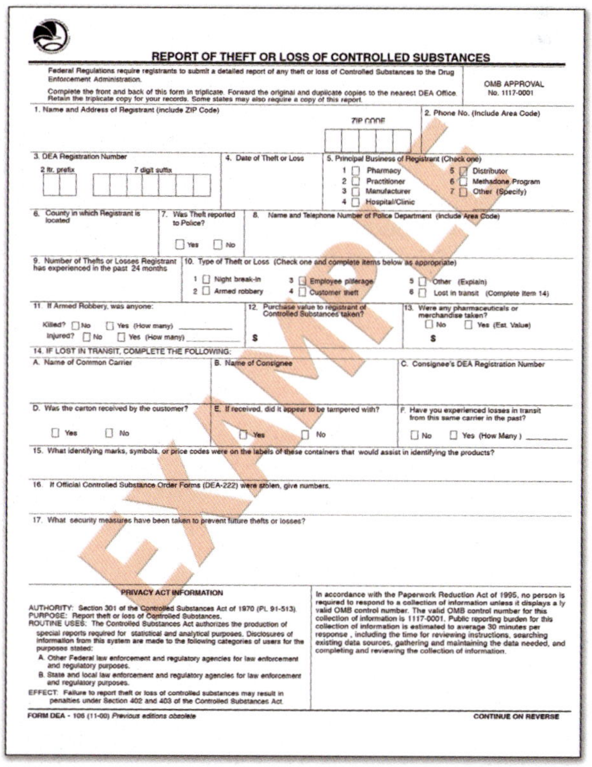

REPORT OF THEFT OR LOSS OF CONTROLLED SUBSTANCES

Federal Regulations require registrants to submit a detailed report of any theft or loss of Controlled Substances to the Drug Enforcement Administration.

Complete the front and back of this form in triplicate. Forward the original and duplicate copies to the nearest DEA Office. Retain the triplicate copy for your records. Some states may also require a copy of this report.

OMB APPROVAL No. 1117-0001

1. Name and Address of Registrant (include ZIP Code) ZIP CODE
2. Phone No. (Include Area Code)
3. DEA Registration Number — 2 ltr. prefix — 7 digit suffix
4. Date of Theft or Loss
5. Principal Business of Registrant (Check one) — 1 ☐ Pharmacy 2 ☐ Practitioner 3 ☐ Manufacturer 4 ☐ Hospital/Clinic 5 ☐ Distributor 6 ☐ Methadone Program 7 ☐ Other (Specify)
6. County in which Registrant is located
7. Was Theft reported to Police? ☐ Yes ☐ No
8. Name and Telephone Number of Police Department (Include Area Code)
9. Number of Thefts or Losses Registrant has experienced in the past 24 months
10. Type of Theft or Loss (Check one and complete items below as appropriate) — 1 ☐ Night break-in 2 ☐ Armed robbery 3 ☐ Employee pilferage 4 ☐ Customer theft 5 ☐ Other (Explain) 6 ☐ Lost in transit (Complete Item 14)
11. If Armed Robbery, was anyone: Killed? ☐ No ☐ Yes (How many) ______ Injured? ☐ No ☐ Yes (How many) ______
12. Purchase value to registrant of Controlled Substances taken? $
13. Were any pharmaceuticals or merchandise taken? ☐ No ☐ Yes (Est. Value) $
14. IF LOST IN TRANSIT, COMPLETE THE FOLLOWING:
A. Name of Common Carrier
B. Name of Consignee
C. Consignee's DEA Registration Number
D. Was the carton received by the customer? ☐ Yes ☐ No
E. If received, did it appear to be tampered with? ☐ Yes ☐ No
F. Have you experienced losses in transit from this same carrier in the past? ☐ No ☐ Yes (How Many) ______
15. What identifying marks, symbols, or price codes were on the labels of these containers that would assist in identifying the products?
16. If Official Controlled Substance Order Forms (DEA-222) were stolen, give numbers.
17. What security measures have been taken to prevent future thefts or losses?

PRIVACY ACT INFORMATION

AUTHORITY: Section 301 of the Controlled Substances Act of 1970 (PL 91-513).
PURPOSE: Report theft or loss of Controlled Substances.
ROUTINE USES: The Controlled Substances Act authorizes the production of special reports required for statistical and analytical purposes. Disclosures of information from this system are made to the following categories of users for the purposes stated:
A. Other Federal law enforcement and regulatory agencies for law enforcement and regulatory purposes.
B. State and local law enforcement and regulatory agencies for law enforcement and regulatory purposes.
EFFECT: Failure to report theft or loss of controlled substances may result in penalties under Section 402 and 403 of the Controlled Substances Act.

In accordance with the Paperwork Reduction Act of 1995, no person is required to respond to a collection of information unless it displays a ly valid OMB control number. The valid OMB control number for this collection of information is 1117-0001. Public reporting burden for this collection of information is estimated to average 30 minutes per response, including the time for reviewing instructions, searching existing data sources, gathering and maintaining the data needed, and completing and reviewing the collection of information.

FORM DEA - 106 (11-00) *Previous editions obsolete*

CONTINUE ON REVERSE

EXAMPLE

This is an example of a **Report of Theft or Loss of Controlled Substances (DEA Form-106)**. The form requests information such as the name and address of the registrant, phone number, name of the police department contacted, type of theft or loss, purchase value to registrant, and name of carrier.

PUBLIC SAFETY

Though the FDA approval process is quite thorough, it is impossible to fully prove that a drug is safe for use.

No matter how many people participate in the clinical trials, the number is always just a fraction of how many will use a drug once it is approved. So there is always the risk that the drug may produce adverse effects when used on a larger population. To monitor this, the FDA maintains a reporting program called MedWatch that encourages health-care professionals to report ***adverse effects*** that occur from the use of an approved drug or other medical product. MedWatch does not monitor vaccines. That is performed by the Vaccine Adverse Event Reporting System (VAERS).

The FDA has several options if it determines that a marketed drug presents a risk of illness, injury, or gross consumer deception.

It may seek an ***injunction*** that prevents the manufacturer from distributing the drug; it may seize the drug; or it may issue a ***recall*** of the drug or certain lots of the drug. Of these, recalls are considered the most effective, largely because they involve the cooperation of the manufacturer, which after all is the only party that knows where the drugs have been distributed. As a result, recalls are the FDA's preferred means of removing dangerous drugs from the market.

A Manufacturer Recall

When in 1982 an as yet unidentified person tampered with a small number of Tylenol® capsule packages, fatally poisoning seven people, Johnson & Johnson immediately recalled the capsules from the market. This swift and responsible action resulted in a highly favorable public response and increased popularity for Tylenol®—and Johnson & Johnson.

adverse effect an unintended side effect of a medication that is negative or in some way injurious to a patient's health.

injunction a court order preventing a specific action, such as the distribution of a potentially dangerous drug.

recall the action taken to remove a drug from the market and have it returned to the manufacturer.

RECALLS

Recalls are, with a few exceptions, voluntary on the part of the manufacturer. However, once the FDA requests a manufacturer recall of a product, the pressure to do so is substantial. The negative publicity from not recalling would significantly damage a company's reputation, and the FDA would probably take the manufacturer to court, where criminal penalties could be imposed. The FDA can also require recalls in certain instances with infant formulas, biological products, and devices that pose a serious health hazard. Manufacturers may, of course, recall drugs on their own and do so from time to time for any number of reasons.

Recall Classifications

There are three classes of recalls:

Class I

Where there is a strong likelihood that the product will cause serious adverse effects or death.

Class II

Where a product may cause temporary but reversible adverse effects, or in which there is little likelihood of serious adverse effects.

Class III

Where a product is not likely to cause adverse effects.

safety you should know

Voluntary MedWatch reports for adverse reactions to drugs may be submitted online at www.accessdata.fda.gov/scripts/medwatch/, by telephone (1-800-FDA-1088), fax, or mail. Forms can be downloaded from www.fda.gov/medwatch/getforms.htm. Adverse reactions to vaccines are reported through the Vaccine Adverse Event Reporting System (VAERS) maintained by the Centers for Disease Control (CDC) and the FDA. The VAERS phone number is 1-800-822-7967; web submissions and downloadable forms are available at vaers.hhs.gov.

THE RECALL PROCESS

Reports of adverse effects

The FDA receives enough reports of adverse effects or misbranding that it decides the product is a threat to the public health. It contacts the manufacturer and recommends a recall.

Manufacturer agrees to recall

If the manufacturer agrees to a recall, they must establish a recall strategy with the FDA that addresses the depth of the recall, the extent of public warnings, and a means for checking the effectiveness of the recall. The depth of the recall is identified by wholesale, retail, or consumer levels. The effectiveness may require anything from no follow up to a complete follow-up check of everyone who should have been notified of the recall. Checks can be made by personal visit, phone calls, or letters.

Customers contacted

Once the strategy is finalized, the manufacturer contacts its customers by telegram, mailgram, or first-class letters with the following information:

- ✔ the product name, size, lot number, code or serial number, and any other important identifying information.
- ✔ reason for the recall and the hazard involved.
- ✔ instructions on what to do with the product, beginning with ceasing distribution.

Recalls listed publicly

Recalls are listed in the weekly FDA Enforcement Report.

LAW AND THE TECHNICIAN

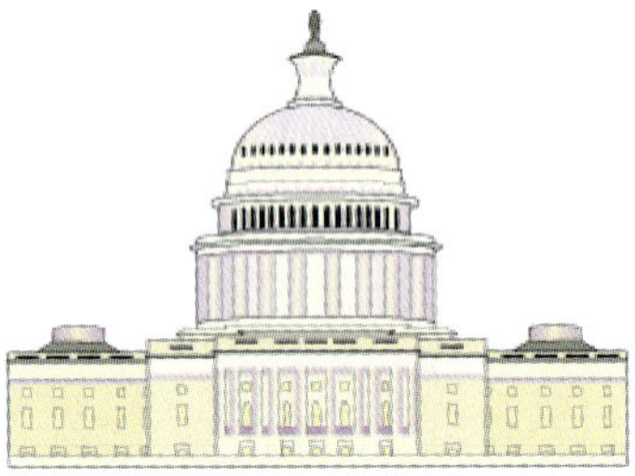

FEDERAL LAW

Federal laws provide a foundation for the state laws that govern pharmacy practice. In addition to the specific drug laws enforced by the FDA and DEA, there are federal laws regulating the treatment of patients (especially in nursing homes) that apply to various aspects of pharmacy practice. These laws guarantee certain patient rights, including privacy and confidentiality, right to file complaints, information necessary for informed consent, and the right to refuse treatment.

A major piece of legislation affecting patients' privacy rights and how health-care providers may or may not use patient health information is the Health Insurance Portability and Accountability Act of 1996. In an effort to streamline health-care costs, this act encourages providers to use electronic transactions and allows a minimum amount of patient health information to be transferred among providers, without patient consent, for purposes of treatment, payment or administrative operations. At the same time, to protect patients' rights, HIPAA makes the health-care provider responsible for maintaining the privacy and security of patient information, informing the patient of their privacy policies and procedures, and allowing the patient to both review and correct any records.

The Affordable Care Act (ACA), also known as Health Care Reform or Obamacare, was signed into law in 2010, with overall goals to improve patient care, quality, and outcomes while reducing cost. In response to the ACA a group of 14 pharmacy organizations worked to develop and advocate the Pharmacy Principles for Health Care Reform that includes three principles: (1) Improve Quality & Safety of Medication Use; (2) Assure Patient Access to Needed Medications & Pharmacy Services; and (3) Promote Pharmacy & Health Information Technology Interoperability.

compliance doing what is required.
protocol specific guideline for practice.

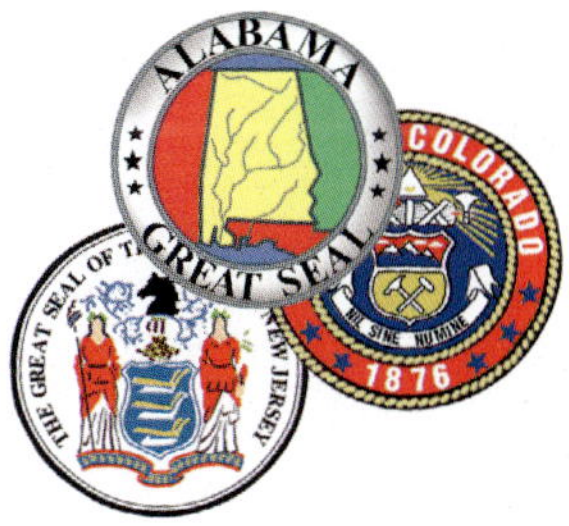

STATE LAW

In each state, departments of professional regulation or state boards are responsible for licensing all prescribers and dispensers. There are also state boards of pharmacy that administer state regulations for the practice of pharmacy in the state. In many cases, state regulations are stricter than federal, and the stricter state regulation must be followed. By definition, this means that the lesser federal requirements are also being met. Following both state and federal regulations is mandatory. When federal and state laws don't agree, the more strict law must be followed.

Each state has specific regulations that may or may not be different from other states. For example, a few states allow pharmacists to prescribe under limited conditions. Many allow nurse practitioners and physician assistants to prescribe. When states allow nonphysicians to prescribe, they limit their scope of authority. That is, a nonphysician prescriber may only prescribe for certain conditions and must follow a strict set of rules called a ***protocol*** that determines the prescription. Nonphysician prescribers include dentists, veterinarians, pharmacists, nurse practitioners, and physician assistants. Since states differ on many aspects of pharmacy practice, including who may and may not prescribe, it is necessary to know your own state's regulations, a copy of which can be obtained from your state's board of pharmacy.

States regulate the work of pharmacy technicians largely by holding the pharmacist supervising a technician responsible for the technician's performance. If a technician fails to observe any relevant law, the supervising pharmacist is subject to a penalty by the state board. As a result, the supervising pharmacist must explain all the regulations (federal, state, and local) that apply to the technician, and must work with the technician to assure ***compliance*** with those regulations.

LAW AND THE TECHNICIAN (cont'd)

OTHER STANDARDS

Besides the FDA, DEA, and the state board of pharmacy, there are various professional bodies and associations that set and maintain pharmacy standards. These include:

- **American Society of Health-System Pharmacists:** The ASHP is a 30,000 member association for pharmacists practicing in hospitals, HMOs, long-term care facilities, home care agencies, and other health- care systems. It is an accrediting organization for pharmacy residency and pharmacy technician training programs.
- **United States Pharmacopeial Convention:** The USP is a voluntary not-for-profit organization that sets standards for the manufacture and distribution of drugs and related products in the United States. These standards are directly referred to by federal and state laws and are published in the *United States Pharmacopeia and the National Formulary*.
- **The Joint Commission:** TJC is an independent non-profit organization that establishes standards and monitors compliance for nearly 20,000 health-care programs in the United States. TJC-accredited programs include hospitals, health-care networks, HMOs, and nursing homes, among others.
- **The American Society for Consultant Pharmacists:** The ASCP sets standards for practice for pharmacists who provide medication distribution and consultant services to nursing homes.

LIABILITY

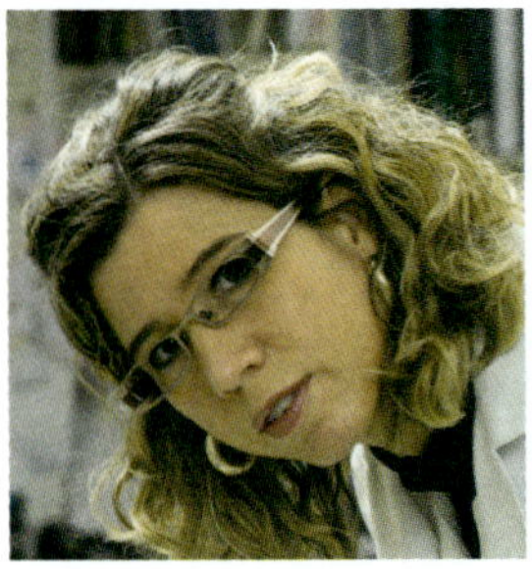

Legal ***liability*** means you can be prosecuted for misconduct. This is true even if you are directed to do it by a supervisor, physician, patient, or customer. Misconduct doesn't necessarily mean you intended to do something, or even that you actively did it. You can be guilty of misconduct by simply failing to do something you should have done. This is called ***negligence***, and is the most common form of misconduct. Here are some ways the pharmacy technician can be negligent:

- incorrectly labeling the prescription;
- failing to maintain patient confidentiality;
- failing to recognize expired drugs;
- calculation errors;
- dispensing the wrong medication;
- incorrect handling of controlled substance;
- inaccurate record keeping.

See Chapter 8 on *Compounding* and Chapter 9 on *Parenterals: Compounding Sterile Formulations* and visit www.usp.org/store/products-services/usp-compounding for more information on USP compounding guidelines.

COMPOUNDING: FEDERAL AND STATE REGULATIONS AND USP GUIDELINES

Federal law 21 USCA 353a defines compounding in pharmacies pursuant to a patient-specific prescription and gives the FDA regulatory authority with regards to the Active Pharmaceutical Ingredients (APIs) used in compounding. State laws regulate compounding practices in their state. In addition to federal and state laws, the United States Pharmacopeia (USP) has published numerous chapters that are standards for compounding, including Chapter <795> on nonsterile compounding and Chapter <797> on sterile preparations. States may adopt some or all of the USP standards or, in some aspects such as licensing requirements, they may have their own standards that are more strict. However, following USP guidelines is considered the standard for pharmacy compounding practice.

A tragedy occurred in 2012 when the New England Compounding Center (NECC) in Massachusetts was found to have dispensed contaminated injectable methylprednisolone acetate to clinics in several different states. State and federal regulators found that NECC was not fully following sterile compounding procedures and that there was "greenish black foreign matter" in some of its methylprednisolone acetate product. Additionally, due to the amount of products that were shipped from NECC, there is concern that NECC may have exceeded the limitations of its Massachusetts state pharmacy compounding license, which requires patient-specific prescriptions for each compounded preparation, and may have been engaging in manufacturing. Manufacturing of pharmaceutical products requires a license from the FDA, and the FDA has more oversight of manufacturers.

Faced with 130 lawsuits and another 270 people who had claimed injury, NECC filed for bankruptcy in December, 2012 and said they hoped to set up a fund to compensate victims of the contaminated products. As of January, 2013 over 675 cases of fungal and other infections, including fungal meningitis, and 44 deaths, had been linked to the contaminated products. The cases spanned 19 states.

In response to the tragedy, Massachusetts Governor Deval Patrick proposed state legislation that would require pharmacies to obtain a special license to compound sterile injectable drugs, designate funds to hire more state inspectors, establish new fines and penalties for those who violate the regulations, offer whistle-blower protection for employees, and possibly re-structure the state's board of pharmacy to include a wider range of health-care professionals such as a nurse, a physician, a pharmacy technician, and a quality improvement officer, as well as three members of the public.

tip

Basic criminal and civil laws also apply to pharmacy technicians, which means that crimes like theft, discrimination, sexual harassment, fraud, etc., are punishable just as they would be outside of your job.

liability legal responsibility for costs or damages arising from misconduct or negligence.

negligence failing to do something that should or must be done.

ETHICS & COMPLIANCE

Ethics is a branch of philosophy that helps determine what should be done, in a principled sense, besides what must be done to comply with laws.

Taking an ethical perspective means examining a situation by moral standards. This means looking at the effects an action can have on others and whether that action could be justified to a higher moral authority.

Dilemmas can occur in day-to-day activities encountered in pharmacy where competing standards make it difficult to determine what is the right thing to do.

Ethical principles can be applied to help determine the best course of action to take. Some organizations adopt codes of conduct or codes of ethics to guide their members and/or employees in making ethical decisions.

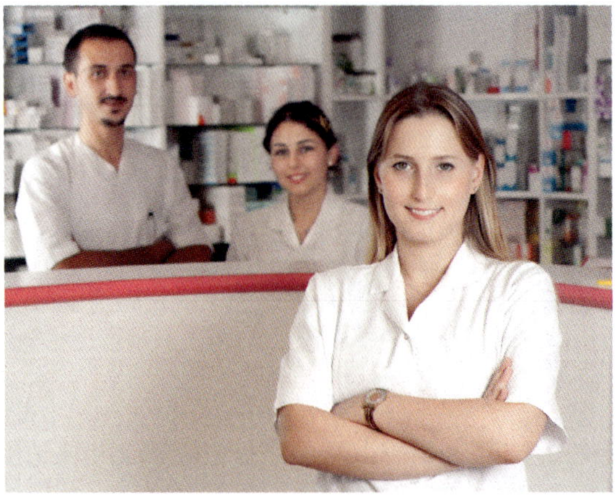

A CODE OF ETHICS

Pharmacy technicians are health-care professionals who assist pharmacists in providing the best possible care for patients. The principles of this code, which apply to pharmacy technicians working in any and all settings, are based on the application and support of the moral obligations that guide the pharmacy profession in relationships with patients, health-care professionals and society.

Principles

- A pharmacy technician's first consideration is to ensure the health and safety of the patient, and to use knowledge and skills to the best of his/her ability in serving patients.
- A pharmacy technician supports and promotes honesty and integrity in the profession, which includes a duty to observe the law, maintain the highest moral and ethical conduct at all times and uphold the ethical principles of the profession.
- A pharmacy technician assists and supports the pharmacists in the safe and efficacious and cost-effective distribution of health services and health-care resources.
- A pharmacy technician respects and values the abilities of pharmacists, colleagues and other health-care professionals. A pharmacy technician maintains competency in his/her practice and continually enhances his/her professional knowledge and expertise.
- A pharmacy technician respects and supports the patient's individuality, dignity, and confidentiality.
- A pharmacy technician respects the confidentiality of a patient's records and discloses pertinent information only with proper authorization.
- A pharmacy technician never assists in dispensing, promoting, or distribution of medication or medical devices that are not of good quality or do not meet the standards required by law.
- A pharmacy technician does not engage in any activity that will discredit the profession, and will expose, without fear or favor, illegal or unethical conduct of the profession.
- A pharmacy technician associates with and engages in the support of organizations, which promote the profession of pharmacy through the utilization and enhancement of pharmacy technicians.

Source: "The American Association of Pharmacy Technicians Code of Ethics," originally published in "White Paper on Pharmacy Technicians 2002: Needed Changes Can No Longer Wait," American Journal of Health-Systems Pharmacists, 60:37-51."

In the past half century, the role of ethics in health care has been increasing with special emphasis in biomedical research.

Universities, colleges, hospitals, and other organizations form committees to provide ethical guidance and ensure legal and ethical standards are followed. The committees are sometimes known as ethical review boards (ERBs) or institutional review boards (IRBs). Additionally, corporations often have compliance officers who report directly to the CEO of the company.

Ethical review boards in hospitals can provide consultation for difficult ethical cases that may arise.

Institutional review boards in hospitals and universities act to review, discuss, approve, and monitor research involving humans.

Corporate compliance officers are responsible to investigate legal or ethical concerns that are identified within a business.

Additionally, corporate compliance officers sometimes perform routine audits to ensure business operations meet legal and ethical standards.

FEDERAL GUIDELINES FOR COMPLIANCE

The Centers for Medicare & Medicaid Services (CMS) provide guidelines for compliance programs to help promote the prevention, detection, and resolution of conduct that does not conform to federal and state law, or to federal health-care program requirements.

The CMS guidelines contain seven suggested elements for a compliance program:

1. Written policies and procedures
2. Designation of a compliance officer and a compliance committee
3. Conducting effective training and education
4. Developing effective lines of communication
5. Auditing and monitoring
6. Enforcement through publicized disciplinary guidelines and policies dealing with ineligible persons
7. Responding to detected offenses, developing corrective action initiatives, and reporting to government authorities

More information about the CMS guidelines for compliance programs can be found at http://www.cms.gov/Medicare/Medicare-Contracting/MedicareContractingReform/Downloads/compliance.pdf.

ethics a branch of philosophy that helps determine what should be done in a principled sense.

Basic Values in Ethical Considerations

Six basic values are commonly applied in ethical considerations:

- **Autonomy:** Patients have the right to choose their treatment.
- **Beneficence:** The actions of the health-care provider should be in the best interest of the patient.
- **Dignity:** The health-care provider should treat the patient with dignity and respect.
- **Non-maleficence:** The health-care provider should do no harm in providing care to the patient.
- **Justice:** Fairness and equality should be applied when providing care to all patients.
- **Truthfulness and honesty:** Health-care providers should be truthful and honest when providing care to patients.

REVIEW

KEY CONCEPTS

DRUG REGULATION

- ✔ In the United States, the leading federal enforcement agency for regulations concerning drug products is the Food and Drug Administration.
- ✔ The distribution of drugs that may be easily abused is controlled by the Drug Enforcement Administration (DEA) within the Justice Department.
- ✔ Manufacturers' containers for prescription drugs must have this legend on the label: "Rx only."

NEW DRUG APPROVAL

- ✔ Before it is approved for marketing, a new drug must be shown to be both safe and effective and that its benefits substantially outweigh its risks.
- ✔ Placebos are inactive substances used to test the effectiveness of drugs.

MARKETED DRUGS

- ✔ Once a patent for a brand drug expires, other manufacturers may copy the drug and release it under its generic name.

BEHIND-THE-COUNTER OTC MEDICATIONS

- ✔ Some OTC medications are kept behind the counter even if they do not require a prescription; these include OTC medications containing ephedrine and pseudoephedrine, exempt narcotics, and emergency contraceptives.

SAMPLE LABELS

- ✔ The minimum requirements on prescription labels for most drugs are as follows: name and address of dispenser, prescription serial number, date of prescription or filling, name of prescriber, name of patient, directions for use, and cautionary statements.

CONTROLLED SUBSTANCES

- ✔ Manufacturers must clearly label controlled drugs with their control classification.
- ✔ All prescribers of controlled substances must be registered with the DEA and are assigned a DEA number that must be used on all controlled drug prescriptions.

ADDITIONAL DEA FORMS

- ✔ Although DEA Form 222 is the most frequently used DEA form, manufacturers, distributors, and dispensers of controlled substances are also required to use other specific DEA forms to register with the DEA and otherwise monitor inventory.

PUBLIC SAFETY

- ✔ Recalls are, with a few exceptions, voluntary on the part of the manufacturer.

LAW AND THE TECHNICIAN

- ✔ Federal laws provide a foundation for the state laws that govern pharmacy practice.
- ✔ State boards of pharmacy are responsible for licensing all prescribers and dispensers and administering regulations for the practice of pharmacy in the state.
- ✔ Legal liability means you can be prosecuted for misconduct, including negligence.

ETHICS AND COMPLIANCE

- ✔ Taking an ethical perspective means examining a situation with moral standards.
- ✔ Institutions form committees such as institutional review boards to provide guidance on ethical issues and ensure compliance.

SELF TEST

the answer key begins on page 569

MATCH THE TERMS

1. adverse effect ____
2. Combat Methamphetamine Epidemic Act (CMEA) ____
3. compliance ____
4. controlled substance mark ____
5. controlled substances ____
6. dual marketing ____
7. ethics ____
8. exempt narcotics ____
9. injunction ____
10. legend drug ____
11. liability ____
12. negligence ____
13. pediatric ____
14. pharmaceutical equivalent ____
15. placebo ____
16. product labeling ____
17. protocol ____
18. recall ____
19. therapeutic equivalent ____

a. medications with habit-forming ingredients that can be dispensed without a prescription by a pharmacist to persons at least 18 years of age.

b. any drug that requires a prescription and this legend on the label: Rx only.

c. failing to do something you should have done.

d. important associated information that is not on the label of a drug product itself.

e. legal responsibility for costs or damages arising from misconduct or negligence.

f. status of medications like Plan B® that are classified as both prescription and OTC drugs.

g. the action taken to remove a drug from the market and have it returned to the manufacturer.

h. the mark (CII–CV) that indicates the control category of a drug with a potential for abuse.

i. Federal law that sets daily and monthly limits on OTC sale of pseudoephedrine and ephedrine.

j. an inactive substance given in place of a medication.

k. having to do with the treatment of children.

l. drug products that contain identical amounts of the same active ingredients in the same dosage form.

m. pharmaceutical equivalents that produce the same effects in patients.

n. five groups of drugs identified by the 1970 Controlled Substances Act (CSA) as having the potential for abuse and whose distribution is therefore strictly controlled by five control schedules set forth in the CSA.

o. an unintended side effect of a medication that is negative or in some way injurious to a patient's health.

p. a court order preventing a specific action, such as the distribution of a potentially dangerous drug.

q. specific guideline for practice.

r. doing what is required.

s. a branch of philosophy that helps determine what should be done in a principled sense.

REVIEW

CHOOSE THE BEST ANSWER

1. The ____________________ prohibited interstate commerce in adulterated or misbranded food, drinks, and drugs.
   a. 1938 Food, Drug, and Cosmetic (FDC) Act
   b. Food and Drug Act of 1906
   c. Harrison Act
   d. 1990 Omnibus Budget Reconciliation Act (OBRA)

2. In response to growing addiction to opiates and cocaine-containing medicines, the Harrison Narcotic Act of 1914 required that all manufacturers, importers, and physicians prescribing narcotics be
   a. licensed.
   b. taxed.
   c. licensed and taxed.
   d. fined.

3. The Food and Drug Administration was initially named the
   a. Food, Drug, and Alcohol Commission.
   b. Food, Drug, and Weapons Administration.
   c. Food, Drug, and Hazardous Substance Regulatory Agency.
   d. Food, Drug, and Insecticide Administration.

4. Because of fatal poisoning from liquid sulfanilamide, the ________________ required new drugs be shown to be safe before marketing.
   a. Food and Drug Act of 1906
   b. 1938 Food, Drug, and Cosmetic Act
   c. 1951 Durham Humphrey Amendment
   d. 1990 Omnibus Budget Reconciliation Act (OBRA)

5. The ______________ required child-proof packaging for most prescription drugs.
   a. Food, Drug, and Cosmetic Act
   b. Poison Prevention Packaging Act
   c. Durham-Humphrey Amendment
   d. Kefauver-Harris Amendment

6. The 1984 Hatch-Watchman Act allowed for
   a. quicker introduction of generic drugs only.
   b. extension of drug patent terms only.
   c. quicker introduction of drugs and extension of drug patent terms.
   d. introduction of generic versions of trade drugs regardless of patent terms.

7. Pharmacists were required to offer counseling to Medicaid patients by the
   a. Durham-Humphrey Amendment.
   b. 1990 Omnibus Budget Reconciliation Act (OBRA).
   c. Kefauver-Harris Amendment.
   d. Harrison Act.

8. Drugs that require prescriptions are ______________ drugs.
   a. Durham
   b. Humphrey
   c. legend
   d. Kefauver

9. Both domestic and imported drugs require approval by (a/the) __________ before they can be marketed in the United States.
   a. FDA
   b. U.S. Marshal
   c. DEA
   d. U.S. Customs

10. An inactive substance given in place of a medication during clinical trials is a
    a. pediatric.
    b. phase 2.
    c. phase 3.
    d. placebo.

11. The FDA requires ____________ phases of testing in humans.
    a. two
    b. three
    c. four
    d. five

12. The main purpose of phase 2 clinical trials is
    a. dosage.
    b. economics.
    c. animals.
    d. effectiveness.

13. Phase 3 clinical trials generally have ________________ participants.
    a. several hundred to several thousand
    b. 20–100 patients
    c. less than 10
    d. up to several hundred patients

14. After a patent has expired for a medication, other manufacturers may copy the drug and release it under the ______________ name.
    a. generic
    b. trade
    c. brand
    d. patent

15. Drugs that do not require a prescription are _____________ drugs.
    a. FDA
    b. OTC
    c. Durham-Humphrey
    d. legend

16. The Combat Methamphetamine Epidemic Act requires that OTC cold and allergy medications containing which of the following drugs be kept behind the counter?
    a. antihistamine
    b. methamphetamine
    c. ephedrine and pseudoephedrine
    d. antitussive

17. Purchasers of exempt narcotics must be at least _____ years of age.
    a. 12
    b. 16
    c. 18
    d. 21

18. There are limits to how many dosage units of an exempt narcotic can be sold in a _____–hour period.
    a. 24
    b. 48
    c. 72
    d. 96

19. A prescription to dispense Plan B®
    a. is not required.
    b. is required for patients under 17.
    c. is required for patients 17 years of age and under.
    d. is required for patients 17 years of age and under unless otherwise allowed by state law.

REVIEW

20. The second set of digits in an NDC represents the
    a. manufacturer.
    b. name of drug and strength.
    c. package size.
    d. lot number.

21. Of the following Schedule of drugs, which one deals with drugs that have no accepted medical use in the United States?
    a. Schedule I
    b. Schedule II
    c. Schedule III
    d. Schedule IV

22. Amphetamines, opium, cocaine, and methadone are in DEA Schedule _____ because they have accepted medical use, but have a high potential for abuse and may lead to physical or psychological dependence.
    a. II
    b. III
    c. IV
    d. V

23. The form for ordering Schedule II controlled substances is DEA Form
    a. 106.
    b. 222.
    c. 224.
    d. 363.

24. The FDA reporting system for adverse effects that occur from use of approved drugs is called
    a. Class I.
    b. MedWatch.
    c. VAERS.
    d. Class II.

25. ________________ drug recalls are issued by manufacturers when there is a strong likelihood that the product will cause serious adverse effects or death.
    a. Class I
    b. Class II
    c. Class III
    d. Class IV

26. Basic criminal and civil laws, like theft, discrimination, sexual harassment, and fraud, apply to pharmacy technicians.
    a. True
    b. False

27. Pharmacies located in health-care institutions (hospitals, etc.) are required to follow regulations of this organization:
    a. ASHP
    b. USP
    c. ASCP
    d. TJC

CRITICAL THINKING QUESTIONS

1. What are the differences between phase I, II, and III clinical drug trials
2. What are the differences between pharmaceutical equivalents and therapeutic equivalents?
3. Discuss how the American Association of Pharmacy Technician's first principle in the *Pharmacy Technician Code of Ethics* can be helpful in guiding ethical practice.

THINKING IT THROUGH WRAP-UP

1. The daily limit is 146 tablets.
2. The monthly limit is 7500 mg so the maximum number of tablets is 250. Only 2 100-count bottles could be sold to the same person in one month.

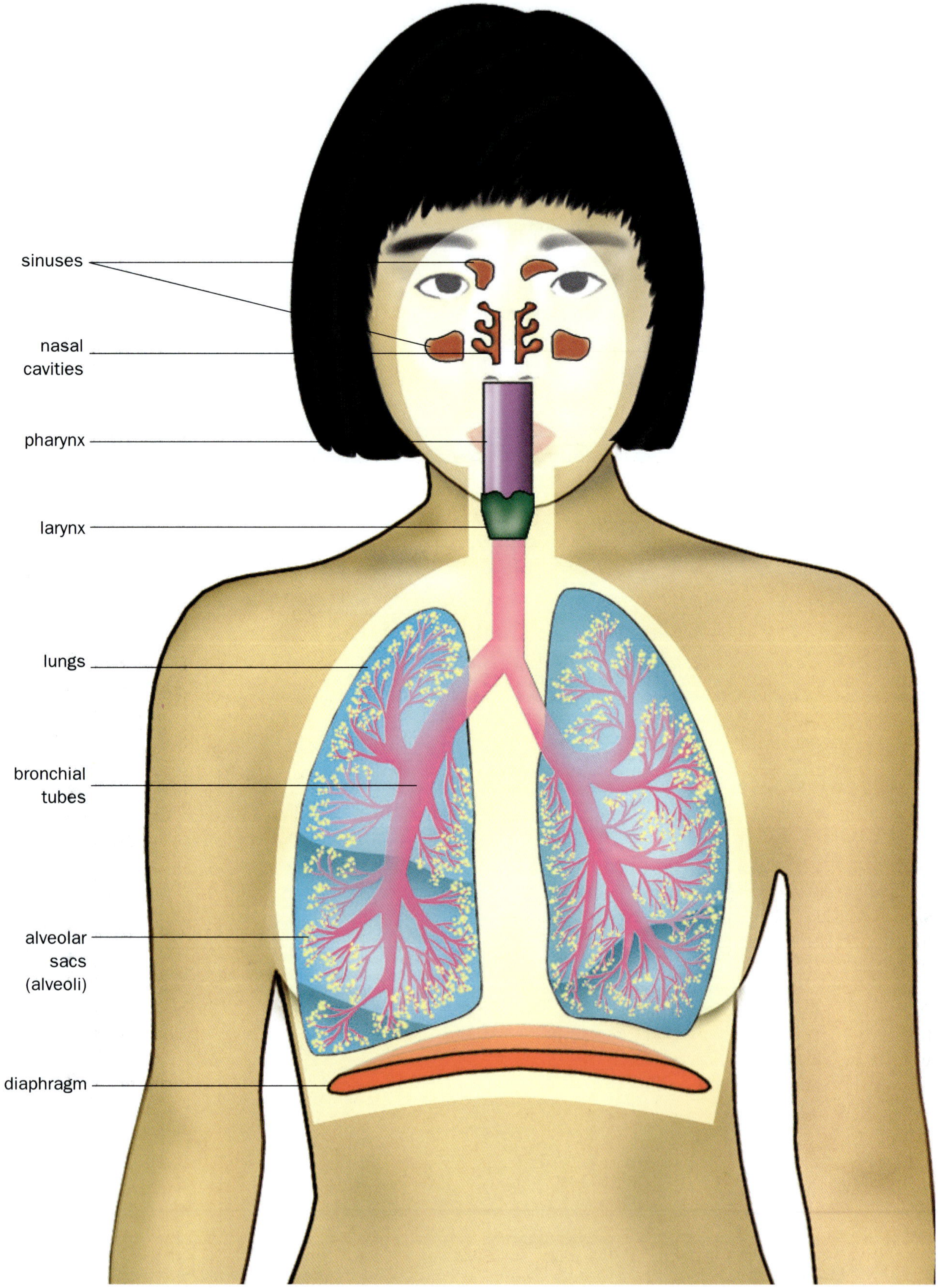
sinuses
nasal cavities
pharynx
larynx
lungs
bronchial tubes
alveolar sacs (alveoli)
diaphragm

4

TERMINOLOGY

LEARNING OBJECTIVES

At the completion of study, the student will:

- ✔ explain the common nomenclature system used in medical science terminology.
- ✔ be familiar with the medical science terminology associated with major body organ systems.
- ✔ recognize how the common nomenclature system is used in naming drug classes.
- ✔ appreciate the complexity of medical abbreviations.

THINKING IT THROUGH

A patient comes to the pharmacy with a prescription for atorvastatin, and tells you that the doctor changed her prescription because she had developed rhabdomyolysis while taking simvastatin. You want to make a note of this information in the patient's profile, and glance through the other information to find the appropriate place to put the new information.

In the patient's medical history, you see that she has hyperlipidemia which is why the simvastatin was prescribed. But the patient also has hyperglycemia, hypertension, COPD, and GERD, and takes an anticoagulant for atrial fibrillation and an antidepressant. The patient was recently discharged from the hospital where she was treated for community acquired pneumonia.

As you read this chapter, see if you can identify the various parts of the medical terms (i.e., root word, prefix, suffix) in the above scenario and then what each whole word means. Also consider the following questions:

1. How are the parts of a medical term combined?
2. Using medical abbreviations can save space on written documentation and can make communication with other professionals faster. What is the major drawback to using abbreviations?
3. The system of learning medical terms associated with an organ system is often used to teach medical terminology. What is an advantage of that learning approach?

TERMINOLOGY

Medical dictionaries contain thousands of words that are used in medicine and pharmacy.

Many of the words don't look like words commonly used in literature or speech, and at first glance they can be quite intimidating. But the secret to learning medical science terminology is to learn that there is a system, or order, to it. The purpose of this chapter is to explain this system.

Medical science terminology is made up of a small number of *root words*.

Most of these root words originate from either Greek or Latin. Words from the Greek language are most often used to refer to diagnosis and surgery. Words from the Latin language generally refer to the anatomy of the body.

Numerous *suffixes* and *prefixes* are attached to the root word.

Suffixes and prefixes give additional meaning to the root word. The suffix is a modifier attached to the end of the root word, and the prefix is attached to the front of the root word. Almost all medical science terms will have at least one root word and a suffix or prefix to complete the meaning. However, it is not required that every root word have both a suffix and a prefix: a root word could have just one. In general, prefixes are used less frequently than suffixes.

***Combining vowels* are sometimes used to connect the prefix, root word, and/or suffix.**

A combining vowel is sometimes also added to make a word easier to pronounce. The most common combining vowel is "o."

combining vowel a vowel used to connect the prefix, root word, or suffix parts of a term.

prefix a modifying component of a term, located at the beginning of the term.

root word the base component of a term which gives it a meaning that may be modified by other components.

suffix a modifying component of a term located at the end of the term.

Root	Prefix
Suffix	C.V.

ROOT WORDS

The root word is the foundation of medical science terminology and can immediately identify a disease or what part of the body a term relates to. For example, consider the following list of common root words and the parts of the body to which they refer:

Root	Part of Body
card	heart
cyst	bladder
derma	skin
dont	teeth
gastr	stomach
glyc	sugar
hemat	blood
hepat	liver
lingu	tongue
mast	breast
my	muscle
nephr	kidney
neur	nerve
ocul	eye
opia	vision
oste	bone
ot	ear
partum	bring forth
pector	chest
pneumon	lung
thorax	chest
thyroid	thyroid
ven	vein

A phrase containing the word *cardiac*, refers to the heart, since *card* is the root word of the word cardiac. The word *ocular* refers to the eye since *ocul* is the root word for the eye.

Medical Term

tip Learning the most popular roots, suffixes, and prefixes will help you to understand a large amount of medical science terminology.

PREFIXES

A prefix is added to the beginning of a root word to clarify its meaning. For example, *derma* is the root word for "skin," or things related to the skin, and *xero* is a prefix used to describe "things that are dry." So:

Prefix	Root
xero (dry)	**derma** (skin)

➥ **xeroderma:** a dry skin condition

Consider another example. The root word for "vision" is *opia,* and the prefix for "double" is *dipl.* So:

Prefix	Root
dipl (double)	**opia** (vision)

➥ **diplopia**: double vision

As another example, *partum* is the root word for "bringing forth", and *post* is the prefix meaning "after."

Prefix	Root
post (after)	**partum** (bringing forth)

➥ **postpartum:** after a baby is born

SUFFIXES

The suffix is added to the end of a root word to clarify the meaning.

Root	Suffix
gastr (stomach)	**itis** (inflammation)

➥ **gastritis**: inflammation of the stomach

Root	Suffix
neur (nerve)	**algia** (pain)

➥ **neuralgia**: pain in the nerve

COMBINING VOWELS

Sometimes a combining vowel (CV) is used to connect two or more root words.

1st Root	CV	2nd Root
pneumon (lung)	**o**	**thorax** (chest)

➥ **pneumothorax**: area of the chest containing the lungs

1st Root	CV	2nd Root	CV	3rd Root
card (heart)	**io**	**my** (muscle)	**o**	**pathy** (disease)

➥ **cardiomyopathy**: disease in heart muscle tissue

COMBINING THE ELEMENTS

A root word may have both a prefix and a suffix.

Prefix	Root	Suffix
hypo (low)	**glyc** (sugar)	**emia** (blood)

➥ **hypoglycemia**: low blood sugar

Prefix	Root	Suffix
hyper (high)	**thyroid** (thyroid)	**ism** (state of)

➥ **hyperthyroidism**: too much thyroid activity

A root word may have a prefix, suffix, and a combining vowel.

Prefix	CV	Root	Suffix
peri (around)	**o**	**dont** (teeth)	**ic** (pertaining to)

➥ **periodontic**: around the teeth

For a final example, consider the prefix *sub* and the root word *lingu. Sub* means "under" or "beneath," and *lingu* is the root word for "tongue." So:

sub + lingu = sublingu

➥ *meaning:* under the tongue

However, there are few English words ending in "u," and so this combination is further modified with the typical suffix *al,* which means "pertaining to," as in:

Prefix	Root	Suffix
sub (under)	**lingu** (tongue)	**al** (pertaining to)

➥ **sublingual***:* pertaining to under the tongue

PREFIXES

Root	Prefix
Suffix	C.V.

Below are common prefixes used in medical science terminology.

Prefix	Meaning
a	without
ambi	both
an	without
ante	before
anti	against
bi	two or both
brady	slow
chlor	green
circum	around
cirrh	yellow
con	with
contra	against
cyan	blue
dia	across or through
dipl	double
dis	separate from or apart
dys	painful, difficult
ec	away or out
ecto	outside
en	in, within
endo	within
epi	upon
erythr	red
eso	inward
eu	good or normal
exo	outside
hemi	half
heter	different
hyper	above or excessive
hypo	below or deficient
im	not
immun	safe, protected
in	not
infra	below or under
inter	between
intra	within
iso	equal
leuk	white

Prefix	Meaning
macro	large
medi	middle
melan	black
meso	middle
meta	beyond, after, changing
micro	small
mid	middle
mono	one
multi	many
neo	new
pachy	heavy, thick
pan	all
para	alongside of or abnormal
peri	around
polio	gray
poly	many
post	after
pre	before
pro	before
pseudo	false
purpur	purple
quadri	four
re	again or back
retro	after
rube	red
semi	half
sub	below or under
super	above or excessive
supra	above or excessive
sym	with
syn	with
tachy	fast
trans	across, through
tri	three
ultra	beyond or excessive
uni	one
xanth	yellow
xer	dry

SUFFIXES

Root	Prefix
Suffix	C.V.

Below are common suffixes used in medical science terminology.

Suffix	Meaning	Suffix	Meaning
ac	pertaining to	oid	resembling
al	pertaining to	ole	small
algia	pain	ology	study of
ar	pertaining to	oma	tumor
ary	pertaining to	opia	vision
asthenia	without strength	opsia	vision
cele	pouching or hernia	osis	abnormal condition, increase
cyesis	pregnancy	osmia	smell
cynia	pain	ous	pertaining to
eal	pertaining to	paresis	partial paralysis
ectasis	expansion or dilation	pathy	disease
ectomy	removal	penia	decrease
edema	swelling	pepsia	digestion
ema	condition	phagia	swallowing
emesis	vomiting	phasia	speech
emia	blood condition	philia	attraction for
esthenia	lack of sensation	phobia	fear
genic	origin or production	plasia	formation, development
gram	record	plasty	surgical repair or reconstruction
graph	recording instrument	plegia	paralysis, stroke
graphy	recording process	pnea	breathing
ia	condition of	rrhage	to burst forth
iasis	condition, formation of	rrhea	discharge
iatry	treatment	sclerosis	hardness
ic	pertaining to	scope	examination instrument
icle	small	scopy	examination
ism	condition of	spasm	involuntary contraction
itis	inflammation	stasis	stop or stand
ium	tissue or structure	tic	pertaining to
lepsy	seizure	tocia	childbirth, labor
lith	stone, calculus	tomy	incision
logy	study of	toxic	poison
lysis	breaking down or dissolution	tropea	to turn
malacia	softening	tropic	stimulate
megaly	enlargement	trophy	nutrition, growth
meter	measuring instrument	ula	small
metry	measuring process	ule	small
mycosis	fungal infection	y	condition, process of

ORGAN SYSTEM TERMINOLOGY

A good way to learn medical science terminology is to learn it based on the different organ systems in the body.

There are names for structures and parts of organ systems that form the root words used in medical science terminology. These names have to be learned. Then they can be applied to understand or to construct words.

CARDIOVASCULAR SYSTEM

The cardiovascular system distributes blood throughout the body using blood vessels called arteries, capillaries, and veins. Blood transports nutrients to the body's cells and carries waste products away from them. Blood is made up of red blood cells, white blood cells, platelets, and plasma. Erythrocytes (red blood cells) transport oxygen from the lungs to the body and carbon dioxide from the body to the lungs. Leukocytes (white blood cells) fight bacterial infections by producing antibodies.

Blood is pumped through the cardiovascular system by the heart. Valves within the heart maintain the flow of blood in only one direction. Conductive nerve tissue unique to the heart muscle is responsible for the heartbeat.

When blood is forced out of the heart, the increased pressure on the system is called the ***systolic phase***. When blood pressure is monitored, this pressure is reported (in mm Hg) as the first number of a two number sequence. The ***diastolic phase***, or relaxation phase, is the second number reported in blood pressure monitoring. Blood pressures are reported as systole/diastole, e.g., 120/80. A sphygmomanometer is used to measure blood pressure.

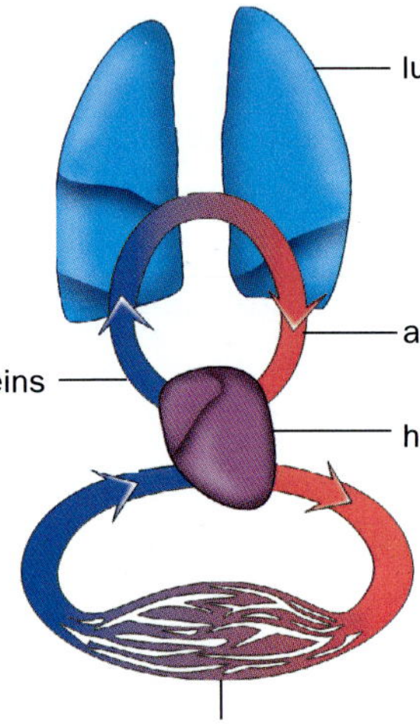

Root	Meaning	Root	Meaning
aneur	widening	oxy	oxygen
angi	vessel	pector	chest
aort	aorta	phleb	vein
arter	artery	stenosis	narrowing
ather	plaque	thromb	clot
card	heart	vas(cu)	blood vessel
cyte	cell	ven	vein
embol	embolus		

Common Cardiovascular System Terminology

Term	Meaning	Term	Meaning
aneur/ism	widening in a blood vessel	fibrilla/tion	a small involuntary muscular contraction
an/gina	chest pain caused by loss of oxygenated blood flow	hyper/tension	high blood pressure
ather/o/sclerosis	hardening of the artery	leuk/o/cyte	white blood cell
brady/card/ia	abnormally slow heart rate	phleb/itis	inflammation of a vein
card/io/my/o/pathy	disease of the heart muscle	tachy/card/ia	abnormally rapid heart rate
embol/ism	obstruction in blood flow	thromb/osis	blood clots in the vascular system
endo/card/itis	inflammation inside the heart muscle	ven/ous	pertaining to the veins

diastolic phase the blood pressure after the heart has completed a pumping stroke.

endocrine system a system of glands that secrete hormones into the bloodstream.

systolic phase the blood pressure as the heart is pumping blood into the cardiovascular system.

ENDOCRINE SYSTEM

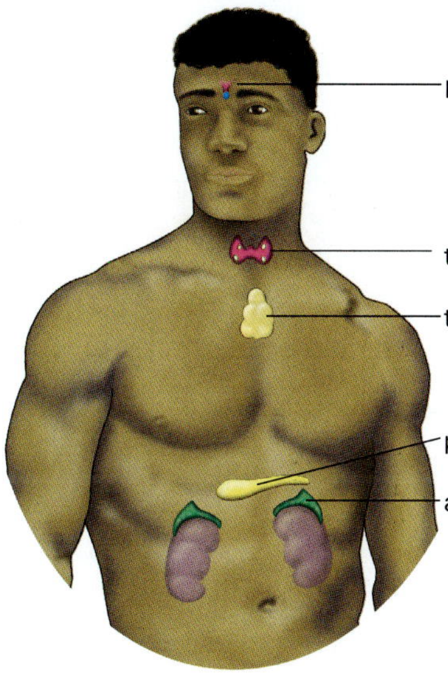

Root	Meaning	Root	Meaning
aden	gland	pancreat	pancreas
adrena	adrenal	plas	development
crine	to secrete	somat	body
glyc	sugar	tetan	tetanus
lipid	fat	thym	thymus
myx	mucus	thyroid	thyroid
nephr	kidney		

The ***endocrine system*** consists of the glands that secrete hormones, chemicals that assist in regulating body functions.

Several organs act as endocrine glands as well as members of other organ systems. For example, the liver, stomach, pancreas, and kidneys are members of the endocrine system as well as other organ systems. Organs that belong primarily to the endocrine system include the pituitary gland, the adrenal glands, the thyroid gland, and the gonads (ovaries and testes).

The pituitary gland produces multiple hormones and is located at the base of the brain. It controls the body's growth and releases hormones into the bloodstream that control much of the activity of the other glands. The thyroid gland is located just below the larynx and releases hormones important for regulating body metabolism. There are four smaller parathyroid glands located on the thyroid gland. The thymus gland is located beneath the sternum. The pancreas is best known for its production of insulin and glucagon. The small adrenal glands are located on top of the kidneys. They produce such hormones as aldosterone, cortisol (hydrocortisone), androgens, and estrogens. The medulla region of the adrenal glands produce the catecholamines adrenaline (epinephrine) and noradrenaline (norepinephrine).

Common Endocrine System Terminology

Term	Meaning	Term	Meaning
aden/oma	benign glandular tumor	hyper/secre/tion	abnormal increased secretion
diabet/ic	pancreatic disorder of insufficient insulin production	hypo/thyroid/ism	a deficiency of thyroid secretion
endo/crine	pertaining to glands that secrete hormones into the bloodstream	myx/edema	adult onset hypothyroidism
eu/thyroid	normal thyroid	pancreat/itis	inflammation of the pancreas
hyper/glyc/emia	high blood sugar	para/thyroid	next to the thyroid gland
hyper/lipid/emia	increase of lipids in the blood	somat/ic	pertaining to the body
hyper/plas/ia	excessive growth or formation	tetan/y	muscle twitches, cramps, convulsions

ORGAN SYSTEM TERMINOLOGY (cont'd)

GASTROINTESTINAL TRACT

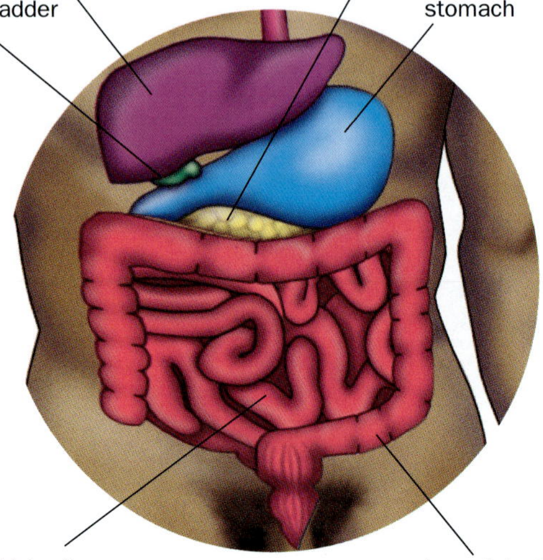

The gastrointestinal (GI) tract is located in the abdomen, and is surrounded by the peritoneal lining. The GI tract contains the organs that are involved in the digestion of foods and the absorption of nutrients. These organs include the stomach, small and large intestine, gallbladder, liver, and pancreas.

The GI tract is sometimes inappropriately referred to as the ***alimentary tract*.** The alimentary tract refers to the system that goes from the mouth to the anus. The alimentary tract contains organs such as lips, tongue, teeth, salivary glands, pharynx, esophagus, rectum, and anus, in addition to the GI tract.

Several organs contribute to the digestion of foods by secreting enzymes into the small intestine when food is present. Ducts carry bile from the liver (hepatic duct) and the gallbladder (cystic duct) to the duodenum. The pancreas is located behind the stomach and also contributes enzymes to the digestive process.

Root	Meaning	Root	Meaning
chol	bile	hepat	liver
col	colon	herni	hernia
duoden	duodenum	lapar	abdomen
enter	intestine	orexia	appetite
esophag	esophagus	pancreat	pancreas
gastr	stomach	pepsia	digestion
hemat	blood	phag	swallow

Common Gastrointestinal Tract Terminology

Term	Meaning	Term	Meaning
an/orexia	loss of appetite	gastr/itis	inflammation of the stomach
a/phag/ia	inability to swallow	gastr/o/enter/itis	inflammation of the stomach and intestinal tract
col/itis	inflamed or irritable colon	hemat/emesis	vomiting of blood
dia/rrhea	liquid or unformed bowel movement	hepat/itis	inflammation of the liver
duoden/al	pertaining to the duodenum	hepat/oma	liver tumor
dys/pepsia	condition of indigestion	herni/a	protrusion of organ or tissue
esophag/itis	inflammation of the esophagus	lapar/o/scopy	operation done in the abdomen

alimentary tract the organs from the mouth to the anus. The GI tract is a portion of the alimentary tract.

integumentary system the body covering, i.e., skin, hair, and nails.

INTEGUMENTARY SYSTEM

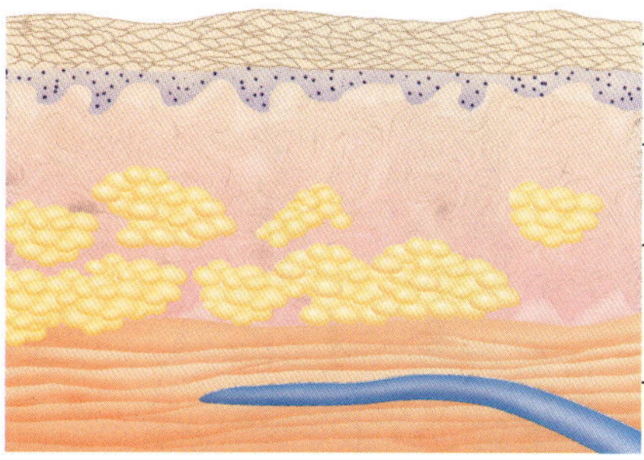

The covering of the body is referred to as the ***integumentary system***. It is the body's first line of defense, acting as a barrier against disease and physical hazards. It also helps control body temperature by releasing heat through sweat or by constricting blood vessels to act as insulation. It includes the skin, hair, and nails.

Hair is made of keratinized cells. Finger nails and toenails are also composed of keratin. The mammary glands, or breasts, are also considered part of the integumentary system.

The skin is composed of the epidermis and dermis. The epidermis has no blood or nerves and is constantly discarding dead cells. The dermis, which is made of living cells, contains capillaries, nerves, and lymphatics. The dermis also contains the sebaceous glands, sweat glands, and hair.

The subcutaneous layer of tissue is beneath the dermis but is closely interconnected to it. It separates the skin from the other organs (for example, the muscular system, as in the illustration).

Root	Meaning	Root	Meaning
adip	fat	mast	breast
cutane	skin	melan	black
derm(at)	skin	necr	death (of cells, etc.)
hist	tissue	onych	nail
kerat	hard		

Common Integumentary System Terminology

Term	Meaning	Term	Meaning
alopec/ia	hair loss	epi/dermis	top layer of the skin
cellul/itis	infection of the skin and subcutaneous tissue	kerat/osis	area of increased hardness
dermat/itis	skin inflammation	melan/oma	black tumor
dermat/o/mycosis	fungal infection of the skin	onych/mycosis	fungal infection of the nails
dia/phoresis	excessive sweating	pachy/derm	abnormal thickness of skin
dys/kerat/osis	abnormal keratin formation in the epidermis	sub/cutane/ous	beneath the skin
ec/zema	chronic skin inflammation	trans/derm/al	through the skin

ORGAN SYSTEM TERMINOLOGY (cont'd)

lymphocyte a type of white blood cell (leukocyte) that helps the body defend itself against bacteria and diseased cells.

LYMPH AND BLOOD SYSTEMS

The lymphatic system is responsible for collecting plasma water that leaves the blood vessels, filtering it for impurities through its lymph nodes, and returning the lymph fluid back to the general circulation. The lymphatic system is the center of the body's immune system.

The largest organ in the system is the spleen. It is responsible for removing old red blood cells from the circulation. It is also a storage organ for ***lymphocytes***, a type of white blood cell that attacks bacteria and disease cells. Lymphocytes release antibodies that destroy disease cells and provide immunity against them.

The thymus, tonsils, spleen, and adenoids are lymphoid organs outside the network of the lymphatic system.

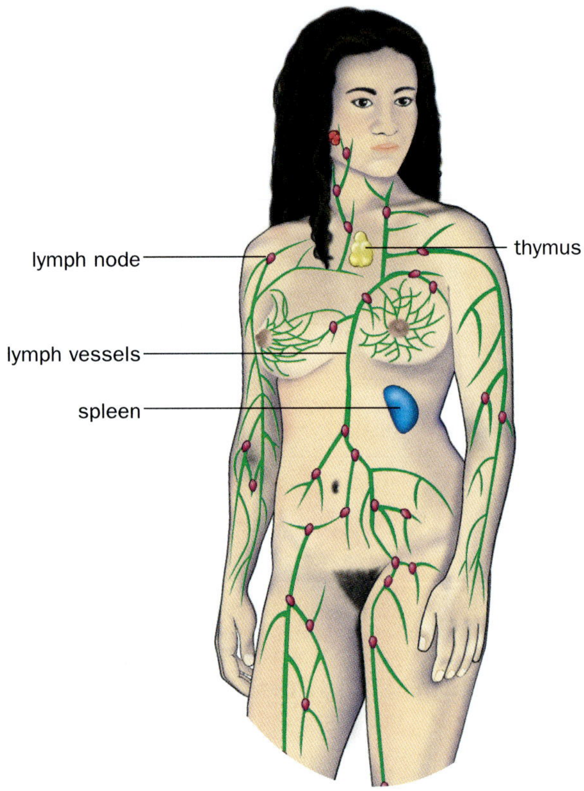

Root	Meaning	Root	Meaning
aden	gland	lymph	lymph
bacter	bacteria	phleb	vein
cyt	cell	splen	spleen
hemat	blood	sepsis	to putrefy
hemo	blood	thromb	clot
leuk	white	thym	thymus

Common Lymph and Blood Systems Terminology

Term	Meaning	Term	Meaning
aden/o/pathy	disease of the lymph nodes	lymph/o/cyte	immune response cell
an/emia	decrease in red blood cells	lymph/o/cyt/o/penia	decreased number of lymphocytes
bacter/emia	presence of bacteria in the bloodstream	lymph/oid	resembling clear lymph fluid
hemat/oma	a collection of blood, often clotted	phlebo/tomy	puncture of vein to draw blood
hemo/philia	a disease in which the blood does not clot normally	septic/emia	systemic blood infection
hyper/uric/emia	excessive level of uric acid in the blood	splen/ec/tomy	removal of the spleen
leuk/emia	increase in white blood cells	thym/oma	tumor of the thymus

flexor movement an expansion or outward movement by muscles.

MUSCULAR SYSTEM

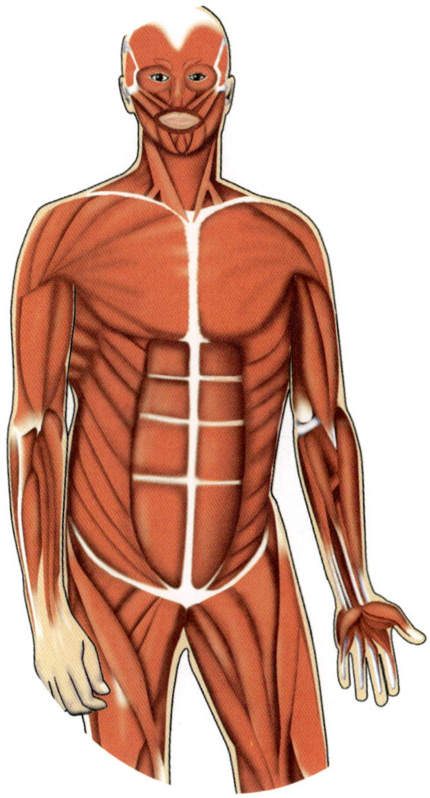

The word *muscle* comes from the Latin *mus* (mouse) and *cle* (little) because muscle movements resemble a mouse moving under a cover.

The body contains more than 600 muscles that give shape and movement to it. The skeletal muscles are attached to the bones by tendons. The muscles themselves are striated, i.e., made up of fibers.

The action of most muscles is called voluntary, because it is controlled consciously. Involuntary muscles operate automatically and are found in the heart, the stomach, or in the walls of blood vessels.

Some muscles produce an outward or ***flexor movement*** and these are called agonist muscles. Antagonist muscles are the ones that contract or bring the limb back to the original position.

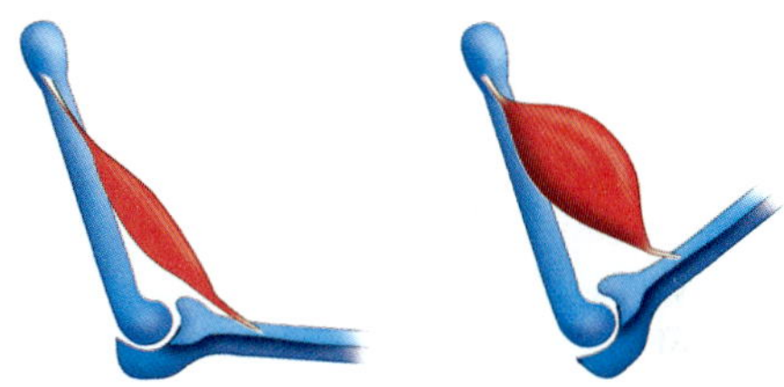

expansion and contraction of muscles

Root	Meaning	Root	Meaning
burs	bursa	my	muscle
chondr	cartilage	rhabdo	rod
fibr	fiber	tendin	tendon

Common Muscular System Terminology

Term	Meaning	Term	Meaning
a/trophy	process of shrinking muscle size	hypo/tonia	decrease in muscle tone
burs/itis	inflammation of the bursa	my/algia	muscle pain
chondr/o/malacia	softening of cartilage	my/asthenia	chronic muscular weakness
dys/trophy	progressive atrophy	my/o/necr/osis	increase in muscle death
fibr/oma	tumor of fibrous tissue	my/o/plasty	plastic surgery of muscle tissue
fibr/o/my/algia	chronic pain in the muscles	rhabdo/my/o/lysis	breaking down of striated muscle
hyper/trophy	process of increase in muscle size	tendin/itis	inflammation of a tendon

ORGAN SYSTEM TERMINOLOGY (cont'd)

NERVOUS SYSTEM

The most complex of the body organ systems is the nervous system, the body's system of communication. The ***neuron*** (nerve cell) is the basic functional unit in this system. There are over 100 billion neurons in the brain alone. Neurons also transmit information from the brain to the entire body.

The primary parts of this system are the brain and the spinal cord, called the central nervous system (CNS). The peripheral nervous system is composed of nerves that branch out from the spinal cord.

There are subdivisions of the peripheral nervous system called the autonomic nervous system and the somatic nervous system. The autonomic nervous system controls the automatic functions of the body, e.g., breathing, digestion, etc. The somatic nervous system controls the voluntary actions of the body, e.g., muscle movements.

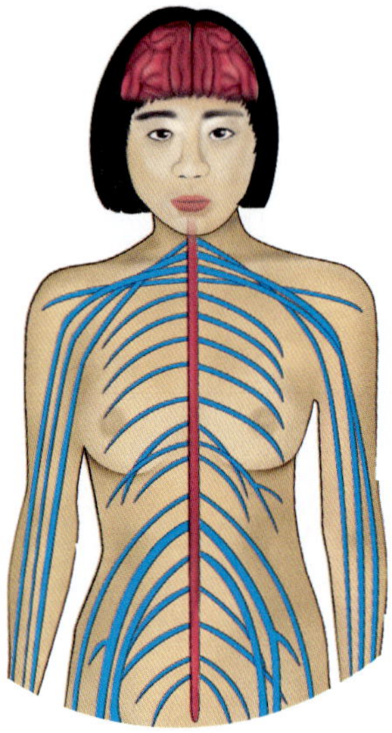

central and peripheral nervous systems

Root	Meaning	Root	Meaning
alges	pain	myel	spinal cord
cerebr	cerebrum	neur	nerve
encephal	brain	phas	speech
esthes	sensation	psycho	mind
mening	meninges	somat	body
ment	mind		

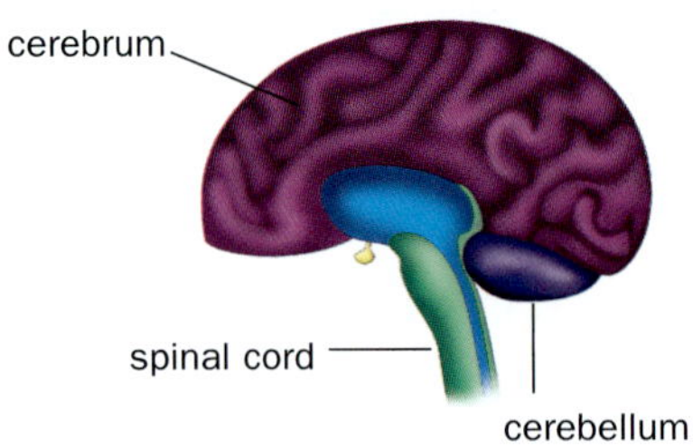

brain and spinal cord

Common Nervous System Terminology

Term	Meaning	Term	Meaning
an/alges/ia	without pain	epi/lepsy	disorder characterized by recurrent seizures
an/esthes/ia	lack of sensation	mening/itis	inflammation of the meninges
anti/depressant	drug that counteracts depression	myel/algia	pain of the spinal cord
auto/nom/ic	pertaining to involuntary actions	neur/algia	severe pain along a nerve
de/ment/ia	disorientation, confusion, loss of memory	neur/oma	tumor of nerve cells
dys/phas/ia	difficulty in speaking	para/lysis	breaking down of motor control
encephal/itis	inflammation of the brain	psych/osis	psychiatric disorder

neuron the functional unit of the nervous system.
osseous tissue the rigid portion of the bone tissue.

SKELETAL SYSTEM

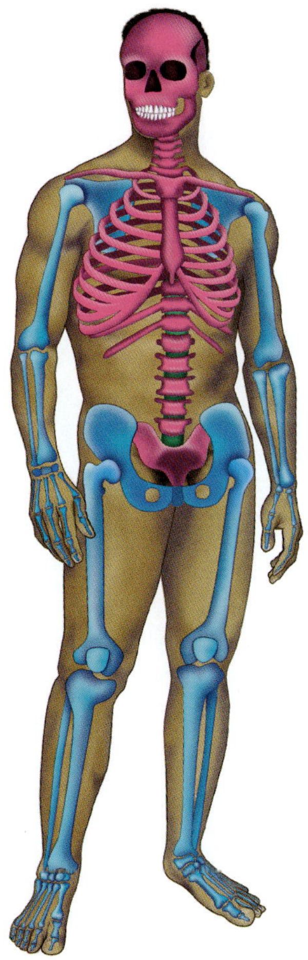

The skeletal system protects soft organs and provides structure and support for the body's organ systems. Made up largely of hard ***osseous tissue***, it is a living system that undergoes dynamic changes throughout life.

The system's 206 bones are called axial (the skull and the vertebra surrounding the spinal column) or appendicular (arms, legs, and connecting bones). They are held together at joints by connective tissue called ligaments and cartilage. Joints range from rigid to those allowing full motion (e.g., the ball and socket joints of the hips and shoulders).

Root	Meaning	Root	Meaning
arthr	joint	oste	bone
carp	wrist	patell	knee cap
crani	skull	ped, pod	foot
dactyl	finger or toe	pelv	pelvis
femor	thigh bone	phalang	bones of fingers and toes
fibul	small lower leg bone	rachi	vertebrae
		scoli	crooked, bent
humer	upper arm bone	spondyl	vertebrae
		stern	sternum, breastbone
lord	curve	tibi	large, lower leg bone

axial and appendicular skeleton

Common Skeletal System Terminology

Term	Meaning	Term	Meaning
arthr/algia	joint pain	osteo/chondr/osis	bone and cartilage disease
arthr/itis	inflammation of the joint	osteo/por/osis	decreased bone density and porosity
carp/al	pertaining to the wrist	peri/oste/itis	inflammation around the bone
crani/o/malacia	softening of the skull	phalang/ia	pain in finger or toe bones
lord/osis	forward curve of spine, swayback	rach/itis	inflammation of the spine
oste/algia	bone pain	scoli/osis	abnormal lateral curvature of the spine
oste/o/arthr/itis	chronic bone and joint disease	spondyl/itis	inflammation of the vertebrae
oste/o/carcin/oma	cancerous bone tumor		

ORGAN SYSTEM TERMINOLOGY (cont'd)

FEMALE REPRODUCTIVE SYSTEM

The female reproductive system produces hormones (e.g., estrogen, progesterone), controls menstruation, and provides for childbearing. The system contains the vagina, uterus, fallopian tubes, ovaries, and the external genitalia.

The mammary glands (located in breast tissue) are also associated with the female reproductive system. The mammary glands produce and secrete milk at childbirth.

The vagina is a muscular tube that leads from an external opening to the cervix and uterus. The uterus is a hollow, pear-shaped organ. The fallopian tubes transport eggs from the ovary to the uterus. The ovaries are located on each side of the uterus. In sexually mature females, the uterus is prepared for the possibility of fertilization and pregnancy each month during the menstrual cycle.

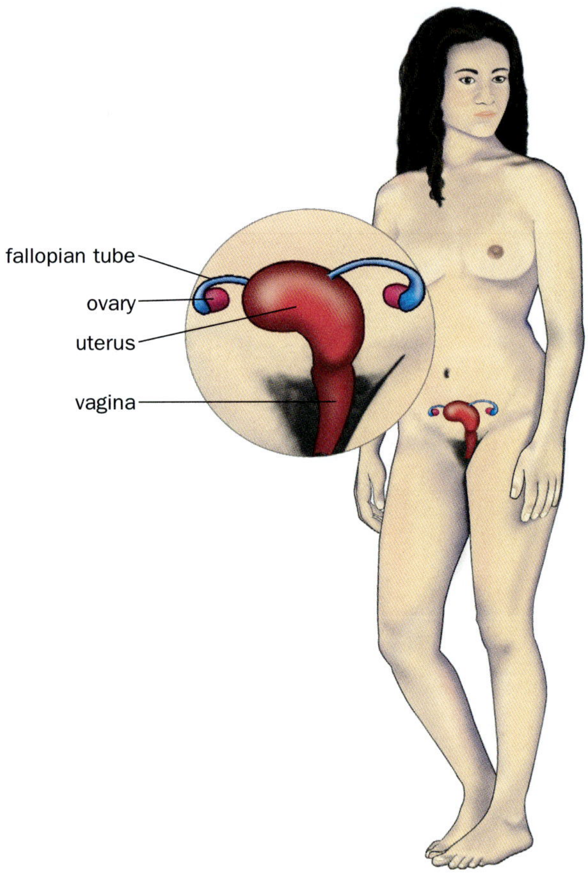

Root	Meaning	Root	Meaning
cervic	cervix	men	menstruation
condyle	knob, knuckle	metr	uterus
eclamps	shining forth	ovari	ovary
gynec	woman	salping	fallopian tube
hyster	uterus	toc	birth
lact	milk	uter	uterine
mamm	breast	vagin	vagina
mast	breast		

Common Female Reproductive System Terminology

Term	Meaning	Term	Meaning
a/men/o/rrhea	absence of menstruation	endo/metr/i/osis	abnormal growth of uteral tissue
an/ovula/tion	absence of ovulation	gynec/o/logy	study of female reproductive organs
cervic/itis	inflammation of the cervix	mamm/o/gram	photographic record of the breast
condyl/oma	genital wart	mast/ectomy	removal of the breast
dys/men/o/rrhea	menstrual pain	mast/itis	inflammation of the breast
dys/toc/ia	difficult childbirth	salping/o/cyesis	pregnancy in fallopian tube
eclamps/ia	severe toxemia during pregnancy	vagin/itis	inflammation of the vagina

MALE REPRODUCTIVE SYSTEM

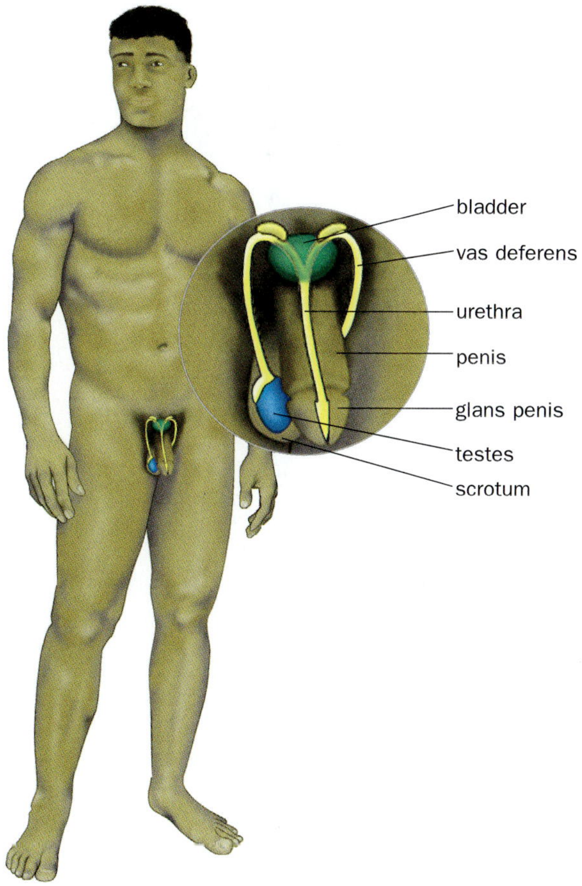

The male reproductive system produces sperm and secretes the hormone testosterone. The primary organs involved in the production of sperm are the testes (also called testicles). They are the oval-shaped organs enclosed in the scrotum.

The seminal glands, located at the base of the bladder, produce part of the seminal fluid. They have ducts that lead into the vas deferens that carry the sperm from the testes. The prostate gland is located at the upper end of the urethra. The penis (glans penis) is the external organ for urination and sexual intercourse. The tip of the penis is covered by the prepuce (foreskin). The urethra, by which urine and semen leave the body, is inside the penis.

Root	Meaning	Root	Meaning
andr	male	semin	semen
balan	glans penis	sperm	sperm
crypt	hidden	vas	vessel, duct
orch	testis	varic	varicose veins
orchid	testis	test	testis, testicle
prostat	prostate gland		

Common Male Reproductive System Terminology

Term	Meaning	Term	Meaning
andr/oid	resembling a male	hemat/o/sperm/ia	blood in semen
andr/o/phobia	morbid dislike of males	prostat/algia	painful prostate
an/orch/ism	absence of testes	prostat/itis	inflammation of the prostate
a/sperm/ia	inability to secrete sperm	test/algia	painful testes
balan/itis	inflammation of the glans penis	varic/o/cele	enlarged swollen vein near the testis
crypt/orchid/ism	failure of testes to drop into the scrotum	vas/ectomy	removal of a segment of the vas deferens

ORGAN SYSTEM TERMINOLOGY (cont'd)

RESPIRATORY SYSTEM

The respiratory system brings oxygen into the body through inhalation and expels carbon dioxide gas through exhalation. It produces sound for speaking and helps cool the body.

Respiratory muscles (especially the diaphragm) expand the lungs automatically, causing air to be inhaled into the upper respiratory tract. The pleural cavity surrounds the lungs and provides lubrication for respiration. The pharynx directs food into the esophagus and air into the trachea. The larynx contains the vocal cords. The trachea, or windpipe, connects to the two bronchi (bronchial tubes) that enter the lungs.

As air enters through the nose, it is warmed, moistened, and filtered. Inside the lungs, the bronchial tubes branch out and lead to the ***alveolar sacs (alveoli)*** that are the sites of gas exchange within the lungs. The alveolar sacs are the specialized tissues responsible for the exchange of gases between the blood and inhaled air.

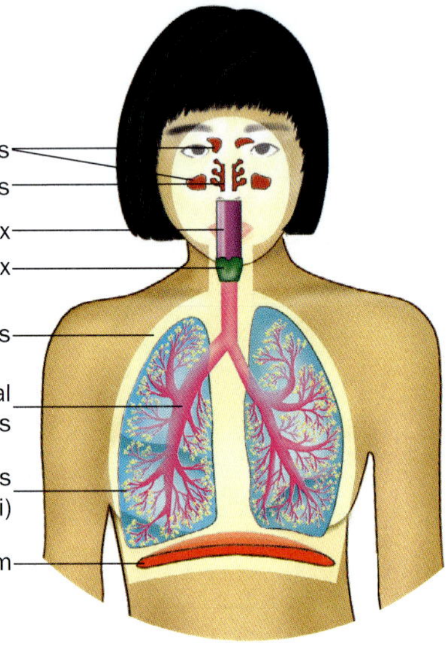

Root	Meaning	Root	Meaning
aer	air	ox	oxygen
aero	gas	pector	chest
bronch	bronchus	pneumon	lung, air
capn	carbon dioxide	pulmon	lung
cyan	blue	respir	breath
laryng	larynx	rhin	nose
nas	nose	sinus	sinus

Common Respiratory System Terminology

Term	Meaning	Term	Meaning
a/pnea	temporary failure to breathe	laryng/itis	inflammation of the larynx
brady/pnea	slow breathing	pector/algia	chest pain
bronch/itis	inflammation of the bronchial membranes	pneumon/ia	bacterial infection of the lungs
cyan/osis	abnormal blue skin color from lack of oxygen in the blood	pulmon/ary	pertaining to the lungs
dys/pnea	labored breathing	respir/a/tion	act or process of breathing
emphys/ema	obstructive pulmonary disease	rhin/itis	inflammation of the nose
hyper/capn/ia	excessive carbon dioxide in the blood	sinus/itis	inflammation of the sinuses

alveolar sacs (alveoli) the small sacs of specialized tissue that transfer oxygen out of inspired air into the blood and carbon dioxide out of the blood and into the air for expiration.

nephron the functional unit of the kidney responsible for removing wastes from the blood and producing urine.

URINARY TRACT

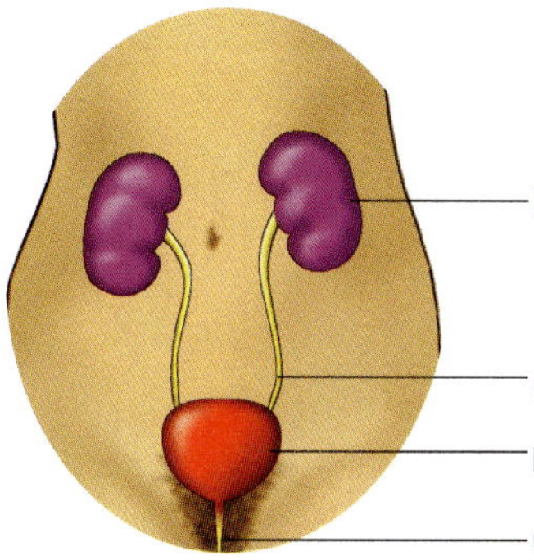

The urinary tract is responsible for removing waste materials from the blood. The urinary tract includes the kidneys, ureters, urinary bladder, and urethra.

The primary organ of the urinary tract is the kidney. The ***nephron*** is the functional unit of the kidney. There are several million nephrons in the kidneys. Urine is produced as plasma water is filtered through the glomerulus and the filtrate is collected in the tubule. Waste materials from the blood may also be filtered into the tubule or may be secreted into the tubule at sites other than the glomerulus. The filtrate that moves along the tubule is called urine.

Urine leaves the kidney through the ureters and collects in the bladder. It is excreted from the bladder through the urethra.

Root	Meaning	Root	Meaning
albumin	protein	ur	kidney
cyst	bladder	uresis	urination
glycos	glucose	ureter	ureter
keto	ketones	urethr	urethra
lith	stone	uria	urine, urination
nephr	kidney	vesic	bladder
ren	kidney		

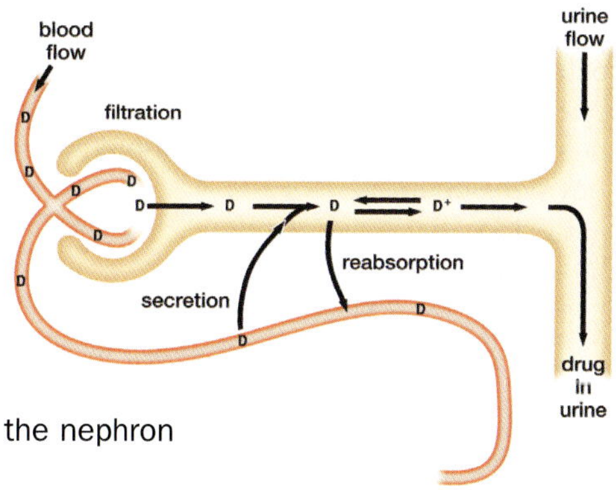

the nephron

Common Urinary Tract Terminology

Term	Meaning	Term	Meaning
albumin/uria	protein in the urine	glycos/uria	glucose in the urine
an/uresis	inability to urinate	hemat/uria	blood in the urine
an/uria	inability to produce urine	keto/uria	ketone bodies in the urine
cyst/itis	inflammation of the bladder	lith/iasis	formation of any stone
dia/lysis	method of filtering impurities from blood	nephr/algia	kidney pain
dys/uria	painful urination	nephr/itis	inflammation of the kidney
en/uresis	involuntary urination	poly/uria	excessive urination

ORGAN SYSTEM TERMINOLOGY (cont'd)

SENSES: HEARING

The sense of hearing, as well as the maintenance of body equilibrium, is performed by the ear. The external ear consists of a funnel-shaped structure that captures sound waves and channels them through an opening to the ***tympanic membrane*** (eardrum). The opening also contains glands that make earwax (cerumen) which protects the external ear.

The middle ear consists of three bony structures (malleus, incus, and stapes) that transmit sound from a vibrating tympanic membrane to the cochlea. The ***eustachian tube*** connects the middle ear to the nose and throat, serving to equalize the air pressure on both sides of the tympanic membrane.

The principal structure in the inner ear is the labyrinth, which consists of the vestibule, the cochlea, and the semicircular canals. The cochlea contains the organ of hearing. When sound waves are transmitted to the cochlea, it converts them into nerve impulses that are sent to the brain for interpretation. The semicircular canals and the vestibule are primarily responsible for body equilibrium.

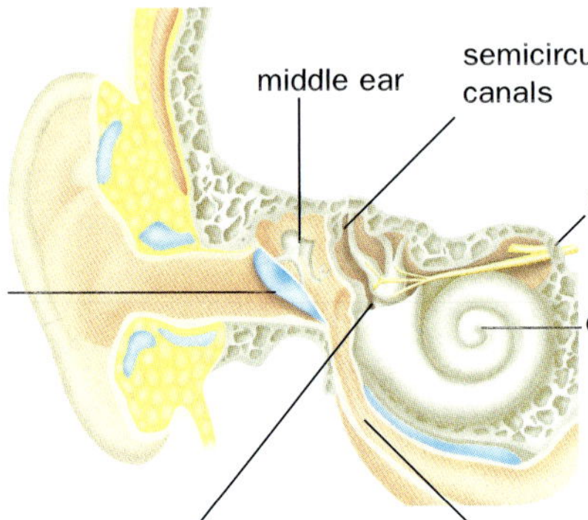

Root	Meaning	Root	Meaning
acous	hearing	myring	eardrum
acusis	hearing condition	ot	ear
audi	hearing	salping	eustachian tube
cerumin	wax-like	tympan	eardrum
labyrinth	inner ear		

Common Hearing Terminology

Term	Meaning	Term	Meaning
an/acusis	without hearing; deafness	ot/o/plasty	plastic surgery on the ear
audi/o/metry	process of measuring hearing	ot/o/rrhag/ia	bleeding of the ear
cerumin/osis	excessive earwax	ot/o/rrhea	ear infection discharge
labyrinth/itis	inflammation of the inner ear	ot/o/sclerosis	abnormal hardening of bone in the middle ear
ot/algia	pain in the ear (earache)	ot/o/scope	instrument for examining the ear
ot/itis	inflammation of the ear	par/acusis	partial hearing loss
ot/o/mycosis	fungal ear infection	tympan/itis	inflammation of the eardrum

conjunctiva the eyelid lining.

cornea the transparent outer part of the eye.

eustachian tube the tube that connects the middle ear to the throat.

lacrimal gland the gland that produces tears for the eyes.

retina thc inncr lining of the eye that translates light into nerve impulses.

tympanic membrane the membrane that transmits sound waves to the inner ear.

SENSES: SIGHT

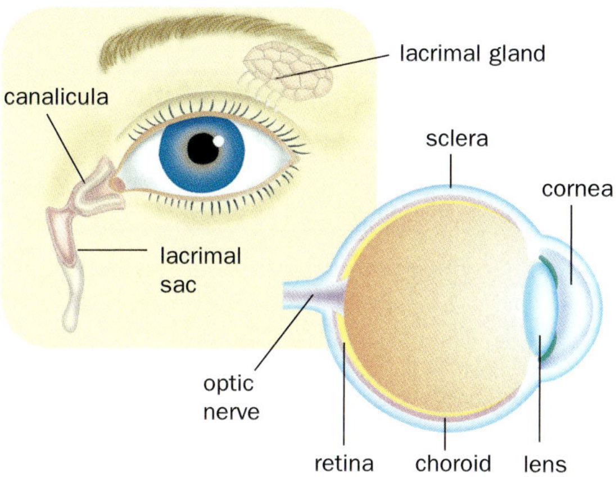

The eyes are the organs that provide sight. The eyelids protect the eye and assist in its lubrication. The ***conjunctiva*** is the blood-rich membrane between the eye and the eyelid. There are several glands that secrete fluids to protect and lubricate the eye: the ***lacrimal glands*** above each eye secrete tears and the meibomian glands produce sebum. Excess fluid drains into the canalicula (tear ducts).

The eye has three layers. The outer layer is composed of the sclera and the cornea. The sclera is the white part of the eye. The ***cornea*** is transparent so the iris (the color of the eye) and the pupil (the opening of the eye) are visible. The middle layer is called the choroid and contains blood vessels that nourish the entire eye. In the third layer, the lens focuses light rays on the ***retina***. The vitreous humor (one of two fluids in the eye) fills the space between the retina and the lens. Rods and cones within the retina are responsible for visual reception. The optic nerve within the retina transmits the nerve impulses to the brain for interpretation.

Root	Meaning	Root	Meaning
ambly	dim, dull	ocul	eye
blephar	eyelid	ophthalm	eye
conjunctiv	conjunctiva	opia	vision
corne	cornea	opt	eye, vision
glauc	gray	retin	retina
irid, ir	iris	stigmat	point(ed)
lacrim	tear duct		

Common Ophthalmic Terminology

Term	Meaning	Term	Meaning
ambly/opia	reduction in vision	eso/tropia	eye turning inward toward the nose
a/stigmat/ism	distorted vision	exo/tropia	eye turning outward away from the nose
blephar/itis	inflammation of the eyelids	glauc/oma	eye disease caused by increased intraocular pressure
blephar/opt/osis	abnormal drooping of the upper eyelid	hyper/opia	farsightedness; difficulty seeing close objects
conjunctiv/itis	inflammation of the conjunctiva	irid/o/plegia	paralysis of the iris
dipl/opia	double vision	ocul/o/mycosis	fungal infection of the eye
end/ophthalm/itis	inflammation of the inside of the eye	retin/itis	inflammation of the retina

DRUG CLASSIFICATIONS

The same system used to interpret medical science terminology can be used to interpret drug classification names.

A classification is a group of drugs that have several therapeutic properties in common.

For example, penicillin, cefoxitine, and ciprofloxacin are used to treat bacterial infections, so they are grouped in a class called anti-infectives.

Each of the drugs mentioned above has unique properties, but they all share the property of being effective against bacterial infections. So the classification name "anti-infective" is created by combining *anti* and *infective* into anti-infective, meaning "against infection." Since much of drug therapy is based on opposing some physiological process in the body, many drug classes begin with the prefix *anti* or *ant*.

Root	Prefix
Suffix	C.V.

Drug classification names can be understood by identifying their components.

THE "AGAINST" CLASSES

Some examples of the "anti" classes of drugs

antacid	relieves gastritis, ulcer pain, indigestion and heartburn
antianginal	relieves heart pain
anticoagulant	dissolves or prevents blood clots
anticonvulsant	prevents seizures
antidepressant	prevents depression
antidiarrheal	stops diarrhea
antiemetic	prevents nausea and vomiting
antihistamine	blocks the effects of histamine
antihyperlipidemic	lowers high cholesterol levels
antihypertensive	reduces high blood pressure
anti-inflammatory	reduces inflammation
antipruritic	prevents or relieves itching
antispasmodic	relieves intestinal cramping
antitussive	relieves coughing by inhibiting cough reflex

OTHER CLASSES

Here are examples of other classification names that can be understood by breaking down the term into its medical terminology components.

bronch + o + dilator	**bronchodilator**:	dilates bronchial tubes in the lung
an + alges + ic	**analgesic**:	without pain, kills pain
hypo + glyc + emic	**hypoglycemic**:	reduces blood sugar levels
hypo + lipid + emic	**hypolipidemic**:	reduces blood lipid (cholesterol) levels
kerat + o + lytic	**keratolytic**:	destroys hard skin layers such as warts
an + orex + ic	**anorexic**:	reduces appetite
psych + o + tropic	**pyschotropic**:	changes mental states
sperm + i + cide	**spermicide**:	destroys sperm

MEDICAL ABBREVIATIONS 4

Many medical terms are abbreviated for ease of communication and record notation.

It has been estimated that about 10,000 abbreviations are used in the medical sciences. Many abbreviations are specific for one institution or one area of the country. It is also possible that one abbreviation may have more than one meaning. When in doubt, the pharmacy technician should verify the meaning of an abbreviation.

Common Medical Abbreviations

ADD	attention deficit disorder
ADR	adverse drug reaction
AIDS	acquired immunodeficiency syndrome
AV	atrial-ventricular
AMI	acute myocardial infarction
ANS	autonomic nervous system
ASAP	as soon as possible
BM	bowel movement
BP	blood pressure
BPH	benign prostatic hyperplasia
BS	blood sugar
BSA	body surface area
CA	cancer
CAD	coronary artery disease
CF	cardiac failure
CHF	congestive heart failure
CMV	cytomegalovirus
CNS	central nervous system
COPD	chronic obstructive pulmonary disease
CVA	cerebrovascular accident (stroke)
DAW	dispense as written
D/C	discontinue
DM	diabetes melitus
DOB	date of birth
DUR	drug utilization review
Dx	diagnosis
EC	enteric coated
ECG, EKG	electrocardiogram
ENT	ears, nose, throat
ER	emergency room
FH	family history
GERD	gastroesophageal reflux disease
GI	gastrointestinal
Gtt	drop
HA	headache
HBP	high blood pressure
HDL	high density lipoprotein
HIV	human immunodeficiency virus
HR	heart rate
IO, I/O	fluid intake and output
IOP	intraocular pressure
IV	intravenous
KVO	keep veins open
LBW	low birth weight
LDL	low density lipoprotein
LOC	loss of consciousness
MI	myocardial infarction
MICU	medical intensive care unit
MRI	magnetic resonance imaging
NKA	no known allergies
NPO	nothing by mouth
NS	normal saline
NVD	nausea, vomiting, diarrhea
OR	operating room
PMH	past medical history
PUD	peptic ulcer disease
PVD	peripheral vascular disease
RA	rheumatoid arthritis
RBC	red blood count or red blood cell
SBP	systolic blood pressure
SOB	shortness of breath
STD	sexually transmitted diseases
T	temperature
T&C	type and cross-match (blood)
TB	tuberculosis
TEDS	thrombo-embolic disease stockings
TPN	total parenteral nutrition
Tx	treatment
U	units
U/A	urinalysis
UCHD	usual childhood diseases
URD	upper respiratory diseases
UTI	urinary tract infection
VD	venereal disease
VS	vital signs
WBC	white blood count or white blood cell
WT	weight

REVIEW

KEY CONCEPTS

TERMINOLOGY

- ✔ Much of medical science terminology is made up of a combination of root words that originated from either Greek or Latin words, suffixes, and prefixes.
- ✔ A prefix is added to the beginning of a root word and a suffix is added to the end of a root word to clarify the meaning.
- ✔ Combining vowels are used to connect the prefix, root word, or suffix parts of the term.
- ✔ It is not necessary that a root word have a prefix, suffix, and combining vowel.

ORGAN SYSTEM TERMINOLOGY

- ✔ The cardiovascular system circulates blood throughout the body in blood vessels called arteries, capillaries, and veins.
- ✔ The endocrine system consists of the glands that secrete hormones (chemicals that assist in regulating body functions).
- ✔ The GI tract contains the organs that are involved in the digestion of foods and the absorption of nutrients.
- ✔ The integumentary system (i.e., the body's covering) is the first line of defense against disease and physical hazards.
- ✔ The lymph and blood systems are the center of the body's immune system.
- ✔ The body contains more than 600 muscles that give it shape and produce movement.
- ✔ The nervous system is the body's system of communication. The neuron (nerve cell) is its basic functional unit.
- ✔ The skeletal system protects soft organs and provides structure and support for the body's organ systems.
- ✔ The female reproductive system produces hormones (estrogens, progesterone), controls menstruation, and provides for childbearing.
- ✔ The male reproductive system produces sperm and secretes the hormone testosterone.
- ✔ The respiratory system brings oxygen into the body through inhalation and expels carbon dioxide gas through exhalation.
- ✔ The primary organ of the urinary tract is the kidney; each kidney has millions of nephrons that help remove waste materials and drugs from the blood.
- ✔ The ear provides the sense of hearing and maintains the body's equilibrium.
- ✔ The eye is the sensitive organ involved in sight. Several body functions are involved in protecting this organ (e.g., tear production, blinking).

DRUG CLASSIFICATIONS/MEDICAL ABBREVIATIONS

- ✔ The same system used in medical science terminology can be applied to the names given to various drug classes.
- ✔ There are an estimated 10,000 abbreviations used in medical science. Many abbreviations are specific to an institution or area of the country.

SELF-TEST

the answer key begins on page 569

MATCH THE TERMS: I

1. through the skin _____
2. blood tumor _____
3. ven _____
4. ot _____
5. gastr _____
6. hardening of the artery _____
7. muscle repair _____
8. otalgia _____
9. liver tumor _____
10. card _____
11. cyst _____
12. derma _____
13. loss of appetite _____
14. hemat _____
15. hepat _____
16. mast _____
17. increase in white blood cells _____
18. nephr _____
19. neur _____
20. ocul _____
21. oste _____
22. brain inflammation _____
23. pector _____
24. pneum _____
25. my _____

a. atherosclerosis
b. kidney
c. chest
d. transdermal
e. eye
f. heart
g. hematoma
h. myoplasty
i. encephalitis
j. bladder
k. blood
l. bone
m. breast
n. ear
o. earache
p. vein
q. liver
r. anorexia
s. lung
t. muscle
u. nerve
v. skin
w. stomach
x. leukemia
y. hepatoma

MATCH THE TERMS: II

1. alimentary tract _____
2. alveoli _____
3. combining vowel _____
4. conjunctiva _____
5. cornea _____
6. diastolic phase _____
7. endocrine system _____
8. eustachian tube _____
9. flexor movement _____

a. the organs from the mouth to the anus.
b. an expansion or outward movement by muscles.
c. the small sacs of specialized tissue that transfer oxygen out of inspired air into the blood and carbon dioxide out of the blood and into the air for expiration.
d. the eyelid lining.
e. a vowel used to connect the prefix, root word, or suffix parts of a term.
f. the blood pressure after the heart has completed a pumping stroke.
g. a system of glands that secrete hormones into the blood stream.
h. the transparent outer part of the eye.
i. the tube that connects the middle ear to the throat.

REVIEW

MATCH THE TERMS: III

1. integumentary system ____
2. lacrimal gland _____
3. lymphocytes _____
4. nephron _____
5. neuron ____
6. osseous tissue ____
7. prefix _____
8. retina ____
9. root word ____
10. suffix ____
11. systolic phase ____
12. tympanic membrane ____

a. the inner lining of the eye that translates light into nerve impulses.
b. the body covering, i.e., skin, hair, and nails.
c. a type of white blood cell (leukocyte) that helps the body defend itself against bacteria and diseased cells.
d. the functional unit of the kidney responsible for removing wastes from the blood and producing urine.
e. the gland that produces tears for the eyes.
f. the base component of a term which gives it a meaning that may be modified by other components.
g. a modifying component of a term located at the end of the term.
h. a modifying component of a term located at the beginning of the term.
i. the blood pressure as the heart is pumping blood into the cardiovascular system.
j. the functional unit of the nervous system.
k. the rigid portion of the bone tissue.
l. membrane that transmits sound waves to the inner ear.

FILL IN THE MEANING

Prefix	Root Word	CV	Suffix	Term	Meaning
tachy	card		ia	tachycardia	1. ________________
endo	crine			endocrine	2. ________________
	hepat		oma	hepatoma	3. ________________
trans	derm		al	transdermal	4. ________________
	hemo		philia	hemophilia	5. ________________
	fibr + my	o	algia	fibromyalgia	6. ________________
dys	phasia			dysphasia	7. ________________
	oste+carcin	o	oma	osteocarcinoma	8. ________________
dys	men	o	rrhea	dysmenorrhea	9. ________________
a	sperm		ia	aspermia	10. ________________
	pector		algia	pectoralgia	11. ________________
	nephr		itis	nephritis	12. ________________
para	acusis			paracusis	13. ________________
	blephar		optosis	blepharoptosis	14. ________________

CHOOSE THE BEST ANSWER

1. Words from the _____ language most often refer to diagnosis and surgery; words from the _____ language generally refer to the anatomy of the body.
   a. Latin, Greek
   b. Greek, Latin
   c. Latin, Latin
   d. Greek, Greek

2. The ________________ is a modifier attached to the end of the root word and the ________________ is a modifier attached to the front of the root word.
   a. prefix, suffix
   b. suffix, prefix
   c. suffix, root
   d. prefix, root

3. The prefix *pseudo* means
   a. true.
   b. with.
   c. false.
   d. across or through.

4. The cardiovascular system distributes blood through the body in
   a. arteries and capillaries.
   b. arteries, capillaries, and veins.
   c. veins and arteries.
   d. veins, glands, and arteries.

5. Pericarditis means
   a. hardening of the arteries.
   b. area of the chest containing the lungs.
   c. movement across the liver.
   d. inflammation around the heart.

6. Chemicals that assist in regulating body functions are called
   a. antibodies.
   b. hormones.
   c. proteins.
   d. catalysts.

7. The gland in the endocrine system that regulates body metabolism is the
   a. thyroid gland.
   b. adrenal gland.
   c. pituitary gland.
   d. thymus gland.

8. Which is not part of the endocrine system?
   a. adrenal glands
   b. lacrimal glands
   c. thymus gland
   d. pituitary gland

9. Hepatitis is inflammation of the
   a. heart.
   b. spleen.
   c. kidneys.
   d. liver.

10. Aphagia means
    a. loss of appetite.
    b. top layer of the skin.
    c. joint pain.
    d. inability to swallow.

11. Which gland(s) is(are) part of the integumentary system?
    a. adrenal glands
    b. pituitary gland
    c. thyroid gland
    d. mammary glands

12. The root word *onych* means ______.
    a. skin
    b. nails
    c. hand
    d. breast

REVIEW

13. The integumentary system
    a. regulates the immune response to bacterial infection.
    b. regulates body temperature and defends against disease.
    c. regulates red blood cell production.
    d. provides structural support for the body.

14. The lymph and blood systems are the center of the ___________ system of the body?
    a. reproductive
    b. nervous
    c. cardiovascular
    d. immune

15. The spleen is the largest organ in the lymph and blood systems and is the storage organ for
    a. leukocytes.
    b. hepatocytes.
    c. lymphocytes.
    d. monocytes.

16. Hematemesis is the vomiting of
    a. partially digested food.
    b. clear colorless liquid.
    c. blood.
    d. bile.

17. Skeletal muscles are attached to the bones by
    a. cartilage.
    b. striated muscles.
    c. tendons.
    d. none of the above.

18. Muscle action that is controlled consciously is called ________ movement.
    a. agonist
    b. antagonist
    c. involuntary
    d. voluntary

19. The root word *somat* refers to the
    a. body.
    b. skin.
    c. abdomen.
    d. neurons.

20. The nerves that branch out from the spinal cord are collectively called the
    a. peripheral nervous system.
    b. autonomic nervous system.
    c. somatic nervous system.
    d. central nervous system.

21. Body functions such as breathing and digestion are controlled by the
    a. cerebrum.
    b. autonomic nervous system.
    c. somatic nervous system.
    d. spinal cord.

22. The body is composed of _____ bones.
    a. 206
    b. 314
    c. 407
    d. more than 500

23. A common skeletal system disease is
    a. dysphasia.
    b. osteoarthritis.
    c. hypercapnia.
    d. meningitis.

24. The female reproductive system
    a. produces hormones.
    b. controls menstruation.
    c. provides for childbearing.
    d. all of the above.

25. The major hormone produced by the male reproductive system is
    a. progesterone.
    b. testosterone.
    c. estrogen.
    d. aldosterone.

26. The root word *andr* means
    a. glans penis.
    b. male.
    c. vessel.
    d. semen.

27. The ________________ surrounds the lungs and provides lubrication for respiration.
    a. pulmonary cavity
    b. pleural cavity
    c. diaphragm
    d. alveolar sacs

28. The functional unit of the kidney is the
    a neuron.
    b. alveoli.
    c. nephron.
    d. axon.

29. Body equilibrium is maintained by the
    a. cochlea.
    b. eustachian tubes.
    c. semicircular canals.
    d. external ear.

CRITICAL THINKING QUESTIONS

1. List five basic combinations of root words, prefixes, and suffixes that are used to make medical terms.

2. What are the reasons for having over 10,000 abbreviations in medical and/or scientific terminology?

THINKING IT THROUGH WRAP-UP

1. Almost all medical terms will have a root word which applies either to a part of the body or a disease or condition. The root word is modified or expanded by adding a prefix (before the root word), or a suffix (after the root word). By knowing the meanings of all these parts, it is possible to understand to what a medical term is referring.
2. Many abbreviations are specific to one institution or one area of the country. Abbreviations may also have more than one meaning. So even though they can help facilitate communication, it is important that everyone has the same interpretation of abbreviations.
3. Patients often have a disease or condition that is confined to one organ system. Knowing the medical terms associated with that organ system help professionals quickly and accurately communicate about the patient's health. For example, in the scenario the patient has hyperlipidemia, hyperglycemia, hypertension, COPD, GERD, atrial fibrillation, and psychosis. So the patient has high blood lipids, high blood sugar, high blood pressure, difficulty breathing, gastrointestinal reflux, a heart condition, and is receiving treatment for altered mental status. In just a few medical terms, you can see what the patient's conditions are and start to understand what they are dealing with in their lives.

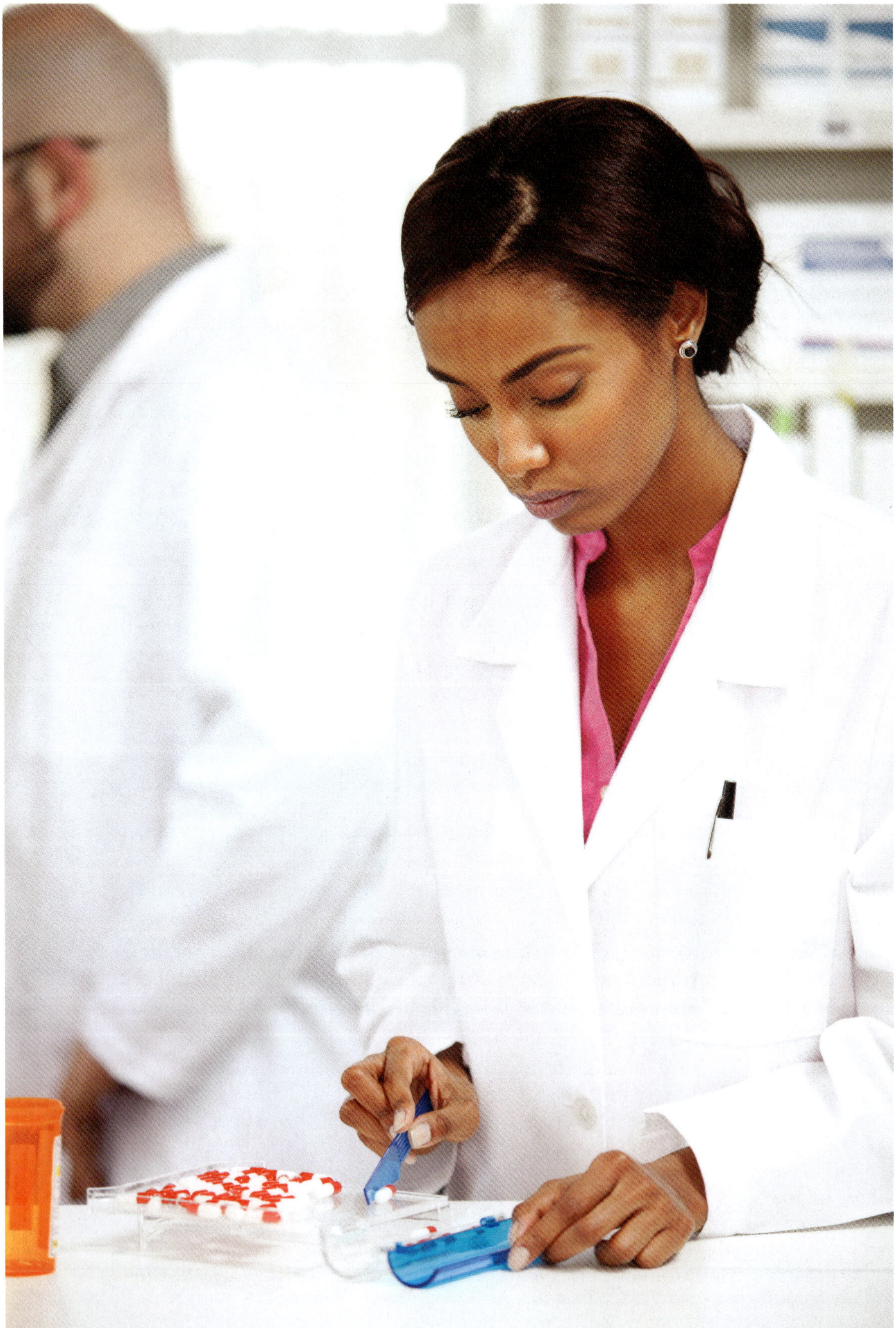

5

PRESCRIPTIONS

LEARNING OBJECTIVES

At the completion of study, the student will:

- ✔ understand the prescription process, including each of the steps involved from the creation of a prescription to patient pick up and counseling.
- ✔ understand the importance of preventing and identifying medication errors at every step of the prescription filling process.
- ✔ understand the differences in responsibilities between pharmacy technicians and pharmacists, as well as the legal and safety reasons for never assuming pharmacist-only responsibilities.
- ✔ understand the importance of protecting patient privacy and treating all patients with respect.

THINKING IT THROUGH

Jenna is a pharmacy technician with eight years experience at a busy pharmacy. On a particularly busy day, Mrs. Harris, who is in a hurry, stops by to pick up two prescriptions. She also needs an over-the-counter cold medication for her husband and asks Jenna for a recommendation.

Jenna has often rung up sales for over-the-counter cough and cold medications that have been recommended to customers by the pharmacist. As you read this chapter, consider whether it is ok for Jenna to show Mrs. Harris some products she knows the pharmacist has recommended to other customers. If it is not ok, how would Jenna explain this to Mrs. Harris?

PRESCRIPTIONS

A ***prescription*** **is an instruction from a medical practitioner that authorizes a patient to be issued a drug or device.**

Medical doctors (MD), doctors of osteopathy (DO), dentists (DDS), and veterinarians (DVM) are the primary practitioners that order prescription drugs. Opticians and podiatrists are also allowed to order prescription drugs relative to their field of practice. In most states, nurse practitioners, physician assistants, and/or pharmacists are also allowed to prescribe medications based on predetermined protocols (specific guidelines for practice) and in collaboration with one of the primary practitioners mentioned above.

Prescriptions are subject to many federal and state rules and regulations.

These regulations have been developed to protect the patient and provide for certain minimum standards of practice. The rules and regulations that govern both community and hospital pharmacy practice are continually evaluated and updated as new technologies, new medications, and new protocols are developed and adopted.

Community pharmacists dispense directly to the patient, who is then expected to administer the medication according to the pharmacist's directions.

This requires clear communication between the pharmacist and the patient. The pharmacist counsels the patient or the patient's representative when the prescription is purchased. In addition, the patient receives information on the prescription label as well as from an information sheet supplied with the medication.

In institutional settings, nursing staff generally administer medications to patients.

As a result, the rules and regulations that govern prescription dispensing in institutional settings are quite different from those that apply to community practice. Labeling is also different and many medications are packaged in individual doses.

Prescription Products

Prescriptions are usually written for commercially available products and are ordered by brand or generic name, strength, and route of administration. The prescription may be filled with that exact product or a chemically equivalent alternative. Prescriptions sometimes require pharmaceutical preparation from raw or individual ingredients (***extemporaneous compounding***). Some insurance companies will cover ***over-the-counter (OTC) drugs*** if ordered by prescription.

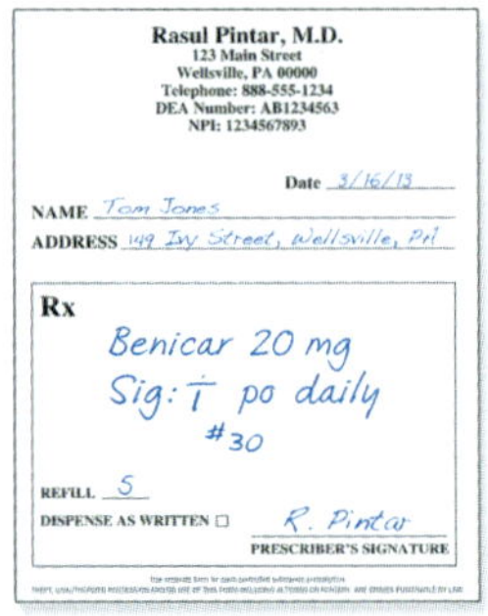

Rasul Pintar, M.D.
123 Main Street
Wellsville, PA 00000
Telephone: 888-555-1234
DEA Number: AB1234563
NPI: 1234567893

Date 3/16/13
NAME Tom Jones
ADDRESS 149 Ivy Street, Wellsville, PA

Rx
Benicar 20 mg
Sig: $\dot{\text{T}}$ po daily
#30

REFILL 5
DISPENSE AS WRITTEN ☐
R. Pintar
PRESCRIBER'S SIGNATURE

1 A prescription is ordered by a prescriber.

The prescriber may give the prescription to the patient or may communicate it to the pharmacy via fax, electronic transmission, or telephone.

10 The pharmacist provides counseling.

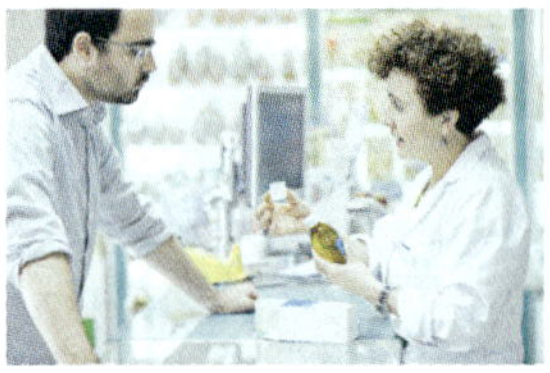

As required by OBRA '90 and other state or provincial statutes, the pharmacist is called to the counter to provide counseling on all new prescriptions. Counseling is sometimes also provided on refill prescriptions, as per the pharmacy's protocol.

Photo courtesy catalina mas sebastian/E+/Getty Images

9 The patient receives the prescription.

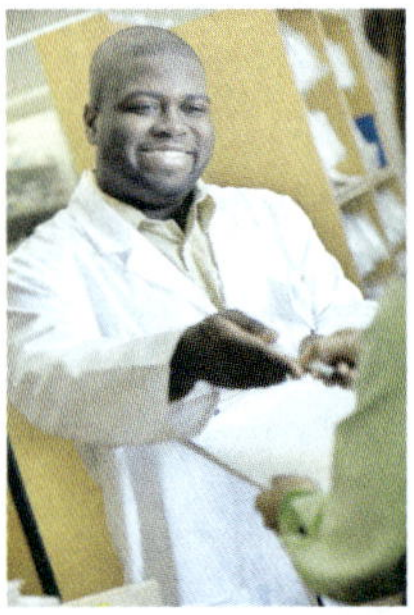

A technician completes his/her final safety and accuracy check by ensuring the correct patient receives the correct drug. The patient or patient's representative then signs the insurance log. If the patient has not yet signed the pharmacy's notice of HIPAA compliance, they are given a copy of the notice and asked to sign that log. The technician then rings the sale through the cash register.

extemporaneous compounding the on-demand preparation of a drug product according to a physician's prescription, formula, or recipe.

over-the-counter (OTC) drugs medications that do not require a prescription but may be filled with a prescription.

prescription an instruction from a medical practitioner that authorizes a patient to be issued a drug or device.

THE PRESCRIPTION PROCESS

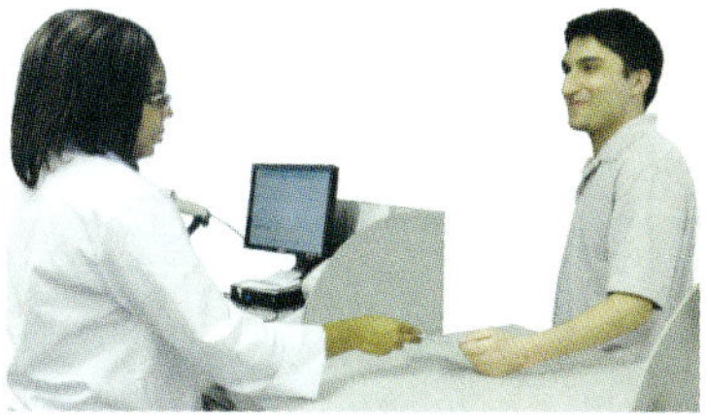

2 The prescription arrives at the pharmacy.

The patient or a representative presents the written prescription at the pharmacy counter. Alternatively, the prescription may be received directly from the prescriber.

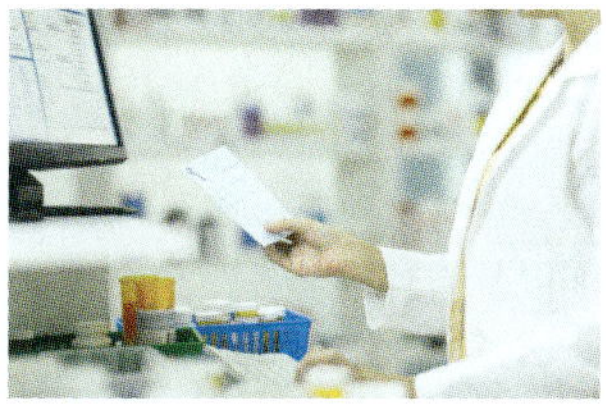

3 Patient and prescriber information is gathered.

The technician collects or confirms the patient's information (e.g., name, address, telephone, allergies, insurance), prescriber's name, and any special instructions (e.g. pick-up time, day's supply).

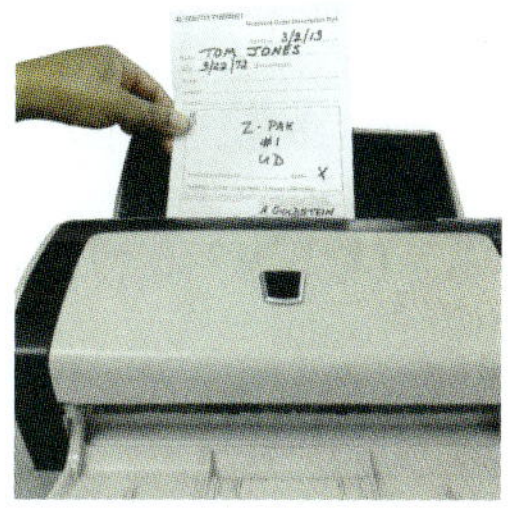

4 The prescription data is entered into the computer system.

The technician scans a copy of the prescription into the system and keys in the data from the prescription, ensuring all safety and accuracy checks are completed as per pharmacy policy.

5 Insurance and billing information is processed.

The computer system evaluates the data against stored information and processes any third-party billing. Messaging may be returned regarding drug utilization review (DUR) edits or the insurance claim. The pharmacist must check all DUR messages.

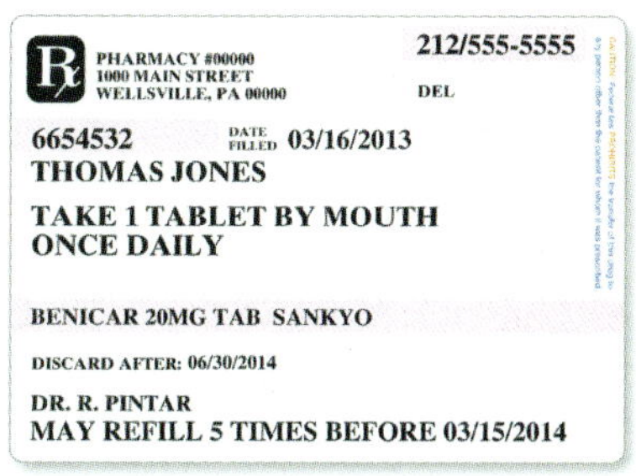
℞ PHARMACY #00000
1000 MAIN STREET
WELLSVILLE, PA 00000
212/555-5555
DEL
6654532 DATE FILLED 03/16/2013
THOMAS JONES
TAKE 1 TABLET BY MOUTH
ONCE DAILY
BENICAR 20MG TAB SANKYO
DISCARD AFTER: 06/30/2014
DR. R. PINTAR
MAY REFILL 5 TIMES BEFORE 03/15/2014

6 The label is generated.

Once the prescription and third-party billing is confirmed, the computer prints the label and receipt. The receipt includes co-payment and/or coinsurance information.

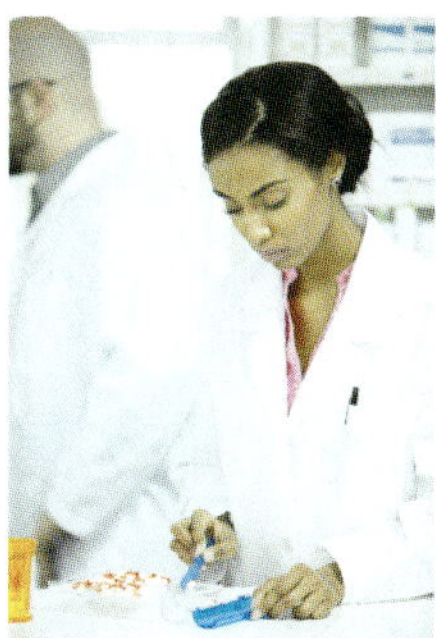

7 The prescription is prepared.

The technician selects the correct product, measures the prescribed amount, places it into a suitable container, and attaches the label. Child-proof containers are required by law unless the patient has on file a request for easy-open caps.

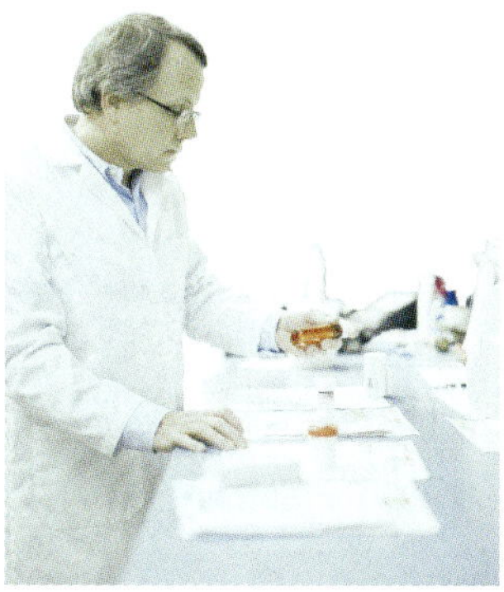

8 The pharmacist checks the prescription.

The pharmacist performs a final check to make sure the prescription is prepared as prescribed and performs a final evaluation for potential clinical issues.

PHARMACY ABBREVIATIONS

Pharmacy abbreviations are often based on Latin words and use Roman numerals for numbers. The prescription *Signa,* or Sig, uses abbreviations to communicate essential information such as the dosage form, dosage regimen (i.e., timing of administration), and route of administration.

COMMON ABBREVIATIONS

	Abbreviation	Meaning	Abbreviation	Meaning
Route of Administration	a.d.	right ear	p.r.	rectally, into the rectum
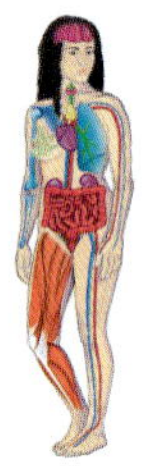	a.s., a.l.	left ear	p.v.	vaginally, into the vagina
	a.u.	each ear	inh	inhalation, inhale
	o.d.	right eye	per neb	by nebulizer
	o.s., o.l.	left eye	SC, subc, subq	subcutaneous
	o.u.	each eye	i.m., IM	intramuscular
	p.o.	by mouth	i.v., IV	intravenous
	S.L.	sublingually, under the tongue	i.v.p., IVP	intravenous push
	top.	topically, locally	IVPB	intravenous piggyback
Dosage Form	tab.	tablet	syr.	syrup
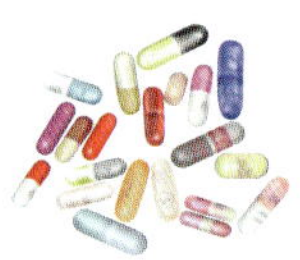	cap	capsule	liq.	liquid
	SR, XR, XL	slow/extended release	supp.	suppository
	sol	solution	crm	cream
	susp	suspension	ung., oint	ointment
Timing of Administration	bid	twice a day	prn	as needed
	tid	three times a day	a.c.	before food, before meals
	qid	four times a day	p.c.	after food, after meals
	a.m./q a.m.	morning/each morning	stat.	immediately, now
	p.m.	afternoon or evening	q__h	every__ hour(s)
	h.s.	at bedtime		
Measurement	i, ii	one, two, etc.	mcg., μg	microgram
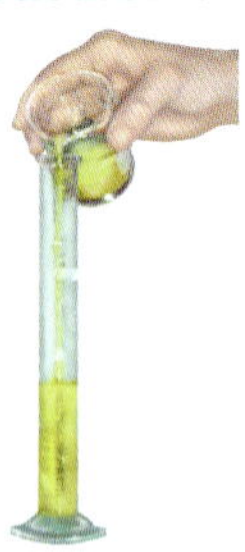	ss	one-half	mg.	milligram
	gtt.	drop	g., G., gm.	gram
	ml., mL	milliliter, millilitre	mEq.	milliequivalent
	tsp.	teaspoon (= 5 mL)	a.a. or aa	of each
	tbsp.	tablespoon (= 15 ml)	ad	to, up to
	fl. oz.	fluid ounce (= 30 mL)	aq. ad	add water up to
	l, L	liter/Litre	qs, q.s. ad	add sufficient quantity to make
Other	UTD	as directed	c̄, w/	with
	NR, ø	no refill	s̄, w/o	without
	DAW	dispense as written		

Note that some prescribers will leave out periods in written abbreviations and that some may use capital letters. Also see the Rx Safety note at right regarding other abbreviations that should not be used.

Signa From the Latin word *signa* meaning "to write." It is abbreviated to Sig or S (or left out entirely). It indicates the directions for use and the administration route.

tip

R_x is an abbreviation of the Latin word *recipe*, which means take. Today it is commonly associated with the word prescription.

LESS COMMON ABBREVIATIONS

Abbreviation	Meaning	Abbreviation	Meaning
aq, aqua	water	per g. button	by/through gastric button
BSA	body surface area	per n.g.t.	by/through naso-gastric tube
c.c.	cubic centimeter (1 cc $\simeq$ 1 ml)	Sig.	write, label
c.c.	with food; with meals	SOB	shortness of breath
D5W	Dextrose 5% in water	troche	lozenge
gr.	grain (1 gr $\simeq$ 65 mg)	tuss.	cough
NS	normal saline		

EXAMPLES

Drug	Rx	Label Directions
Synthroid® 100 mcg tablets	i tab po q a.m.	➥ Take one tablet by mouth once daily, in the morning
azithromycin 250 mg tablets	ii tabs po today, i tab po daily days 2—5	➥ Take two tablets by mouth today, then take one tablet once daily on days 2 through 5.
Alphagan-P® 0.1% eye drops	i gtt ou q8h	➥ Instill one drop into each eye every 8 hours.
Advair Diskus® 100/50	Inh i po BID	➥ Inhale the contents of one blister, by mouth, twice daily. [Rinse mouth after use.]—Optional.
Enbrel® 50 mg SC injection	inject 50 mg SC weekly	➥ Inject the contents of one syringe, subcutaneously, once weekly.*

** Check with your pharmacist—sometimes "as directed" is added for complex drug products such as injections.*

safety you should know

➥ To help prevent costly and potentially tragic medication errors, technicians must be alert throughout the prescription filling process to identify any possible prescribing or filling errors. For example, ask yourself, "Does the route of administration make sense for this drug? What about the dosage form and the timing of doses?" Never guess. Ask your supervising pharmacist if in doubt.

➥ While abbreviations are helpful, misinterpretations can be very dangerous. In the interests of safety, The Joint Commission has created a Do Not Use List of abbreviations, which can be downloaded from the Patient Safety Page at www.jointcommission.org/.

PRESCRIPTION INFORMATION

The written prescription has stringent requirements designed to inform the pharmacist and protect the patient.

Prescription regulations vary from state to state and province to province, but generally a prescription for a community pharmacy will contain the information illustrated below.

ELEMENTS OF THE PRESCRIPTION

Prescriber information: Name, title, office address, and telephone number.

Drug Enforcement Administration (DEA) prescriber registration number: A number assigned to the prescriber by the DEA that is required on all controlled substance prescriptions.

Name and address of patient: Other patient information such as date of birth is optional, but sometimes important, e.g., a child's weight

National Provider Identifier (NPI): The prescriber's unique national identification number, mandated by HIPAA and administered by the National Plan and Provider Enumeration System (NPPES).

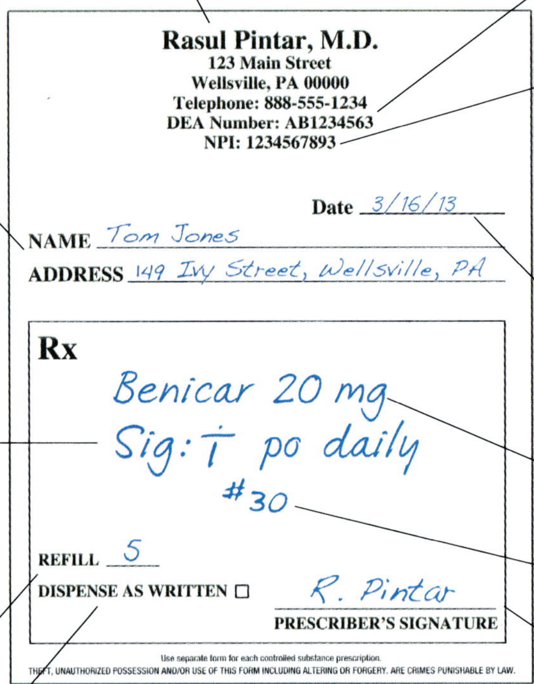

Rasul Pintar, M.D.
123 Main Street
Wellsville, PA 00000
Telephone: 888-555-1234
DEA Number: AB1234563
NPI: 1234567893

Date 3/16/13

NAME Tom Jones

ADDRESS 149 Ivy Street, Wellsville, PA

Rx

Benicar 20 mg
Sig: i po daily
#30

REFILL 5

DISPENSE AS WRITTEN ☐

R. Pintar
PRESCRIBER'S SIGNATURE

Use separate form for each controlled substance prescription.
THEFT, UNAUTHORIZED POSSESSION AND/OR USE OF THIS FORM INCLUDING ALTERING OR FORGERY ARE CRIMES PUNISHABLE BY LAW.

Date: The date the prescription was written.

Signa: The directions for use. Note: If a compound is prescribed, a list of ingredients and directions for mixing is also included.

Drug name and strength

Quantity

Refill instructions

Signature of prescriber: Required on written prescriptions.

***DAW*/PSC**: Dispense As Written/Product Select Code—generic substitution instructions (optional).

Additional Information

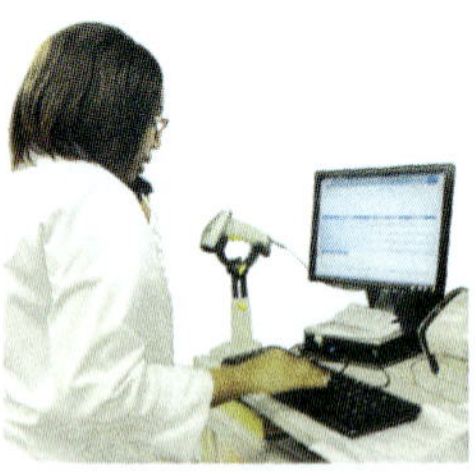

The information on the right must also be included with the prescription data. Some information is automatically assigned by the computer (e.g., prescription number), while other information, such as the product being dispensed, is added by the pharmacist or pharmacy technician. This information is stored in the computer and is printed out with the prescription label.

- Date the product is dispensed
- Identity of the product by manufacturer and NDC (National Drug Code)—DIN (Drug Identification Number) in Canada
- Prescription origin code (e.g., written, electronic)
- Prescription and/or transaction number
- Insurance information for the patient
- Price charged
- Initials of the technician and pharmacist involved in the filling of the prescription

DAW (Dispense as Written) a code specifying that the brand name drug, rather than its generic equivalent, is to be dispensed.

Schedule II drugs drugs that have a high potential for abuse or addiction but that also have safe and accepted medical uses; they require special handling.

PRESCRIPTION INFORMATION SAFETY CHECKLIST

Consider these Factors	Take this Action
Is the patient's full name clearly written on the prescription? Has a nickname or initial been used?	✔ **Determine the exact name** so that multiple files are not created for one patient and to ensure the prescription is assigned to the correct patient.
Is the patient's date of birth, street address, telephone number, insurance information, preference for brand or generic drugs, and allergy information already on file in the pharmacy?	✔ **Always confirm the information on file is current.** Record the patient's date of birth on the prescription to use as a double check when filling the prescription.
Is the medication for an over-the-counter product that the patient can receive without a prescription?	✔ **Check with the pharmacist on all OTC prescriptions.** Only the pharmacist should recommend an OTC medicine or determine which OTC medicine is requested on the prescription.
Is the prescription for a *Schedule II drug*? Schedule II drugs have a high potential for abuse and are subject to special prescription requirements (e.g., tamper-proof prescription blanks and short expiration dates).	✔ **Check with the pharmacist on all Schedule II prescriptions.** Complete Schedule II perpetual inventory log, as appropriate.
When was the prescription written? How many days or weeks has it been since it was written?	✔ **Check with the pharmacist to determine if the prescription can be filled if it is more than a few days old.** Some prescriptions may be valid for months, but others must be verified if they are more than a few days old.
Is the drug available in the quantity written? Does it require compounding?	✔ **Inform the patient if there may be a delay in filling the prescription.**
Is the prescription suspicious in any way? Is it written on a legitimate prescription blank and all in the same hand writing and with the same ink? Are there any signs of alteration of quantities, strength, or the name of the drug? Is this a drug with the potential for abuse and if so do the quantities and directions seem appropriate?	✔ **Alert the pharmacist to any potential forgeries.** Let the pharmacist follow through with the patient, the prescriber, and law enforcement, if necessary.

THE FILL PROCESS

Once prescription information is finalized in the computerized prescription system, a label and receipt are printed out.

At this point, the correct medication must be selected from pharmacy stock and the prescribed amount measured or counted and packaged. If the prescription calls for a compounded product, the technician must follow pharmacy policy in its preparation.

The pharmacy technician completes the fill process by placing the correct amount of medication into an appropriate container and labeling it correctly.

This includes placing the computer-generated label on the container so it sticks firmly, is straight, and is easy to read and placing the appropriate auxiliary labels on the container (see page 107). In addition, some medications such as oral contraceptives require Patient Package Inserts (PPI). Medication Guides (MedGuides) may also be provided voluntarily by some manufacturers. Both PPIs and MedGuides provide information on how to safely use medications and are part of FDA-approved labeling.

A pharmacist must check the final product and its label.

When finished with preparation, the technician initials the pharmacy copy of the label and organizes the finished product, prescription order, and the stock bottle that the medication was taken from for the pharmacist to check. The pharmacist signs off on the prescription via computer or by initialing the pharmacy copy of the label information, indicating the prescription was correctly filled. At this point the prescription may be released to the patient.

℞ safety you should know: common errors

Being aware that serious medication errors can happen is the first step in preventing them. Medication errors include, but are not limited to, dispensing:

- ✔ the wrong medication
- ✔ the wrong strength, dosage form, or quantity
- ✔ the wrong directions
- ✔ the medication to the wrong patient
- ✔ a medication on a forged or altered prescription

ISMP, The Institute for Safe Medication Practices, is an excellent resource for drug safety information. Visit www.ismp.org for a list of commonly confused drug names and more.

SAFETY CONSIDERATIONS

The technician should consider these factors when filling prescriptions:

Is the prescription for a high-alert medication?
High-alert medications are medications that are known to cause significant harm to the patient if an error is made. Examples of high-alert medications can be found online at http://www.ismp.org/tools/highalertmedications.pdf.

Are the instructions logical?
Are the directions, quantity, and strength typical for this medication? For example, is the dosing schedule q pm or prn? Does the Sig. read: 4 ml or .4 ml?

Are the directions clear?
Are the directions clearly translated in an unambiguously, avoiding any misinterpretation by the patient? For example, does "Take two tablets daily" mean "Take one tablet twice daily" or "Take two tablets once daily"?

Are there look-alike names?
Are there any look-alike drug names that could be confused with the intended medication? For example, did the prescriber write Janumet® or Sinemet®; Zovirax® or Zyvox®?

Pay attention to warnings!
When a DUR warning screen appears, such as a high-alert medication, a high-dose alert, or a drug interaction, the pharmacist must be notified as per pharmacy's rules—some pharmacies allow warnings to be printed for review with the final check, while others require immediate pharmacist review.

Check against the original!
During the fill process, always refer to the original prescription first and then refer to the label.

Don't add information!
Never add information based on what you assume the prescriber meant.

Rx tip

A number of drugs have moved from prescription-only to over-the-counter status. Many insurance companies have responded by agreeing to pay for select OTC medications with a valid prescription. Examples of over-the-counter medications that were previously available by prescription only are: Allegra®, Prevacid OTC®, and Zaditor® eye drops.

THE PHARMACY TECHNICIAN'S ROLE

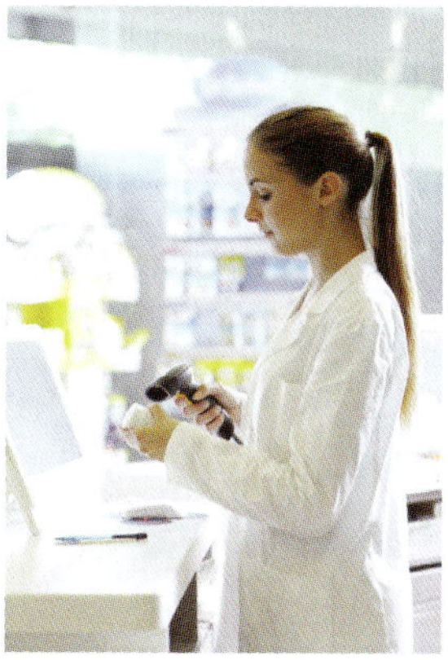

The pharmacy technician's responsibilities include:

- ✔ assisting the pharmacist in routine, technical aspects of prescription filling
- ✔ treating each patient, their personal information, and their medications with respect
- ✔ accepting new prescriptions from patients, obtaining all necessary information, and keying it into the computer in an efficient, and accurate manner
- ✔ alerting the pharmacist whenever a DUR warning screen appears while filling a prescription
- ✔ faxing or telephoning refill and clarification requests to prescribers
- ✔ consulting formularies and responding appropriately to third-party adjudication messaging such as: non-preferred drug, prior authorization or step-edit required
- ✔ quickly locating the correct medication for dispensing, calculating quantities, repackaging medication, and locating the corresponding patient medication guide
- ✔ compounding a prescription under supervision
- ✔ recording the dispensing of controlled drugs
- ✔ checking the work of other technicians, as instructed by a pharmacist
- ✔ referring patients to a pharmacist for counseling on the use of prescription and over-the-counter medications, or any other question requiring judgement
- ✔ ALWAYS ensuring the accuracy and safety of the prescription by incorporating quality control checks into every step in the process

THE PHARMACIST'S ROLE

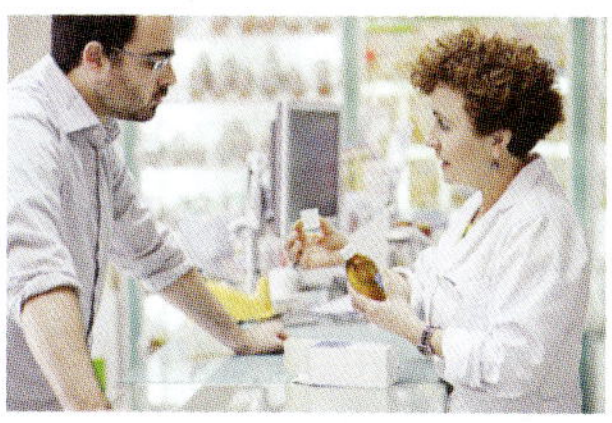

Photo courtesy catalina mas sebastian/ E+/Getty Images

The pharmacist uses his/her expertise to ensure physicians' orders are carried out accurately and safely by checking that:

- ✔ the correct medication, strength, and dosage form is dispensed to the correct patient
- ✔ the directions for the patient are clear, accurate, and unambiguous
- ✔ the patient knows how to take the medication and how and when to refill it
- ✔ there are no potential problems with drug allergies, drug-drug, or drug-disease interactions. Information from DUR warnings are essential to this process.
- ✔ the patient understands the expected beneficial effects of the medication and any potential side effects the patient should be aware of
- ✔ the prescriber has been contacted regarding the prescription if appropriate
- ✔ the prescription has been accurately billed to the patient and/or the appropriate third party

In addition:

- ✔ only a pharmacist may counsel patients on the use of OTC medications
- ✔ only a pharmacist may receive telephone requests for new prescriptions

LABELS

The prescription label provides information for the patient regarding the dispensed medication and how to take it.

The label also includes information about the pharmacy, the patient, the prescriber, as well as the prescription or transaction number. Requirements for prescription labels vary from state to state (and in Canada from province to province). Generally, however, a prescription label contains the information indicated below.

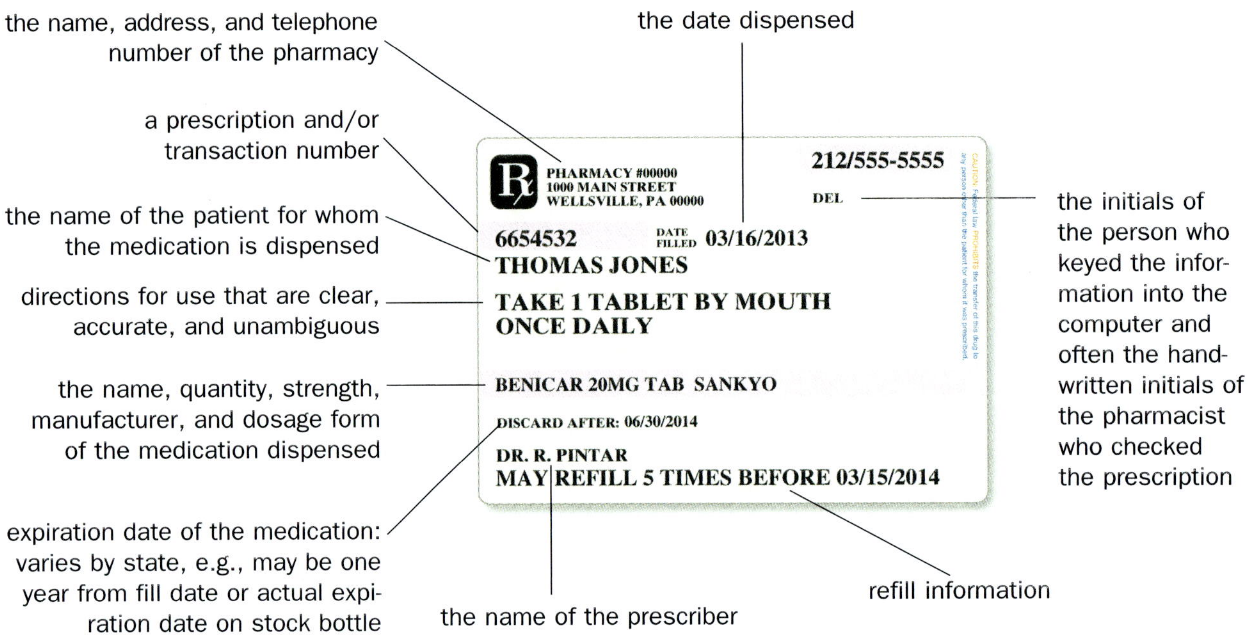

DIRECTIONS FOR USE

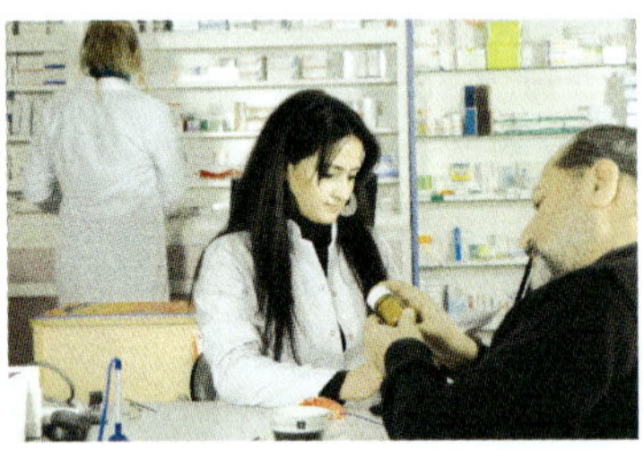

- ✔ **Directions should start with a verb** (take, instill, inhale, insert, apply) **and completely, clearly, and accurately describe the administration of the medication.**
- ✔ **Indicate the route of administration.** For example, "take one capsule by mouth," "apply to affected area," "insert rectally," "place one tablet under the tongue," etc.
- ✔ **Use whole words, not abbreviations.** For example, use "tablets" not "tabs."
- ✔ **Use familiar words, especially in measurements.** For example, use "two teaspoonfuls" or "10 ml" as most measuring droppers and spoons are calibrated in teaspoons and ml. Double check that the units listed on the label match the units on the measuring spoon or dropper supplied.

safety you should know

Tall man lettering has been encouraged by the FDA, ISMP and TJC to help distinguish soundalike, look-alike drugs from one another and avoid medication errors. The distinguishing part of the drug's name is printed in upper case letters (e.g., hydrALAZINE vs. hydrOXYzine).

AUXILIARY LABELS

Colored auxiliary labels may be applied to the prescription container to provide additional information to the patient (e.g., Shake Well, Keep Refrigerated, Take With Food or Milk). Many computerized prescription systems will automatically print out the appropriate labels to use.

For many drugs, the timing of the dose is almost as important as taking the dose. For example, taking with food or milk enhances the absorption of some drugs but greatly diminishes the effectiveness of others.

Prescriptions for controlled substances from Schedules II, III and IV must carry the following warning, which is preprinted on the label: *Caution: Federal law prohibits the transfer of this drug to any person other than the patient for whom it was prescribed.*

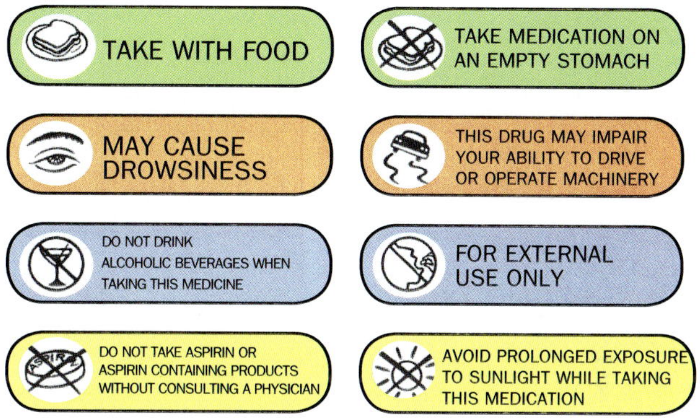

PLACING THE LABEL

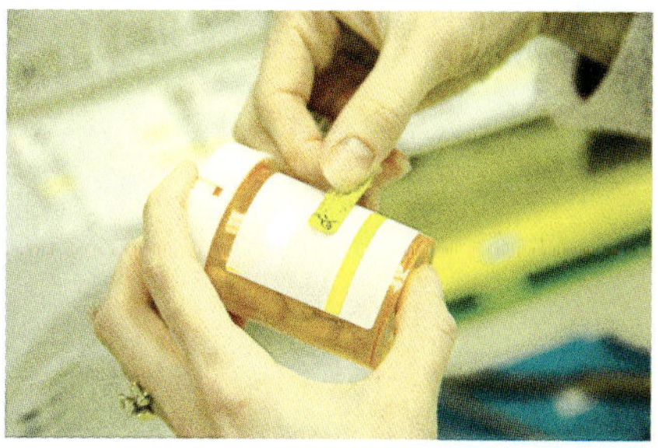

Labeling the container correctly includes:

- ✔ placing the computer-generated label on the container so it is parallel to the edges of the container, easy to locate, and easy to read
- ✔ making sure the label sticks adequately to the container without creases. (Some pharmacies place transparent tape over the label to protect the label from spills or accidental smudging.)
- ✔ placing the appropriate auxiliary labels on the container
- ✔ placing labels on prescription vials containing eye drops, ear drops and eye ointments
- ✔ in some states, placing the label on the actual container rather than the box in which it is packaged

UNIT DOSE LABELS

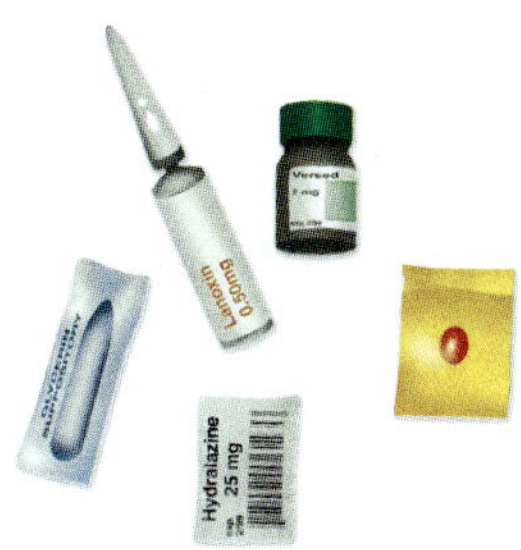

Unit dose packaging is widely used in institutional pharmacy. Although rules for institutional pharmacy prescription labels vary by institution, they often contain only the name, strength, manufacturer, lot number, expiration date, and dosage form of the medication. Since the condition of a patient in an institutional setting may change relatively quickly, patient medication orders are regularly updated. As a result, the nursing staff refer to the most recent physician's instructions in the patient's chart to verify prescribing information.

EXAMPLES

PRESCRIPTION TO LABEL

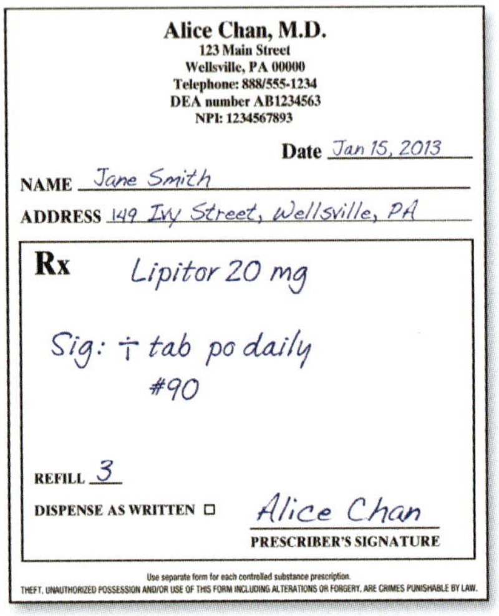
Alice Chan, M.D.
123 Main Street
Wellsville, PA 00000
Telephone: 888/555-1234
DEA number AB1234563
NPI: 1234567893

Date Jan 15, 2013

NAME Jane Smith

ADDRESS 149 Ivy Street, Wellsville, PA

Rx Lipitor 20 mg

Sig: i tab po daily
#90

REFILL 3

DISPENSE AS WRITTEN ☐ Alice Chan
PRESCRIBER'S SIGNATURE

Use separate form for each controlled substance prescription.
THEFT, UNAUTHORIZED POSSESSION AND/OR USE OF THIS FORM INCLUDING ALTERATIONS OR FORGERY, ARE CRIMES PUNISHABLE BY LAW.

- Lipitor® is a brand name for atorvastatin.
- 20 mg is the strength.
- Sig means "the directions are..."
- i tab means "take one tablet."
- p.o. means "by mouth."
- daily means "daily" or "once daily.""
- # 90 means a "quantity of 90."
- There are 3 refills.
- Generic substitution may be used.

Therefore, the prescription is for a 90 day supply of atorvastatin 20 mg tablets: 90 tablets, one tablet to be taken each day.

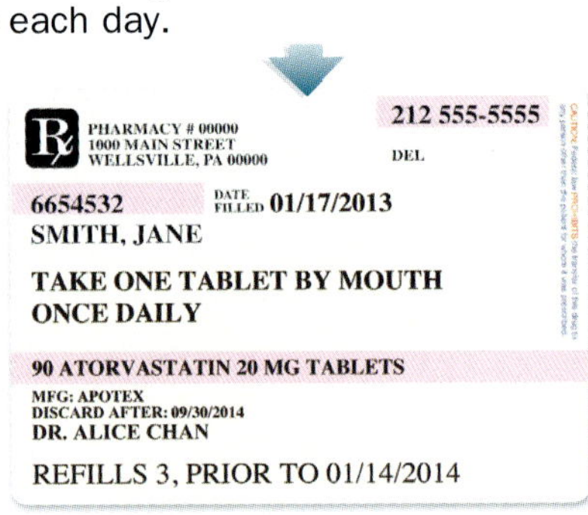
PHARMACY # 00000
1000 MAIN STREET
WELLSVILLE, PA 00000
212 555-5555
DEL
6654532 DATE FILLED 01/17/2013
SMITH, JANE
TAKE ONE TABLET BY MOUTH
ONCE DAILY
90 ATORVASTATIN 20 MG TABLETS
MFG: APOTEX
DISCARD AFTER: 09/30/2014
DR. ALICE CHAN
REFILLS 3, PRIOR TO 01/14/2014

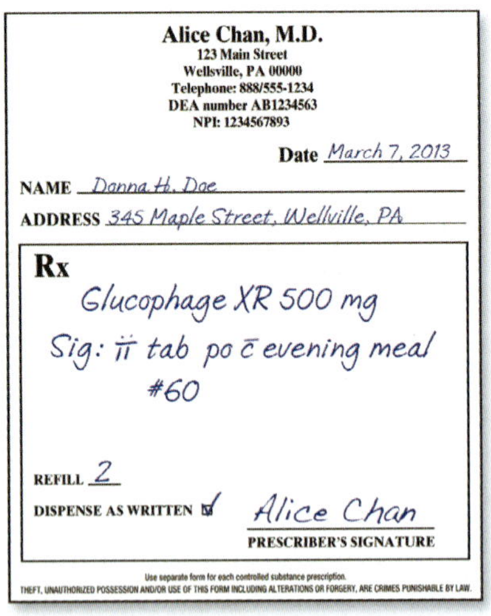
Alice Chan, M.D.
123 Main Street
Wellsville, PA 00000
Telephone: 888/555-1234
DEA number AB1234563
NPI: 1234567893

Date March 7, 2013

NAME Donna H. Doe

ADDRESS 345 Maple Street, Wellville, PA

Rx Glucophage XR 500 mg

Sig: ii tab po $\overline{c}$ evening meal
#60

REFILL 2

DISPENSE AS WRITTEN ☑ Alice Chan
PRESCRIBER'S SIGNATURE

Use separate form for each controlled substance prescription.
THEFT, UNAUTHORIZED POSSESSION AND/OR USE OF THIS FORM INCLUDING ALTERATIONS OR FORGERY, ARE CRIMES PUNISHABLE BY LAW.

- The drug is Glucophage XR®.
- 500 mg is the strength.
- ii tab means "take two tablets."
- p.o. means "by mouth."
- $\overline{c}$ evening meal means to take with supper.
- # 60 means a "quantity of 60."
- There are 2 refills.
- Dispense as written: generic substitution not allowed.

Therefore, the prescription is for a 30 day supply of Glucophage XR® 500 mg tablets, two tablets to be taken together each day with the evening meal.

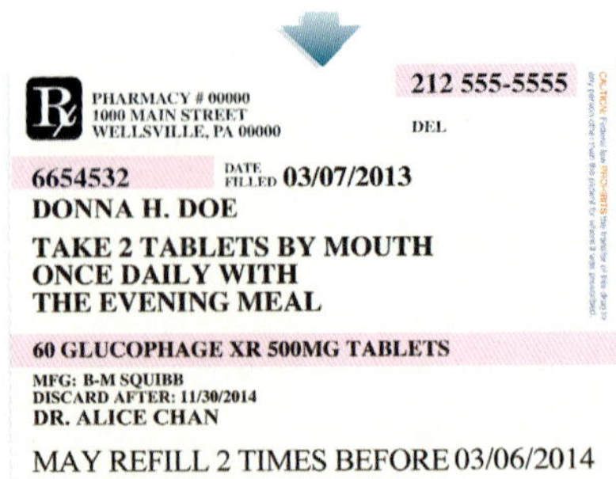
PHARMACY # 00000
1000 MAIN STREET
WELLSVILLE, PA 00000
212 555-5555
DEL
6654532 DATE FILLED 03/07/2013
DONNA H. DOE
TAKE 2 TABLETS BY MOUTH
ONCE DAILY WITH
THE EVENING MEAL
60 GLUCOPHAGE XR 500MG TABLETS
MFG: B-M SQUIBB
DISCARD AFTER: 11/30/2014
DR. ALICE CHAN
MAY REFILL 2 TIMES BEFORE 03/06/2014

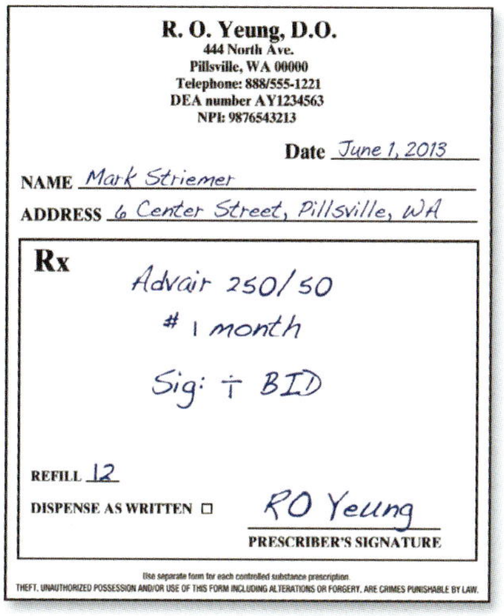
R. O. Yeung, D.O.
444 North Ave.
Pillsville, WA 00000
Telephone: 888/555-1221
DEA number AY1234563
NPI: 9876543213

Date June 1, 2013

NAME Mark Striemer

ADDRESS 6 Center Street, Pillsville, WA

Rx
Advair 250/50
1 month
Sig: i BID

REFILL 12

DISPENSE AS WRITTEN ☐ RO Yeung
PRESCRIBER'S SIGNATURE

Use separate form for each controlled substance prescription.
THEFT, UNAUTHORIZED POSSESSION AND/OR USE OF THIS FORM INCLUDING ALTERATIONS OR FORGERY, ARE CRIMES PUNISHABLE BY LAW.

- The drug is Advair® Diskus Inhaler.
- It is a combination of two drugs and the strength is 250 mcg of one ingredient and 50 mcg of the other.
- #1 month means "dispense a one month supply."
- i BID means "inhale the contents of one blister twice daily."

Note: There are 60 "blisters" in the diskus. Each blister is punctured just before use and the contents are inhaled.

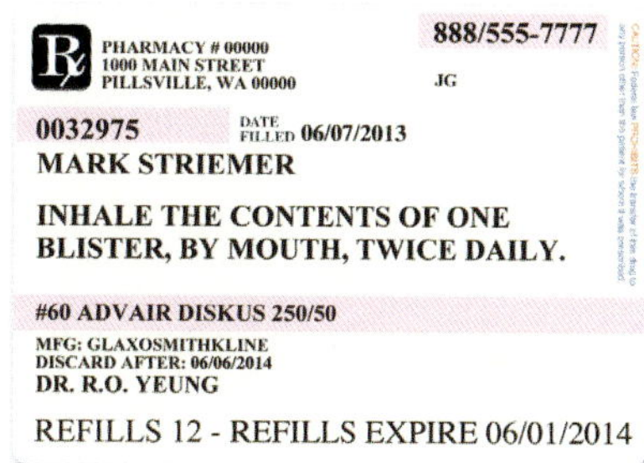
PHARMACY # 00000
1000 MAIN STREET
PILLSVILLE, WA 00000
888/555-7777
JG
0032975 DATE FILLED 06/07/2013
MARK STRIEMER
INHALE THE CONTENTS OF ONE BLISTER, BY MOUTH, TWICE DAILY.
#60 ADVAIR DISKUS 250/50
MFG: GLAXOSMITHKLINE
DISCARD AFTER: 06/06/2014
DR. R.O. YEUNG
REFILLS 12 - REFILLS EXPIRE 06/01/2014

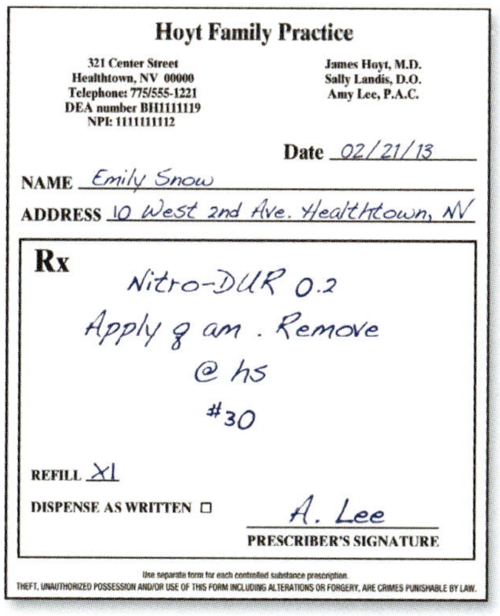
Hoyt Family Practice
321 Center Street
Healthtown, NV 00000
Telephone: 775/555-1221
DEA number BH1111119
NPI: 1111111112

James Hoyt, M.D.
Sally Landis, D.O.
Amy Lee, P.A.C.

Date 02/21/13

NAME Emily Snow

ADDRESS 10 West 2nd Ave. Healthtown, NV

Rx
Nitro-DUR 0.2
Apply q am. Remove
@ hs
#30

REFILL X1

DISPENSE AS WRITTEN ☐ A. Lee
PRESCRIBER'S SIGNATURE

Use separate form for each controlled substance prescription.
THEFT, UNAUTHORIZED POSSESSION AND/OR USE OF THIS FORM INCLUDING ALTERATIONS OR FORGERY, ARE CRIMES PUNISHABLE BY LAW.

- The drug is Nitro-DUR® Transdermal Patches.
- The strength is 0.2 mg/h.
- The directions are to apply one patch in the morning, and to remove the patch at bedtime.
- # 30 means a "quantity of 30."
- There is one refill.

Note: "As directed" is added to the label to encourage the patient to ask for more information if they are unclear about how to apply the patch.

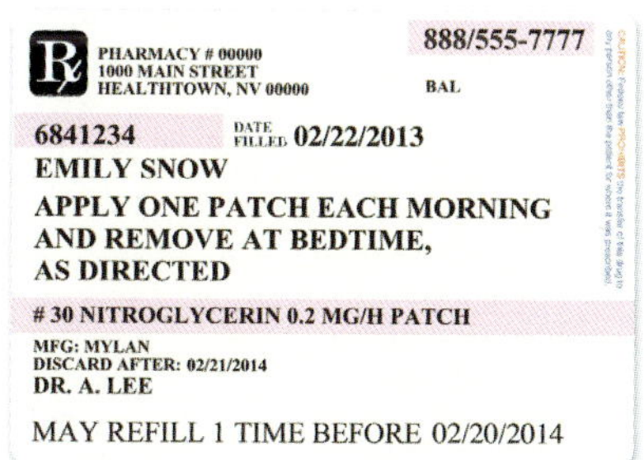
PHARMACY # 00000
1000 MAIN STREET
HEALTHTOWN, NV 00000
888/555-7777
BAL
6841234 DATE FILLED 02/22/2013
EMILY SNOW
APPLY ONE PATCH EACH MORNING AND REMOVE AT BEDTIME, AS DIRECTED
30 NITROGLYCERIN 0.2 MG/H PATCH
MFG: MYLAN
DISCARD AFTER: 02/21/2014
DR. A. LEE
MAY REFILL 1 TIME BEFORE 02/20/2014

EXAMPLES (cont'd)

MEDICATION ORDERS

There are various formats used for medication orders in institutional settings. Some common aspects of the medication order are:

- patient identification information (name, ID#, date of birth)
- patient allergy information
- patient location (room and bed number)
- multiple orders are written on one sheet
- date and time of day are indicated, with the most recent entry listed last
- orders are often read from the bottom up so as to read the most recent information first
- orders may also include requests for lab work, physical therapy, or drug items stocked in the nursing station

These and other aspects of medication orders reflect the special characteristics of the institutional environment.

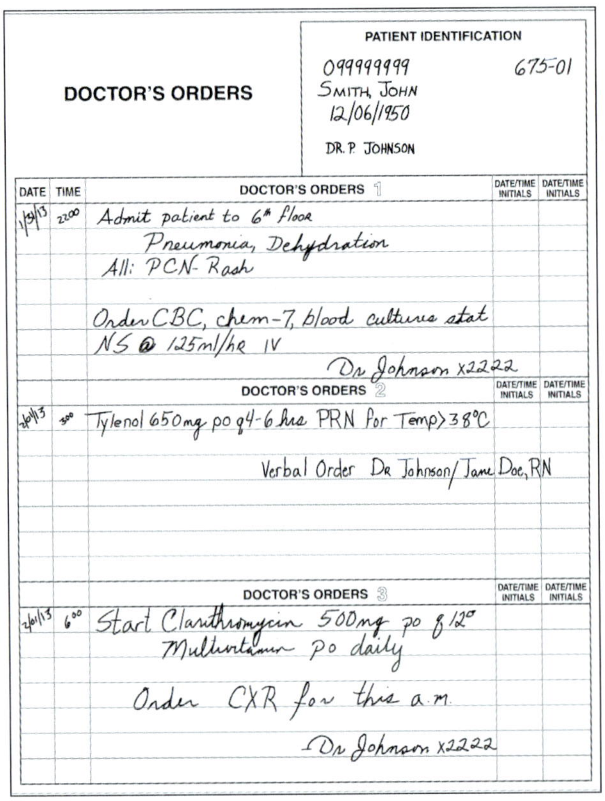

DOCTOR'S ORDERS

PATIENT IDENTIFICATION
099999999 675-01
SMITH, JOHN
12/06/1950
DR. P. JOHNSON

DATE	TIME	DOCTOR'S ORDERS 1	DATE/TIME INITIALS	DATE/TIME INITIALS
1/31/13	2200	Admit patient to 6th floor		
		Pneumonia, Dehydration		
		All: PCN- Rash		
		Order CBC, chem-7, blood cultures stat		
		NS @ 125ml/hr IV		
		Dr Johnson x2222		

DATE	TIME	DOCTOR'S ORDERS 2	DATE/TIME INITIALS	DATE/TIME INITIALS
2/1/13	300	Tylenol 650mg po q4-6 hrs PRN for Temp>38°C		
		Verbal Order Dr Johnson/Jane Doe, RN		

DATE	TIME	DOCTOR'S ORDERS 3	DATE/TIME INITIALS	DATE/TIME INITIALS
2/1/13	600	Start Clarithromycin 500mg po q12°		
		Multivitamin po daily		
		Order CXR for this a.m.		
		Dr Johnson x2222		

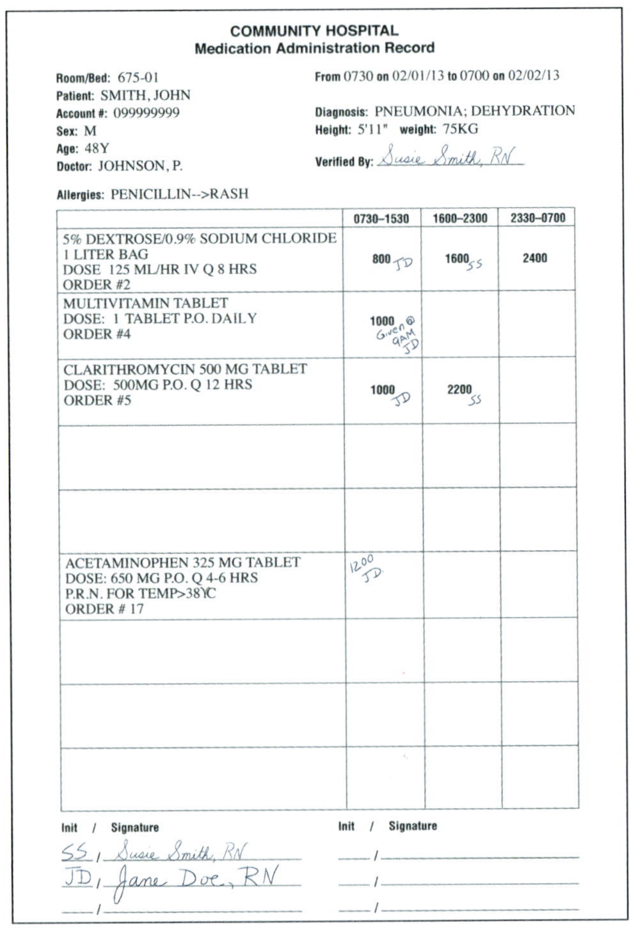

COMMUNITY HOSPITAL
Medication Administration Record

Room/Bed: 675-01
Patient: SMITH, JOHN
Account #: 099999999
Sex: M
Age: 48Y
Doctor: JOHNSON, P.

From 0730 on 02/01/13 to 0700 on 02/02/13
Diagnosis: PNEUMONIA; DEHYDRATION
Height: 5'11" weight: 75KG
Verified By: Susie Smith, RN

Allergies: PENICILLIN-->RASH

	0730–1530	1600–2300	2330–0700
5% DEXTROSE/0.9% SODIUM CHLORIDE 1 LITER BAG DOSE 125 ML/HR IV Q 8 HRS ORDER #2	800 JD	1600 SS	2400
MULTIVITAMIN TABLET DOSE: 1 TABLET P.O. DAILY ORDER #4	1000 Given @ 9AM JD		
CLARITHROMYCIN 500 MG TABLET DOSE: 500MG P.O. Q 12 HRS ORDER #5	1000 JD	2200 SS	
ACETAMINOPHEN 325 MG TABLET DOSE: 650 MG P.O. Q 4-6 HRS P.R.N. FOR TEMP>38°C ORDER # 17	1200 JD		

Init / Signature	Init / Signature
SS / Susie Smith, RN	/
JD / Jane Doe, RN	/
/	/

tip

There are rules for written information on institutional documents. For example, red ink may be required for information such as patient allergies.

HIPAA

HIPAA: The Health Insurance Portability and Accountability Act

The ***Health Insurance Portability and Accountability Act (HIPAA)*** of 1996 has wide reaching consequences for health-care professionals. HIPAA is a large statute that primarily concerns the continuation of health insurance coverage for workers who leave their jobs. However, there are a number of regulations that all health-care providers ("covered entities"), including pharmacies, must follow.

HIPAA requires the use of a National Provider Identifier (NPI) for all health-care providers. The NPI is a ten-digit number, with a check digit in the last position to help detect keying errors. Each provider may receive only one unique NPI, which is expected to stay with that provider for life. HIPAA mandates that all covered entities, such as health plans, physicians, and pharmacies, must use their NPI for all standard transactions covered by HIPAA.

Rules also have been established to regulate how and when pharmacies and other covered entities may use and disclose a patient's ***protected health information (PHI)***. Other rules require administrative, physical, and technical safeguards to prevent illicit access to patient information while it is stored or transmitted electronically. Examples of PHI are the patient's name and address, date of birth, Social Security number, payment history, account number, and medical/prescription drug histories.

Under HIPAA, pharmacies and other covered entities are required to provide a written notice of their privacy practices to their patients. This notice must describe the pharmacy's privacy procedures and patients' privacy rights, and must describe how the pharmacy intends to use and disclose patients' PHI. Each pharmacy must make a good faith effort to have every patient sign an "acknowledgement" that the patient has received its notice of privacy practices. This acknowledgement may be signed when the patient picks up his or her medication. The acknowledgement must be maintained separately from the consultation log that all patients sign when picking up their medication. Acknowledgement signatures must remain on file for six years from the last date of service to the patient.

HIPAA also states that a pharmacy may disclose PHI, without patient approval, to business associates that perform services on behalf of the patient. Examples of such business associates would be physicians' offices and pharmacy benefits management (prescription insurance) companies. However, these disclosures must follow the "minimum necessary" requirement, which means that covered entities may use, disclose and request only the minimum necessary amount of PHI to other covered entities.

All personnel who have access to PHI must be formally trained regarding HIPAA on an annual basis. This includes pharmacists, pharmacy technicians, pharmacy clerks, and any other employee who may come into contact with PHI. Even the computer specialists who come to the pharmacy to service computers must be HIPAA trained and HIPAA compliant.

Health Insurance Portability and Accountability Act (HIPAA) a federal act that protects the privacy of individuals and the sharing of protected health information.

protected health information (PHI) any personal information that could be used to identify an individual or their health history.

REVIEW

KEY CONCEPTS

PRESCRIPTIONS

- ✔ A prescription is a written or verbal order from a practitioner for the preparation and administration of a medicine or a device.
- ✔ Medical doctors (MD), doctors of osteopathy (DO), dentists (DDS), and veterinarians (DVM) are the primary practitioners who write prescriptions. Podiatrists and optometrists are also allowed to write prescriptions. All practitioners must write within the scope of their practice.
- ✔ In many states, nurse practitioners, physicians assistants and/or pharmacists are also allowed limited rights to prescribe medications.
- ✔ In community pharmacies, pharmacy technicians generally receive the prescription, collect patient data (correct spelling of name, address, allergy, and insurance information, etc.) and enter it into a computerized prescription system.

PRESCRIPTION INFORMATION

- ✔ The pharmacist should be consulted on all OTC and Schedule II prescriptions.
- ✔ The prescription is entered into the computer and drug-drug, drug-disease, and drug-allergy information is automatically checked by the pharmacy software. If third-party billing is involved, this is done online simultaneously.

THE FILL PROCESS

- ✔ Once the prescription and third-party billing is confirmed by the online computer system, the label and receipt are printed and the prescription is prepared.
- ✔ Since the patient is expected to self-administer the medication, the label's directions for use must be clear, unambiguous, and concise.
- ✔ Pharmacists must provide counseling to patients on all new prescriptions and on any refilled prescriptions where clarification is required. A patient may refuse counseling.
- ✔ In institutional settings, nursing staff generally administer medications to patients.
- ✔ Technicians must request the advice of the pharmacist whenever judgment is required.

LABELS

- ✔ Many computerized prescription systems will automatically indicate which auxiliary labels to use with each drug.

HIPAA

- ✔ The Health Insurance Portability and Accountability Act (HIPAA) contains regulations related to privacy and protected health information (PHI).
- ✔ Examples of PHI are name and address, date of birth, Social Security number, payment history, account number, name and address of health-care provider and/or health plan, and medical or prescription history.
- ✔ Under HIPAA, pharmacies and other covered entities are required to provide a written notice of their privacy practices to their patients.
- ✔ A pharmacy may disclose PHI to business associates that perform services for the patient.
- ✔ All personnel who have access to PHI must be formally trained regarding HIPAA.

SELF TEST

the answer key begins on page 569

MATCH THE TERMS: I

1. DAW ____
2. extemporaneous compounding ____
3. HIPAA _____
4. OTC drugs ____
5. prescription ____
6. protected health information (PHI) _____
7. Schedule II drugs ____
8. Signa _____

a. an instruction from a medical practitioner that authorizes a patient to be issued a drug or device.
b. medications that do not require a prescription but may be filled with a prescription.
c. a federal act that protects the privacy of individuals and the sharing of protected health information.
d. mechanism by which a prescriber indicates that only the brand product, and not an equivalent generic, must be dispensed.
e. drugs that have been shown to be subject to abuse and require special handling.
f. the on-demand preparation of a drug product according to a physician's prescription, formula, or recipe.
g. any personal information that could be used to identify an individual or their health history.
h. the directions for use and route of administration to be printed on the prescription label.

MATCH THE TERMS: II

1. subcutaneously ____
2. drop ____
3. twice a day ____
4. right ear ____
5. four times a day ____
6. as needed ____
7. each eye ____
8. every morning _____
9. under the tongue ____
10. at bedtime ____
11. microgram ____
12. vaginally ____
13. immediately, now ____
14. every 12 hours ____
15. before food, before meals ____
16. by mouth ____

a. prn
b. gtt
c. ac
d. bid
e. hs
f. SL
g. stat
h. po
i. sc
j. qid
k. q 12h
l. ad
m. mcg, µg
n. pv
o. o.u.
p. q am

REVIEW

CHOOSE THE BEST ANSWER

1. Counseling, as required by OBRA '90, is provided by
   a. physicians.
   b. pharmacy technicians.
   c. pharmacists.
   d. nurses.

2. When the directions for a prescription are unclear, the pharmacy technician should
   a. fax the doctor for clarification.
   b. ask the pharmacist.
   c. ask the patient.
   d. do their best to fill the prescription without assistance.

3. The directions on a prescription medication are: i gtt ou hs. This medication is
   a. an eye drop.
   b. dosed twice a day.
   c. taken in the morning.
   d. used by injection.

4. For the prescription: Glucophage XR® 500 mg, ii BID x 90 days, how many tablets are dispensed?
   a. 90
   b. 180
   c. 360
   d. not enough information is given to fill the prescription.

5. The unique identifying number of a drug is the
   a. DEA.
   b. PHI.
   c. DAW.
   d. NDC.

6. For the prescription: Clarithromycin 500 mg #20 i po b.i.d., what is the Sig?
   a. i po b.i.d
   b. 500
   c. Clarithromycin 500 mg
   d. #20

7. A medication error may involve
   a. the wrong dosage form.
   b. the wrong directions.
   c. the wrong patient.
   d. all of the above.

8. The two drug names Accupril® 40 mg and Accutane® 40 mg exemplify
   a. Signa.
   b. extemporaneous compounding.
   c. look-alike names.
   d. OTC medications.

9. Which of the following may be performed only by a pharmacist?
   a. accepting a return call from a prescriber's office approving refills
   b. accepting a return call from a prescriber's office clarifying a prescription
   c. calling a prescriber's office on behalf of a patient to request refills
   d. calling an insurance company to verify a patient's eligibility

10. All of the following duties may be performed by a pharmacy technician except
    a. requesting PHI from a patient such as date of birth, address, allergy, and insurance information.
    b. selecting an OTC product for a patient.
    c. inputting and updating patient information in the computer.
    d. placing the medication in a vial and attaching the prescription label to it.

11. Directions for use should start with a/an
    a. adjective.
    b. verb.
    c. noun.
    d. adverb.

Questions 12 and 13 are based on this information from a prescription:

Cefzil® 125 mg/5 ml
Sig: i tsp bid x10d
qs

12. The medication should be taken
    a. twice daily.
    b. every 10 hours.
    c. three times daily.
    d. none of the above.

13. The amount of medication to be dispensed is:
    a. 100 ml.
    b. 150 ml.
    c. 250 ml.
    d. the amount of medication is not indicated.

14. For the prescription "methotrexate 2.5 mg tab vi po q week # 24," the day's supply is
    a. 28 days.
    b. 34 days.
    c. 42 days.
    d. 90 days.

15. What is the number of tablets to dispense for the following prescription?

    prednisone 5 mg tab
    Sig: 5 bid x 2 days, 4 bid x 2 days, 3 bid x 2 days, 2 bid x 2 days, 1 bid x 2 days, then stop
    qs

    a. 15.
    b. 30.
    c. 45.
    d. 60.

16. For the prescription "ProAir HFA® # 1, Sig: ii puff q 6h prn" there are 200 doses in one inhaler. The day's supply would be
    a. 15.
    b. 25.
    c. 30.
    d. 50.

17. The directions on a prescription read "1 tbsp QID, ac and hs." The quantity to be dispensed for a 30-day supply is
    a. 600 ml.
    b. 1,000 ml.
    c. 1,800 ml.
    d. 2,000 ml.

18. Medication orders in institutional settings may
    a. be administered by nursing staff.
    b. contain only one request per sheet.
    c. not be used in place of label directions for dosing information.
    d. all of the above.

REVIEW

19. All of the following are examples of PHI except the
    a. patient's insurance identification number.
    b. patient's address.
    c. pharmacy address.
    d. patient's date of birth.

20. All of the following pharmacy personnel must be formally trained regarding HIPAA except
    a. the pharmacist.
    b. the pharmacy technician.
    c. custodial personnel.
    d. none of the above.

CRITICAL THINKING QUESTIONS

1. Kyle, a pharmacy technician, answers the pharmacy telephone. The caller says she is Dr. Smith's nurse and is reviewing a refill request the pharmacy had faxed to her regarding a diabetes medication for Mr. Hoyt, a patient. The nurse would like to know when Mr. Hoyt last picked up his blood pressure medications. Is Kyle allowed to share this information with the nurse?

2. A new customer presents a prescription for a narcotic pain medication at Lemon Bay Pharmacy. Amy, a pharmacy technician, receives the prescription and, per pharmacy protocol, checks the patient's photo ID and records his address, allergy, and insurance information in the computer. As she is finishing, Amy notices the quantity on the prescription seems to have been changed from # 12 to # 120. What should Amy do?

3. Marie is entering a prescription order in the computer when a red warning screen appears with the following message: "Therapeutic Duplication—pravastatin 20 mg/simvastatin 20 mg." She prints the screen for the pharmacist to review and continues filling the prescription. Did she do the right thing?

THINKING IT THROUGH WRAP-UP

Jenna must not recommend a product to Mrs. Harris. Jenna should explain that she is not trained to provide advice on the use of over-the-counter products, but the pharmacist is. For example, the pharmacist would be able to consider potential interactions between cold medications and the patient's health history or with any other medications the patient may be taking. Jenna should add that the pharmacist would be happy to recommend a product and should offer to call the pharmacist over.

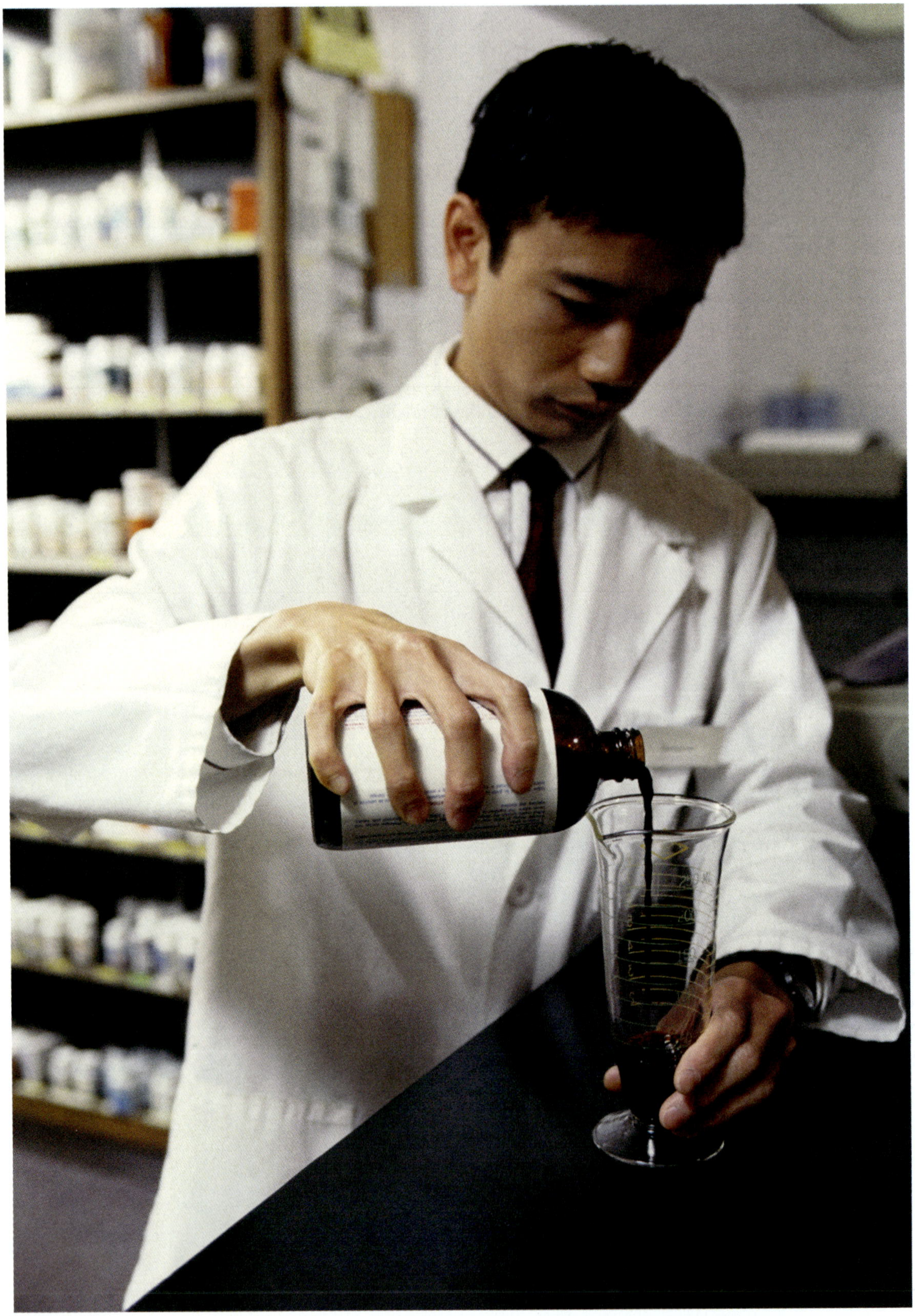

Photo courtesy Keith Brofsky/Photodisc/Getty Images

6

CALCULATIONS

LEARNING OBJECTIVES

At the completion of study, the student will:

- ✔ define numerator, denominator, and fractions.
- ✔ perform mathematical operations to solve problems with fractions.
- ✔ perform mathematical operations to solve problems with decimals and percents.
- ✔ describe measurement systems used in pharmacy.
- ✔ perform mathematical operations to solve problems that involve different units of measurement.
- ✔ use ratio and proportion to solve problems in pharmacy.
- ✔ use the alligation method to solve problems involving two different strengths of the same ingredient.
- ✔ use powder volume to solve problems with powders for reconstitution.
- ✔ describe considerations for children's doses of medications.
- ✔ perform basic calculations associated with the business aspect of pharmacy.

THINKING IT THROUGH

Michelle has worked as a pharmacy technician in a community pharmacy for five years and is now starting to work as a pharmacy technician in a hospital. She was confident in her skills for performing the necessary calculations in the community pharmacy, but she knows she will need to develop skills to solve different types of problems in the hospital.

As you read this chapter keep in mind the following questions:

1. What are some types of calculations commonly performed by pharmacy technicians in community pharmacies?
2. What types of calculations are commonly performed by pharmacy technicians in hospital pharmacies?
3. Why is accuracy in calculations important in both environments?

NUMBERS

The amount of a drug in its manufactured or prescribed form is always stated numerically—that is, with numbers.

Knowing how to work with numbers is essential to the proper handling of drugs and preparation of prescriptions. This involves understanding the different number forms, measurement units, and mathematical operations that are regularly used. In pharmacy we use two different number systems: Arabic (such as 1, 1/2, 0.5, or 50%) and Roman (such as I, V, X, L, C, D, or M). Most of the time we use Arabic numerals, although Roman numerals are often used to indicate quantities in prescription order writing.

Roman Numerals

Roman numerals are letters that represent numbers. They were originally developed and used by the Roman Empire. They can be capital or lowercase letters, and are:

ss = 1/2	L or l = 50
I or i = 1	C or c = 100
V or v = 5	D or d = 500
X or x = 10	M or m = 1,000

When grouped together, these few letters can express a large range of numbers, using a simple ***positional notation***. That means the position of the letters has a mathematical importance, as determined by these rules:

When the second of two letters has a value equal to or smaller than that of the first, add their values together.

Example—Converting Roman Numerals I

xxx = 30	or	10 plus 10 plus 10
dc = 600	or	500 plus 100
lxvi = 66	or	50 plus 10 plus 5 plus 1

When the second of two letters has a value greater than that of the first, subtract the smaller from the larger.

Example—Converting Roman Numerals II

ix = 9	or	1 subtracted from 10
xxxix = 39	or	30 plus (1 subtracted from 10)
xc = 90	or	10 subtracted from 100

Note: Answers for all the exercises in this chapter are included in the answer key, beginning on page 571.

—I V X L D C M—

PRACTICE PROBLEMS—ROMAN NUMERALS

Write the following in Roman numerals:

1. 18 ________
2. 64 ________
3. 72 ________
4. 126 ________
5. 100 ________
6. 7 ________
7. 28 ________

Write the following in Arabic numbers:

8. xxxiii ________
9. CX ________
10. mc ________
11. iss ________
12. XIX ________
13. xxiv ________

Interpret the quantity in each of these phrases taken from prescriptions:

14. Caps. no. xiv. ________
15. Gtts. ix. ________
16. Tabs. no. XLVIII. ________
17. Tabs. no. xxi ________

positional notation a system used in Roman numerals whereby the the position of the numeral signifies its mathematical value.

FRACTIONS

1/4

FRACTIONS

Fractions are commonly used in the Arabic system. A fraction is a numerical representation (such as 3/4, 5/8, 3.234) indicating a part of a whole. A fraction also represents the division of two numbers.

NUMERATORS AND DENOMINATORS

In a fraction, the ***denominator*** (number below the bar) tells us how many parts the whole is divided into, and the ***numerator*** (number above the bar) tells us how many of those parts exist.

The numerator can be zero, but the denominator cannot be zero. Division by zero is undefined, therefore no denominator can be zero.

One way to think of a fraction is as division that hasn't been completed.

Fractions can be used to indicate equal parts of a whole unit.

Example—Reading Fractions
We can read 2/5 as two-fifths, two over five or two divided by five.

Every fraction can be converted to a decimal by dividing. Using a calculator to divide 2 by 5:

2/5 = 0.4

Here are some other fractions and their decimal equivalents. Remember, you can find the decimal equivalent of any fraction by dividing.

1/8 = 0.125

1/2 = 0.5

3/4 = 0.75

denominator the bottom or right number in a fraction.
numerator the top or left number in a fraction.

RECIPROCALS

Reciprocals are two different fractions that equal 1 when multiplied together. Every fraction has a reciprocal (except those fractions with zero in the numerator). The easiest way to find the reciprocal of a fraction is to switch the numerator and denominator, or just turn the fraction over.

To find the reciprocal of a whole number, just put 1 over the whole number.

Example—Finding Reciprocals

The reciprocal of 2 is 1/2.

The reciprocal of 3 is 1/3.

The reciprocal of 4 is 1/4.

The reciprocal of 2/3 is 3/2.

PRACTICE PROBLEMS—NUMERATORS, DENOMINATORS, AND RECIPROCALS

Use a calculator to convert the following fractions to decimals:

1. 1/3 = ________
2. 1/2 = ________
3. 1/4 = ________
4. 3/10 = ________
5. 1/10 = ________

Determine the reciprocal of the following fractions:

6. 1/5 is ________
7. 2/3 is ________
8. 2/5 is ________
9. 2/9 is ________
10. 1/15 is ________

FRACTIONS (cont'd)

1/4

Adding and Subtracting Fractions

In order to add or subtract fractions the fractions must have the same denominator or common denominators. Addition and subtraction of like fractions is easy. To add or subtract like fractions just add or subtract the numerators and write the sum or difference over the common denominator.

To add or subtract fractions with different denominators, you must first find equivalent fractions with common denominators: First find the smallest multiple for the denominator of both numbers. Then rewrite the fractions as equivalent fractions with the smallest multiple of both numbers as the denominator. The smallest multiple of both numbers is called the *least common denominator*.

Example—1/3 + 3/5

The smallest multiple for the denominator of both numbers is 15:

$$1/3 = \frac{1 \times 5}{3 \times 5} = 5/15$$

$$3/5 = \frac{3 \times 3}{5 \times 3} = 9/15$$

The problem can now be rewritten:

$$5/15 + 9/15$$

Since the denominators are equal, we only have to add the numerators to get the answer:

$$\frac{5 + 9}{15} = 14/15$$

Practice Problems—Adding and Subtracting Fractions

Add or subtract the following fractions.

1. 1/4 + 1/4 = ________
2. 3/8 + 5/8 = ________
3. 2/5 - 1/5 = ________
4. 7/8 - 3/8 = ________
5. 2/5 + 3/5 = ________
6. 1/8 + 3/8 = ________
7. 1/4 + 1/5 = ________
8. 4/15 + 1/5 = ________
9. 1/4 + 3/16 = ________
10. 5/8 - 1/4 = ________

least common denominator smallest possible denominator for an equivalent fraction so that two fractions can be added or subtracted and have the same denominator.

tip

Multiplying fractions is frequently stated by using the word "of." If you must determine 1/2 of 10, you would multiply 1/2 X 10. 1/2 X 10 = 5.

MULTIPLYING AND DIVIDING FRACTIONS

To multiply fractions, first multiply the numerators of the fractions to get the new numerator. Then multiply the denominators of the fractions to get the new denominator.

Example—2/3 of 24

Multiply the numerators and denominators:

2/3 x 24/1 = 48/3

Reduce 48/3:

48/3 reduces to 16

To divide a number by a fraction multiply the number by the reciprocal of the fraction.

Example—24 ÷ 1/3

Find the reciprocal of the fraction:

The reciprocal of 1/3 is 3.

Multiply the number by the reciprocal of the fraction:

24 x 3 = 72

Example—1/3 ÷ 8

First, find the reciprocal of the fraction:

The reciprocal of 8 is 1/8.

Second, multiply the number by the reciprocal of the fraction:

1/3 x 1/8 = 1/24

PRACTICE PROBLEMS—MULTIPLYING AND DIVIDING FRACTIONS

Multiply the following fractions:

1. 1/4 of 1/4 = ________
2. 1/3 of 3/8 = ________
3. 2/3 of 1/3 = ________
4. 3/8 of 5/8 = ________

Divide the following fractions:

5. 1/3 divided by 1/2 = ________
6. 1/4 divided by 3/4 = ________
7. 2/5 divided by 1/5 = ________
8. 3/8 divided by 3/8 = ________

DECIMAL NUMBERS

0.1

Adding and Subtracting Decimals

To add decimal numbers, first put the numbers in a vertical column, aligning the decimal points. Then add each column of digits, starting on the right and working left. If the sum of a column is more than 10, "carry" digits to the next column on the left. Place the decimal point in the answer directly below the decimal points in the terms.

Example—Adding Decimals

Add 324.5678 to 1.2345

Step 1:

$$\begin{array}{r} 324.5678 \\ +\ 1.2345 \\ \hline 3 \end{array}$$ (carry the 1)

Step 2:

$$\begin{array}{r} 324.5678 \\ +\ 1.2345 \\ \hline 23 \end{array}$$ (carry the 1)

Step 3:

$$\begin{array}{r} 324.5678 \\ +\ 1.2345 \\ \hline 023 \end{array}$$ (carry the 1)

Step 4:

$$\begin{array}{r} 324.5678 \\ +\ 1.2345 \\ \hline .8023 \end{array}$$

Step 5:

$$\begin{array}{r} 324.5678 \\ +\ 1.2345 \\ \hline 5.8023 \end{array}$$

Step 6:

$$\begin{array}{r} 324.5678 \\ +\ 1.2345 \\ \hline 25.8023 \end{array}$$

Step 7:

$$\begin{array}{r} 324.5678 \\ +\ 1.2345 \\ \hline 325.8023 \end{array}$$

Practice Problems—Adding Decimals

Add the following decimal fractions:

1. 0.6 + 0.4 + 0.3 = ________
2. 4 + 3.1 + 0.3 = ________
3. 0.39 + 3.92 + 0.03 = ________
4. 3.365 + 15.432 + 5.001 = ________
5. 37.02 + 25 + 6.4 + 3.89 = ________
6. 4.0086 + 0.034 + 0.6 + 0.05 = ________
7. 43.766 + 9.33 + 17 + 206 = ________

8. $$\begin{array}{r} 354.2312 \\ +\ 5.1092 \\ \hline \end{array}$$

9. $$\begin{array}{r} 224.0021 \\ +\ 6.4444 \\ \hline \end{array}$$

10. $$\begin{array}{r} 5223.2312 \\ +\ 65.3217 \\ \hline \end{array}$$

tip
Decimal numbers are another way to express fractions. Working with fractions can be challenging, and performing calculations with decimal numbers can be less challenging.

To subtract decimal numbers, first put the numbers in a vertical column, aligning the decimal points. Then subtract each column, starting on the right and working left. If the digit being subtracted in a column is larger than the digit above it, "borrow" a digit from the next column to the left. Place the decimal point in the answer directly below the decimal points in the terms.

Example—Subtracting Decimals

Subtract 1.203 from 32.255

Step 1:

$$\begin{array}{r} 32.255 \\ -\ 1.203 \\ \hline 2 \end{array}$$

Step 2:

$$\begin{array}{r} 32.255 \\ -\ 1.203 \\ \hline 52 \end{array}$$

Step 3:

$$\begin{array}{r} 32.255 \\ -\ 1.203 \\ \hline .052 \end{array}$$

Step 4:

$$\begin{array}{r} 32.255 \\ -\ 1.203 \\ \hline 1.052 \end{array}$$

Step 5:

$$\begin{array}{r} 32.255 \\ -\ 1.203 \\ \hline 31.052 \end{array}$$

PRACTICE PROBLEMS—SUBTRACTING DECIMALS

Subtract the following decimal fractions:

1. 3.2 – 3.36 = ________
2. 14.33 – 5.7 = ________
3. 25.5 – 11.21 = ________
4. 1.0026 – 0.03 = ________
5. 75.013 – 3.048 = ________
6. 30.313 – 15.721 = ________

7. $\begin{array}{r} 254.2311 \\ -\ 3.1082 \\ \hline \end{array}$

8. $\begin{array}{r} 24.0032 \\ -\ 3.3333 \\ \hline \end{array}$

9. $\begin{array}{r} 523.2309 \\ -\ 63.3467 \\ \hline \end{array}$

10. $\begin{array}{r} 372.21 \\ -\ 3.89 \\ \hline \end{array}$

tip
When adding and subtracting decimals it is very important to line up the terms so that all the decimal points are in a vertical line.

DECIMAL NUMBERS (cont'd)

0.1

MULTIPLYING DECIMALS

To multiply decimal numbers, first multiply the numbers just as if they were whole numbers. Then line up the numbers on the right (do not align the decimal points). Next, starting on the right, multiply each digit in the top number by each digit in the bottom number. Then add the products.

Finally, place the decimal point in the answer by starting at the right and moving the point the number of places equal to the sum of the decimal places in both numbers that were multiplied together.

Example—Multiply 47.2 by 5.5

47.2	(has 1 decimal place)
x 5.5	(has 1 decimal place)
2360	
2360	
259.60	(has 2 decimal places)

Example—Find the product (9.683)(6.1)

9.683	(has 3 decimal places)
x 6.1	(has 1 decimal place)
9683	
58098	
59.0663	(has 3 + 1 = 4 decimal places)

PRACTICE PROBLEMS—MULTIPLYING DECIMALS

Multiply the following decimals:

1. (0.5)(0.7) = ________
2. (0.4)(0.8) = ________
3. (0.3)(0.3) = ________
4. (0.5)(0.3) = ________
5. 6(3.7) = ________
6. 5.3(0.03) = ________
7. 7.2(0.02) = ________
8. 0.22(0.12) = ________
9. 25.24 x 23.02
10. 123.444 x 3.1

SIGNIFICANT FIGURES

SIGNIFICANT FIGURES

In pharmacy, we usually use a calculator to perform calculations. Calculators are useful because they help us to avoid mathematical errors. We use decimal fractions when we use calculators.

We also often perform calculations using measured amounts. For example, we may need to measure 80 ml of water to prepare an oral suspension. The actual value that we can use in our calculations that contain measured amounts depends on the sensitivity of the measuring device. When we multiply and divide decimal fractions using calculators, we must be careful to *include only the significant figures in our calculations* and answers. That is to say, we must be careful to keep in mind the sensitivity of the measuring device that is used when we perform the calculations.

A significant figure (or significant digit) is one that is actually measured using the measuring device. For instance, in the example above of measuring 80 ml of water, if the sensitivity of the graduate used to measure the water measures to the nearest ml, the measurement should be expressed as 80 ml and not 80.0 ml. Numbers that are not measured (for example a count of 30 capsules) are not affected by the sensitivity of a measuring device, and therefore are not subject to the rules of significant figures. When a calculation (addition, subtraction, multiplication, etc.) involves several measurements, and each measurement has a different number of significant digits, the final answer should have the same number of significant figures as the measured item that has the least number of significant figures. Also, if a calculation contains both numbers that are measured and numbers that are not measured, only the numbers that are measured should be considered when determining the number of significant figures for the answer.

RULES FOR ASSIGNING SIGNIFICANT FIGURES

1. Digits other than zero are always significant.
2. Final zeros after a decimal point are always significant.
3. Zeros between two other significant digits are always significant.
4. Zeros used only to space the decimal are never significant.

Example—Determining the Number of Significant Figures

1.40 g of hydrocortisone powder are needed to compound a prescription.

Question: How many significant figures are in this measured amount?

Answer: Since final zeros after a decimal point are always significant, the number of significant figures is 3.

MEASUREMENT

There are different systems of measurement used in pharmacy: metric, English, apothecary, and avoirdupois.

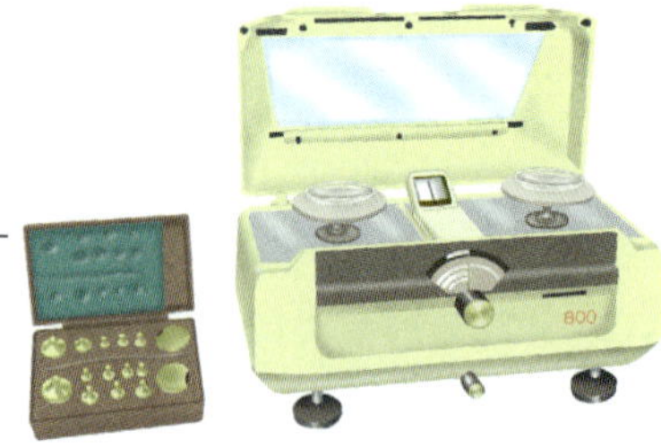

The metric system is the primary system used. Within these systems there are different measurements for weight, volume, and length, as well as for liquids and solids. There are also different measurement systems for temperature. It is necessary to know how to perform *conversions*—i.e., how to convert one type of measurement to another so that both amounts are equal.

Metric System

The major system of weights and measures used in medicine is the metric system. It was developed in France in the late 18th century and is based on a decimal system. That is, *different measurement units are related by measures of ten.* Technicians need to know metric measures for both liquids and solids.

Liquids

Liquids (including lotions) are measured by volume. The most widely used metric volume measurements are liters or milliliters.

Unit	Symbol	Liquid Conversions				
liter	l	1 l	=	10 dl	=	1,000 ml
deciliter	dl	1 dl	=	0.1 l	=	100 ml
milliliter	ml	1 ml	=	0.001 l	=	0.01 dl

Note: deciliters are rarely used in pharmacy, but are included here for reference and to illustrate the decimal relationship of these measures.

Solids

Solids (pills, granules, ointments, etc.) are measured by weight.

Unit	Symbol	Solid Conversions				
kilogram	kg	1 kg	=	1,000 g		
gram	g	1 g	=	0.001 kg	=	1,000 mg
milligram	mg	1 mg	=	0.001 g	=	1,000 mcg
microgram	mcg or µg	1 mcg	=	0.001 mg	=	0.000001 g

Rx tip

Milliliters are sometimes referred to as cubic centimeters (cc). They are not precisely the same but are quite close and are sometimes used interchangeably. Milliliter is the preferred usage for pharmacy.

tip

To convert milligrams to grams, move the decimal 3 places to the left (1 mg = 0.001 g).

AVOIRDUPOIS SYSTEM

The avoirdupois system is the system of weight (ounces and pounds) that we commonly use. However, one avoirdupois unit used in pharmacy is rarely used elsewhere. It is the grain.

Unit	Symbol	Conversions		
pound	lb	1 lb	=	16 oz
ounce	oz	1 oz	=	437.5 gr
grain	gr	1 gr	=	64.8 mg

THE GRAIN

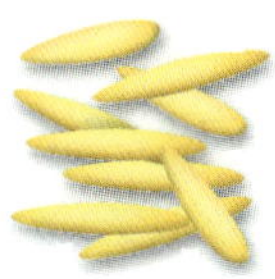

The grain is the same weight in several different measurement systems: apothecary, avoirdupois, and troy. It is said to have been established as a unit of weight in 1266 by King Henry III of England when he required the English penny to weigh the equivalent of 32 dried grains of wheat. On the metric scale, one grain equals 64.8 milligrams. However, this is often rounded to 65 milligrams.

APOTHECARY SYSTEM

The apothecary system is sometimes used in prescriptions, primarily with liquids. It includes the fluid ounce, pint, quart, and gallon. Although there are apothecary weight units, they are generally not used, with the exception of the grain. The fluid ounce is a volume measure and is different than the weight ounce. It is always indicated by "fl oz."

Unit	Symbol	Conversions		
gallon	gal	1 gal	=	4 qt
quart	qt	1 qt	=	2 pt
pint	pt	1 pt	=	16 fl oz
ounce	fl oz	1 fl oz	=	8 fl dr
fluid dram	fl dr	1 fl dr	=	60 min
minim	min or M_x			

Note: drams and minims are rarely used in pharmacy today, but are included here for reference.

conversions changing one unit of measure into another so that both amounts remain equal.

MEASUREMENT (cont'd)

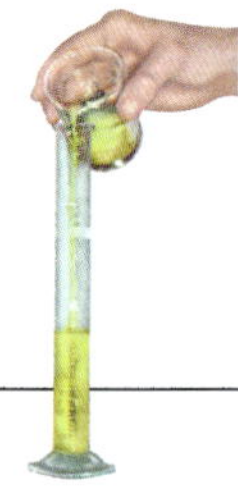

Household Units

The teaspoon and tablespoon are common household measurement units that are regularly used in liquid prescriptions. Note that home teaspoons and tablespoons are not accurate for use in measuring medications.

Unit	Abbreviation	Conversion
teaspoon	tsp	1 tsp = 5 ml
tablespoon	tbsp	1 tbsp = 3 tsp = 15 ml
cup	cup	1 cup = 8 fl oz

Temperature

The Celsius scale, which is also called centrigrade, is used to measure temperature. The relationship of Celsius (C) to Fahrenheit (F) is:

F temperature = ($1\frac{4}{5}$ times number of degrees C) + 32

Example—Converting Celsius to Fahrenheit

Question: What is 100°C in Fahrenheit?

Answer: $1\frac{4}{5} \times 100 = 180$ and $180 + 32 = 212$°F

C temperature = 5/9 x (number of degrees F – 32)

Example—Converting Fahrenheit to Celsius

Question: What is 212°F in Celsius?

Answer: $\frac{5}{9} \times (212 - 32) = \frac{5}{9} \times 180 = 100$°F

Note that the temperature of water freezing is 0°C and 32°F.

Some people find the following formula easier to remember and use:

9°C = 5°F – 160

Conversions

Following are some commonly used unit conversions. See page 165 for additional conversions.

1 L	=	33.8 fl oz	1 oz	=	28.35 g
1 pt	=	473.167 ml	1 g	=	15.43 gr
1 fl oz	=	29.57 ml	1 gr	=	64.8 mg
1 kg	=	2.2 lb	1 tsp	=	5 ml
1 lb	=	453.59 g	1 tbsp	=	15 ml

℞ tip

Some medications orders and prescriptions use military time for dosing. See page 434 in Chapter 16 for more information on military time.

PRACTICE PROBLEMS—METRICS

Provide the abbreviation for these:

1. microgram ________
2. liter ________
3. milliliter ________
4. gram ________
5. milligram ________
6. kilogram ________

Convert these units to equivalents:

7. 1 kg = _____ g
8. 1 mg = _____ mcg
9. 2 gr = _____ mg
10. 1 L = _____ ml
11. 1 ml = _____ l
12. 1 mg = _____ g

PRACTICE PROBLEMS—CONVERSIONS

Convert these numbers using the conversions provided on the preceding pages as well as your knowledge of decimals:

1. 7 mg = _____ mcg
2. 3.2 g = _____ mg
3. 1 gr = _____ g
4. 2 tbsp = _____ ml
5. 0.3 L = _____ ml
6. 7 kg = _____ g
7. 1 oz = _____ gr
8. 0.5 kg = _____ lb
9. 10 ml = _____ tsp
10. 15 ml = _____ tbsp
11. 0°C = _____ °F
12. 250 ml = _____ l

Calculating Daily Dosage from Common Pharmacy Sigs

Sig	Meaning	Interpret As
i tab q.d.	Take one tablet every day	1 tablet/dose X 1 dose/day = 1 tablet/day
i tab b.i.d.	Take one tablet twice a day	1 tablet/dose X 2 doses/day = 2 tablets/day
i tab t.i.d.	Take one tablet three times a day	1 tablet/dose X 3 doses/day = 3 tablets/day
i tab q.i.d.	Take one tablet four times a day	1 tablet/dose X 4 doses/day = 4 tablets/day
i tab q.o.d.	Take one tablet every other day	1 tablet/dose X 1/2 dose/day = 1/2 tablet/day
ss tab q.d.	Take one-half tablet every day	1/2 tablet/dose X 1 dose/day = 1/2 tablet/day
i tab a.m.	Take one tablet in the morning	1 tablet/dose X 1 dose/day = 1 tablet/day
i tab h.s.	Take one tablet at bedtime	1 tablet/dose X 1 dose/day = 1 tablet/day
i tab a.c.	Take one tablet before meals	1 tablet/dose X 3 doses/day = 3 tablets/day
i tab p.c.	Take one tablet after meals	1 tablet/dose X 3 doses/day = 3 tablets/day
i tsp q.d.	Take one teaspoonful every day	5 ml/dose X 1 dose/day = 5 ml/day

EQUATIONS & VARIABLES

x

EQUATIONS AND VARIABLES

In the calculations of pharmacy related problems there is often an unknown value that needs to be determined. Solving the unknown value involves setting up a mathematical statement between the known amounts and the unknown. This statement is called an equation. The unknown fact in an equation is called a ***variable***. The variable is often indicated by the letter x.

An equation is a mathematical statement in which two terms are equal.

Equations use the equal sign (=) to indicate equivalence. The following are equations:

$$1 = 1/2 + 1/2$$

$$1 = 1/2 \times 2$$

Example—Converting ml into Fluid Ounces

You have a prescription for 120 ml of theophylline liquid and want to know how many fluid ounces is equal to 120 ml.

In this case, the number of fluid ounces is the variable x that you want to determine.

x = number of fluid ounces needed

Step 1: Since there are 29.57 ml in each fluid ounce, one way to state this problem mathematically is the following equation:

x = (total prescribed ml) ÷ (ml/fl oz conversion rate)

or

$$x = \frac{\text{total prescribed ml}}{\text{ml/fl oz conversion rate}}$$

Step 2: Solve the equation with the known information:

$$x = \frac{120 \text{ ml}}{29.57 \text{ ml}}$$

x = 4 fl oz

variable an unknown value in a mathematical equation.

Example—Filling a Capsule Prescription

A prescription reads: amoxicillin 250 mg, one capsule orally, three times a day for seven days.

Question: How many capsules will be needed to fill this prescription?

In this case, the number of capsules needed is the unknown variable that you want to determine.

x = capsules needed
x = (capsules per dose) x (doses per day) x (days)
x = (1 capsule per dose) x (3 doses per day) x (7 days)
x = 21

Answer: You need 21 capsules of amoxicillin 250 mg to fill the prescription.

Example—Preparing an Intravenous Solution of Potassium Chloride

You are preparing an intravenous solution (IV) that requires the addition of potassium chloride (KCl). You have a vial of KCl containing a concentration of 20 mEq per 10 ml.

Question: How many ml of this solution should you add to the IV if the IV should have a total of 50 mEq of KCl in it?

Step 1: This is made easier by first solving for the number of KCl per ml:

20 mEq divided by 10 ml = 2 mEq per ml
x (ml of KCl solution) = mEq KCl needed ÷ mEq KCl per ml
x = (50 mEq) ÷ (2 mEq/ml)
x = 25 m

Answer: You need to add 25 ml of KCl solution to the IV.

RATIO & PROPORTION

Ratio and Proportion

Understanding ratios and proportions is important for pharmacy technicians. If you understand ratios and proportions, you will be able to perform most of the calculations necessary for your job.

A ratio states a relationship between two quantities.

The ratio of a to b can be stated as: $\frac{a}{b}$

Two equal ratios form a proportion: $\frac{a}{b} = \frac{c}{d}$

Example—Ratio and Proportion I

An example of this is the equation: $\frac{1}{2} = \frac{2}{4}$

$\frac{1}{2}$ and $\frac{2}{4}$ are equivalent ratios. 1 has the same relationship to 2 as 2 has to 4. Therefore, the equation is a proportion.

Example—Ratio and Proportion II

If one person has a bottle containing 5 tablets and another has 3 bottles each containing 5 tablets, one person may have more tablets than the other but they both have the same proportion of tablets to bottles.

$$\frac{5 \text{ tablets}}{1 \text{ bottle}} = \frac{15 \text{ tablets}}{3 \text{ bottles}}$$

Each person has fives times as many tablets as bottles. The ratios are equivalent.

Example—Ratio and Proportion III

A solution of 5 g of a substance in 100 ml of water is equivalent to 50 g of the same substance in 1,000 ml of water.

$$\frac{5 \text{ g}}{100 \text{ ml}} = \frac{50 \text{ g}}{1{,}000 \text{ ml}}$$

Both numerators can be divided into their denominators 20 times. Therefore, the ratios are equivalent.

SOLVING RATIO AND PROPORTION PROBLEMS

In a proportion equation, all four terms are related to each other and the relationship of each term to the others can be stated in different ways:

$\frac{a}{b} = \frac{c}{d}$ *can be stated as* $\frac{b}{a} = \frac{d}{c}$

You can also state the equation for any one term by multiplying both sides of the equation by one of the other terms.

$$b \times \frac{a}{b} = b \times \frac{c}{d}$$

$$\cancel{b} \times \frac{a}{\cancel{b}} = b \times \frac{c}{d}$$

➡ *cancel out equal values*

$$a = \frac{bc}{d}$$

These are also true: $b = \frac{ad}{c}$ $c = \frac{ad}{b}$ $d = \frac{bc}{a}$

Therefore, if three of the four terms in a proportion problem are known, an unknown fourth term (x) can also be calculated.

When you know the values of three of the four terms in a proportion equation, the unknown term is indicated by x, and the proportion equation can be written as:

$\frac{x}{b} = \frac{c}{d}$ ➡ *ratio you want = ratio you have*

Multiplying both sides of the equation by the value of **b** will then establish the relationship of the known terms to x.

$$b \times \left(\frac{x}{b}\right) = b \times \left(\frac{c}{d}\right)$$

$$\cancel{b} \times \frac{x}{\cancel{b}} = b \times \frac{c}{d}$$

➡ *cancel out equal values*

$$x = \frac{bc}{d}$$

You can then solve for the value of x by simple multiplication and division of the known values of b, c, and d.

$$x = (b \times c) \div d$$

RATIO & PROPORTION (cont'd)

$\frac{a}{b}$ $\frac{x}{b}$

Example—Using Ratio and Proportion

Question: In one bottle there are 30 capsules. If every bottle contains the same number of capsules, how many capsules are in six bottles?

Step 1: Define the variable and the correct ratios.

a. define the unknown variable ➡ x (total capsules)

b. establish the known ratio ➡ 30 capsules/1 bottle

c. establish the unknown ratio ➡ x capsules/6 bottles

Step 2: Set up the proportion equation $\left(\frac{x}{b} = \frac{c}{d}\right)$.

$$\frac{x \text{ capsules}}{6 \text{ bottles}} = \frac{30 \text{ capsules}}{1 \text{ bottle}}$$

➡ Note that the units must be the same in both the numerator and denominator: numerator units are capsules and denominator units are bottles

Step 3: Establish the x equation.

$$6 \text{ bottles} \times \frac{x \text{ capsules}}{6 \text{ bottles}} = 6 \text{ bottles} \times \frac{30 \text{ capsules}}{1 \text{ bottle}}$$

$$6 \text{ bottles} \times \frac{x \text{ capsules}}{6 \text{ bottles}} = 6 \text{ bottles} \times \frac{30 \text{ capsules}}{1 \text{ bottle}}$$

➡ *cancel out equal values and units*

$$x \text{ capsules} = 6 \times 30 \text{ capsules}$$

Step 4: Solve for x.

$$x \text{ capsules} = 180 \text{ capsules}$$

Step 5: Express solution in correct units.

There are 180 capsules in the six bottles.

CONDITIONS FOR USING RATIO AND PROPORTION

1. Three of the four values must be known.
2. Numerators must have the same units.
3. Denominators must have the same units.

Example—A Prescription for Tablets

Question: You receive a prescription for KTabs® one tablet b.i.d. x 30 days. How many tablets are needed to fill this prescription?

Step 1: Define the variable and correct ratios.

a. define the unknown variable ➡ x = total tablets needed
b. establish the known ratio ➡ 2 tablets/1 day
c. establish the unknown ratio ➡ x tablets/30 days

Step 2: Set up the proportion equation.

$$\frac{x \text{ tablets}}{30 \text{ days}} = \frac{2 \text{ tablets}}{1 \text{ day}}$$

Step 3: Establish the x equation.

$$x \text{ tablets} = 30 \text{ days} \times \frac{2 \text{ tablets}}{1 \text{ day}}$$

Step 4: Solve for x.

$$x \text{ tablets} = 30 \cancel{\text{days}} \times \frac{2 \text{ tablets}}{1 \cancel{\text{day}}} = 60 \text{ tablets}$$

$$x \text{ tablets} = 60 \text{ tablets}$$

Step 5: Express solution in correct units.

60 tablets of KTabs® are needed to fill the prescription.

RATIO & PROPORTION (cont'd)

Example—A Liquid Prescription

You receive a prescription for amoxicillin 75 mg 4 times a day for 10 days. You have available amoxicillin 250 mg/5 ml 150 ml.

Question 1: What is the correct individual dose?

Step 1: Define the variable and correct ratios.

a. define the unknown variable ➡ x = ml per dose
b. establish the known ratio ➡ 5 ml/250 mg
c. establish the unknown ratio ➡ x ml/75 mg

Step 2: Set-up the proportion equation.

x ml/75 mg = 5 ml/250 mg

Step 3: Establish the x equation.

$$x \text{ ml} = 75 \text{ mg} \times \frac{5 \text{ ml}}{250 \text{ mg}}$$

Step 4: Solve.

$$x \text{ ml} = 75 \cancel{\text{mg}} \times \frac{5 \text{ ml}}{250 \cancel{\text{mg}}} = \frac{375 \text{ ml}}{250} = 1.5 \text{ ml}$$

Step 5: Express solution in correct units.

The dose is 1.5 ml of amoxicillin.

Question 2: How many mls of amoxicillin do you need for 10 days?

Step 1: A simple equation can determine this. Note that it is often useful to state the equation first in words, and then restate it in numbers. Using words to describe mathematical operations helps you to visualize and better understand the mathematics involved.

Word Equation: amount needed = dose amount x doses day x number of days
➡ amoxicillin needed = 1.5 ml x 4 x 10 = 60 ml

Step 2: Double check your answer.

$$1.5 \text{ ml of } \frac{250 \text{ mg}}{5 \text{ ml}} = 75 \text{ mg}$$

Example—A Mixture Dose

Question: If an antidiarrheal mixture contains 3 ml of paregoric in each 30 ml of mixture, how many ml of paregoric would be contained in a teaspoonful dose of mixture?

conversion: 1 tsp = 5 ml

Step 1: Define the variable and correct ratios.

a. define the unknown variable ➡ x ml of paregoric

b. establish the known ratio ➡ 3 ml/30 ml (mix)

c. establish the unknown ratio ➡ x ml/5 ml (mix)

Step 2: Set up the proportion equation.

x ml paregoric/5 ml mix = 3 ml paregoric/30 ml mix

Step 3: Establish the x equation.

$$x \text{ ml} = 5 \text{ ml mix} \times \frac{3 \text{ ml paregoric}}{30 \text{ ml mix}}$$

Step 4: Solve.

$$x \text{ ml paregoric} = 5 \text{ ml mix} \times \frac{3 \text{ ml paregoric}}{30 \text{ ml mix}} =$$

$$\frac{1.5 \text{ ml paregoric}}{30 \text{ ml mix}} = 0.5 \text{ ml paregoric}$$

Step 5: Express solution in correct units.

There are 0.5 ml of paregoric in a teaspoon.

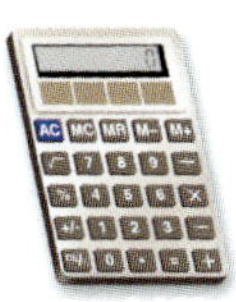

USING CALCULATORS

Though most of these examples can be solved without the use of a calculator, the use of calculators is essential in the correct computation of many dosage calculations. Their answers are precise and provided in decimals. Since it is relatively easy to make entry mistakes on a calculator, always recheck answers. Also, use judgment. If an answer doesn't appear to make sense, check it.

RATIO & PROPORTION (cont'd)

IV Flow Rate

In the pharmacy setting, you may be asked to provide information on *flow rate,* or rate of administration, for an IV solution. Flow rates are calculated using ratio and proportion equations. They are generally done in ml/hour, but for pumps used to dispense IV fluids to the patient, the calculation may need to be done in ml/min.

Example—IV Flow Rate

Question: If you have an order for KCl 10 mEq and K Acetate 15 mEq in D5W 1,000 ml to run at 80 ml/hour, you would determine the administration rate in ml/min as follows:

Step 1: Define the variable and correct ratios.

a. define the unknown variable ➡ x = ml

b. establish the known ratio ➡ 80 ml/60 min

c. establish the unknown ratio ➡ x ml/1 min

Step 2: Set up the proportion equation.

$$x \text{ ml/1 min} = 80 \text{ ml/60 min}$$

Step 3: Establish the x equation.

$$x \text{ ml} = 1 \text{ min} \times \frac{80 \text{ ml}}{60 \text{ min}}$$

Step 4: Factor and solve.

$$x \text{ ml} = 1 \cancel{\text{min}} \times \frac{80 \text{ ml}}{60 \text{ min}} = 1.33 \text{ ml}$$

➡ *80 divided by 60 = 1.33*

Step 5: Express solution in correct units.

The flow rate would be 1.33 ml/min.

Note: IV Flow Rate calculations may involve drops per ml or drops per minute or involve calculating the amount of time before an IV bag will empty and require replacement. Using simple ratio and proportion equations will solve these problems.

flow rate the rate (in ml/hour or ml/min) at which a solution is administered to a patient; also known as *rate of administration.*

STEPS FOR SOLVING PROPORTION PROBLEMS

1. Define the variable and correct ratios.
2. Set up the proportion equation
3. Establish the x equation
4. Solve for x.
5. Express solution in correct units.

DAY'S SUPPLY

Especially in the community pharmacy setting, technicians often need to be able to calculate how long the prescription should last the patient when taken as prescribed, i.e., a day's supply.

Example—Day's Supply

Question: A customer gives you a prescription written for clofibrate 600 mg #60 i tab b.i.d. What is the day's supply?

Step 1: Determine how many dosage units (i.e., tablets) are taken each day from the directions.

i tab b.i.d. means 2 tablets/day

Step 2: Set up the proportion equation.

60 tablets/x days = 2 tablets/1 day

Step 3: Establish the x equation.

x days = 60 tablets x 1 day/2 tablets

Step 4: Factor and solve.

x days = 60 tablets x 1 day 2 tablets = 30 days

PRACTICE PROBLEMS—RATIO AND PROPORTION

1. A prescription calls for 100 mg of a drug that you have in a 250 mg/5 ml concentration. How many ml of the liquid do you need?

2. A prescription calls for 400 mg of a drug that you have in a 50 mg/ml concentration. How many ml of the liquid do you need?

3. A prescription calls for 10 mg of a drug that you have in a 2 mg/15 ml concentration. How many ml of the liquid do you need?

4. KCl 10 mEq and K Acetate 15 mEq in D5W 1,000 ml is ordered to be administered over 8 hours. What would the rate be in ml/min?

5. A prescription calls for 0.24 mg of a drug that you have in a 50 mcg/ml concentration. How many ml of the liquid do you need?

PERCENTS & SOLUTIONS

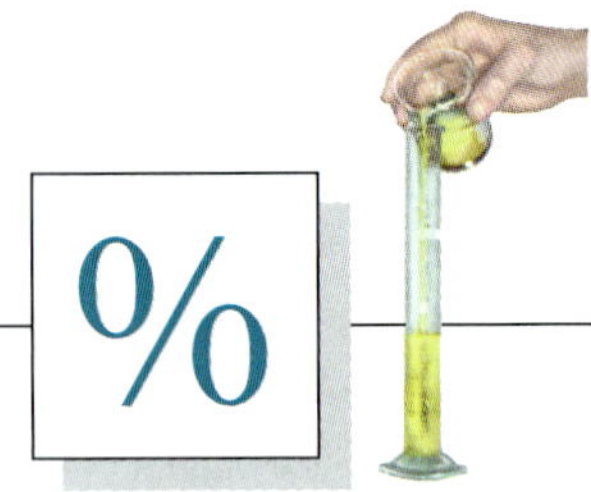

PERCENTS AND SOLUTIONS

Percents are used to indicate the amount, or ***concentration,*** of something in a solution. Concentrations are indicated in terms of weight-to-volume or volume-to-volume.

Weight-to-Volume: grams per 100 milliliters ➡ g/100 ml

Volume-to-Volume: milliliters per 100 milliliters ➡ ml/100 ml

Example—IV Solution

Question: If there is 50% dextrose in a 1,000 ml IV bag, how many grams of dextrose are there in the bag?

Step 1: You can solve this by developing a proportion equation. Since 50% dextrose means there are 50 grams of dextrose in 100 ml, the equation would be:

$$x \text{ g} \div 1{,}000 \text{ ml} = 50 \text{ g} \div 100 \text{ ml}$$

Step 2: The x equation:

$$x \text{ g} = 1{,}000 \cancel{\text{ml}} \times \frac{50 \text{ g}}{100 \text{ ml}} = 10 \times 50 \text{ g} = 500 \text{ g}$$

➡1,000 ÷ by 100 = 10

Answer: There are 500 grams of dextrose in the bag.

Another way to solve this is to convert the percent to a decimal.

Step 1: In a 50% solution, there are .5 g per ml:

$$50 \text{ g}/100 \text{ ml} = 0.5 \text{ g/ml}$$

Step 2: You can then multiply 0.5 g by the total number of milliliters.

$$x = 0.5 \text{ g} \times 1{,}000 = 500 \text{ g}$$

Question: Now how many ml will give you a 10 g of dextrose?

Step 1: The proportion equation:

$$x \text{ ml}/10 \text{ g} = 100 \text{ ml}/50 \text{ g}$$

Step 2: The x equation:

$$x \text{ ml} = 10 \cancel{\text{g}} \times \frac{100 \text{ ml}}{50 \cancel{\text{g}}} = \frac{1{,}000 \text{ ml}}{50} = 20 \text{ ml}$$

Answer: 20 ml of 50% solution contain 10 g of dextrose.

concentration the strength of a solution as measured by the weight-to-volume or volume-to-volume of the substance being measured.

PRACTICE PROBLEMS—PERCENTS

Convert the following fractions to percents:

1. 60/100 = ________%
2. 80/100 = ________%
3. 12/100 = ________%

Convert the following percents to decimals:

4. 50% = ________
5. 12.5% = ________
6. 99% = ________

You have a 70% dextrose solution. How many grams in:

7. 50 ml of solution ________
8. 75 ml of solution ________
9. 20 ml of solution ________

You have a 50% dextrose solution, how many ml will give you:

10. 25 g of dextrose ________
11. 35 g of dextrose ________
12. 10 g of dextrose ________

13. You have a liquid that contains 12 mg /10 ml. What percent is this liquid? ________
    (Hint: To solve, you will need to convert mg to g per 100 ml using decimals.)

PERCENTS & SOLUTIONS (cont'd)

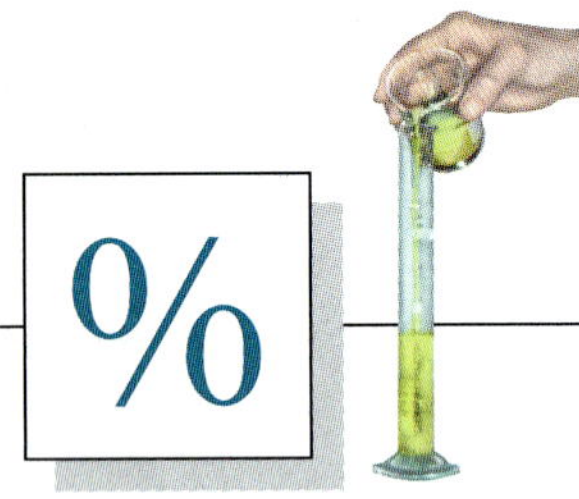

A Percent Solution Formula

It is possible to set up a proportion equation specifically to convert concentrations for preparation of special intravenous solutions known as hyperalimentation, or *total parenteral solutions (TPNs)*.

$$\frac{x \text{ volume needed}}{\text{want \%}} = \frac{\text{volume prescribed}}{\text{have \%}}$$

Example—A Dilution

Question: A physician wants a 35% solution of dextrose 1,000 ml. You have a 50% solution of dextrose 1000 ml. How will you make up what the physician wants?

Step 1: The terms for the formula are:

volume needed	➡	x ml
want %	➡	35% dextrose
volume prescribed	➡	1,000 ml
have %	➡	50% dextrose

Step 2: The formula is:

$$x \text{ ml}/35\% = 1000 \text{ ml}/50\%$$

Step 3: The x equation is:

$$x \text{ ml} = 35\not\% \times \frac{1{,}000 \text{ ml}}{50\not\%} = 35 \times 20 \text{ ml} = 700 \text{ ml}$$

➡ *1,000 ÷ 50 = 20*

Step 4: 700 ml of dextrose 1,000 ml will give you the 350 g of dextrose you will need in your solution. However, you will still need to add sterile water *qs ad* until you have a total solution of 1,000 ml as ordered by the physician. (qs ad means quantity needed to make total volume).

Total Volume	1,000 ml
Dextrose 50% Solution	– 700 ml
Sterile Water (qs ad)	300 ml

Answer: You need to add 300 ml of sterile water to 700 ml of 50% dextrose to create 1,000 ml of 35% dextrose.

milliequivalent (mEq) the unit of measure for electrolytes in a solution.

qs ad the quantity needed to make a prescribed amount.

total parenteral nutrition administration of all nutrients intravenously; also known as hyperalimentation.

valence the number of positive or negative charges on an ion.

℞ **tip**

In order to calculate mEq for an electrolyte, the atomic weight and valence of the electrolyte must first be known. The weight is then divided by the valence.

MILLIEQUIVALENTS: MEQ

Electrolyte solutions are often used in hospitals. Electrolytes are substances that conduct an electrical current and are found in the body's blood, tissue fluids, and cells. Salts are electrolytes, and saline solutions are commonly used electrolyte solutions.

The concentration of electrolytes is expressed as ***milliequivalents (mEq)*** per milliliter or milliequivalents per liter.

A milliequivalent is a specific unit of measurement that cannot be converted into the metric system. A 0.9% solution of one electrolyte will have a different mEq value than a 0.9% solution of another because mEq values are different for different electrolytes. Milliequivalents are based on each electrolyte's atomic weight and electron properties known as ***valence***.

Example—Milliequivalents

Question: A solution calls for 5 mEq of sodium that you have in a 1.04 mEq/ml solution of NaCl. How many ml of it do you need?

$$x \text{ ml}/5 \text{ mEq} = 1 \text{ ml}/1.04 \text{ mEq}$$

$$x \text{ ml} = 5 \cancel{\text{mEq}} \times \frac{1 \text{ ml}}{1.04 \cancel{\text{mEq}}} = \frac{5 \text{ ml}}{1.04} = 4.8 \text{ ml}$$

Answer: 4.8 ml of the solution is needed.

Common Electrolytes		Common Saline Solutions	
NaCl	➡ Sodium Chloride	0.9% NaCl	➡ Normal Saline
MgSO4	➡ Magnesium Sulfate	0.45% NaCl	➡ 1/2 Normal Saline
KCl	➡ Potassium Chloride	0.2% NaCl	➡ 1/4 Normal Saline
K Acetate	➡ Potassium Acetate	3% NaCl	➡ Hypertonic Saline
Ca Gluconate	➡ Calcium Gluconate		
Na Acetate	➡ Sodium Acetate		

PERCENTS & SOLUTIONS (cont'd)

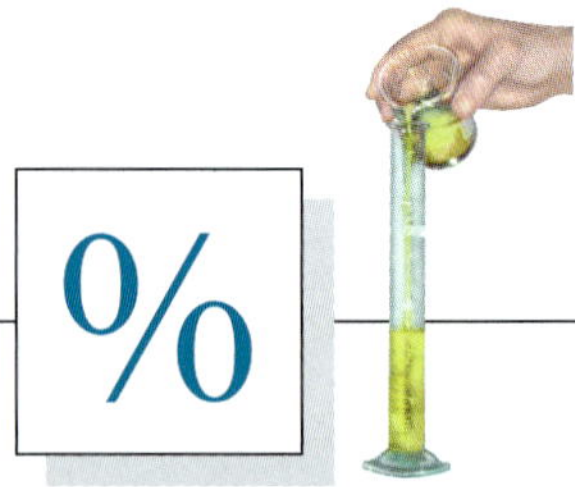

Example—Total Parenteral Nutrition

A TPN order calls for the amounts on the left, including additives, to be made from the items you have on hand, on the right. The total volume is to be 1,000 ml.

TPN Order		What You Have On Hand
Aminosyn 4.25%		Aminosyn 8.5% 1,000 ml
Dextrose 25%		Dextrose 70% 1,000 ml
Additives:		
KCl	20 mEq	KCl 2 mEq/ml 10 ml
MVI	10 ml	MVI 10 ml
NaCl	24 mEq	NaCl 4.4 mEq/ml 20 ml

Question 1: How much aminosyn do you need to prepare this TPN?

Step 1: Using the percent solutions formula:

$$x \text{ ml}/4.25\% = 1{,}000 \text{ ml}/8.5\%$$

$$x \text{ ml} = 4.25\cancel{\%} \times \frac{1{,}000 \text{ ml}}{8.5\cancel{\%}} = 1{,}000 \text{ ml} \times 0.5$$

➡ *4.25 ÷ 8.5 = 0.5*

$$x \text{ ml} = 500 \text{ ml}$$

Answer: 500 ml of aminosyn 8.5% is needed.

Question 2: How much dextrose do you need?

Step 1: Using the percent solutions formula:

$$x \text{ ml}/25\% = 1{,}000 \text{ ml}/70\%$$

$$x \text{ ml} = 25\cancel{\%} \times \frac{1{,}000 \text{ ml}}{70\cancel{\%}} = \frac{25{,}000 \text{ ml}}{70}$$

$$x \text{ ml} = 357.14 \text{ ml dextrose} \rightarrow 357 \text{ ml}$$

Answer: 357 ml of dextrose 70% is needed.

Rx safety you should know

Generally, amounts less than 0.5 are rounded down and amounts greater than 0.5 are rounded up. However, some drugs may be rounded and others may not. You will need to know when you must be precise and when you may round for each drug.

Example—Total Parenteral Nutrition (cont'd)

Question 3: How much KCl do you need ?

Step 1: Using a proportion equation:

$$x \text{ ml}/20 \text{ mEq} = 1 \text{ ml}/2 \text{ mEq}$$

$$x \text{ ml} = 20 \cancel{\text{mEq}} \times \frac{1 \text{ ml}}{2 \cancel{\text{mEq}}} = 10 \text{ ml KCl}$$

Answer: 10 ml KCl are needed.

Question 4: How much MVI do you need?

Step 1: Add the 10 ml MVI on hand.

Question 5: How much NaCl do you need?

Step 1: Using a proportion equation:

$$x \text{ ml}/24 \text{ mEq} = 1 \text{ ml}/4.4 \text{ mEq}$$

$$x \text{ ml} = 24 \cancel{\text{mEq}} \times \frac{1 \text{ ml}}{4.4 \cancel{\text{mEq}}} = 5.45 \text{ ml}$$

Answer: 5.45 ml of NaCl is needed.

Question 6: How much sterile water is needed?

Step 1: Using a word equation, water needed = 1,000 ml – total ml of other ingredients.

Aminosyn	500 ml
Dextrose	357 ml
KCl	10 ml
MVI	10 ml
NaCl	5.45 ml
total	882.45 ml

Step 2: Water needed = 1,000 – 882.45 = 117.55

Answer: 117.55 ml sterile water is needed to fill the TPN order.

PERCENTS & SOLUTIONS (cont'd)

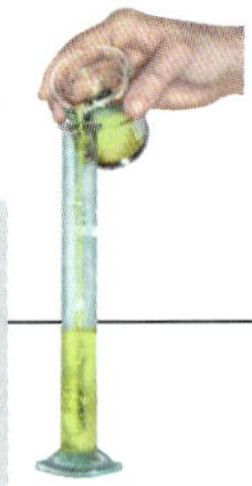

PERCENT SOLUTION FORMULA

$$\frac{x \text{ volume needed}}{\text{want \%}} = \frac{\text{volume prescribed}}{\text{have \%}}$$

PRACTICE PROBLEMS—TPN SOLUTIONS

A TPN order calls for the amounts on the left (including additives) to be made from the items you have on hand on the right. The total volume is to be 250 ml. How much of each ingredient do you need to prepare this TPN?

TPN Order	What You Have On Hand
Aminosyn 2.5%	Aminosyn 8.5%
Dextrose 7.5%	Dextrose 50%
Additives	
KCl 4 mEq	KCl 2 mEq/ml
Ca Gluconate 2 mEq	Ca Gluconate 4.4 mEq/ml
Ped MVI 5 ml	Ped MVI

Use the space to work out the answers.

1. Aminosyn 8.5% Answer: _____ ml

2. Dextrose 50% Answer: _____ ml

3. KCl 2 mEq/ml Answer: _____ ml

4. Ca Gluconate 4.4 mEq/ml Answer: _____ ml

5. Pediatric MVI 10 ml Answer: _____ ml

6. Sterile Water (qs ad) Answer: _____ ml

ALLIGATION

ALLIGATION

Alligation is a way to solve problems associated with mixing preparations of two different strengths of the same ingredient to obtain a strength in-between the starting preparations. The problems could also be solved using algebra, but using the alligation method is often easier.

To use the alligation method, set up a grid with three rows and three columns. Place the strength of the lower-strength component in the upper left corner, place the strength of the higher-strength component in the lower left corner, and place the desired strength of the product in the middle.

Strength of lower-strength component (L)		
	Desired strength of product (P)	
Strength of higher-strength component (H)		

Then subtract the lower value from the higher value on each diagonal to find the amounts needed of the lower-strength (L) and higher-strength (H) components:

Strength of lower-strength component (L)		H − P = Relative amount of L needed to prepare P
	Desired strength of product (P)	
Strength of higher-strength component (H)		P − L = Relative amount of H needed to prepare P

Example—Alligation I

Question: What are the relative amounts of 70% alcohol and 40% alcohol needed to prepare 60% alcohol?

In this example, since the value of P is higher than that of L, you will be subtracting L from P rather than P from L.

Strength of lower-strength component (L): 40		70 − 60 (H − P) = 10 parts needed of L
	Desired strength of product (P): 60	
Strength of higher-strength component (H): 70		60 − 40 (P − L) = 20 parts needed of H

10 + 20 = 30 total parts P. ➡

		10/30 of the final volume is L
		20/30 of the final volume is H

The proportion of each component in the final product is found by first adding the part values in the right-hand column (10 + 20) to get the total part value of the product (30) and then dividing each part value by the total part value. Thus the amount of 70% alcohol will be 20/30 of the product and the amount of 40% alcohol will 10/30.

In practice, it is necessary to know how to convert relative amounts to real values that can be measured. This requires using addition, subtraction, multiplication, division, and fractions.

Example—Alligation II

Question: Using the alligation above, how many ml of 70% alcohol should be mixed with how many ml of 40% alcohol to prepare 300 ml of 60% alcohol?

Step 1: In the example above, we determined the ratio of H to P is 20 H/30 P. Ratio and proportion can be used to solve for the volume. 20 ml H/30 ml P = x ml H/300 ml P. To solve for the volume of H:

300 ml P x 20 ml H/30 ml P = 200 ml H

Step 2: In the example above, we determined the ratio of L to P is 10 L/30 P. Ratio and proportion can be used to solve for the volume. 10 ml L/30 ml P = x ml L/300 ml P. To solve for the volume of L:

300 ml P x 10 ml L/30 ml P = 100 ml L

Answer: When 200 ml of 70% alcohol are mixed with 100 ml of 40% alcohol, the resulting solution is 300 ml of 60% alcohol.

ALLIGATION (cont'd)

Example—Alligation III

Question: How many grams of 1% hydrocortisone cream and 5% hydrocortisone cream are needed to prepare 30 grams of 2.5% hydrocortisone cream?

Strength of lower-strength component (L): 1		5 − 2.5 (H − P) = 2.5 parts needed of L
	Desired strength of product (P): 2.5	
Strength of higher-strength component (H): 5		2.5 − 1 (P − L) = 1.5 parts needed of H

2.5 + 1.5 = 4 total parts. So if the final weight of the 2.5% cream is 30 grams, you can solve for the weight needed of L and H. ➡

		2.5/4 x 30 g = 18.75 g needed of L
		1.5/4 x 30 g = 11.25 g needed of H

Step 1: To solve for total parts of P:

2.5 (L) + 1.5 (H) = 4 total parts of P

Step 2: To solve for grams of 1% hydrocortisone cream:

30 g P x 2.5 g L/4 g P = 18.75 g L

Step 3: To solve for grams of 5% hydrocortisone cream:

30 g P x 1.5 g H/4 g P = 11.25 g H

Answer: When 11.25 g of 5% hydrocortisone cream are mixed with 18.75 g of 1% hydrocortisone cream, the resulting product is 30 g of 2.5% hydrocortisone cream.

Example—Alligation IV

Question: How many grams of 20% zinc oxide ointment and petrolatum should be mixed to prepare to prepare 60 grams of 3% zinc oxide ointment? (Hint: petrolatum has 0% zinc oxide.)

Strength of lower-strength component (L): 0		20 − 3 (H − P) = 17 parts needed of L
	Desired strength of product (P): 3	
Strength of higher-strength component (H): 20		3 − 0 (P − L) = 3 parts needed of H

17 + 3 = 20 total parts. So if the final weight of the 3% ointment is 60 grams, you can solve for the weight of L and H needed. ➡

		17/20 x 60 g = 51 g needed of L
		3/20 x 60 = 9 g needed of H

Step 1: To solve for total parts P:

17 + 3 = 20 total parts P

Step 2: To solve for grams of petroleum:

60 g P x 17 g L/20 g P = 51 g L

Step 3: To solve for grams of 20% zinc oxide ointment:

60 g P x 3 g H/20 g P = 9 g H

Answer: When 9 g of 20% zinc oxide ointment are mixed with 51 g of petrolatum, the resulting product is 60 g of 3% zinc oxide ointment.

The alligation method is a little tricky at first. With practice, the alligation method can be mastered. Once the method is mastered, it becomes an easy and quick way to perform difficult calculations that involve mixing different strengths of the same ingredient.

POWDER VOLUME

Powder Volume

Some medications that are dispensed in liquid dosage form are manufactured and provided to the pharmacy as powders. The powders are then constituted or mixed with a specific volume of liquid to produce a desired strength of the liquid dosage form.

There may be a need to perform two different types of calculations with powders for constitution:

1. Determining the strength or concentration of a product when different volumes of diluent are added.
2. Determining how to change the concentration or strength of the constituted dosage form by varying the amount of diluent.

For either type of calculation, it is necessary to make an assumption that when the powder is constituted or mixed, the volume occupied by the powder portion of the final product is a constant. The portion of the volume of the final mixed product that is attributed to the powder is called the powder volume.

For calculations with powders for constitution, the following relationship exists:

The final volume of the constituted product (FV)
=
The volume of the diluent (D) + the powder volume (PV)

FV = D + PV

Additionally, it is important to keep in mind the total amount of drug in the manufacturer's bottle remains constant no matter how much diluent is added. For example, if a manufacturer packages 7,500 mg of a drug in a bottle for constitution, the amount of drug in the bottle will always be 7,500 mg (unless some medication is removed from the bottle).

Example—Powder Volume

Question: The directions for mixing a liquid antibiotic state when 80 ml of water are added to the contents of the bottle, the resulting volume is 150 ml. Determine the powder volume.

FV = D + PV
150 ml = 80 ml + PV
PV = 150 ml − 80 ml = 70 ml

Example—Using Powder Volume to Calculate Concentration

Question: The directions for mixing a 250 mg/5 m liquid antibiotic state when 80 ml of water are added to the contents of the bottle, the resulting volume is 150 ml. Determine what the concentration of drug in mg/5 ml would be if only 40 ml of water were added.

Step 1: Determine the total mg of drug in the bottle (recall, this amount is a constant):

250 mg drug/5 ml FV x 150 ml FV = 7,500 mg drug

Step 2: Determine the powder volume for the drug in the bottle:

FV = D + PV

150 ml = 80 ml + PV

PV = 150 ml – 80 ml

PV = 70 ml

Step 3: Determine the volume of the new product (NP):

(NP) = D + PV

NP = 40 ml + 70 ml

NP = 110 ml

Answer: The new concentration is:

Total mg drug in bottle/volume of the new product (NP)

7,500 mg/110 ml = 68.2 mg/ml = 341 mg/5 ml

CHILDREN'S DOSES

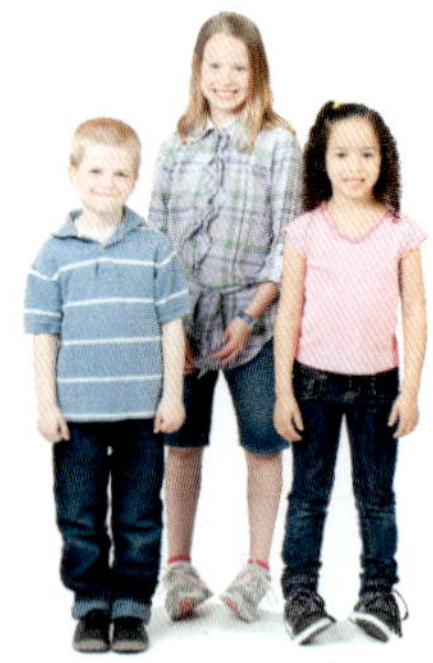

Calculation of Children's Doses

The average doses in the U.S.P. (United States Pharmacopoeia) and other drug reference sources are for adults. Doses for drugs that can be taken by a child are often provided by the manufacturer. When children's doses are not provided, the adult dose needs to be lowered. Two formulas for this are Clark's Rule and Young's Rule.

Clark's Rule

$$\frac{\text{weight of child}}{150 \text{ lb}} \times \text{adult dose} = \text{dose for child}$$

Young's Rule

$$\frac{\text{age of child}}{\text{age} + 12} \times \text{adult dose} = \text{dose for child}$$

For Clark's Rule, 150 lbs is considered an average weight for an adult. This is not a very precise way to calculate pediatric doses since there are many factors besides weight that may need to be taken into account: height, age, condition, etc. Another approach is based upon multiplying the adult dose by a ratio of the child's size to that of an average adult:

Body Surface Area Formula

$$\frac{\text{child bsa times adult dose}}{\text{average adult bsa}} = \text{child's dose}$$

The ***body surface area (bsa)*** of a person is based on their height and weight. It is always given in square meters (m^2). 1.73 m^2 is commonly used as an average bsa for adults. A chart called a ***nomogram*** has been traditionally used to manually calculate bsa. Body surface area nomograms contain three columns of numbers: height, body surface, and weight. The bsa is identified by the intersection of a line drawn between the weight and height columns with the bsa column, which is in the middle. Body surface area formulas are generally solved by computer. For comparison, the average bsa for adults is 1.73 m^2 while the bsa for a nine-year-old child who is 44 in tall and weighs 50 lbs would be 0.83 m^2.

Using Body Weight to Calculate Children's Dosage

Because of the many variables, however, conversion formulas for pediatric doses are not always appropriate and can lead to incorrect doses with some medications. Although doses are generally given by the physician, the pharmacy should always use a suitable drug information resource to check children's doses. Children's doses are stated by kg of body weight (dose/kg). Since 1 kg = 2.2 lb, you can solve for the prescribed dose by using a proportion equation if you know the child's body weight. See the example at right.

body surface area a measure used for dosage that is calculated from the height and weight of a person and measured in square meters.

nomogram a chart showing relationships between measurements.

Example—Infant Dose

Question: An antibiotic IV is prescribed for an infant. The dose is to be 15mg/kg twice a day. The baby weighs 18 lbs. How much drug is to be given for one dose?

Step 1: Calculate the infant's weight in kilograms.

$$x \text{ kg}/18 \text{ lb} = 1 \text{ kg}/2.2 \text{ lb}$$

$$x \text{ kg} = 18 \cancel{\text{lb}} \times \frac{1 \text{ kg}}{2.2 \cancel{\text{lb}}} = \frac{18 \text{ kg}}{2.2} = 8.18 \text{ kg}$$

You can also easily solve this with a calculator:

- ➥ enter 18
- ➥ press divide (/) key
- ➥ enter 2.2
- ➥ press equal (=) key
- ➥ answer 8.18

Step 2: You can solve the next part of this problem with a proportion equation or you can set up a simple word equation.

$$\text{one dose} = (\text{amount of drug}) \times (\text{number of kg of infant weight})$$

$$\text{one dose} = \frac{15 \text{ mg}}{\text{kg}} \times 8.18 \text{ kg}$$

With a calculator:

- ➥ enter 15
- ➥ press multiplication (*) key
- ➥ enter 8.18
- ➥ press equal (=) key
- ➥ answer 122.7 mg

CALCULATIONS FOR BUSINESS

$

Determining Selling Prices for Prescriptions

The selling, or retail, prices for prescriptions are typically determined at the corporate level, and pharmacy computers are usually programmed to automatically calculate them. However, prices are sometimes determined at the time the prescription is filled by using the following formula:

average wholesale price (AWP) + professional fee = selling price of prescription

AWP costs are provided on stock containers for the amount of drug originally provided in a given stock bottle. Ratio and proportion is used to determine the AWP for the amount of medication needed for a prescription. For instance, if a stock bottle has a price of $20 for 100 capsules, then the cost for 25 capsules would be 1/4 the cost of the stock bottle price since 25 is 25% or 1/4 of 100.

The professional fee is the amount of money pharmacies add on to the AWP to cover their processing costs. Professional fees for the examples and problems in this chapter are determined using the following chart:

Average Wholesale Price (AWP)	Professional Fee
less than $20.00	$4.00
$20.01–$50.00	$5.00
$50.01 and higher	$6.00

Example—Determining the Selling Price for a Prescription

Question: If the AWP for 100 capsules of amoxicillin 250 mg is $11.67, what will be the retail price of a prescription for 30 amoxicillin 250 mg?

Step 1: Use ratio and proportion to calculate the AWP for the prescription of 30 capsules:

30/100 x 11.67 = $3.50

Step 2: Use the chart above to find the professional fee for the prescription:

Since the AWP for the prescription is less than $20.00, the professional fee is $4.00.

Step 3: Use the formula above to calculate the prescription price:

AWP + professional fee = selling price of prescription
$3.50 + $4.00 = $7.50

Some pharmacies sell certain medications at a price lower than the acquisition cost (i.e, what the pharmacy paid for it). Therefore, the selling price may be less than the average wholesale price (AWP) or less than the acquisition cost. Third-party plans usually reimburse pharmacies based on the lowest amount, whether that is the AWP, acquisition cost, or amount paid by the patient.

PRACTICE PROBLEMS—SELLING PRICES

Calculate the retail price of the following prescriptions:

	Prescription	Stock/AWP	Retail Price
1.	Verapamil SR Tabs #30	100/$135.85	________
2.	Glyburide 5 mg Tabs #30	1,000/$480.15	________
3.	Dexamethasone 4 mg Tabs #12	100/$62.50	________
4.	Danazol 200 mg Caps #100	100/$322.38	________
5.	Doxepin 150 mg Caps #30	100/$73.50	________

DISCOUNTS

Pharmacies sometimes give a 5% or 10% discount on the price of prescriptions to certain patients such as senior citizens that do not participate in third-party programs. State pharmacy regulations or third-party contractual agreements may prohibit discounting prescriptions that are covered by third-party programs. Sometimes the discount is restricted to prescriptions purchased on certain days of the week.

Example—Discounts

A senior citizen is paying for a prescription for amoxicillin 250 mg #30. The selling price is $8.49; however this patient qualifies for a 10% discount. How much will the patient pay?

$$\$8.49 - 10\%(\$8.49) = \$8.49 - (0.1)(\$8.49) = \$8.49 - \$0.85 = \$7.64$$

PRACTICE PROBLEMS—DISCOUNTS

Calculate the price after a 5% discount for each of the following retail prescription prices:

1. $8.99 ______
2. $18.41 ______
3. $39.20 ______
4. $99.99 ______
5. $128.50 ______

Calculate the price after a 10% discount for each of the following retail prescription prices:

6. $8.99 ______
7. $18.49 ______
8. $39.30 ______
9. $9.99 ______
10. $180.55 ______

CALCULATIONS FOR BUSINESS (cont'd)

$

Gross profit and Net Profit

Gross Profit

The gross profit is the difference between the selling price and the acquisition cost. To calculate gross profit, no consideration is given for any expenses associated with filling the prescription.

Gross profit = Selling price – Acquisition cost

The gross profit can be expressed as a percent.

Example—Gross Profit

A prescription for amoxicillin 250 mg #30 has a selling price of $8.49. The acquisition cost of amoxicillin 250 mg #30 is $2.02.

Question: What is the gross profit?

Gross profit = Selling price – Acquisition cost
Gross profit = $8.49 – $2.02 = $6.47

Net Profit

The net profit is the difference between the selling price of the prescription and the sum of all the costs associated with filling the prescription. All the costs associated with filling the prescription include the cost of the medication, the cost of the container, the cost of the label, the cost of the bag, the cost of the labor to dispense the prescription, a portion of the rent, etc. For practical purposes, all the other costs can be grouped together and considered as a dispensing fee. Since the costs associated with operation of a pharmacy vary, the dispensing fee can vary.

Net profit = Selling price – Acquisition cost – Dispensing fee

or

Net profit = Gross profit – Dispensing fee

Net profit can also be expressed as a percent.

Example—Net Profit

A prescription for amoxicillin 250 mg #30 has a usual and customary price of $8.49. The acquisition cost of amoxicillin 250 mg #30 is $2.02.

Question: What is the net profit if the dispensing fee/professional fee is $5.50?

Net profit = Selling price – Acquisition cost – Dispensing fee
Net profit = $8.49 – $2.02 – $5.50 = $0.97

PRACTICE PROBLEMS—GROSS PROFIT AND NET PROFIT

Use this table to determine the dispensing/professional fee

AWP	Professional Fee
less than $20.00	$4.00
$20.01–$50.00	$5.00
$50.01 and higher	$6.00

and then calculate the gross profit and the net profit for the following prescriptions.

1. **Zocor® 5 mg, 60 tablets**
   acquisition cost = $85.47 AWP = $106.84 selling price = $109.93
   Gross profit = __________ Net profit = __________
2. **Prilosec® 20 mg, 30 cap.**
   acquisition cost = $99.20 AWP = $108.90 selling price = $116.38
   Gross profit = __________ Net profit = __________
3. **Norvasc® 5 mg, 90 tablets**
   acquisition cost = $97.92 AWP = $125.66 selling price = $117.82
   Gross profit = __________ Net profit = __________
4. **Procardia® XL 30 mg, 100 tab.**
   acquisition cost = $105.05 AWP = $131.31 selling price = $134.36
   Gross profit = __________ Net profit = __________
5. **Vasotec® 10 mg, 100 tab.**
   acquisition cost = $85.56 AWP = $102.94 selling price = $109.19
   Gross profit = __________ Net profit = __________
6. **Relafen® 500 mg, 100 tab.**
   acquisition cost = $88.88 AWP = $111.10 selling price = $120.27
   Gross profit = __________ Net profit = __________
7. **Zoloft® 50 mg, 100 tab.**
   acquisition cost = $172.44 AWP = $215.55 selling price = $226.50
   Gross profit = __________ Net profit = __________
8. **Fosamax® 10 mg, 30 tablets**
   acquisition cost = $50.91 AWP = $51.88 selling price = $57.62
   Gross profit = __________ Net profit = __________
9. **Cardizem CD® 240 mg, 90 tablets**
   acquisition cost = $154.10 AWP = $165.42 selling price = $179.69
   Gross profit = __________ Net profit = __________
10. **Ticlid® 250 mg, 60 tablets**
   acquisition cost = $99.44 AWP = $108.90 selling price = $122.07
   Gross profit = __________ Net profit = __________

REVIEW

PROBLEM SOLVING SUMMARY

Positional Notation Rules for Roman Numerals

1. When the second of two letters has a value equal to or larger than that of the first, their values are to be subtracted.
2. When the second of two letters has a value equal to or smaller than that of the first, their values are to be added.

Rules for Assigning Significant Figures

1. Digits other than zero are always significant.
2. Final zeros after a decimal point are always significant.
3. Zeros between two other significant digits are always significant.
4. Zeros used only to space the decimal are never significant.

Conditions for Using Ratio and Proportion

1. Three of the four values must be known.
2. Numerators must have the same units.
3. Denominators must have the same units.

Steps for Solving Proportion Problems

1. Define the variable and correct ratios.
2. Set up the proportion equation
3. Establish the x equation.
4. Solve for x.
5. Express solution in correct units.

Percent Solution Formula

$$\frac{x \text{ volume needed}}{\text{want } \%} = \frac{\text{volume prescribed}}{\text{have } \%}$$

Conversions

Liquid Metric

1 l	=	10 dl	=	1,000 ml
1 dl	=	0.1 l	=	100 ml
1 ml	=	0.001 l	=	0.01 dl

Solid Metric

1 kg	=	1,000 g		
1 g	=	0.001 kg	=	1,000 mg
1 mg	=	0.001 g	=	1,000 mcg
1 mcg	=	0.001 mg		

Avoirdupois

1 lb	=	16 oz
1 oz	=	437.5 gr
1 gr	=	64.8 mg (0.0648 g)

Apothecary

1 gal	=	4 qt
1 qt	=	2 pt
1 pt	=	16 fl oz
1 fl oz	=	8 fl dr
1 fl dr	=	60 m

Household

1 tsp	=	5 ml		
1 tbsp	=	3 tsp	=	15 ml
1 cup	=	8 fl oz		

Temperature

9°C = 5°F - 160

Conversions Between Systems

1 l	=	33.8 fl oz	1 lb	=	453.59 g
1 pt	=	473.167 ml	1 oz	=	28.35 g
1 fl oz	=	29.57 ml	1 g	=	15.43 gr
1 kg	=	2.2 lb	1 gr	=	64.8 mg

REVIEW

KEY CONCEPTS

NUMBERS

- ✔ The amount of a drug in its manufactured or prescribed form is always stated numerically—that is, with numbers.
- ✔ In pharmacy we use two different number systems: Arabic (such as 1, 1/2, 0.5, or 50%) and Roman (such as I, V, X, L, C, D, or M). Most of the time, Arabic numerals are used; however, sometimes Roman numeral are used in prescriptions.

FRACTIONS

- ✔ Fractions have numerators and denominators; the denominator of a fraction cannot be zero.
- ✔ Reciprocals are two different fractions that equal 1 when multiplied together.
- ✔ The least common denominator is needed when adding or subtracting fractions.

DECIMAL NUMBERS

- ✔ Decimal numbers are another way to express fractions.
- ✔ Calculations with decimal numbers can be less challenging than fractions with numerators and denominators.

SIGNIFICANT FIGURES

- ✔ When working with measured amounts, significant figures provide us with information about the sensitivity of equipment used.

MEASUREMENT

- ✔ Common systems of measurement in pharmacy include the metric, English, apothecary, and avoirdupois systems.
- ✔ The metric system is the primary system used in pharmacy.

EQUATIONS & VARIABLES

- ✔ Equations are used to calculate unknown amounts that are needed to fill prescriptions or calculate dosages.
- ✔ An equation is a mathematical statement in which two terms are equal.

RATIO & PROPORTION

- ✔ A ratio states the relationship between two quantities, while a proportion can be used when there are two equal ratios.
- ✔ Ratio and proportion is often used to determine a quantity that is needed to fill or prepare a prescription, especially for compounded medications.

PERCENTS & SOLUTIONS

- ✔ Percents can be used to indicate the amount or concentration of something in solution.
- ✔ The units for weight-to-volume percents are g/100 ml.
- ✔ The units for volume-to-volume percents are ml/100 ml.
- ✔ Milliequivalents are sometimes used for expressing the concentration in electrolyte solutions such as solutions containing potassium.

ALLIGATION

- ✔ Alligation is a way to solve problems associated with mixing two different strengths of the same ingredient to make a strength that is in between the two starting preparations.
- ✔ Once the alligation method is mastered, it becomes an easy and quick way to perform difficult calculations that involve mixing different strengths of the same ingredient.

POWDER VOLUME

- ✔ Some medications are provided to the pharmacy in powder form but are constituted by the pharmacy so they are dispensed in liquid form.
- ✔ The final volume of the constituted liquid is equal to the volume of the diluent plus the powder volume of the medication.

CHILDREN'S DOSES

- ✔ Clark's Rule, Young's Rule, and the Body Surface Area formula are formulas to calculate children's doses based on the adult dose.
- ✔ Dosing for children based on body weight is a preferred method when mg/kg dose information is known.

CALCULATIONS FOR BUSINESS

- ✔ Formulas based on a medication's acquisition cost and professional fee can be used to calculate what the selling price should be for a prescription.
- ✔ Gross profit and net profit calculations are important when considering the costs associated with a pharmacy business.

SELF TEST

the answer key begins on page 569

MATCH THE TERMS: I

1. body surface area ____
2. concentration _____
3. conversions ____
4. denominator ____
5. flow rate _____
6. least common denominator ____
7. milliequivalent (mEq) _____

a. the bottom (or right) number in a fraction; it indicates how many parts the whole is divided into.

b. the unit of measure for electrolytes in a solution.

c. the rate (in ml/hour or ml/minute) at which a solution is administered; also known as rate of administration.

d. smallest possible denominator for an equivalent fraction so that two fractions can be added or subtracted and have the same denominator.

e. the strength of a solution as measured by its weight-to-volume or volume-to-volume.

f. the change from one unit of measure to another so that both amounts are equal.

g. a measure for dosage calculated from the height and weight of a person and measured in square meters.

REVIEW

MATCH THE TERMS II

1. nomogram ____
2. numerator ____
3. positional notation ____
4. qs ad ____
5. total parenteral nutrition ____
6. valence ____
7. variable ____

a. a system used in Roman numerals whereby the position of a numeral signifies its value.
b. the top (or left) number in a fraction; it indicates how many parts of the whole exist.
c. an unknown value in a mathematical equation.
d. administration of all nutrients intravenously; also known as hyperalimentation.
e. adding a sufficient quantity of an ingredient to make the prescribed amount.
f. the number of positive or negative charges on an ion.
g. a chart showing relationships between measurements.

CHOOSE THE CORRECT ANSWER

1. The doctor orders 1/2 gr codeine. How many milligrams is this equivalent to?
   a. 16.2 mg
   b. 32.4 mg
   c. 64.8 mg
   d. 97.6 mg

2. If the temperature in the refrigerator is 45° Fahrenheit, to the nearest whole degree, what is the temperature in degrees Celsius?
   a. 5° Celsius
   b. 6° Celsius
   c. 7° Celsius
   d. 10° Celsius

3. A solution of halperidol (Haldol®) contains 2 mg/ml of active ingredient. How many grams would be in 240 ml of this solution?
   a. 4.8 grams
   b. 0.48 grams
   c. 0.048 grams
   d. 0.0048 grams

4. The physician orders ferrous sulfate 300 mg po qd. You have on the shelf ferrous sulfate 220 mg/5 ml. How many ml are required for one dose?
   a. 5.4 ml
   b. 8.4 ml
   c. 6.8 ml
   d. 13.4 ml

5. Using the information from the previous problem, approximately how many ml are required to fill this prescription for a 30 day supply?
   a. 162 ml
   b. 252 ml
   c. 205 ml
   d. 402 ml

6. What volume of solution that is 25 mg/ml should be measured to deliver a dose of 20 mg?
   a. 1.25 ml
   b. 0.8 ml
   c. 0.20 ml
   d. 0.25 ml

7. A patient is taking 2 teaspoonfuls of sucralfate suspension four times a day. How much suspension will the patient use in 72 hours?
   a. 3 oz
   b. 100 ml
   c. 4 oz
   d. 150 ml

8. Phos-Flur® rinse contains sodium fluoride 0.044% (w/v). How many mg of sodium fluoride are in a 10 ml dose?
   a. 0.044 mg
   b. 0.44 mg
   c. 4.4 mg
   d. 44 mg

9. If 0.44 mg of sodium fluoride is equal to 0.2 mg of fluoride, how many mg of fluoride are in 2.2 mg of sodium fluoride?
   a. 1 mg
   b. 2 mg
   c. 5 mg
   d. 20 mg

10. You have an ampule of digoxin injection that contains 500 mcg in 2 ml. What volume is needed to deliver a dose of 0.125 mg?
    a. 0.124 ml
    b. 0.25 ml
    c. 0.5 ml
    d. 0.75 m

11. The doctor changes a prescription for 150 ml of amoxicillin 250 mg/5 ml to 250 mg chewable tablets. How many chewable tablets should be dispensed?
    a. 15 tablets
    b. 30 tablets
    c. 45 tablets
    d. 60 tablets

12. If the dose of a drug is 500 mg and the drug is available as 400 mg/5 ml, how many teaspoonfuls are needed for the required dose?
    a. 1.25 teaspoonfuls
    b. 2.5 teaspoonfuls
    c. 4 tcaspoonfuls
    d. 5 teaspoonfuls

13. How many tablets should be dispensed if a prescription is written as follows:
    Tabs iss b.i.d. for 10 days
    a. 10 tablets
    b. 15 tablets
    c. 30 tablets
    d. 45 tablets

14. How many ounces of medication are needed to last eight days if the dose of medication is one and one-half teaspoonfuls four times a day?
    a. 4 oz
    b. 6 oz
    c. 8 oz
    d. 12 oz

REVIEW

15. How many 4 oz bottles can be filled from a gallon of Coke™ Syrup?
    a. 32 bottles
    b. 48 bottles
    c. 64 bottles
    d. 72 bottles

16. You receive a prescription for metronidazole (Flagyl®) 250 mg/5 ml po qid 240 ml. You find that you will have to compound this using 500 mg tablets. How many tablets will be needed to fill this order completely?
    a. 22 tablets
    b. 24 tablets
    c. 42 tablets
    d. 48 tablets

17. How much hydrocortisone powder is needed to compound 60 g of hydrocortisone cream 1%?
    a. 0.6 mg
    b. 600 mg
    c. 0.06 g
    d. 6 mg

18. You are asked by the pharmacist to add 45 mEq of Ca gluconate in an IV bag of D5%W 1,000 ml. You have a concentrated vial of Ca gluconate 4.4 mEq/ml 50 ml. How many ml of this concentrated vial needs to be added to the IV bag?
    a. 1.2 ml
    b. 10.2 ml
    c. 0.12 ml
    d. 2.4 ml

19. An IV contains 5 mg of drug per ml and the patient needs to receive 50 mg per hour. What is the infusion rate in ml/hr?
    a. 5 ml/hr
    b. 10 ml/hr
    c. 16.7 ml/hr
    d. 0.167 ml/hr

20. The infusion rate of an IV is over 12 hours. The total volume is 1,000 ml. What would the infusion rate be in ml per minute?
    a. 83.3 ml/minute
    b. 8.3 ml/minute
    c. 16.7 ml/minute
    d. 1.4 ml/minute

21. You receive an order for vancomycin (Vancocin®) 10 mg/kg 500 ml to be infused over 90 minutes. The patient is five foot eleven inches tall and weighs 165 lb. What dose is needed for this patient?
    a. 750 mg
    b. 500 mg
    c. 250 mg
    d. 125 mg

22. A child's dose for cefadroxil is 30 mg/kg body weight once a day for 14 days. What is the smallest bottle that will provide enough medication to last 14 days if the child weighs 44 pounds?
    a. 50 ml bottle of 125 mg/5 ml
    b. 50 ml bottle of 250 mg/5 ml
    c. 75 ml bottle of 500 mg/5 ml
    d. 100 ml bottle of 500 mg/5 ml

23. You have a 70% solution of dextrose 1,000 ml. How many kg of dextrose is in 400 ml of this solution?

    a. 280 kg
    b. 28 kg
    c. 2.8 kg
    d. 0.28 kg

24. You have diluted 40 ml of a 50% dextrose solution with water so the volume of the resulting solution is 100 ml. What is the concentration of dextrose in the resulting solution?

    a. 12%
    b. 20%
    c. 24%
    d. 40%

25. How many ml of 70% alcohol should be mixed with 20% alcohol to prepare 50 ml of 50% alcohol?

    a. 20 ml
    b. 30 ml
    c. 40 ml
    d. 50 ml

26. How many grams of 1% hydrocortisone cream should be mixed with 2.5% hydrocortisone cream to make 15 grams of 2% hydrocortisone cream?

    a. 2 g
    b. 5 g
    c. 10 g
    d. 13 g

27. The mixing instructions for a liquid antibiotic call for 45 ml of water for constitution to make a 150 ml suspension. The final concentration of the suspension is 250 mg/5 ml. What is the powder volume?

    a. 45 ml
    b. 90 ml
    c. 105 ml
    d. 205 ml

28. What is the cost for 30 tablets of a drug if the cost for 100 tablets is $75?

    a. $19.65
    b. $21.83
    c. $22.50
    d. $24.23

29. The retail price for a prescription is $37.50. What amount should be charged if the patient is to receive a 10% discount?

    a. $34.50
    b. $34.00
    c. $33.75
    d. $31.95

REVIEW

CONVERT THE FOLLOWING:

1. 5 g	=	_____	mg	6. 102 kg	=	_____	lb
2. 10 kg	=	_____	g	7. 2.2 kg	=	_____	g
3. 300 ml	=	_____	l	8. 473 ml	=	_____	l
4. 600 mg	=	_____	g	9. 145 lb	=	_____	kg
5. 120 mcg	=	_____	mg	10. 0.01 kg	=	_____	mg

SOLVE THE FOLLOWING PROBLEMS IN THE SPACE PROVIDED

1. Oral polio virus vaccine (Poliovax®) should be stored in a temperature not to exceed 46° Fahrenheit. What is this temperature in Celsius?

2. A prescription reads for erythromycin 100 mg every six hours for ten days. You have on hand erythromycin 250 mg/5 ml. How much erythromycin is needed for one dose?

3. You have an IV that needs $MgSO_4$ (magnesium sulfate) 10 mEq. You have on hand a bottle of $MgSO_4$ 4 mEq/ml. How much $MgSO_4$ do you need to inject into this IV bag?

4. You have an order for 20% dextrose 500 ml. You have a 1000 ml bag of dextrose 70%. How much of the dextrose 70% do you need to use to make dextrose 20% 500 ml? How much sterile water do you need?

CRITICAL THINKING QUESTIONS

1. Discuss reasons why pharmacy technicians need to perform calculations using the metric system.
2. Discuss reasons why electrolytes are dosed in mEq.
3. Discuss reasons why special care is needed when performing calculations for children's medications.

THINKING IT THROUGH WRAP-UP

1. Calculations to determine the amount of medications needed to fill a prescription, calculations to determine how long medications will last, and calculations to determine the cost of medications are three of the most common types of calculations in community pharmacies.
2. Calculations to determine the amount of medications needed to fill a medication order are very common in the hospital environment. Additionally, pharmacy technicians need to perform careful calculations when preparing intravenous medications.
3. There is no room for error when preparing medications for prescriptions or medication orders. Appropriate amounts of medications are critical to obtain the desired effects. Also, toxicity and even death can result if there is a miscalculation leading to an overdose.

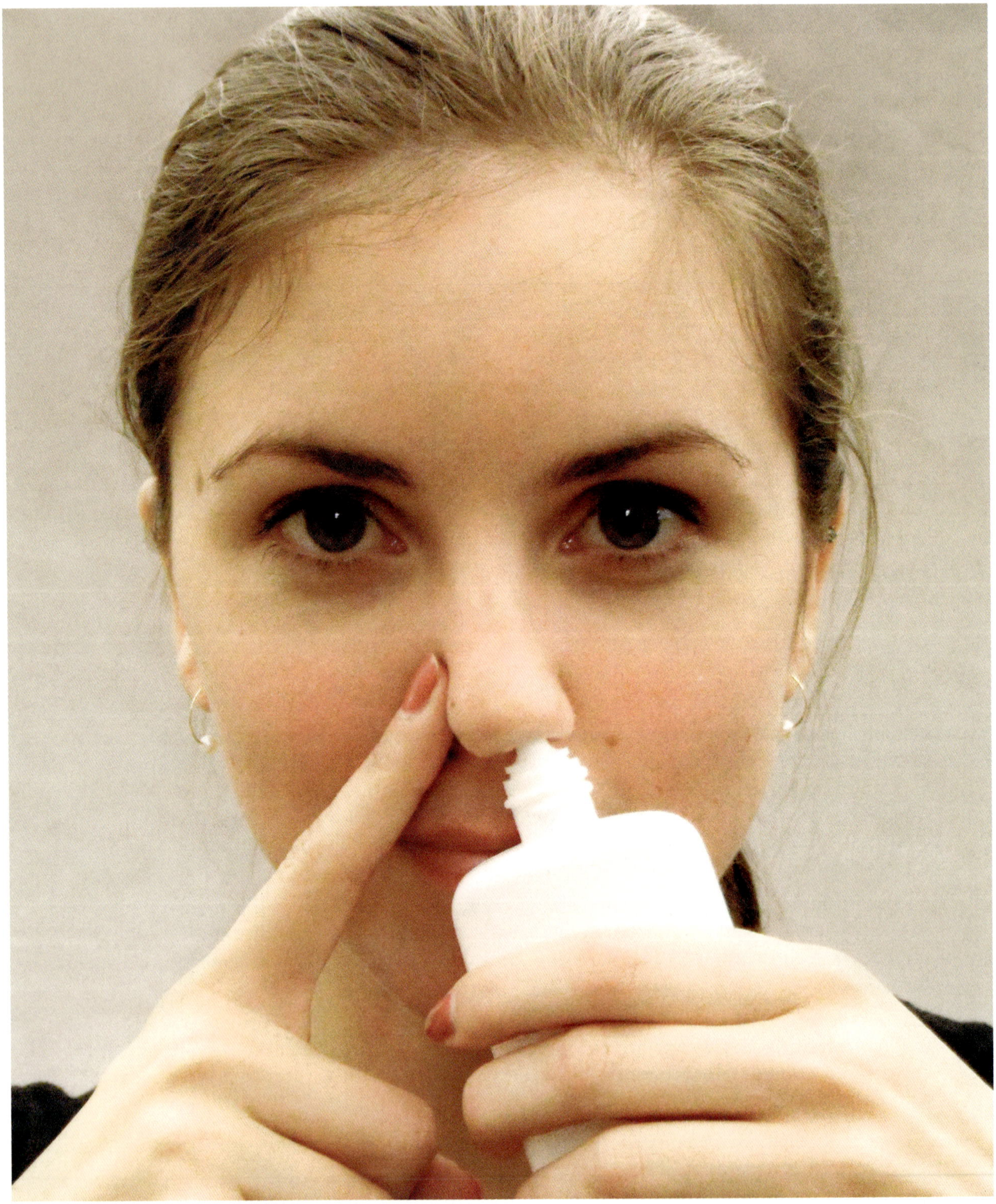

7

ROUTES & FORMULATIONS

LEARNING OBJECTIVES

At the completion of study, the student will:

- ✔ distinguish between enteral and parenteral routes of administration.
- ✔ know the common dosage forms used in enteral and parenteral routes of administration.
- ✔ understand the unique characteristics or limitations of dosage forms used in enteral and parenteral routes of administration.

THINKING IT THROUGH

There are different routes of administration and there are different drug formulations. But not all drug formulations are manufactured for all routes of administration. For example, many neonatal solutions are dosed orally, but an oral solution of a given drug may not be available from the manufacturer.

Suppose you are a technician for the afternoon shift in a hospital's special care nursery and are responsible for drawing up neonatal solution doses. You need to prepare oral caffeine citrate for Babygirl Stone. There is no manufactured oral solution product of caffeine citrate, but there is an intravenous solution product in the IV room.

As you read through this chapter, think about the following questions:

1. Can you substitute an intravenous solution for an oral solution?
2. If you were to give an intravenous solution of caffeine citrate orally, would you expect the caffeine absorption to be different than if you used an oral solution?
3. If the situation were reversed and you had only the oral version of the product but needed to give it intravenously, should you do that?

ROUTES & FORMULATIONS

The way in which the body absorbs and distributes drugs varies with the route of administration and the dosage form used.

Drugs are contained in dosing units called formulations or dosage forms. There are many dosage forms and many different routes of administration.

Routes of administration are classified as enteral or parenteral.

Enteral refers to anything involving the alimentary tract, i.e., from the mouth to the rectum. This tract is involved with digesting foods, absorbing nutrients, and eliminating unabsorbed wastes. There are four enteral routes of administration: oral, sublingual, buccal, and rectal.

Any route other than oral, sublingual, buccal, or rectal is considered a parenteral route.

The term parenteral means next to, or beside, the enteral. It refers to any sites of administration that are outside of or beside the alimentary tract.

For each route of administration, there are various formulations used to deliver the drug via that route.

Different dosage forms affect onset times, duration of action, or concentrations of a drug in the body. Some drugs are formulated in more than one dosage form, each of which has different characteristics. A consideration for selecting a particular route of administration or dosage form is the type of effect desired. A *local effect* occurs when the drug activity is at the site of administration (e.g., eyes, ears, nose, skin). A *systemic effect* occurs when the drug is introduced into the circulatory system from the route of administration and carried by the blood to the site of activity.

local effect when drug activity is at the site of administration.

systemic effect when a drug is introduced into the venous (circulatory) system and carried to the site of activity.

DOSAGE FORMS

Enteral Route	Dosage Form
Oral	Tablets Capsules Bulk powders Solutions Suspensions Elixirs Syrups Emulsions
Buccal	Tablets Solutions
Sublingual	Tablets Lozenges
Rectal	Solutions Ointments Suppositories

Parenteral Route	Dosage Form
Intraocular	Solutions Suspensions Ointments Inserts
Intranasal	Solutions Suspensions Ointments Gels
Inhalation	Solutions Aerosols Powders
Intravenous **Intramuscular** **Intradermal**	Solutions Suspensions Colloids Emulsions
Dermal	Solutions Tinctures Collodions Liniments Suspensions Ointments Creams Gels

ROUTES OF ADMINISTRATION

Enteral Routes are in red. Parenteral routes are in blue.
The term is followed by the organ(s) of absorption.

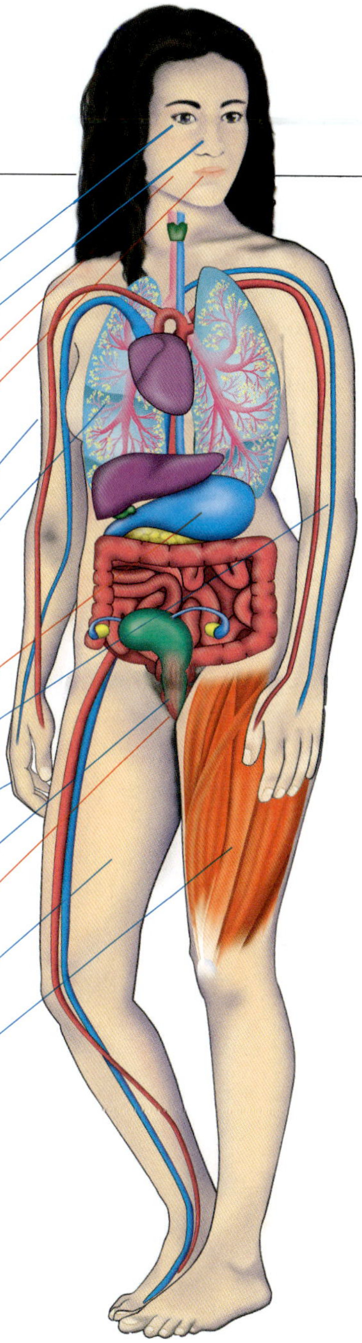

Intraocular	Eye
Intranasal	Nose
Buccal	Inside the cheek
Sublingual	Under the tongue
Dermal	Through or on the skin*
Inhalation	Lungs
Oral	Stomach and intestine
Intravenous	Venous circulatory system
Intradermal	Dermal layer of the skin*
Vaginal	Vagina
Rectal	Rectum
Subcutaneous	Subcutaneous layer of the skin*
Intramuscular	Muscle*

**this route has various administration sites*

Parenteral Route	Dosage Form
Dermal (cont'd)	Lotions Pastes Plasters Powders Aerosols Transdermal patches
Subcutaneous	Solutions Suspensions Emulsions Implants
Vaginal	Solutions Ointments Creams

Parenteral Route	Dosage Form
Vaginal (cont'd)	Aerosol foams Powders Suppositories Tablets IUDs

ORAL FORMULATIONS

Oral administration is the most frequently used route of administration.

Oral dosage forms are easy to carry, use, and administer. The term used to specify oral administration is peroral or PO (per os). This indicates that the dosage form is to be swallowed and that absorption will occur primarily from the stomach and the intestine.

When formulations are orally administered, they enter the stomach, which is very acidic.

The stomach has a ***pH*** around 1–2. Certain drugs cannot be taken orally because they are degraded (chemically changed to a less effective form) or destroyed by stomach acid and intestinal enzymes. Additionally, the absorption of many drugs is affected by the presence of food in the stomach.

Drugs administered in liquid dosage forms generally reach the circulatory system faster than drugs formulated in solid dosage forms.

This is because the processes of ***disintegration*** and ***dissolution*** are not required. Oral liquids include solutions, suspensions, gels, and emulsions. Solid oral dosage forms include tablets, capsules, and bulk powders.

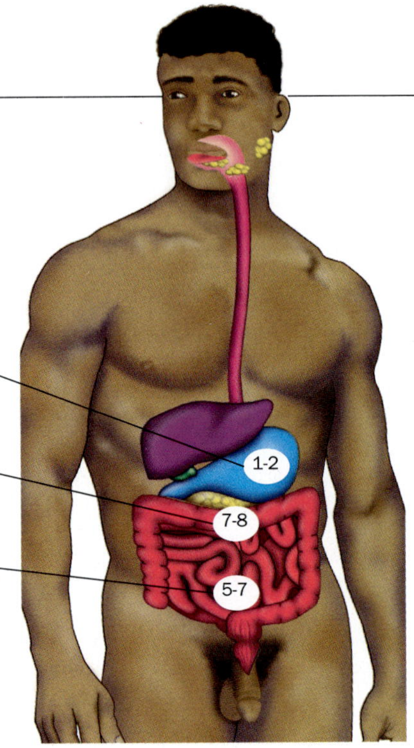

gastrointestinal organs and their pH

Gastrointestinal Action

The disintegration and dissolution of tablets, capsules, and powders generally begins in the stomach, but will continue to occur when the stomach content empties into the intestine. Enteric coated tablets are used when the drug can be degraded by the stomach acid. The enteric coating will not let the tablet disintegrate until it reaches the higher pHs of the small intestine.

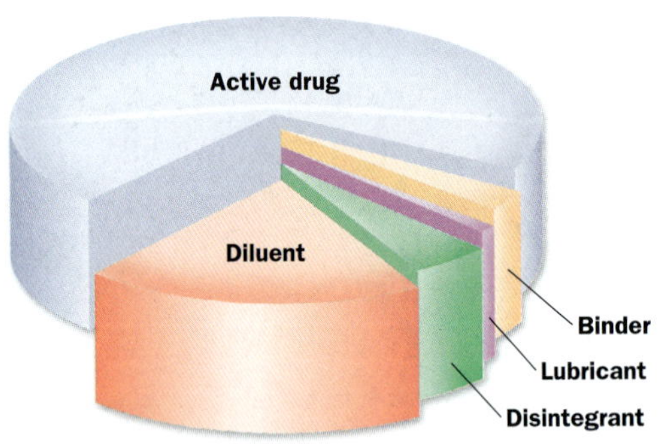

Inactive Ingredients

Oral formulations contain various ingredients besides the active drug. These include binders, lubricants, fillers, diluents, and disintegrants. They are added to help manufacture the formulation and to help the dosage form disintegrate and dissolve when administered. A sample breakdown of ingredients is illustrated at right. (Note, however, that the breakdown for each formulation is different.)

disintegration the breaking apart of a tablet into smaller pieces.

dissolution when the smaller pieces of a disintegrated tablet dissolve in solution.

pH the pH scale measures the acidity or the opposite *(alkalinity)* of a substance. Seven is the neutral midpoint of the scale, values below which represent increasing acidity, and above which represent increasing alkalinity.

Rx tip
Most oral dosage forms are intended for systemic effect, but not all. For example, antacids have a local effect confined to the gastrointestinal tract.

SOLID FORMULATIONS

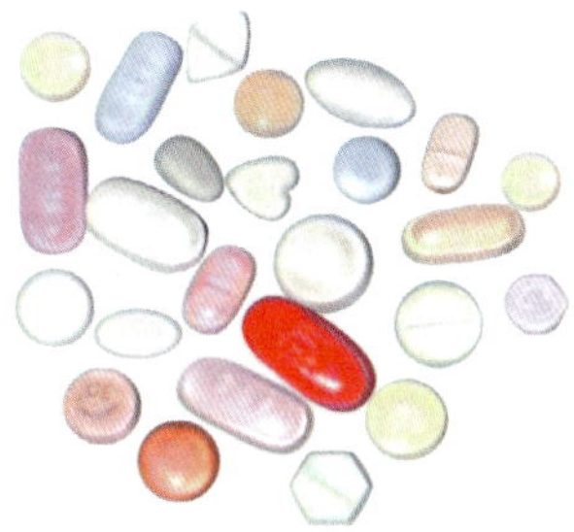

Tablets are hard formulations in which the drug and other ingredients are machine compressed under high pressure into a shape. Tablets vary in size, weight, hardness, thickness, and disintegration and dissolution characteristics, depending upon their intended use. Most tablets are manufactured for oral use, and many are coated on the formulation to give an identifying color or logo. Sugar-coated tablets are coated with a sweet glaze. Film-coated tablets are coated with a non-sweet coating. Multiple compressed tablets contain one drug in an inner layer and another drug (or the same drug) compressed at a lower pressure around it as an outer layer. A multiple compressed tablet can also have the two layers adjacent to each other. Repeat action tablets initially release one dose of the drug and then release a second dose sometime later. Other popular tablets are chewable and effervescent.

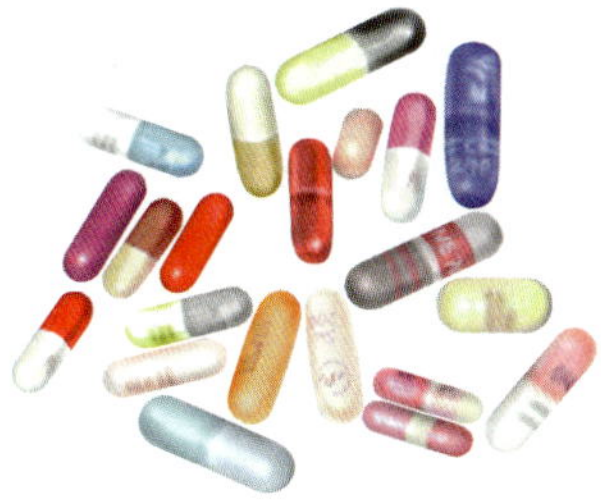

Capsules contain the drug and the other ingredients packaged in a gelatin shell. There are several capsule sizes. The capsule size used in any formulation is based on the amount of material to be placed inside the capsule. The gelatin shell dissolves in the stomach and releases the contents of the capsule. The freed contents must still undergo disintegration and dissolution before the drug is absorbed into the circulatory system. There are some capsule formulations that contain liquid instead of powders inside the gelatin shell; these are called "soft" or "soft-gel" capsules. The active drug is already dissolved in the liquid.

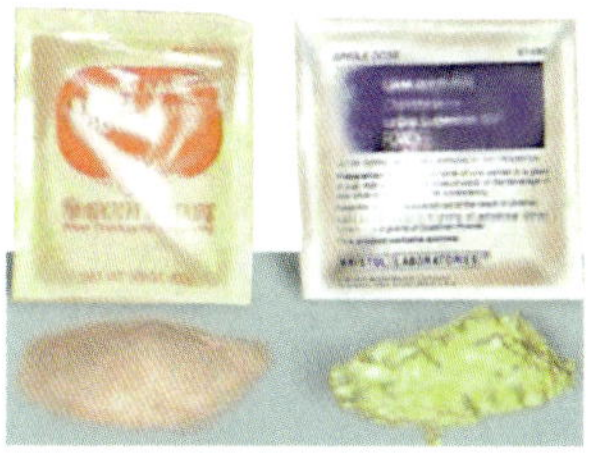

Bulk powders (e.g., Goody's BC powders) contain the active drug in a small powder paper or foil envelope. The patient empties the envelope into a glass of water or juice and drinks the contents. Most of the drug and ingredients dissolve in the water before the patient takes it.

MODIFIED RELEASE FORMULATIONS

Several oral formulations release the drug so that a longer duration of action is achieved compared to a conventional tablet, capsule, or powder. These are called modified release drug products. The primary goal of these products is to reduce the number of doses a patient needs to take during a day (i.e., reduce the frequency of dosing). Some modified release products also control the blood concentrations of the drug better than conventional dosage forms.

Through the years, many terms have been used to identify these kinds of products. Examples include sustained release (SR), sustained action (SA), extended release (ER or XR), prolonged action (PA), controlled or continuous release (CR), time release (TR), and long acting (LA).

ORAL FORMULATIONS (cont'd)

LIQUID FORMULATIONS

Solutions

A ***solution*** is a clear, not necessarily colorless, liquid made up of one or more ingredients dissolved in a solvent. A solvent is a liquid that can dissolve another substance to form a solution.

Aqueous solutions are the most common kind of oral solution. ***Aqueous*** means that water was used as the solvent.

Nonaqueous solutions are those solutions that predominately contain solvents other than water, either alone or in addition to water. Only a few nonaqueous solvents such as glycerin, alcohol, and propylene glycol can be used in oral solutions.

Syrups are concentrated or nearly saturated solutions of sucrose (i.e., sugar) in water. They are more viscous (thicker) than water, and contain less than 10% alcohol. Syrups containing flavoring agents are known as flavoring syrups (e.g., Wild Cherry Syrup), and medicinal syrups are those that contain drugs (e.g., Guaifenesin Syrup).

Elixirs are clear, sweetened, hydroalcoholic liquids intended for oral use. They can contain either alcohol soluble or water soluble drugs. Elixirs are usually less sweet and less viscous than syrups, and are generally less effective in masking taste. Their alcohol content ranges from 5–40% (10–80 proof), though a few commercial elixirs contain no alcohol.

Spirits or **essences** are alcoholic or hydroalcoholic solutions of volatile substances (usually volatile oils) with alcohol contents ranging from 62–85% (124–170 proof). They are most frequently used as flavoring agents (e.g., Peppermint Spirit) but some spirits are used for their medicinal effect.

Tinctures are alcoholic or hydroalcoholic solutions of nonvolatile substances. Tinctures of potent drugs have 10 grams of the drug in each 100 ml of tincture; they are called 10% tinctures. Nonpotent tinctures generally have 20 grams of the drug per 100 ml of tincture.

Suspensions

Suspensions are formulations in which the drug does not completely dissolve in the solvent. The drug particles are suspended in the formulation. Since they are intended for oral administration, suspensions are sweetened and flavored.

The primary concern in formulating suspensions is that they tend to settle over time, leading to a lack of dose uniformity. A well-formulated suspension will remain suspended or settle very slowly, and can be easily redispersed with shaking.

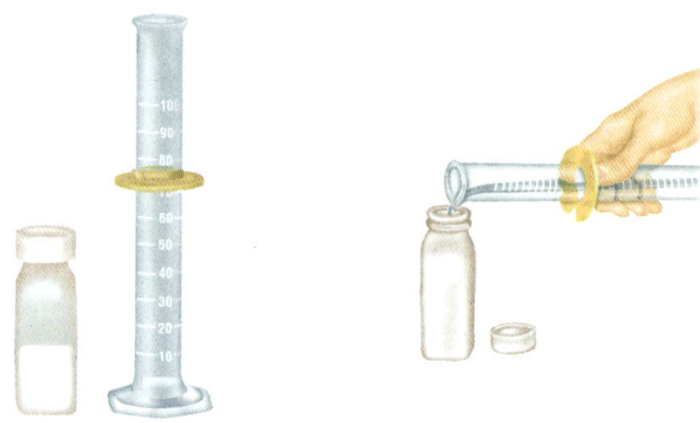

Some commercial suspensions are packaged as lyophilized powder. The suspension is made by adding water to the container. This process is called reconstitution.

Advantages of Solutions	Disadvantages of Solutions
➥ Completely homogenous doses	➥ Drugs and chemicals are less stable in solution than in dry dosage forms.
➥ Immediately available for absorption	➥ Some drugs are not soluble in solvents that are acceptable for therapeutic use.
➥ For patients who cannot swallow tablets or capsules	➥ May require special additives or techniques to mask objectionable taste.
➥ Doses can be easily adjusted	➥ More difficult to handle, transport, and store because of bulk and weight.
	➥ Solutions in bulk containers require dosage measurement devices.

aqueous water based.

solution a clear liquid made up of one or more substances dissolved in a solvent.

Emulsions

It is well known that "oil and water don't mix." Yet, some formulations contain both aqueous and oleaginous (oil based) components. These two non-mixable components can be formulated into a homogenous mixture when an emulsifying agent (***emulsifier***) is used. Emulsifiers dispense one of the components into the other in the form of tiny droplets or globules. If the oleaginous component is present as droplets, the ***emulsion*** is called an oil-in-water (o/w) emulsion. If the aqueous component is present as droplets, the emulsion is called a water-in-oil (w/o) emulsion.

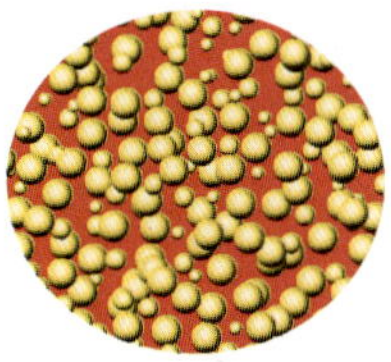

droplets in an emulsion

Emulsions are used in many routes of administration. Oral administration can be used, but patients generally object to the oily feel of emulsions in the mouth. But sometimes emulsions are the formulation of choice to mask the taste of a very bitter drug or when the oral solubility or bioavailability of a drug is to be dramatically increased. More typically, emulsions are used for topical administration as creams, lotions, or ointment bases.

Emulsions used for oral administration are physically unstable and tend to separate into two distinct phases over time. Creaming occurs when dispersed droplets merge and rise to the top or fall to the bottom of the emulsion. A creamed emulsion can be easily redispersed by shaking. Coalescence (breaking or cracking) is the irreversible separation of the dispersed phase.

Gels

Gels are made using substances called gelling agents that increase the viscosity of the medium in which they are placed. The gelling agents form an interlacing three-dimensional network of particles that restricts the movement of the solvent. Gelling agents are most often added as an ingredient to liquid formulations.

There are many gelling agents. Some of the common ones are acacia, alginic acid, Carbopols® (now known as carbomers), gelatin, methylcellulose, tragacanth, and xanthan gum. Though each gelling agent has some unique properties, there are some generalizations that can be made.

- Most gelling agents require 12–24 hours to reach maximum viscosity and clarity.
- Gelling agents are used in concentrations of 0.5% up to 10%, depending on the agent.
- It is easier to add the active drug before the gel is formed, if the drug doesn't interfere with the gel formation.
- Only Carbopol® 934P, methylcellulose, hydroxypropylmethyl cellulose, and sodium caboxymethyl cellulose are recommended for oral administration.

emulsifier a stabilizing agent in emulsions.

emulsions mixture of two liquids that do not mix with each other in which one liquid is dispersed through the other by using a stabilizer called an emulsifier.

Advantages of Suspensions	Disadvantages of Suspensions
Can orally administer drugs that are insoluble in acceptable solvents	Tend to settle over time, leading to a lack of dose uniformity
Can be taken or administered to patients who cannot swallow tablets or capsules	Unpleasant oral texture
Masks objectionable taste of some drugs	
Drugs are chemically more stable than in solution	

SUBLINGUAL & BUCCAL

The mouth is the route of administration for certain drugs when a rapid action is desired.

Formulations used in the mouth are generally fast dissolving uncoated tablets that contain highly ***water soluble*** drugs. These tablets are placed under the tongue (***sublingual*** administration). When the drug is released from the tablet, it is quickly absorbed into the circulatory system since the membranes lining the mouth are very thin and there is a rich blood supply to the mouth.

Nitroglycerin is the best known example of a sublingual tablet formulation.

Nitroglycerin is sublingually administered since it is degraded in the stomach and intestine. Nitroglycerin is also available in a translingual aerosol that permits a patient to spray droplets of nitroglycerin under the tongue. There are also some steroid sex hormones that are sublingually administered.

Sublingual administration has certain limitations.

For instance, the bitter taste of most drugs makes holding a tablet in the mouth for almost any period of time unpleasant, so lozenges, which are generally formulated with sweetening agents, are sometimes used instead of tablets for sublingual administration. For various reasons (including the condition of the mouth, the patient, etc.), other routes of administration are considered more convenient for many drugs that would otherwise be candidates for sublingual administration.

The *buccal* cavity is also in the mouth and refers to the insides of the cheek and on the tongue.

Buccal tablets and lozenges are placed in the pouch between the cheeks and the teeth to dissolve. Rapidly dissolving tablets or strips such as M-Tab® and orally disintegrating tablets dissolve when placed on the tongue; they use only the moisture in the mouth so the patient does not have to drink a liquid to take it. Like the sublingual administration route, the buccal cavity allows for rapid absorption of drugs and bypasses first-pass metabolism in the liver.

Using Sublingual Tablets

Sublingual tablets are highly water soluble, so patients should first take a sip of water to wet their mouth if it is dry.

The tablet is then placed far under the tongue and the mouth is closed and must remain closed until the tablet dissolves and is absorbed. No food or beverages should be placed in the mouth until the drug is fully absorbed.

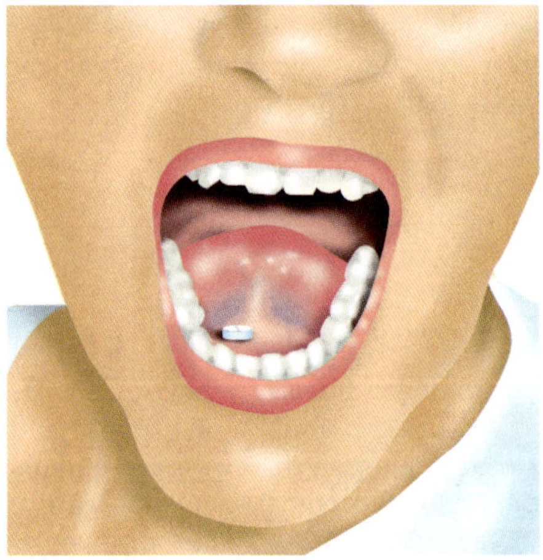

Rx tip

Like many medical terms, *sub*, *trans*, and *lingua* are Latin words. They mean under, across or over, and tongue, respectively.

buccal pouch between the teeth and cheek in the mouth.

sublingual under the tongue.

water soluble the property of a substance being able to dissolve in water.

RECTAL

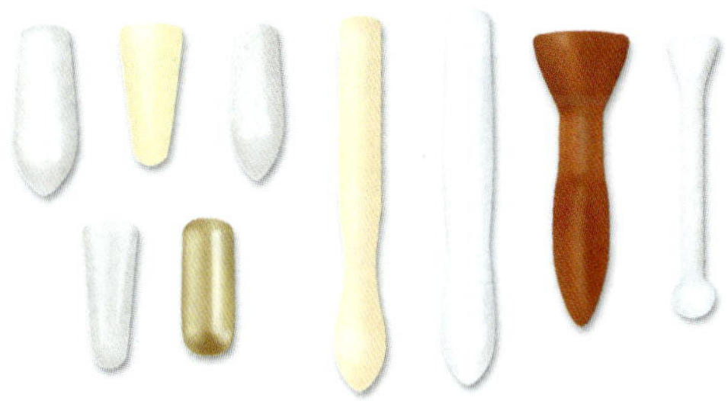

various suppository sizes and shapes

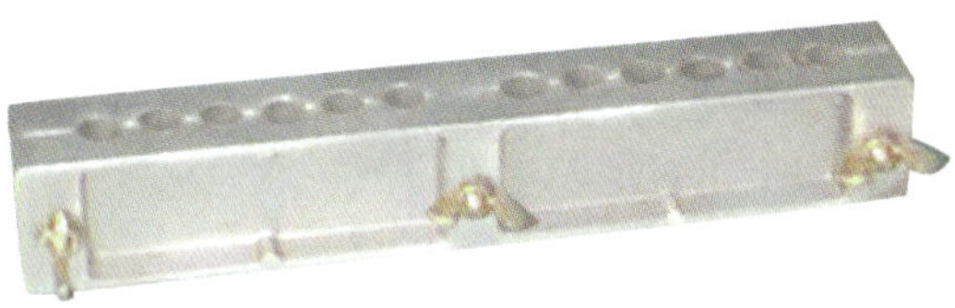

aluminum mold for making suppositories

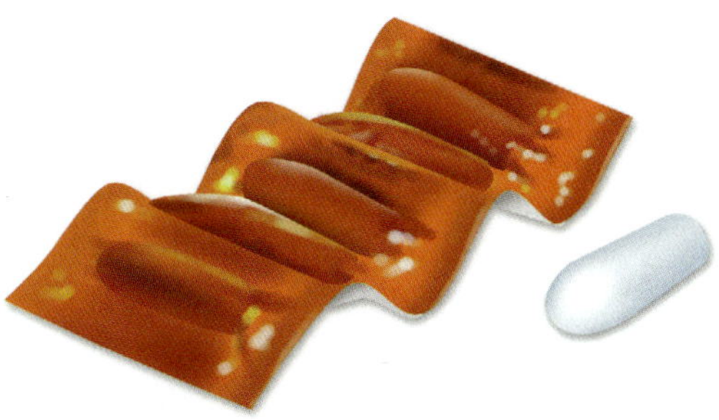

suppository in plastic mold

Drugs are administered via the rectum either for a local effect or to avoid degradation after oral administration.

Local effects may include the soothing of inflamed *hemorrhoidal* tissues or promoting laxation. Rectal administration for systemic activity is preferred when the drug is degraded by stomach acid or intestinal enzymes, or if oral administration is unavailable (if the patient is vomiting, unconscious, or incapable of swallowing oral formulations). Rectal administration is used to achieve a variety of systemic effects, including asthma control, anti-nausea, motion sickness, and anti-infective therapy.

The most common rectal administration dosage forms are suppositories, solutions, and ointments.

Suppositories are semisolid dosage forms that dissolve or melt when inserted into the rectum. Suppositories are manufactured in a variety of shapes and are also used in other routes of administration such as vaginal or urethral. Most rectal solutions are used as enemas or cleansing solutions. Rectal ointments are intended to be spread around the anal opening and are most often used to treat inflamed hemorrhoidal tissues.

Rectal dosage forms have significant disadvantages.

They are not preferred by most patients. They are inconvenient. Moreover, rectal absorption of most drugs is frequently erratic and unpredictable.

Enemas

Enemas create an urge to defecate due to the placement of fluid into the rectum. A cleansing enema uses water or a cleansing solution. A retention enema uses an oil that is held in the rectum to soften the stool. Frequent use of enemas is discouraged because it can have significant adverse effects.

hemorrhoid painful swollen veins in the anal/rectal area, generally caused by strained bowel movements from hard stools.

PARENTERAL ROUTES

Parenteral routes of administration are used for a variety of reasons.

If an orally administered drug is poorly absorbed, or is degraded by stomach acid or intestinal enzymes, then a parenteral route may be indicated. Some parenteral routes are also preferred when a rapid drug response is desired, as in an emergency situation. Parenteral routes of administration are also useful when a patient is uncooperative, unconscious, or otherwise unable to take a drug by an enteral route.

There are disadvantages to giving formulations by parenteral routes.

One is cost. Many parenterals are more expensive than enteral route formulations. Another is that many parenterals require skilled personnel to administer them. A third disadvantage is that once a parenteral drug is administered, it is most difficult to remove the dose if there is an adverse or toxic reaction. Finally, some types of parenteral administration have risks associated with invading the body with a needle (e.g., infection, thrombus, etc.).

Injection dependent parenteral routes require a needle and some type of propelling device (syringe, pump) to administer a drug.

The injectable routes are intravenous, intramuscular, intradermal, subcutaneous, epidural, and intrathecal. The formulations for these routes have several characteristics in common: They are limited to solutions, suspensions, and emulsions because any other dosage formulation cannot pass through a syringe; they must be ***sterile*** (bacteria-free) since they are placed in direct contact with the internal body fluids or tissues where infection can easily occur; the pH of the formulation must be carefully maintained, usually by adding ingredients to create a ***buffer system***; and only limited volumes can be injected since too much volume can cause pain and increased cell death (***necrosis***).

PARENTERAL ROUTES OF ADMINISTRATION

Injection Independent

ophthalmic
intranasal
inhalation
dermal
vaginal
otic

Injection Dependent

intravenous
intramuscular
intradermal
subcutaneous
epidural
intrathecal

Route of Administration	Needle Gauge	Needle Length
Intravenous (IV)	16–20	1–1.5″
Intramuscular (IM)	19–22	1–1.5″
Subcutaneous (SC)	24–27	3/8–1″
Intradermal (ID)	25–26	3/8″

syringe needle recommendations for injection dependent routes of administration

buffer system ingredients in a formulation designed to control the pH.

necrosis increase in cell death.

sterile a sterile condition is one which is free of *all* microorganisms, both harmful and harmless.

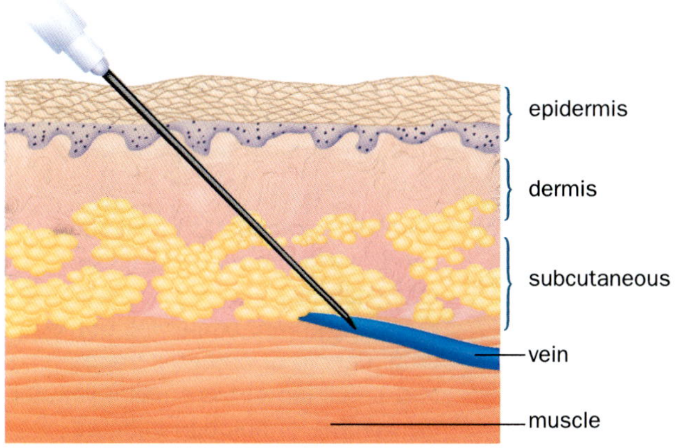

Intravenous

Intravenous injections are administered directly into veins. They may be large volume, slow infusions with aqueous solutions such as D5W (dextrose 5% in water) or NS (0.9% sodium chloride in water), or small volume single injections (e.g., furosemide, metoprolol, or morphine). Fat emulsions, blood transfusions, and patient-controlled analgesia (PCA) solutions are also intravenously administered.

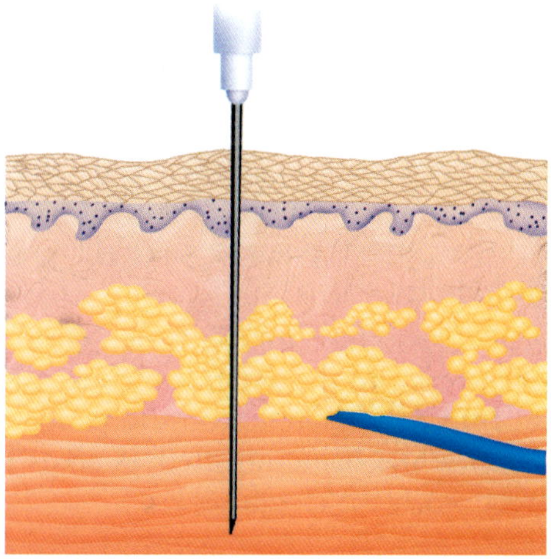

Intramuscular

Intramuscular injections are administered into muscle tissue and generally result in a slower onset but longer duration of action compared to IV administration. Drugs that can be given by IM administration include haloperidol, prochlorperazine, iron dextran, olanzapine, ziprasidone, and metoclopramide.

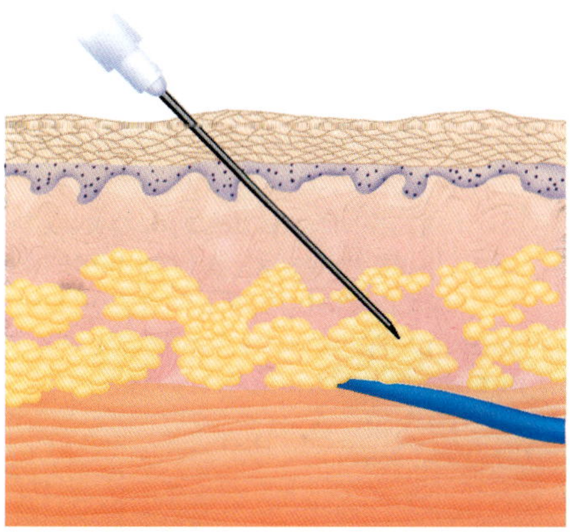

Subcutaneous

Subcutaneous injections are administered into the subcutaneous tissue of the skin. Subcutaneous administration generally provides slower absorption compared to IM administration, but faster absorption compared to oral administration. It is also the preferred route of administration for implants. Common drugs given by SC administration include the insulins, heparin, enoxaparin, and several vaccines.

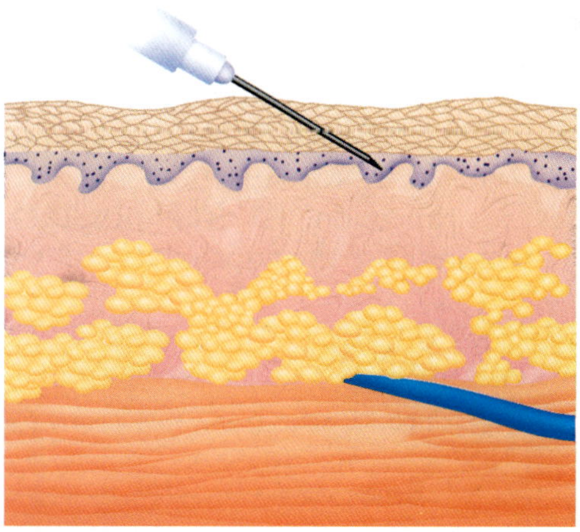

Intradermal

Intradermal injections are administered into the top layer of the skin at a slight angle using short needles. Most of the drugs administered by this route are for diagnostic determinations, desensitization, or immunization.

INTRAVENOUS FORMULATIONS

Intravenous dosage forms are administered directly into a vein and therefore directly into the circulating blood.

It takes about 20 seconds for intravenously administered drugs to circulate throughout the body. Solutions are the most common intravenously administered formulations. Most solutions are aqueous, but they may also have glycols, alcohols, or other nonaqueous solvents in them.

Injectable suspensions are difficult to formulate because they must possess suitable syringeability and injectability.

Syringeability refers to the ease with which the suspension can be drawn from a container into a syringe. ***Injectability*** refers to the properties of the suspension while being injected, such as flow evenness, freedom from clogging, etc.

Emulsions are formulations that contain both aqueous and nonaqueous (oil) components.

Fat emulsions in total parenteral nutrition (TPN) solutions are used to provide triglycerides, fatty acids, and calories for patients who cannot absorb them from the gastrointestinal tract.

Dry powder formulations are manufactured for intravenous use, but must be reconstituted with a suitable diluent to make a liquid formulation.

Many drugs that are not stable in liquid form can be lyophilized (freeze-dried) into a powder. The powder is reconstituted just prior to use with a solvent called a ***diluent***. The most common diluents are Sterile Water for Injection and Bacteriostatic Water for Injection. A drug product's package insert will indicate the appropriate diluent to use.

COMPLICATIONS

There are a number of complications that can occur from intravenous administration such as thrombus formation, phlebitis, air emboli, and particulate material.

- Thrombus (blood clot) formation can result from many factors: extremes in solution pH, particulate material, irritant properties of the drug, needle or catheter trauma, and selection of too small a vein for the volume of solution injected.
- Phlebitis, or inflammation of the vein, can be caused by the same factors that cause thrombosis.
- Air emboli occur when air is introduced into the vein. The human body is generally not harmed by very small amounts of air injected into the venous system, but excess air injected into the veins can be fatal, so it is necessary to remove all air bubbles from formulation and administration sets before use.
- Particulate material can include small pieces of glass that chip from the product's vial or rubber pieces that come from the closure on the vials. Although great care is taken to eliminate the presence of particulate material, a final filter in the administration line just before entering the venous system is an important precaution.

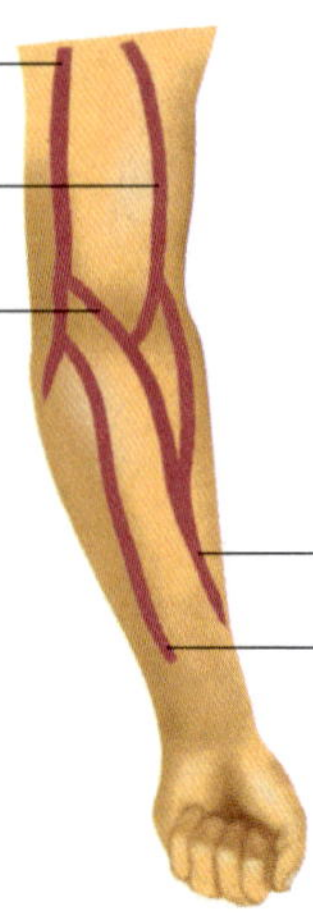

Intravenous Sites

Several sites on the body are used to intravenously administer drugs: the veins of the antecubital area (in front of the elbow), the back of the hand, and some of the larger veins in the foot. On some occasions, a vein must be exposed by a surgical cut.

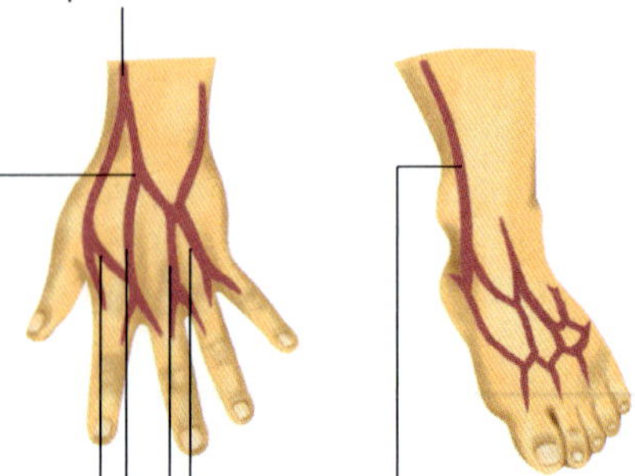

diluent a solvent that dissolves a freeze-dried powder or dilutes a solution.
injectability the ease of flow when a suspension is injected into a patient.
syringeability the ease with which a suspension can be drawn from a container into a syringe.

DEVICES

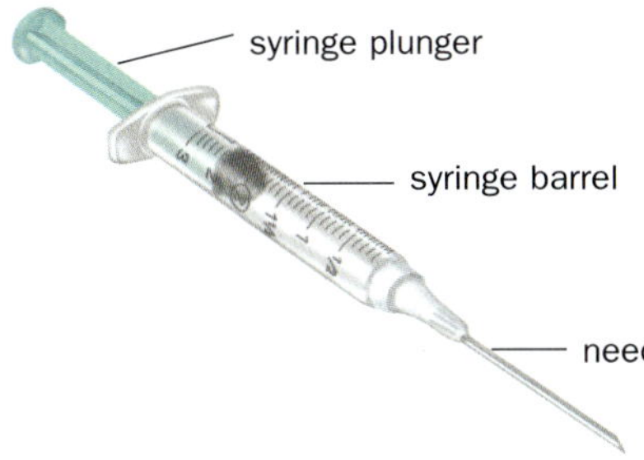

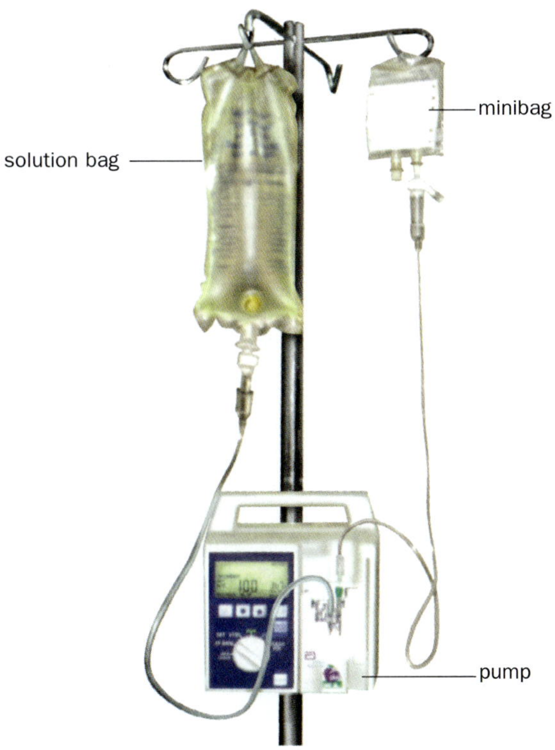

a solution bag and a minibag connected to an infusion pump

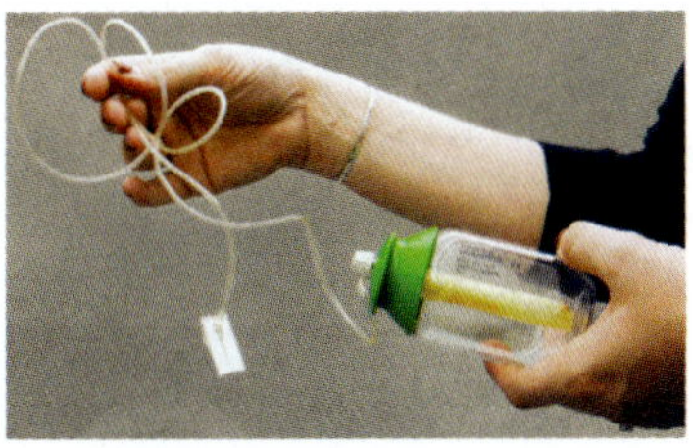

an elastomeric pump

Syringes

Simple syringe and needle setups can be used to inject formulations over a short period of time (generally up to 2 minutes). There are a variety of syringe sizes and needle sizes; syringe size is selected based on the volume of the formulation to inject. The needle size is generally based on the route of administration being used (IV, IM, SC, ID). Some products come from the manufacturer with syringes and needles already assembled and prefilled.

Infusion

Infusion is the gradual intravenous injection of a volume of fluid into a patient. The infusion solution is generally a large volume (500 ml to 1,000 ml) of electrolyte solution such as D5W (dextrose 5% in water) or 1/2NS (one-half normal saline, 0.45% sodium chloride in water). It is infused at a rate of 2 ml to 3 ml per minute.

The solution bag has two ports: an administration set port and a medication port. The administration set provides the connection between the solution bag and the needle in the patient. The administration set may also be connected to an infusion pump to control the flow rate. A simple syringe and needle may be used to inject a drug through the medication port into the solution bag. Sometimes a second small bag containing the drug (called a minibag) can be piggybacked onto the administration set or through an infusion pump.

Infusion Pumps

Administration devices that are dependent upon gravity flow have been shown to have a variable delivery rate. To ensure a constant delivery rate, controlled rate infusion pumps are used. Infusion pumps controlled by patients are called PCA (patient-controlled anesthesia) pumps. The newer "smart pumps" have drug libraries to pre-program drug administration rates and provide additional safety at the point-of-care.

Elastomeric Pumps

Elastomeric pumps are useful for intermittent or very slow, continuous infusions. They are balloon-like reservoirs filled with medication that is forced out of the reservoir through a flow restrictor.

INTRAMUSCULAR

Drugs are often given by the intramuscular route to patients who are unable to take them by oral administration.

This route is also used for drugs that are poorly absorbed from the gastrointestinal tract. It is generally considered less hazardous and easier to use than the intravenous route. However, patients generally experience more pain from intramuscular administration than intravenous administration.

Intramuscular (IM) injections are made into the muscle fibers that are under the subcutaneous layer of the skin.

Needles used for the injections are generally 1 inch to 1.5 inches long and 19 to 22 gauge in size. The principal sites of injection are the gluteus maximus (buttocks), deltoid (upper arm), and vastus lateralis (thigh) muscles. When giving intramuscular injections into the gluteus maximus, one must be aware of the thickness of gluteal fat, particularly in female patients. An appropriate size needle must be used or the injection will not reach the muscle.

The site of injection should be as far as possible from major nerves and blood vessels to avoid nerve damage and accidental intravenous administration.

Injuries that can occur following intramuscular injection are abscesses, cysts, embolism, hematoma, skin sloughing, and scar formation. To avoid injury when a series of injections are given, the injection site is changed or rotated. Generally only limited volumes can be given by intramuscular injection: 2 ml in the deltoid and thigh muscles, and up to 5 ml in the gluteus maximus.

Intramuscular injections usually result in lower but longer lasting blood concentrations compared to intravenous administration.

Part of the reason is that intramuscular injections have an absorption step that delays the time to peak concentration. Also, when a formulation is injected, a *depot* forms inside the muscle tissue where the drug is injected. Absorption from this depot is dependent on many factors such as muscle exercise, particle size of the drug, and the salt form of the drug used in the formulation.

FORMULATIONS

Drugs for intramuscular injection are formulated as:

- solutions;
- suspensions;
- ***colloids*** in aqueous and oleaginous (oil-based) solvents;
- oil-in-water emulsions;
- water-in-oil emulsions.

Colloids and suspensions both contain insoluble particles in solution, but the particles in colloids are about 100 times smaller than those in suspensions.

Emulsions are mixtures of two liquids, one aqueous and the other oleaginous, which are not miscible in each other. One liquid is dispersed through the other by using a stabilizing agent called an emulsifier.

Different salt forms of the drug may also be used to take advantage of a slower dissolution rate or a lower solubility.

So, particle size, the type of emulsion, and the salt form of the drug can all be varied to achieve the desired absorption rate. In general, aqueous solutions have a faster absorption rate than oleaginous solutions. Both have a faster absorption rate than colloids or suspensions.

colloids particles up to a hundred times smaller than those in suspensions that are, however, likewise suspended in a solution.

depot the area in the muscle where the formulation is injected during an intramuscular injection.

INJECTION SITES

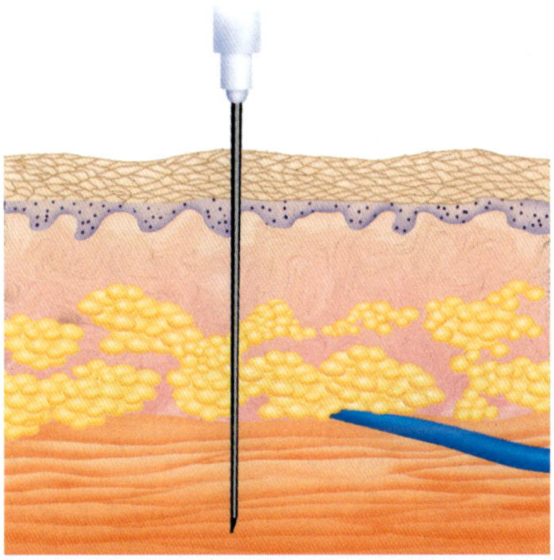

When administering intramuscular injections, it is necessary to adjust the needle size for any layers of body fat (especially in the gluteal area) and to use a size of needle that will penetrate to the muscle.

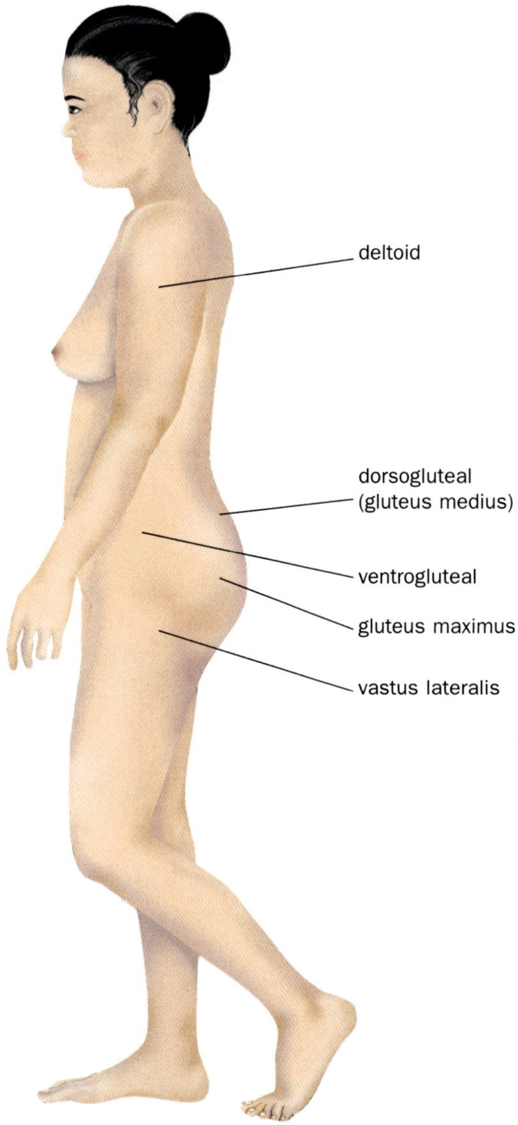

sites for intramuscular injection

Z-Tract Injection

This is a technique used for medications that stain the skin (e.g., iron dextran injection) or irritate tissues (e.g., diazepam). The skin is pulled to one side prior to injection. Then the needle is inserted and the injection is performed. Once the needle is removed, the skin is released so that the injection points in the skin and muscle are no longer aligned. This keeps the drug from entering the subcutaneous tissue and staining or irritating the skin. A Z-track injection is generally 2 to 3 inches deep.

Rx tip
Intramuscular injections are generally more painful than intravenous injections.

SUBCUTANEOUS

The subcutaneous (SC, SQ) route is a versatile route of administration that can be used for both short term and very long term therapies. The injection of a drug or the implantation of a device beneath the surface of the skin is made in the loose tissues of the upper arm, the front of the thigh, or the lower portion of the abdomen. The upper back also can be used as a site of subcutaneous administration. The site of injection is usually rotated when injections are given frequently. The maximum amount of medication that can be subcutaneously injected is about 2 ml. Needles are generally 3/8 to 1 inch in length and 24 to 27 gauge.

Absorption of drugs from the subcutaneous tissue is influenced by the same factors that determine the rate of absorption from intramuscular sites.

However, there are fewer blood vessels in the subcutaneous tissue than in muscle, and absorption may be slower than with intramuscular administration. On the other hand, absorption after subcutaneous administration is generally more rapid and predictable than with oral administration. There are several additional ways to change the absorption rate. Using heat or massaging the site have been found to increase absorption rates of many drugs. Also, there are various co-administered drugs that have been shown to increase absorption rate. By contrast, epinephrine decreases regional blood flow, which in turn decreases the absorption rate.

Many different solutions and suspensions are given subcutaneously, but insulin is the most common drug routinely administered by this route.

Insulin comes in many different formulations, each having a characteristic rate of absorption. The rate is controlled by the same factors used for intramuscular formulations: slowly soluble salt forms, suspensions versus solutions, differences in particle size, ***viscosity*** (thickness) of the media, etc. Other drugs commonly administered by subcutaneous injection include heparin and enoxaparin.

In spite of the advantages of this route of administration, there are some precautions to observe.

Drugs that are irritating or that are in very viscous suspensions may produce serious adverse effects, including abscesses and necrosis, and be painful to the patient.

INJECTION SITES

- lower abdomen
- front of thigh
- upper back
- back of upper arm

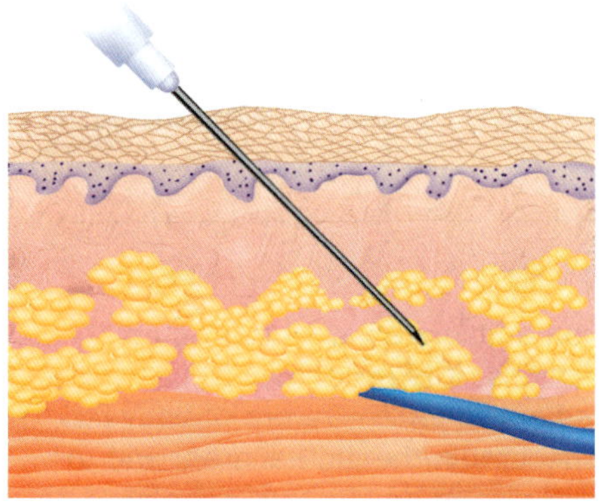

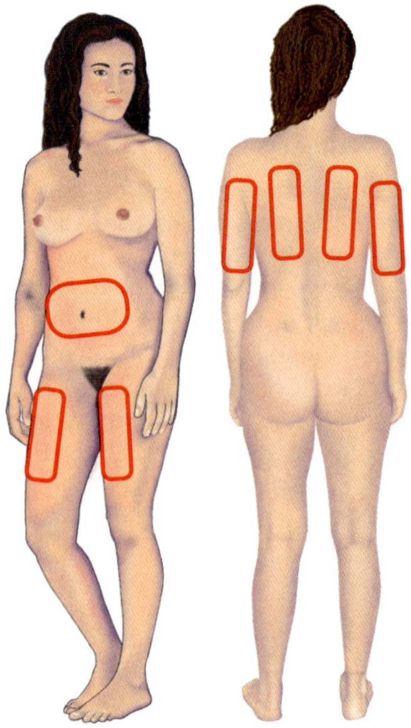

biocompatibility not irritating; does not promote infection or abscess.

viscosity the thickness of a liquid. A measure of a liquid's resistance to flow.

IMPLANTS

One of the most popular ways to achieve very long-term drug release is to place the drug in a delivery system or device that is implanted into a body tissue. The subcutaneous tissue is the ideal tissue for implantation of such devices. Implantation generally requires a surgical procedure or a specialized injection syringe. Because the device will be in constant contact with the subcutaneous tissue, implant materials must be ***biocompatible*** (i.e., nonirritating) and must not promote infection or sterile abscess. An advantage of using subcutaneous tissue for the implantation is that the device can be easily removed if necessary.

There are many devices used for subcutaneous implantation. Viadur™ Duros® implants are made of titanium alloy and are capable of delivering a drug for up to one year. Supprelin LA® implants last one year and are used to treat precocious puberty in children. Implanon® and Nexplanon® release a drug for three years and are used to prevent pregnancy.

Sometimes ports and pumps are placed in subcutaneous tissue and an attached delivery catheter is placed in a vein, cavity, artery, or CNS system. This allows for the continuous infusion of chemotherapy agents or antibiotics.

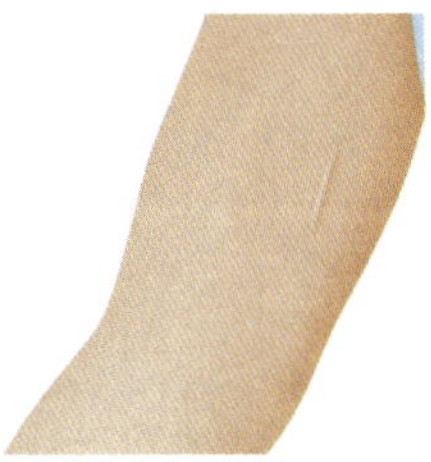

a subcutaneous implant

INTRADERMAL 7

Intradermal injections involve small volumes that are injected into the top layer of skin.

They are used for diagnostic reasons, desensitization, or immunization. Their effects can be both local and systemic.

An intradermal injection forms a *wheal*, or raised blister-like area, from which the drug will slowly be absorbed into the dermis.

The dermis is the layer of the skin just beneath the epidermis. It contains more blood vessels than the epidermis but fewer than most other injection sites. As a result, absorption is gradual.

The usual site for intradermal injections is the anterior surface of the forearm.

Needles are generally 3/8 inches long and 25 to 26 gauge. The needle is inserted horizontally into the skin with the bevel facing up. The injection is made when the bevel just disappears into the skin. For this route of administration, 0.1 ml of solution is the maximum volume that can be administered.

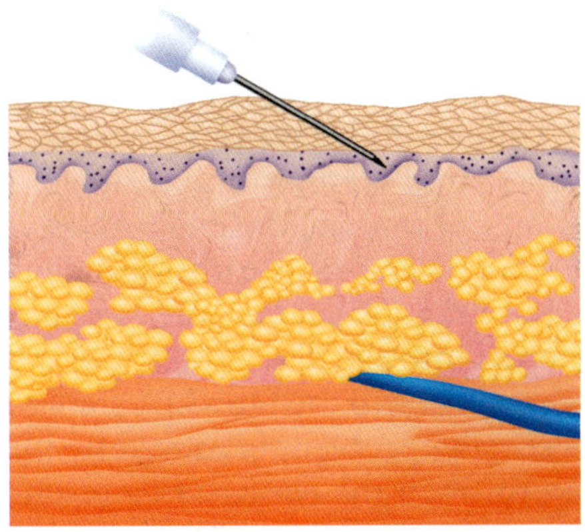

wheal a raised, blister-like area on the skin caused by an intradermal injection.

OPHTHALMIC FORMULATIONS

Drugs are administered to the eye for local treatment of various eye conditions and for anesthesia.

Formulations that are used include aqueous solutions, aqueous suspensions, ointments, and implants. Every *ophthalmic* product must be manufactured to be sterile in its final container. Also, because of the sensitivity of the eye, various elements of the formulation, including pH and viscosity, must be carefully controlled.

A major problem of ophthalmic administration is the immediate loss of a dose by natural spillage from the eye.

The normal volume of tears in the eye is estimated to be 7 microliters, and if blinking occurs, the eye can hold up to 10 microliters without spillage. The normal commercial eyedropper dispenses 50 microliters of solution. As a result, about 80% of a dose will be lost from the eye by overflow. The ideal volume of drug solution to administer would be 5 to 10 microliters. However, microliter dosing eyedroppers are not generally available to patients.

Other problems include lacrimal (tear) drainage and very rapid absorption by the eyelid lining.

Tears that wash the eyeball flow from the *lacrimal gland* across the eye and drain into the *lacrimal canalicula* (tear ducts). The rate of tear production is approximately 2 microliters per minute, so the entire tear volume in the eye turns over every 2 to 3 minutes. This rapid washing and turnover accounts for loss of an ophthalmic dose in a relatively short period of time. It can also cause systemic absorption since the drug drains into the lacrimal sac and is then emptied into the gastrointestinal tract where it can be absorbed into the blood. A similar and frequently occurring problem is caused by absorption of the drug through the *conjunctiva* (eyelid lining). The drug is then rapidly carried away from the eye by the circulatory system.

℞ **tip**

Ophthalmic administration is used to deliver a drug on the eye or onto the conjunctiva. Drug penetration into the eye is not considered an effective process because only one-tenth of a dose penetrates into the eye.

OPHTHALMIC ADMINISTRATION

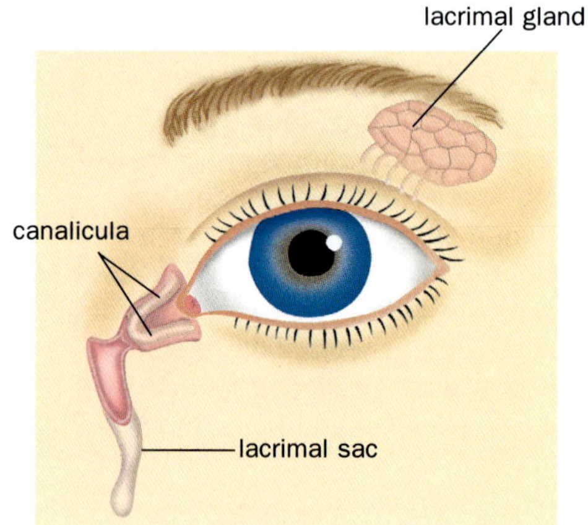

anatomy of the eye

How to Use Ophthalmic Drops

1. Wash your hands thoroughly with soap and warm water.
2. If the product container is transparent, check the solution before using it. If it is discolored or has changed in any way (e.g., particles in the solution, color change), don't use it.
3. If the product container has a depressible rubber bulb, draw up a small amount of medication into the eyedropper by first squeezing, then relieving, pressure on the bulb.
4. Tilt your head back with your chin up, and look toward the ceiling.
5. With both eyes open, gently draw down the lower lid of the affected eye with your index finger.
6. In the "gutter" formed, place one drop of the solution. Hold the dropper or administration tip as close as possible to the lid without actually touching your eye. Do not allow the dropper or administration tip to touch any surface.
7. If possible, hold your eyelid open, and don't blink for 30 seconds.

tip

Ophthalmic ointment tubes are typically small, holding approximately 3.5 g of ointment and fitted with narrow gauge tips that permit the extrusion of a narrow ribbon of ointment.

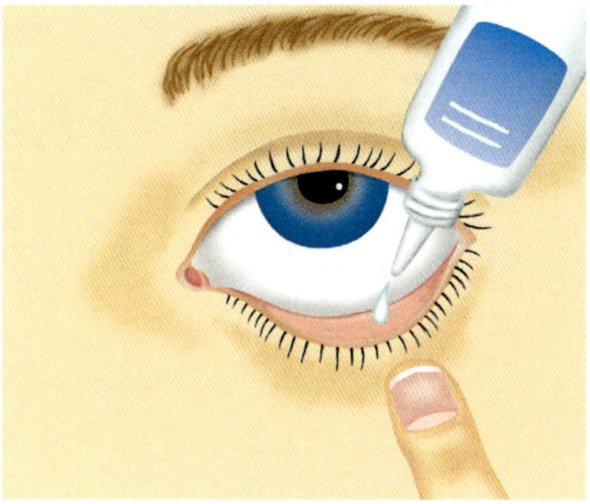

using an eyedropper

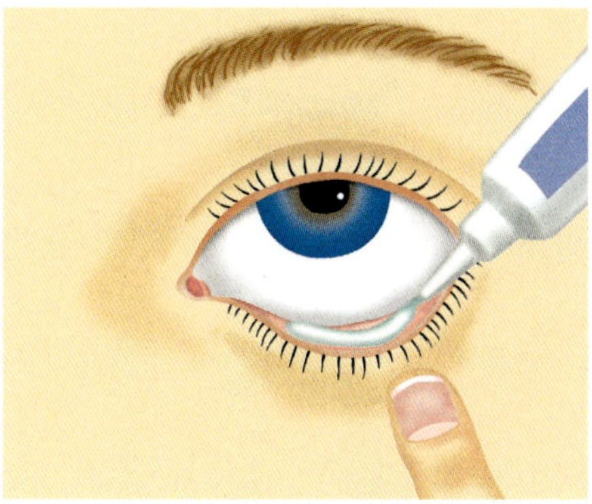

using an ointment

8. Press your finger against the inner corner of your eye for one minute to keep the medication in your eye.
9. Cap the bottle tightly.

Additional Tips

- Keep in mind that this is a sterile solution. Contamination of the dropper or eye solution can lead to a serious eye infection.
- If irritation persists or increases, discontinue use immediately.
- Avoid eye makeup while using eye solutions.
- Use a mirror when applying the drops, or have someone help instill the eyedrops.

Most ophthalmic solutions and suspensions are dispensed in eyedropper bottles.

Because of the unique characteristics of this route, patients must be shown how to properly instill the drops in their eyes, and every effort should be made to emphasize the need for instilling only one drop, not two or three.

To maintain longer contact between the drug and the surrounding tissue, suspensions and ointments have been developed.

Ophthalmic suspensions are aqueous based, with the drug's particle size kept to a minimum to prevent irritation of the eye. Ointments tend to keep the drug in contact with the eye longer than suspensions. Most ophthalmic ointment bases are a mixture of mineral oil and white petrolatum and have a melting point close to body temperature. But ointments tend to blur patient vision as they remain viscous and are not removed easily by the tear fluid. Therefore, ointments are generally used at night as additional therapy to eyedrops used during the day.

Contact lenses and soluble inserts can be used to deliver ophthalmic dosages.

Hydrogel contact lenses are placed in a solution containing a drug such as an antibiotic, and the lenses absorb some of the drug. The lenses are then placed in the eye and the drug will be released from the lenses over a period of time. Soluble ophthalmic drug inserts are dried solutions that have been fashioned into a film or rod. These solid inserts are placed between the eyeball and the lower eyelid, and as they absorb tears, they slowly erode away. Lacrisert® is a soluble insert used in the treatment of moderate to severe dry eye syndrome.

conjunctiva the eyelid lining.

lacrimal canalicula the tear ducts.

lacrimal gland the gland that produces tears for the eye.

ophthalmic related to the eye.

INTRANASAL FORMULATIONS

The adult *nasal cavity* has a capacity of about 20 ml, a very large surface area for absorption, and a very rich blood supply.

The most common drugs used for intranasal administration are used for their decongestant activity on the ***nasal mucosa***, the cellular lining of the nose. Other drugs that are typically used are antihistamines and corticosteroids.

The intranasal absorption of some drugs produces blood concentrations similar to when the drug is intravenously administered.

Because of this, intranasal administration is being investigated as a possible route of administration for insulin in the treatment of diabetes mellitus and for glucagon in the treatment of hypoglycemia. Intranasal administration also serves as a possible alternate route for drugs that are seriously degraded or poorly absorbed after oral administration.

Intranasal formulations include solutions, suspensions, ointments, and gels.

Generally solutions or suspensions are administered by drops or as a fine mist from a nasal spray or aerosol container. Nasal sprays are preferred to drops because drops are more likely to drain into the back of the mouth and throat and be swallowed. Plastic squeeze bottles were commonly used to administer nasal mists but have been largely replaced by glass containers with a metered dose inhaler (MDI) actuator.

If the drug is sufficiently volatile, it can be administered in a nasal inhaler.

The ***nasal inhaler*** is a cylindrical tube with a cap that contains fibrous material impregnated with a volatile drug. The cap is removed and the inhaler tip is placed just inside the nostril. As the patient inhales, air is pulled through the tube and the vaporized drug is pulled into the nasal cavity.

nasal cavity the cavity behind the nose and above the roof of the mouth that filters air and moves mucus and inhaled contaminants outward and away from the lungs.

nasal inhaler a device that contains a drug that is vaporized by inhalation.

nasal mucosa the cellular lining of the nose.

DEVICES

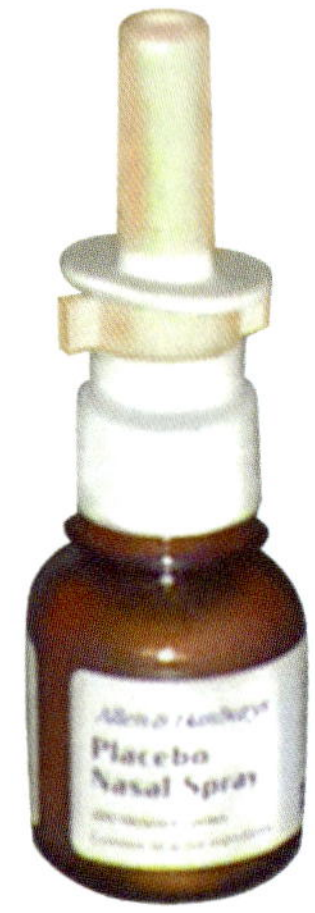

nasal spray with MDI actuator

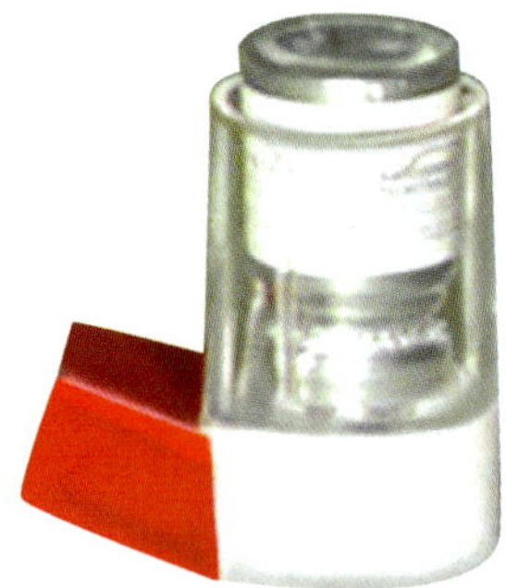

nasal aerosol

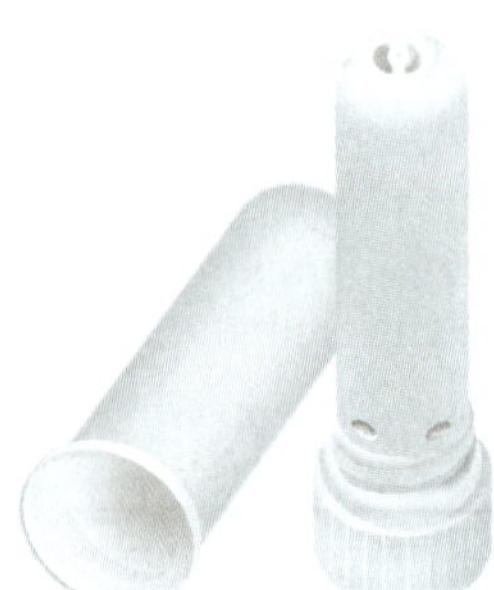

nasal inhaler

USING A NASAL SPRAY

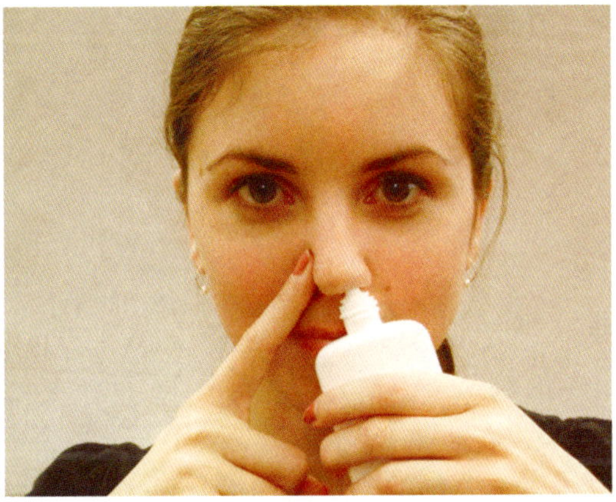

using a nasal spray

How to Use Intranasal Sprays

1. Blow your nose gently to clear the nostrils.
2. Wash your hands with soap and warm water.
3. Hold your head upright.
4. Close one nostril with one finger.
5. With the mouth closed, insert the tip of the spray into the open nostril. Breathe in through the nostril while quickly and firmly squeezing the spray container or activating the MDI actuator.
6. Hold your breath for a few seconds, and then breathe out through your mouth.
7. Repeat this procedure for the other nostril only if directed to do so.
8. Rinse the spray or MDI tip with hot water, and replace the cap tightly on the container.
9. Wash your hands.

There are three ways a dosage can be lost following nasal administration.

The nasal lining contains enzymes that can metabolize and degrade some drugs. In addition, normal mucus flow, which protects the lungs by moving mucus and inhaled contaminants away from the lungs and out of the nostril, will carry the drug with it as well. Finally, nasal administration often causes amounts of the drug to be swallowed. In some cases, the amount of drug swallowed will equal an oral dose which may lead to a systemic effect from the drug.

Intranasal dosage forms should not be used for prolonged periods.

This may lead to chronic swelling (edema) of the nasal mucosa, which aggravates the symptoms the dosage forms were intended to relieve. As a result, intranasal administration should be for short periods of time (no longer than 3 to 5 days). Patients should be advised not to exceed the recommended dosage and frequency of use.

Ways Intranasal Dosage Is Lost

- ✔ Enzymes in the mucosa metabolize certain drugs.
- ✔ Normal mucus flow removes the drug.
- ✔ An amount of the drug can be swallowed.

℞ **safety you should know**

Intranasal administration is generally kept to limited volumes for short periods of time because it can lead to irritation and swelling.

INHALATION FORMULATIONS

Inhalation dosage forms are intended to deliver drugs to the pulmonary system (lungs).

The lungs have a large surface area for absorption and a rich blood supply. This route avoids the problems of degradation and poor absorption found with oral administration. However, there is enough inconsistency in the absorption of drugs from the lungs that this route is not considered an alternative to intravenous administration.

Gaseous or volatile anesthetics are the most important drugs administered via this route.

Other drugs administered affect lung function, act as bronchodilators, or treat allergic symptoms. Examples of drugs administered by this route are adrenocorticoid steroids (beclomethasone), bronchodilators (isoproterenol, metaproterenol, albuterol), and antihistamines (cromolyn sodium).

Most inhalation dosage forms are MDI aerosols that depend on the power of compressed or liquefied gas to expel the drug from a container.

Aerosols are easy to use and have no danger of contamination. However, they are not very effective in delivering a drug to the respiratory tract because of the physical barriers of the airway and lungs.

Particle size is the critical factor with inhalation dosage forms.

Large particles (about 20 microns) hit in the back of the mouth and throat and are eventually swallowed rather than inhaled. Particles from 1 to 10 microns reach the bronchioles. Smaller particles (0.6 micron) penetrate to the ***alveolar sacs (alveoli)*** of the lungs where absorption is rapid, but retention is limited since a large fraction of the dose is exhaled. The particles that reach the alveolar sacs and remain there are responsible for providing systemic effects. Breathing patterns and the depth of breathing also play important roles in the delivery of drugs into the lung by inhalation aerosols.

alveolar sacs (alveoli) the small sacs of specialized tissue that transfer oxygen out of inspired air into the blood and carbon dioxide out of the blood and into the air for exhalation.

ABSORPTION

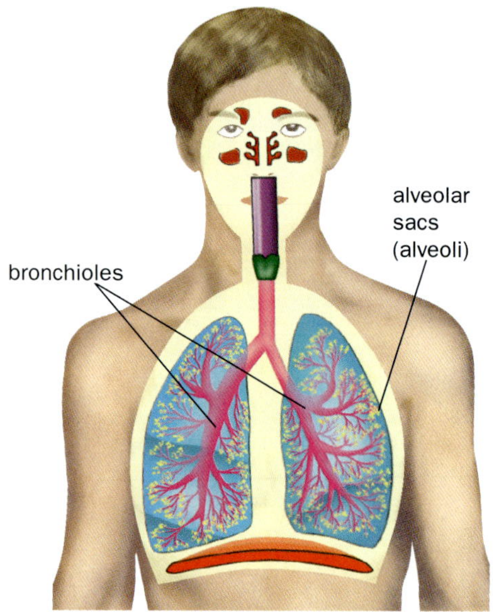

For an inhalation dosage to reach the alveolar sacs of the lungs, it has to pass through a series of twists, turns, and increasingly smaller passageways. When the drug reaches the alveolar sacs, it will be absorbed directly into the circulatory system. Because of the difficult route from the mouth to the alveoli, varying amounts of inhaled drug are lost along the way.

DEVICES

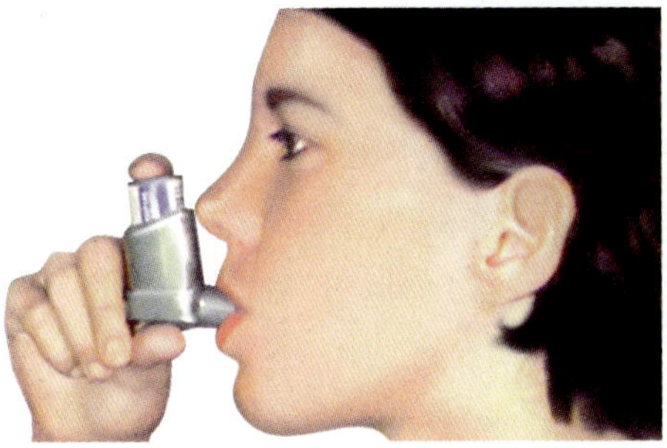

using an MDI aerosol

Metered Dose Inhaler (MDI) Aerosols

MDI aerosols used to administer drugs by inhalation have special metering valves that deliver a fixed dose when the aerosol is actuated. The amount of drug released with each actuation is regulated by a valve that has a fixed capacity or fixed dimensions.

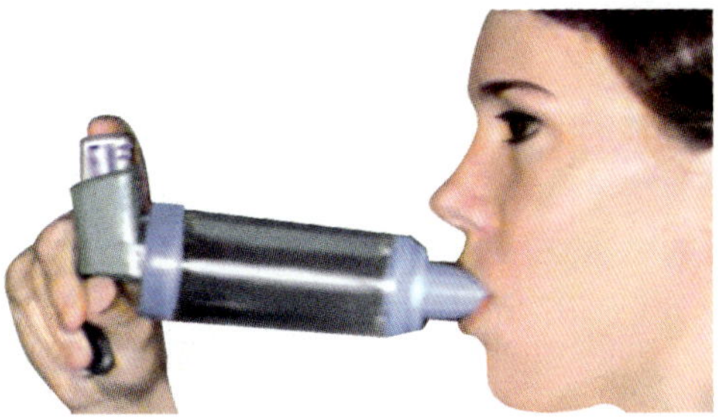

using an MDI aerosol with spacer

Adapters and Spacers

Coordination is required on the part of the patient between breathing in (inspiration) and actuation of the aerosol. Extender devices or spacers have been developed to assist patients who cannot coordinate these two actions. The spacer goes between the aerosol's mouthpiece and the patient's mouth. The spacer allows the patient to separate actuation of the aerosol from inhalation by 3 to 5 seconds.

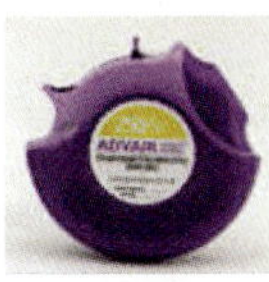

ADVAIR DISKUS® 250/50 inhaler device

Dry Powder Inhalers

Some drugs are administered in powder form using a special inhalation device**.** The device automatically releases the drug when the user inhales. The powdered drug is supplied in hard gelatin capsules, cartridges, or foil blister strips (e.g., ADVAIR®) and is loaded into the inhalation device.

Atomizers and Nebulizers

Atomizers are devices that break up a liquid into a spray. One type of atomizer uses a squeeze bulb to blow air across a liquid solution, causing the liquid to vaporize. As the liquid vaporizes, the air stream created by the bulb also carries the spray out of the device and into the mouth. A nebulizer contains an atomizing unit inside a chamber. When the rubber bulb is squeezed, the drug solution is drawn up the dip tube and aerosolized by the passing air stream. Most commercially available nebulizers have an automatic air supply so that aerosolization is continuous.

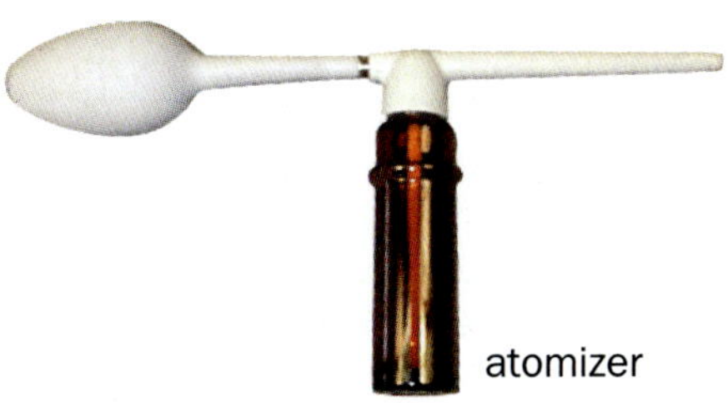

atomizer

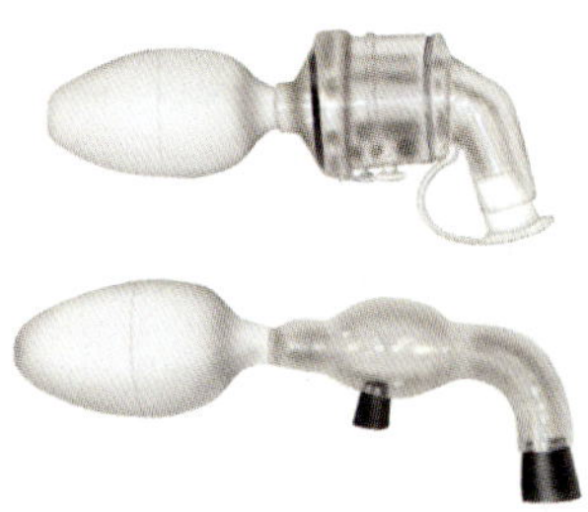

nebulizers

DERMAL FORMULATIONS

The skin is the largest and heaviest organ in the body and accounts for about 17% of a person's weight.

It forms a barrier that protects the underlying organ systems from trauma, temperature, humidity, harmful penetrations, moisture, radiation, and microorganisms. Dosage forms that are applied to the skin are called dermal or topical dosage formulations.

Most dermal dosage forms are used for local effects on or within the skin.

Dermal formulations are used as protectants, lubricants, emollients, drying agents, or as a delivery vehicle for a drug. Examples of treatments using dermal formulations include minor skin infections, itching, burns, diaper rash, insect stings and bites, athlete's foot, corns, calluses, warts, dandruff, acne, psoriasis, and eczema. Some dermal formulations promote ***percutaneous absorption*** (i.e., absorption through the skin).

Dermal administration has a number of advantages.

It provides an ease of administration not found in other routes, and usage by patients is generally good. It can also provide continuous drug delivery. In addition, dermal formulations can be easily removed if necessary. The major disadvantage of this route of administration is that drug absorption is limited to about 2 mg/hour. This is often a significant limitation if the route is being considered for systemic therapy.

Basic rules of percutaneous absorption:

- More drug is absorbed when the formulation is applied to a larger surface area.
- Formulations or dressings that increase the hydration of the skin generally improve absorption.
- The greater the amount of rubbing in (inunction) of the formulation, the greater the absorption.
- The longer the formulation remains in contact with the skin, the greater will be the absorption.

THE SKIN

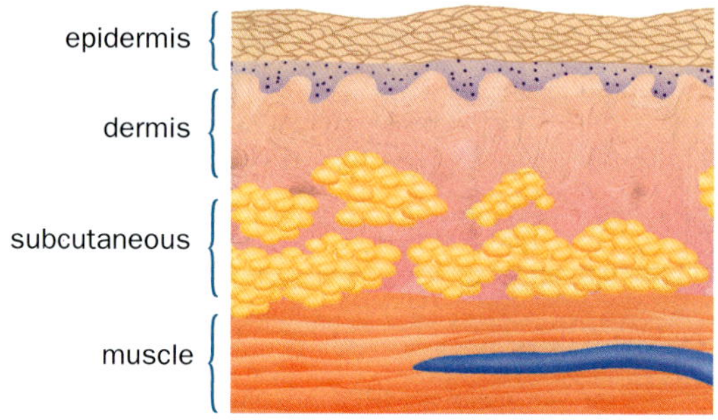

The skin is composed of three layers of tissue:

- epidermis;
- dermis;
- and subcutaneous tissue.

The skin is generally 3–5 millimeters thick, though it is thicker in the palms and soles of the feet and thinner in the eyelids and genitals. Within the skin are several structures: hair follicles, sebaceous glands, sweat glands, and nails.

The outer layer of epidermis is called the ***stratum corneum***. In normal skin, this layer is continually replaced by new cells from underneath. The turnover time from cell development to shedding of dead cells (sloughing) is about 21 days.

The stratum corneum is the primary barrier to drug penetration. It is about 10 micrometers thick, but can swell to approximately three times that size by absorbing as much as five times its weight in water. When the stratum corneum absorbs water (***hydrates***), it becomes easier for drugs to penetrate. For that reason, certain dressings are designed to hydrate the skin. Also, some skin conditions, such as eczema and psoriasis, cause the stratum corneum to hydrate and increase the absorption of some drugs.

FORMULATIONS

Solutions, Tinctures, Collodions, and Liniments

Dermal solutions and tinctures are generally used as anti-infective agents. Both are dispensed in small volumes, and should be packaged in containers that are convenient to use. Dropper bottles (glass bottles with an applicator tip) are most often used. Examples of solutions and tinctures are Coal Tar Solution, Hydrogen Peroxide, Povidone Iodine Tincture, and Compound Benzoin Tincture.

Collodions are liquid preparations of pyroxylin dissolved in a solvent mixture of alcohol and ether. Pyroxylin looks like raw cotton and is slowly but completely soluble in the solvent mixture. When applied to the skin, the solvent rapidly evaporates, leaving a protective film on the skin that contains a thin layer of the drug. Liniments are alcoholic or oleaginous solutions generally applied by rubbing.

Ointments, Creams, and Lotions

Ointments, creams, and lotions are the most popular dermal formulations. Physically, they appear to be very similar in consistency and texture, but there are differences. Ointments have drugs that have been incorporated into a base. There are several different types of bases, ranging from petrolatum to polyethylene glycols. Creams are semisolid emulsions, and are less viscous and softer in texture than ointments. Creams have an added feature in that they "vanish" or disappear with rubbing. Lotions are suspensions of solid drugs in an aqueous vehicle.

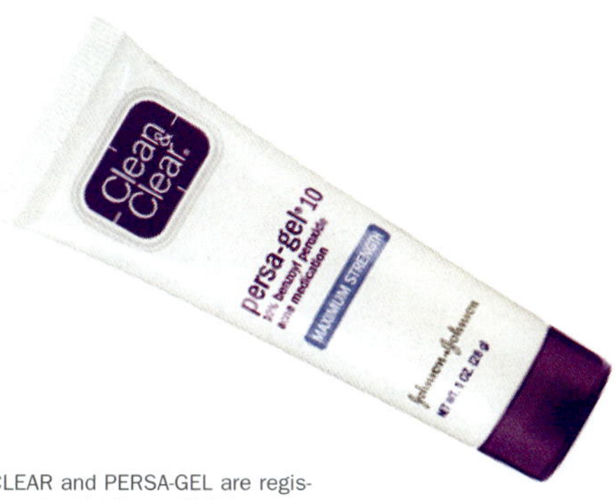

CLEAN & CLEAR and PERSA-GEL are registered trademarks of Johnson & Johnson. Used with permission.

Pastes, Plasters, and Powders

Pastes are generally used for their protective action and for their ability to absorb secretions from skin lesions. Pastes contain more solid material than ointments, and are stiffer and less penetrating. Plasters are solid or semisolid adhesive masses that are spread on a suitable backing material. They provide prolonged contact at the site of application. Some of the common backing materials used are paper, cotton, felt, linen, muslin, silk, and moleskin. The backing is cut into different shapes appropriate to cover the affected area. Medicated dermal powders are a mixture of drug and an inert (inactive) base such as talcum or corn starch. Powders have different dusting and covering capability.

Transdermal Patches, Tapes, and Gauzes

Transdermal systems (patches, tapes, and gauzes) deliver drugs through the skin for a systemic effect. The systems can be divided into two kinds: those that control the rate of drug delivery to the skin, and those that allow the skin to control the rate of drug absorption. The first type is for potent drugs that must have their absorption rate controlled by a device. The second type is for less potent drugs. The largest problems with transdermal patches are skin sensitivity experienced by some patients, and technical difficulties associated with the adhesiveness of the systems to different skin types and under various conditions.

Aerosols

Dermal aerosols are generally used to apply anesthetic and antibiotic drugs for local effect.

hydrates absorbs water.

percutaneous absorption the absorption of drugs through the skin, often for a systemic effect.

stratum corneum the outermost cell layer of the epidermis.

VAGINAL FORMULATIONS

Vaginal administration has many of the same characteristics found with other parenteral routes of administration.

It avoids the degradation that occurs with oral administration; doses can be retrieved if necessary; and it has the potential of providing long term drug absorption. However, vaginal administration leads to variable absorption since the vagina is a physiologically and anatomically dynamic organ with pH and absorption characteristics changing over relatively short periods of time. Another disadvantage of this route is that administration of a formulation during menstruation could predispose the patient to toxic shock syndrome. There is also a tendency of some dosage forms to be expelled after insertion into the vagina.

Formulations for this route of administration are solutions, powders for solutions, ointments, creams, aerosol foams, suppositories, tablets, and IUDs.

Powders are used to prepare solutions for vaginal douches used to cleanse the vagina. The powder is supplied either as bulk or unit dose packages and is dissolved in a prescribed amount of water prior to use. Most douche powders are used for their hygienic effects, but a few contain antibiotics.

contraceptive device or formulation designed to prevent pregnancy.

intrauterine device (IUD) an intrauterine contraceptive device that is placed in the uterus for a prolonged period of time.

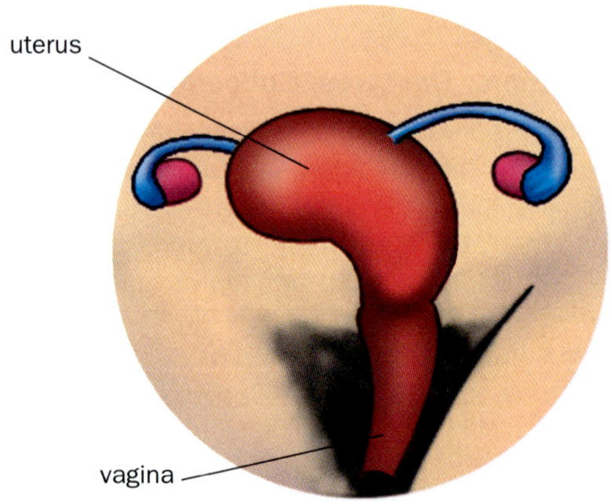

The Vagina

The vagina is a cylinder-like organ that leads from the cervix and uterus to an external opening. It is used for intercourse, releasing menstrual fluids, and is the lower portion of the birth canal.

Toxic Shock Syndrome (TSS)

Toxic shock syndrome is a rare and potentially fatal disease that results from a severe bacterial infection of the blood. In women, it can be caused when bacteria natural to the vagina move into the bloodstream. Though primarily associated with the use of superabsorbency tampons, it has also been associated with various vaginal dosage forms. TSS symptoms include a high fever, nausea, skin rash, faintness, and muscle ache. It is treated with antibiotics and other medicines.

FORMULATIONS

Tablets (Inserts)

Vaginal tablets, also called inserts, have the same activity and are inserted in the same manner as vaginal suppositories. Patients should be instructed to dip the tablet into water before insertion. Also, because tablets are generally used at bedtime and can be messy if the formulation is an oleaginous base, it should be recommended to patients that they wear a sanitary napkin to protect nightwear and bed linens. These same instructions should be given to patients receiving vaginal suppositories.

Ointments, Creams, and Aerosol Foams

Vaginal ointments, creams, and aerosol foams typically contain antibiotics, estrogenic hormonal substances, or ***contraceptive*** agents.

Creams and foams are placed in a special applicator tube, and the tube is then inserted high in the vaginal tract. The applicator plunger is depressed to deposit the formulation.

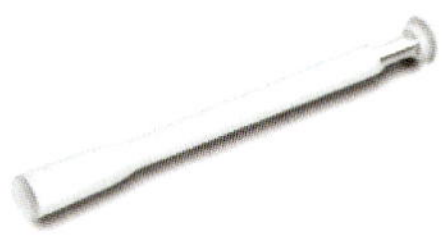

Suppositories

Vaginal suppositories are used as contraceptives, feminine hygiene antiseptics, bacterial antibiotics, or to restore the vaginal mucosa. They are inserted high in the vaginal tract with the aid of a special applicator. The suppositories are usually globe, egg, or cone-shaped and weigh about 5 grams.

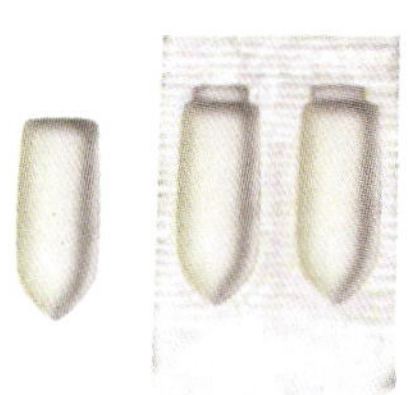

Suppositories are made from a variety of bases. Glycerinated gelatin (70% glycerin, 20% gelatin, 10% water) suppositories are translucent, resilient, and have a soft, rubbery texture. They are the preferred base for vaginal suppositories because they slowly dissolve over about 30 minutes in the vaginal mucus secretions, giving a prolonged local effect of the drug. These suppositories require refrigeration.

Polyethylene glycol suppositories also dissolve in vaginal mucous secretions but do so faster than glycerinated gelatin suppositories. Polyethylene glycol suppositories can be formulated so that no refrigeration is required.

Intrauterine Devices (IUDs)

Vaginal administration provides an opportunity for long-term drug therapy. This potential has been explored in the area of contraception protection using intrauterine devices (IUDs).

Precursors to present day IUDs were first mentioned in scientific literature in the early 1900s. Many of the early prototypes were made of stainless steel and produced high rates of infection and high failure rates.

The first plastic, T-shaped IUDs were available in the 1970s. These devices had a lower rate of vaginal expulsion due to their similarity to the uterine shape. They also had higher surface areas of copper and were effective at a rate of greater than 99%. ParaGard® is an IUD that has been shown to be effective for up to 10 years.

Another category of IUDs is based on the release of the hormone progesterone. Progestasert® was the first hormonal uterine device. It was developed in 1976 and manufactured until 2001. It released an average of 60 micrograms of progesterone per day and had a failure rate of 2% per year.

Currently, Mirena® is the only hormone based IUD available that can be left in the uterus long term. First introduced in 1990, it releases levonorgestrel and is effective for five years in preventing pregnancy.

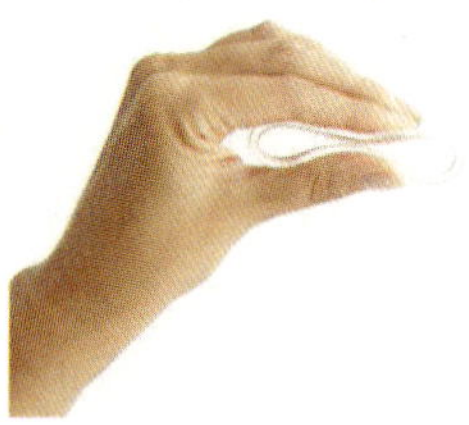

The vaginal ring is also a hormone based IUD, but is used in one month cycles. The ring is inserted into the vagina for 3 weeks, removed for 7 days, and then reinserted. NuvaRing® is an example of such a device.

REVIEW

KEY CONCEPTS

ROUTES AND FORMULATIONS

- ✔ The way in which the body absorbs and distributes drugs varies with the route of administration and the dosage form used.
- ✔ Enteral refers to anything involving the alimentary tract from the mouth to the rectum. There are four enteral routes: oral, sublingual, buccal, and rectal.
- ✔ Parenteral refers to anything next to or beside the enteral route. Some parenteral routes use formulations that are injected. Other parenteral formulations do not require injection.
- ✔ A local effect occurs when the drug activity is at the site of administration (e.g., eyes, ears, nose, skin).
- ✔ A systemic effect occurs when the drug is introduced into the circulatory system and carried to the site of activity.

ENTERAL ROUTES AND FORMULATIONS

- ✔ Oral administration means the dosage form is to be swallowed.
- ✔ Drugs administered in liquid dosage forms generally reach the circulatory system faster than drugs formulated in solid dosage forms.
- ✔ The primary goal of modified release dosage forms is to reduce the number of doses a patient must take per day.
- ✔ The mouth has two enteral routes of administration: sublingual (under the tongue) and buccal (in the cheek pouch).
- ✔ Rectal administration is used for both systemic and local effects. Suppositories, ointments, and solutions are common dosage forms.

PARENTERAL ROUTES AND FORMULATIONS

- ✔ Some parenteral routes requiring injection for administration are intravenous, intramuscular, intradermal, and subcutaneous. Intravenous solutions must be sterile (bacteria-free) and free of particulate material.
- ✔ Intramuscular injections generally result in lower but longer lasting blood concentrations than with intravenous administration.
- ✔ The subcutaneous (SC, SQ) route can be used for both short-term and very long-term therapies. Insulin is the most important drug routinely administered by this route.
- ✔ Intradermal administration is used for diagnostics, desensitization, and immunization.
- ✔ Ophthalmic administration can lead to a significant loss of dose due to spillage and drainage.
- ✔ Intranasal administration of some drugs produce blood concentrations similar to intravenous administration.
- ✔ Inhalation dosage forms deliver drugs to the lungs. MDI aerosols, dry powder inhalers, and nebulizers are common devices used to administer drugs by this route.
- ✔ Dermal formulations vary from solutions and lotions to aerosols, ointments, and pastes. Transdermal patches are also common dosage forms.
- ✔ Vaginal dosage forms (e.g., suppositories, tablets, solutions) are most often used for local effect. However, long-term systemic effects can be achieved with IUDs.

SELF TEST

the answer key begins on page 569

MATCH THE TERMS: I

1. alveolar sacs (alveoli) ____
2. aqueous ____
3. biocompatibility ____
4. buccal ____
5. buffer system ____
6. colloids ____
7. conjunctiva ____
8. contraceptive ____
9. depot ____
10. diluent ____
11. disintegration ____
12. dissolution ____
13. emulsifier ____
14. emulsions ____
15. hemorrhoid ____
16. hydrates ____
17. injectability ____
18. intrauterine device (IUD) ____
19. lacrimal canalicula ____
20. lacrimal gland ____
21. local effect ____
22. nasal cavity ____
23. nasal inhaler ____
24. nasal mucosa ____

a. absorbs water.
b. ingredients in a formulation designed to control the pH.
c. mixture of two non-miscible liquids where one is dispersed throughout the other as tiny droplets.
d. water based.
e. when drug activity is at the site of administration.
f. pouch between the teeth and cheek in the mouth.
g. painful swollen veins in the anal/rectal area, generally caused by strained bowel movements from hard stools.
h. solvent that dissolves a freeze-dried powder or dilutes a solution.
i. the ease of flow when a suspension is injected into a patient.
j. the area in the muscle where the formulation is injected during an intramuscular injection.
k. particles up to a hundred times smaller than those in suspensions that are, however, also suspended in a solution.
l. not irritating; does not promote infection or abscess.
m. the gland that produces tears for the eye.
n. the tear ducts.
o. the eyelid lining.
p. the small sacs of specialized tissue that transfer oxygen out of inspired air into the blood and carbon dioxide out of the blood and into the air for exhalation.
q. an intrauterine contraceptive device that is placed in the uterus for a prolonged period of time.
r. device or formulation designed to prevent pregnancy.
s. the cavity behind the nose and above the roof of the mouth that filters air and moves mucus and inhaled contaminants outward and away from the lungs.
t. a device that contains a drug that is vaporized by inhalation.
u. the cellular lining of the nose.
v. the breaking apart of a tablet into smaller pieces.
w. when the smaller pieces of a disintegrated tablet dissolve in solution.
x. a stabilizing agent in emulsions.

REVIEW

MATCH THE TERMS: II

1. necrosis ____
2. ophthalmic ____
3. percutaneous absorption ____
4. pH ____
5. solution ____
6. sterile ____
7. stratum corneum ____
8. sublingual ____
9. syringeability ____
10. systemic effect ____
11. viscosity ____
12. water soluble ____
13. wheal ____

a. a condition that is free of all microorganisms.
b. the absorption of drugs through the skin, often for a systemic effect.
c. related to the eye.
d. a measure of a liquid's thickness or resistance to flow.
e. under the tongue.
f. when a drug is introduced into the circulatory system and carried to the site of activity.
g. measures the acidity or the opposite (alkalinity) of a substance.
h. the ease with which a suspension can be drawn from a container into a syringe.
i. a raised, blister-like area on the skin caused by an intradermal injection.
j. the outermost cell layer of the epidermis.
k. able to dissolve in water.
l. increase in cell death.
m. a clear liquid made up of one or more substances dissolved in a solvent.

CHOOSE THE BEST ANSWER

1. Which route of administration is not a parenteral route?
   a. intranasal
   b. buccal
   c. inhalation
   d. ophthalmic

2. A local effect occurs
   a. at the site of administration.
   b. throughout the body.
   c. only after intravenous administration.
   d. only within the alimentary tract.

3. The stomach has a pH of
   a. 3–4.
   b. 7–8.
   c. 5–6.
   d. 1–2.

4. A dissolution step would not be necessary for drug absorption from a/an
   a. tablet.
   b. enteric coated tablet.
   c. oral syrup.
   d. bulk powder.

5. Modified release tablets might be called
   a. extended release.
   b. prolonged action.
   c. long acting.
   d. all of the above.

6. Nonaqueous solutions often contain glycerin, alcohol, and
   a. polyethylene glycol.
   b. polyvinyl alcohol.
   c. propylene glycol.
   d. chloroform.

7. Which oral formulation is characterized by a high sucrose content?
   a. solution
   b. syrup
   c. elixir
   d. suspension

8. An oral liquid formulation in which one non-miscible liquid is dispersed throughout another in the form of small droplets is called
   a. an emulsion.
   b. a suspension.
   c. a gel.
   d. a solution.

9. ___________ tablets are placed under the tongue.
   a. Enteric coated
   b. Buccal
   c. Sublingual
   d. Sugar coated

10. Which statement is false?
    a. Rectal administration can be used for systemic effect.
    b. Drug absorption from rectal administration is erratic and unpredictable.
    c. Rectal suppositories are intended to spread around the anal opening.
    d. Rectal enemas create an urge to defecate.

11. Which statement is true?
    a. Parenteral formulations containing active drug(s) also serve as buffers.
    b. Parenteral formulations can be administered in non-enteral routes.
    c. Parenteral formulations must be administered through a syringe.
    d. All of the above.

12. Which is not an injection dependent parenteral route?
    a. subcutaneous
    b. inhalation
    c. intramuscular
    d. epidural

13. Which will not be caused by particulate material in an intravenous injection?
    a. air emboli
    b. thrombus
    c. phlebitis
    d. blood clots

14. The gradual intravenous injection of a volume of fluid into a patient is called
    a. bolus.
    b. infiltration.
    c. infusion.
    d. Z-tracking.

15. Which order of the absorption rate (from fastest to slowest) is correct when considering IM administration?
    a. aqueous solutions > oleaginous solutions > colloids > suspensions
    b. oil-in-water emulsions > oleaginous solutions > aqueous solutions > suspensions
    c. colloids > suspensions > oleaginous solutions > aqueous solutions
    d. oleaginous solutions > colloids > aqueous solutions > suspensions

REVIEW

16. Needles for subcutaneous injection are generally ____ inches long and ____G.
    a. 3/8 to 1, 18 to 20
    b. 1 to 1.5, 24 to 27
    c. 3/8 to 1, 24 to 27
    d. 1 to 1.5, 18 to 20

17. A raised, blister-like area on the skin caused from an intradermal injection is called a
    a. thrombus.
    b. pachyderma.
    c. wheal.
    d. phlebitis.

18. Which ophthalmic formulation will maintain drug contact with the eye for the longest period of time?
    a. solution
    b. suspension
    c. gel
    d. ointment

19. When administering ophthalmic drops, why is instilling two drops at a time not recommended?
    a. The eye only holds about 10 microliters.
    b. The second drop will be lost due to spillage.
    c. The average drop size is 50 microliters.
    d. The second drop will cause corneal abrasion.

20. Do not use an ophthalmic solution if it is/has
    a. particles.
    b. discolored.
    c. developed gas bubbles.
    d. all of the above.

21. What percent of an administered ophthalmic solution is delivered to the eye?
    a. 5%
    b. 20%
    c. 50%
    d. 75%

22. When administering a nasal spray,
    a. lay on the bed with the head hanging over the edge.
    b. keep both nostrils open.
    c. breathe through the nostril while spraying the solution.
    d. exhale immediately.

23. A drug is administered by inhalation using a metered dose inhaler (MDI) aerosol. Which pathway will the drug follow?
    a. mouth, trachea, alveoli, bronchioles
    b. mouth, bronchioles, trachea, alveoli
    c. mouth, trachea, bronchioles, alveoli
    d. bronchioles, alveoli, nasal cavity, trachea

24. Which is the barrier to drug absorption after dermal administration?
    a. stratum corneum layer
    b. epidermis layer
    c. dermis layer
    d. subcutaneous tissue

25. Dermal formulations can deliver about ______mg/hr of active drug.
    a. 2
    b. 4
    c. 6
    d. 10

26. Plasters are generally used with the ________ route of administration.
    a. dermal
    b. rectal
    c. intranasal
    d. vaginal

27. The primary reason to use a vaginal applicator is to
    a. prevent a "mess" during application.
    b. prevent patients from using oral tablets by the route.
    c. place the formulation high in the vaginal tract.
    d. enable patients to retrieve the formulation if needed.

CRITICAL THINKING QUESTIONS

1. Why are drugs available in dosage forms or formulations instead of just the pure drug by itself?
2. Why would you want a dosage formulation to provide a local effect rather than a systemic effect?
3. Why is the most common route of drug administration the oral route?

THINKING IT THROUGH WRAP-UP

1. Technically, the answer is yes. But there are considerations. IV solutions are more expensive than oral solutions because IV solutions must be sterile. Also, the IV solution will have no flavoring; this would probably not be an issue with neonates, but it might be a consideration with older patients.
2. You would expect the absorption to be the same with either formulation since caffeine citrate is already in solution and disintegration and dissolution will not be factors. One possible problem is if the IV solution has a buffer system to control its pH. This could make the pH of the IV solution stronger than that of the stomach and small intestine, which may affect the absorption. However, since the volume of the dose for a neonate will be very small compared to the volume of the neonate's alimentary tract, the difference in pH will probably not affect the absorption.
3. You would not do that. Intravenous solutions must be sterile, and oral solutions are not sterile. In addition, oral solutions would have additional ingredients such as sugars, flavorings, etc. that are not suitable for IV administration. Using an oral solution intravenously would have serious and possibly fatal consequences.

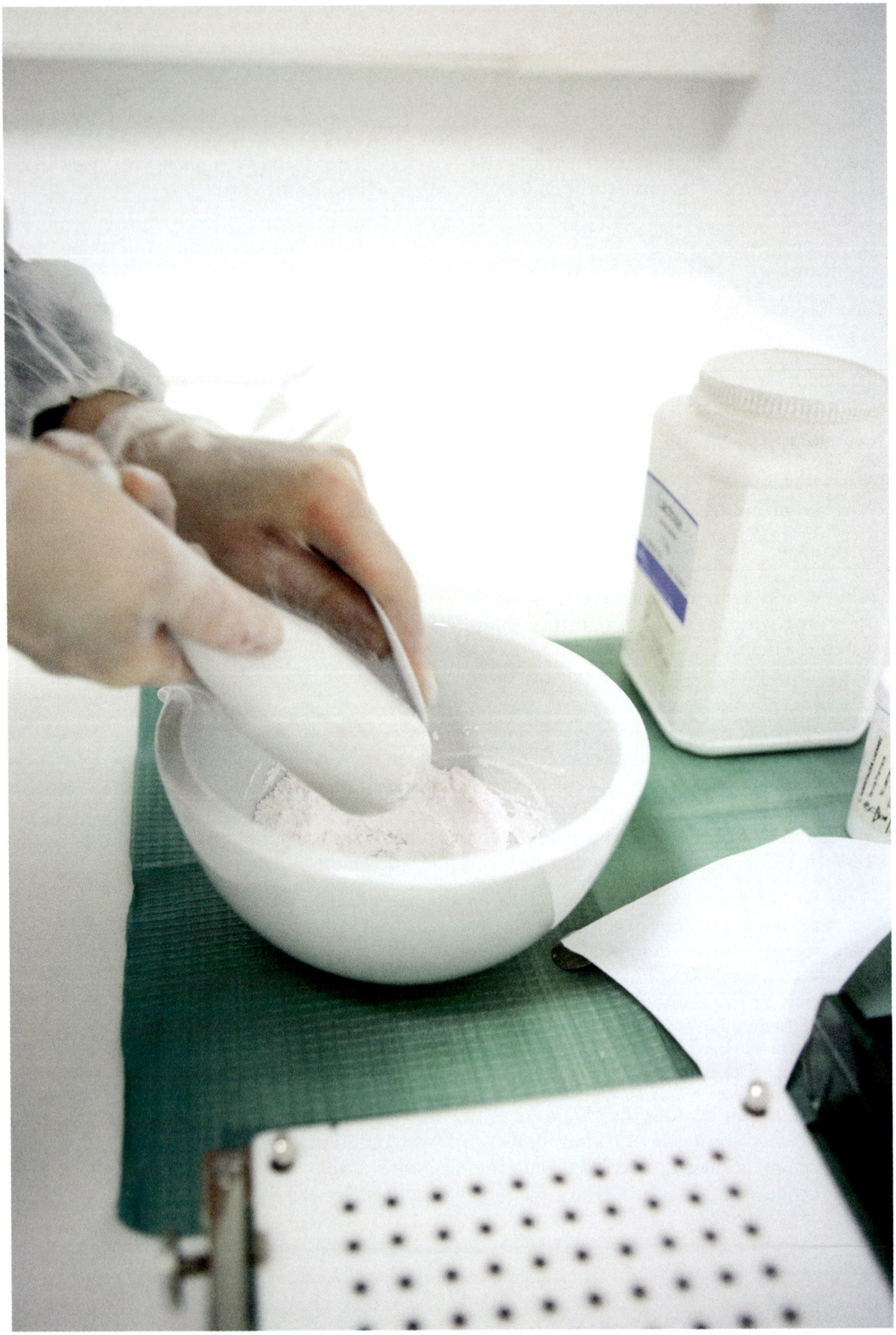

Photo courtesy BSIP/Universal Images Group/Getty Images

8

COMPOUNDING

LEARNING OBJECTIVES

At the completion of study, the student will:

- ✔ explain the need for compounded formulations.
- ✔ know the role of state boards of pharmacy, the USP–NF, and the FDA in regulating a compounding pharmacy practice.
- ✔ understand factors that must be considered before a formulation is compounded.
- ✔ explain how to determine a beyond-use date for a compounded formulation.
- ✔ describe common equipment used in compounding formulations.
- ✔ understand the difference in volumetric and non-volumetric glassware.
- ✔ know how to measure a liquid in volumetric glassware.
- ✔ explain how to properly mix solids and semisolids.
- ✔ describe common compounding techniques for a variety of formulations.
- ✔ appreciate the complexity of flavoring and sweetening in compounded liquids.

THINKING IT THROUGH

A patient is prescribed levothyroxine because of a low T3 level. After six weeks he tells his doctor that he feels extremely tired all the time but does not tell the doctor that he quit taking the levothyroxine about 5 weeks ago. A thyroid function test shows that the patient's T3 level has not changed at all since the last test six weeks ago. Upon further questioning by the doctor, the patient admits he quit taking the levothyroxine tablets because they caused nausea and vomiting. As you read this chapter, consider the following questions:

1. How could a compounded dosage form be useful in this patient's situation?
2. What compounded dosage forms might the pharmacist recommend?
3. If the doctor prescribed a suppository dosage form, what decisions would be involved in compounding that dosage form?

COMPOUNDING

Extemporaneous compounding is the on-demand preparation of a prescribed drug product to meet the unique needs of an individual patient.

Compounding has always been a component of pharmacy. There is an art involved in using raw ingredients to formulate a drug product that meets the special needs of a patient. It requires specialized knowledge of the physical and chemical properties of drugs and their vehicles. It also requires proper training and skill. This chapter will focus on the terminology, equipment, and basic principles of extemporaneous compounding.

There are various aspects of compounding.

It can mean the preparation of suspensions, dermatologicals, and suppositories; the conversion of one dosage form into another; the preparation of select dosage forms from bulk chemicals; the preparation of intravenous admixtures, parenteral nutrition solutions, and pediatric dosage forms from adult dosage forms; the preparation of radioactive isotopes; or the preparation of cassettes, syringes, and other devices for administering drugs in the home.

The demand for pharmaceutical compounding has grown substantially.

Reasons include the growth of home health care, the unavailability of certain drug products, orphan drugs, veterinary compounding, and biotechnology derived drug products. Newly evolving dosage forms and therapies also suggest that compounding will become more common in pharmacy practice.

Technicians, under pharmacist supervision, are increasingly involved in compounding.

Specific responsibilities will vary from environment to environment. Therefore, it is necessary to know and understand the specific responsibilities and requirements that apply to your job.

Chapter <795> regulations from USP–NF pertaining to compounding nonsterile formulations.

Chapter <797> regulations from USP–NF pertaining to compounding sterile formulations.

COMPOUNDING FOR SPECIAL NEEDS

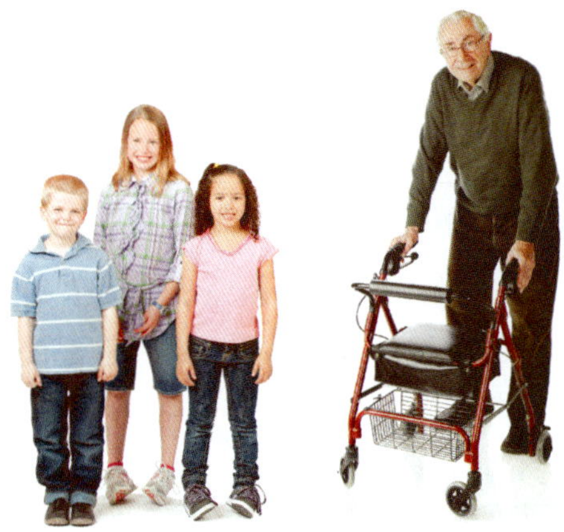

Compounding is done for many special reasons, including:

- pediatric patients requiring diluted adult strengths of drugs;
- patients who need an oral solution or suspension of a product that is only available in another form;
- patients with sensitivity to dyes, preservatives, or flavoring agents;
- dermatological formulations with fortified (strengthened) or diluted concentrations;
- specialized dosages for therapeutic drug monitoring;
- special care for hospice patients in pain management;
- providing medications that are no longer commercially available;
- drugs being used off-label, which might involve dosages that are not commercially available;
- preparing total parenteral nutrition (TPN) solutions;
- preparing radiopharmaceuticals;
- preparing special versions or doses of drugs for animals.

MANUFACTURING VS. COMPOUNDING

Manufacturing and compounding are not the same.

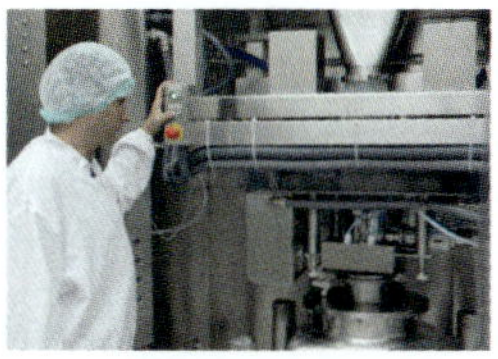

As defined by the USP–NF, manufacturing is "the production, propagation, conversion, or processing of a drug or device, either directly or indirectly, by extraction of the drug from substances of natural origin or by means of chemical or biological synthesis. Manufacturing also includes any packaging or repackaging of the substance(s) or labeling or relabeling of containers for re-sale to pharmacies, practitioners, or other persons."

The USP–NF defines compounding as "the preparation, mixing, assembling, altering, packaging, and labeling of a drug or device in accordance with a licensed practitioner's prescription, medication order, or an initiative based on the practitioner/patient/pharmacist/compounder relationship in the course of professional practice."

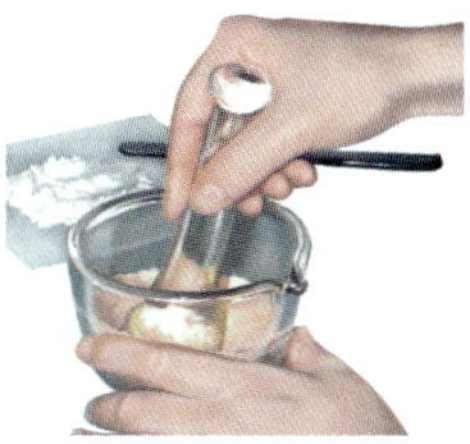

By USP definition, pharmacies are allowed to make formulations in anticipation of prescription drug orders, on the basis of routine, regularly-observed prescribing patterns, if a state has adopted USP guidelines. But "inordinate amounts" would be considered manufacturing. The 2012 FDA Safety and Innovation Act also allows hospitals and health systems to, for a limited time, repack and share drugs on an FDA published shortage list. Finally, some state laws have provisions so pharmacies can provide to prescribers, for administration to patients in their practices, limited amounts of compounded drugs that are not commercially available.

Compounding is regulated by the individual state boards of pharmacy.

Some states have their own regulations. But many states accept the standards of the United States Pharmacopeia-National Formulary (USP–NF) as their standards for compounding. The USP–NF is a scientific, nonprofit organization that has been granted federal authority to set standards pertaining to both manufacturing and compounding. The USP–NF standards are published annually, and are available online.

The USP–NF standards are published in numbered chapters.

Chapters with numbers less than 1000 are legally enforceable by the FDA, and those with numbers greater than 1000 are guidelines or informational chapters. The enforcement of the USP–NF compounding standards by the FDA has not always been a clear-cut matter since jurisdiction for pharmacy compounding rests with the state. However, the FDA has responded on a case-by-case basis to issues or violations where the public's health safety has been jeopardized, or where compounding practices appear to be of a manufacturing nature.

The USP has been extremely active in setting standards for compounding.

Expert committees develop standards, ranging from the definition of compounding to equipment specifications, personnel training, and compounding nonsterile and sterile products. *Chapter <795>* sets the legal standards for nonsterile compounded preparations and *Chapter <797>* sets the legal standards for sterile preparations. Other examples are Containers <661>, Good Compounding Practices <1075>, Pharmaceutical Stability <1150>, and Pharmaceutical Dosage Forms <1151>.

The USP–NF also contains monographs of the most commonly compounded preparations used in pharmacy practice.

These official formulations have the advantage of USP–NF's testing, quality assurance, and beyond-use date assignment. When a formulation is compounded according to a monograph, it's stability and time for a beyond-use assignment can be assumed to be identical to what is stated in the monograph.

REGULATIONS

The USP–NF establishes standards of quality, strength, purity, packaging, and labeling for medications.

Currently, the USP–NF provides standards for more than 3,700 prescription and non-prescription drugs, nutritional and dietary supplements, and medical devices. It also provides additional standards for personnel, facilities, and record keeping. Following are summaries of significant parts of these standards that apply to compounding; the technician should consult the USP–NF for further information and additional regulations.

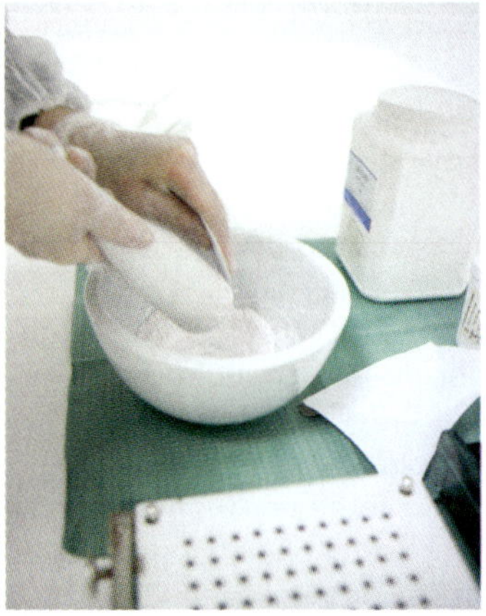

Photo courtesy BSIP/Universal Images Group/Getty Images

Personnel

These standards give the pharmacist responsibility and authority for managing the compounding area. They outline the duties of the pharmacist and the pharmacist's responsibilities for other personnel. These standards also list the qualifications a pharmacist or technician must have to compound and they recommend further training and continuing education responsibilities.

Facilities and Equipment

These standards go into great detail about the physical design and maintenance of the compounding area. They specify that the compounding area, either nonsterile or sterile, should be a designated area away from the "routine dispensing and counseling functions and high traffic areas" of the pharmacy. The standards also recommend compounding equipment that should be in the compounding area.

Ingredients

Raw chemicals are supplied in many levels of purity. The following table summarizes some of the purity classifications (from least pure to most pure). The minimum grade of purity that should be used is USP or NF; if that grade is not available, then a higher grade can be used if deemed acceptable by the pharmacist.

Grade of Chemical	Description
Technical (commercial)	Commercial or industrial quality, generally of indeterminate quality
CP (chemically pure)	More refined than technical grade, but still of unknown quality; only partial analytical information available
USP or NF	Meets standards set by the USP–NF
FCC	Meets specifications of Food Chemical Codex
ACS reagent	High purity; meets specifications of the Reagent Chemicals Committee of the American Chemical Society
AR (analytical reagent)	Very high purity
HPLC	Very high purity; used in high pressure chromatography
Spectroscopic grade	Very high purity
Primary standard	Highest purity; used in standard solutions for analytical purposes

compounding record a record of what actually happened when the formulation was compounded.

formulation record formulas and procedures (i.e., recipes) for what should happen when a formulation is compounded.

Quality Assurance (QA) and Quality Control (QC)

QA is a program of activities used to assure that the compounded formulation meets specifications and satisfies standards. QC is a set of testing procedures that determine the quality of the compounded formulation.

Packaging and Storage

The pharmacist is responsible for the appropriate packaging of compounded formulations. The appropriate container choice depends on the physical and chemical properties of the formulation and its intended use. Packaging materials should not chemically react with any drug or ingredient in the formulation. Other packaging considerations include strength, visibility, moisture protection, ease of use, and cost.

The pharmacist is also responsible for the storage of all ingredients, drugs, supplies, and formulations in the compounding area. Materials should be stored according to the manufacturer's labeling or USP–NF requirements; marked with the date of receipt and the date the container is opened; rotated to use the oldest stock first; and not used beyond their expiration date. Storage temperature requirements are defined in the table below.

Documentation and Record Keeping

Documentation and record keeping provides for consistency when the same formulation is compounded multiple times. They also provide a way to review procedures and ingredients if there is a problem with the formulation. Finally, they are important in any liability cases.

Four sets of records must be kept for each formulation:

- a ***formulation record***: formulas and procedures, a master sheet, a "recipe"—what should happen when the formulation is compounded;
- a ***compounding record***: what actually happened when the formulation was compounded;
- standard operating procedures (SOPs) for equipment maintenance, equipment calibration, handling and disposal of supplies, etc.;
- an ingredients record with certificates of purity and Material Safety Data Sheets (MSDS).

Sample document templates for a formulation record, a compounding record, and standard operating procedures are in Chapter Eight of *The Pharmacy Technician Workbook and Certification Review, Fifth Edition*, that accompanies this text.

Storage Temperature Definitions	
Freezer	-20°C to -10°C
Protect from Freezing	Store above 0°C
Cold	Any temperature not exceeding 8°C
Refrigerator	Between 2°C and 8°C
Cool	Between 8°C and 15°C
Room Temperature	Temperature in the work area
Controlled Room Temperature	Thermostatically controlled at 20°C to 25°C
Warm	Between 30°C and 40°C
Excessive Heat	Any temperature above 40°C

STABILITY & BEYOND-USE DATES

Stability is defined as the extent to which a dosage form retains, within specified limits, and throughout its period of storage and use (i.e., its shelf life), the same properties and characteristics it possessed when it was made.

A ***beyond-use date*** is different than an expiration date. Expiration dates are required on commercially manufactured products and are determined after extensive study of the product's stability. Most expiration dates are in the order of years. Beyond-use dates are used only for compounded preparations and are generally in the order of days or months.

Assigning a Beyond-Use Date

A manufacturer's expiration date should not be used to extrapolate or estimate a beyond-use date for a compounded formulation. Compounded formulations have different drug concentrations, use different diluents, have a different fill volume, and/or are packaged in a different container than the manufactured drug product.

When assigning a beyond-use date, follow these guidelines:

1. If the formulation is an official USP–NF compounded preparation, the beyond-use date and packaging requirements are given in the monograph.
2. If it is not an official USP–NF formulation, beyond-use dates can be determined using the manufacturer's label, provided the compounded drug is formulated according to the manufacturer's directions or uses the same concentration of drug, in the same diluent, in the same packaging, for the same intended period of use, etc.
3. When either of the above is not possible, use drug-specific stability documentation from reference books or primary literature.
4. If published references do not evaluate the exact same formulation, or if a study has not examined the stability for a long enough period of time, use the USP–NF recommendations in the tables below.

USP–NF Chapter <795> Maximum Beyond-Use Dates for Nonsterile Compounded Products

➥ Oral formulations containing water	Not later than 14 days stored at a controlled cold temperature
➥ Topical, dermal, mucosal liquid or semi-solid formulations containing water	Not later than 30 days
➥ Nonaqueous formulations	The earliest expiration date of any active principal ingredient (API) or 6 months, whichever is earlier

USP–NF Chapter <797> Maximum Beyond-Use Dates for Sterile Compounded Drug Products Not Tested for Sterility

Risk Level	Room Temperature	Refrigeration	Freezer
Low	48 hours	14 days	45 days
Medium	30 hours	9 days	45 days
High	24 hours	3 days	45 days

beyond-use date a date assigned to compounded prescription beyond which the formulation should not be used.

stability the extent to which a dosage form retains the same properties and characteristics it possessed when it was made.

COMPOUNDING CONSIDERATIONS

Compounding considerations are questions to ask before, during, and after compounding a prescription. For example, there must be an initial decision if it is even necessary to compound the prescription. Then there are numerous factors to consider as the prescription is compounded. Finally, records and checks must be completed at the end of the process. Below is a summary of these considerations. The pharmacy technician will be involved in each.

Whether to Compound

- ✔ Is there a commercial product already available?
- ✔ If yes, are its ingredients different from the prescribed ingredients, such that the commercial product cannot be used?
- ✔ If no, the pharmacist should determine whether the purpose of the prescription can be achieved without having to compound a product.

Before Beginning the Compounding Process

- ✔ Read and interpret the prescription.
- ✔ Prepare a formulation record.
- ✔ Is the pharmacy personnel qualified to prepare this formulation?
- ✔ Are the proper equipment and supplies available?
- ✔ Can the drug and the ingredient identity, quality, and purity be assured?
- ✔ Is there literature information about the formulation to help determine an appropriate beyond-use date?
- ✔ What basic quality control measures will assure the formulation is compounded correctly?
- ✔ Does the patient have the necessary skills to use and store the formulation?

As the Prescription is Being Compounded

- ✔ Collect and prepare the required ingredients, drugs, supplies, equipment, and clothing.
- ✔ Compound the formulation according to the instructions stated on the formulation record.
- ✔ Package the formulation in an appropriate container and affix appropriate labels.
- ✔ Perform quality control procedures.

After Compounding

- ✔ Recheck all work.
- ✔ If the compounded formulation is new to the pharmacy, keep a sample or make a second batch to assess its stability or appearance over the expected time of therapy.
- ✔ Document the compounding process on a compounding record.
- ✔ Deliver the formulation to the patient with appropriate consultation.
- ✔ Return ingredients, supplies, etc., to their proper locations.
- ✔ Perform required equipment maintenance.

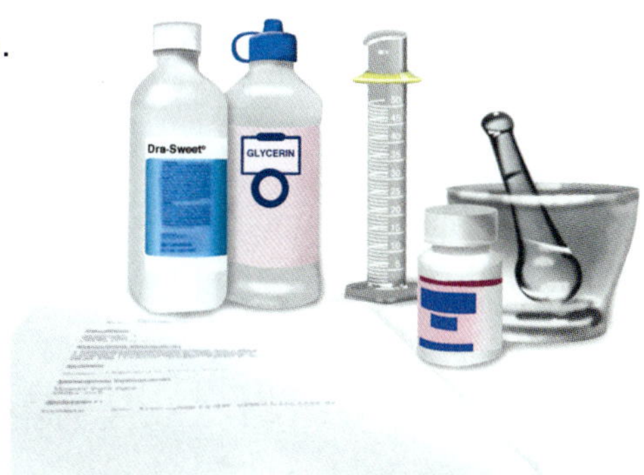

EQUIPMENT

Each compounding process—measuring, mixing, molding, and packaging—has its own set of tools or equipment.

Measuring equipment includes balances, weights, weighing containers, and volumetric glassware such as graduates, pipets, flasks, and syringes. Mixing uses beakers, Erlenmeyer flasks, spatulas, funnels, sieves, and mortar and pestles. Hot plates, suppository molds, capsule shells, and ointment slabs are used for molding. Finally, packaging includes prescription bottles, capsule vials, suppository boxes, and ointment jars. We will discuss these types of equipment and their use in compounding processes over the next several pages; then we will discuss compounding select dosage forms.

One of the most fundamental pieces of compounding equipment is a balance.

A balance is used to determine the weight of a powder, dosage form, liquid, etc. Most pharmacies have a Class A torsion balance, which is a two-pan balance that uses both internal and external weights. The balance has a rider that adds the internal weights to the right-hand pan. The rider is always *calibrated* in the metric system (grams), though some riders also have calibration marks in the apothecary system (grains).

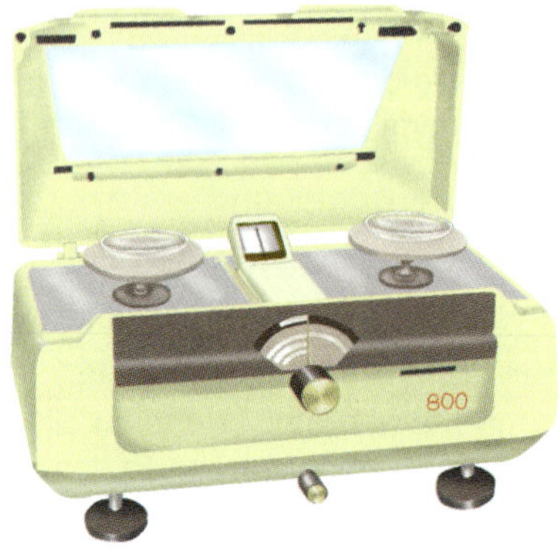

a Class A torsion balance

Class A torsion balances have a sensitivity requirement of up to 6 mg.

The *sensitivity* of a balance is the amount of weight that will move the balance pointer one division mark on the marker plate.

aliquot a portion of a mixture.

calibrate to set, mark, or check the graduations of a measuring device.

sensitivity the amount of weight that will move the balance pointer one division mark on the marker plate.

Weights

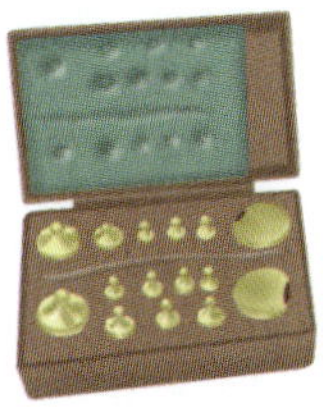

A proper set of metric weights is essential for prescription compounding. These are usually brass cylindrical weights ranging from 1 gram to 50 grams and fractional weights of 10 mg to 500 mg. Weights should be stored in their box. They must be handled with forceps (not with fingers!) to prevent soiling and erosion of the weights.

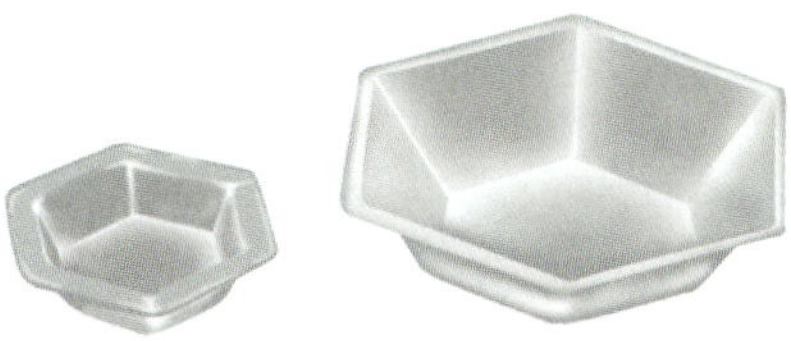

Weighing Papers or Weighing Boats

Weighing papers or weighing boats should always be placed on the balance pans before any weighing is done. These protect the pans from damage and also provide a convenient way to transfer the weighed material from the balance to another vessel. Weighing papers are made of nonabsorbable glassine paper and weighing boats are made of polystyrene. When using weighing papers, the paper should be diagonally creased from each corner and then flattened and placed on the pans. This ensures a collection trough in the paper. New weighing papers or weighing boats should be used with each new drug weighing to prevent cross contamination.

Class A torsion balances have a minimum weighable quantity of 120 mg with a 5% error.

Generally, five percent error is considered an acceptable performance with most torsion compounding balances. Allowing for this error, the minimum weighable quantity is 120 mg. The maximum weighable quantity for most Class A balances is 60 grams, but some will weigh up to 120 grams.

Sometimes a prescription calls for less than 120 mg of an ingredient.

When this happens, the ingredient is mixed with an inert (inactive) powder so that the resulting mix will contain the precise amount of drug needed and also weigh at least 120 mg. A portion of mixed powders is called an ***aliquot***.

Another method for weighing quantities smaller than 120 mg is to use an analytical balance.

Analytical balances come in a variety of sizes and shapes. Most are top-loading and have sensitivities around 1 mg. Analytical balances may be found in some pharmacies, but are generally only found in research laboratories. They are designed to weigh small milligram and microgram quantities of materials.

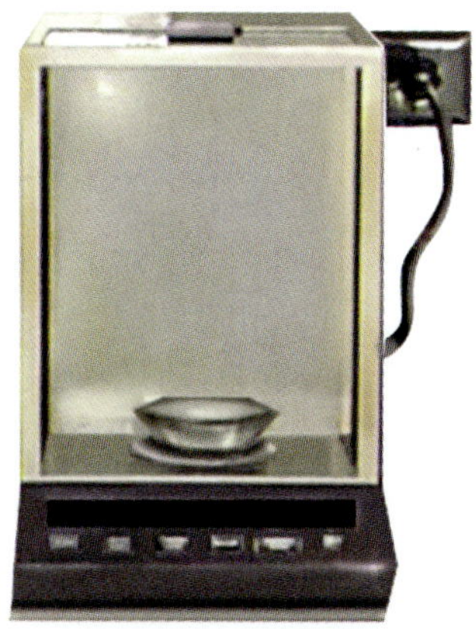

an analytical balance

USING A BALANCE

Following are general rules for using a balance and maintaining it in top condition.

- ✔ Always use the balance on a level surface and in a draft free area.
- ✔ Always use weighing papers or weighing boats. These protect the pans from abrasions, eliminate the need for repeated washing, and reduce loss of drug to porous surfaces.
- ✔ A clean weighing paper or boat should be used for each new ingredient to prevent cross contamination of components.
- ✔ The balance must be readjusted after a new weighing paper or boat has been placed on a pan. Weighing papers taken from the same box can vary as much as 30 mg in weight. Larger weighing boats can vary as much as 200 mg.
- ✔ Always arrest the balance before adding or removing weight from either pan. Although the balance is noted for its durability, repeated jarring of the balance will ultimately damage the working mechanism of the balance and reduce its accuracy.
- ✔ Use a spatula to add or remove ingredients from the balance instead of pouring ingredients out of the bottle.
- ✔ Always clean the balance, close the lid, and arrest the pans before storing the balance between uses.

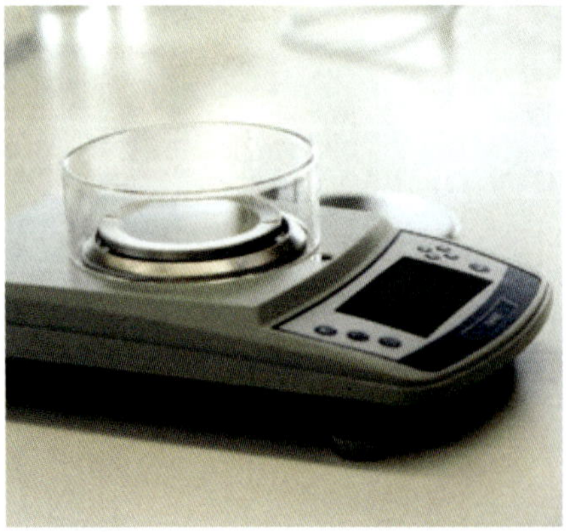

an electronic balance

USING AN ELECTRONIC BALANCE

Electronic balances have digital displays and may have internal calibration capabilities. These may either be top-loading or encased to protect the balance from dust and drafts. To use an electronic balance, follow these guidelines:

- ✔ Move the balance to a place in the compounding area where it won't be moved again during the day.
- ✔ Turn the leveling feet all the way into the balance and then move them in the same direction until the level bubble is within the black circle of the sight glass. If needed, turn the leveling feet in opposite directions to center the bubble.
- ✔ Turn on the balance.
- ✔ For the first use of the day, check internal weight calibration.
- ✔ Remove the top ring of the draft shield (if present) and place the weighing boat in the center of the weighing pan. Replace the draft shield ring. Press the TARE key and the balance should read 0.000 g.
- ✔ Add the ingredients to be weighed through the top ring of the draft shield or, if necessary, remove the ring to add or remove the ingredients, and then replace the ring before reading the weight measurement.
- ✔ Use a lint-free towelette to clean any spills off the weighing pan.
- ✔ Turn off the balance at the end of the day.

arrest knob the knob on a balance that prevents any movement of the balance pans.

USING A TORSION BALANCE

Specific techniques must be used to obtain an accurate weight of ingredients using a torsion balance. Always take the following steps to ensure accuracy.

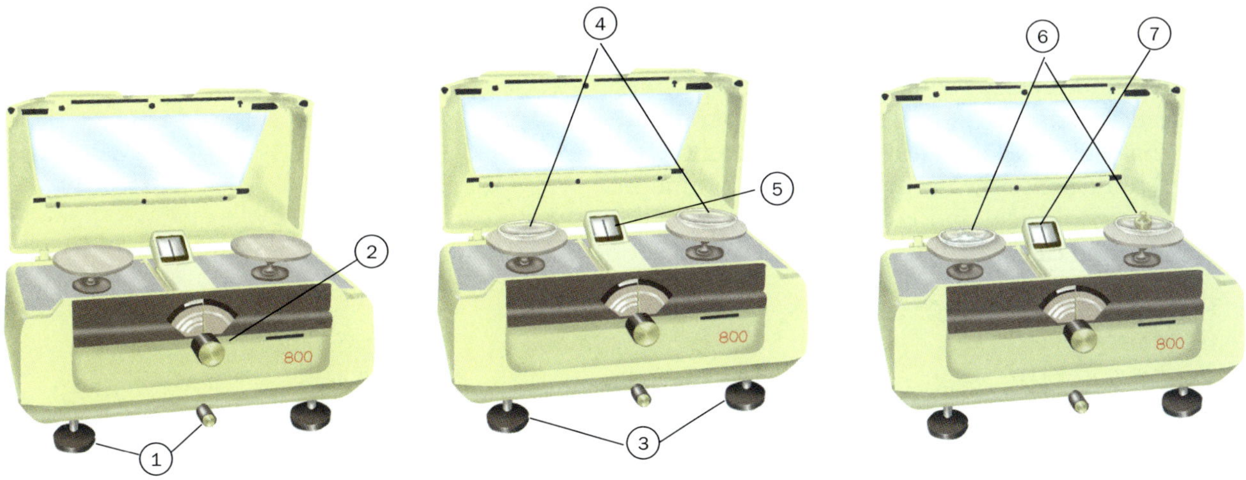

1. Lock the balance by turning the ***arrest knob***. Level the balance front to back by turning the leveling screw feet all the way into the balance and then moving them the same direction until the 4 bottom sides of the balance are equidistant from the bench top. If the balance has a leveling bubble, move the leveling screw feet until the bubble is in the middle of the tube.

2. Set the internal weights to zero. This is done by turning the calibrated dial (i.e., rider) to zero.

3. Unlock the balance and level it left to right by adjusting the leveling screw feet in opposite directions. To shift the pointer left, rotate the feet inward. To shift to the right, rotate the feet outward. Continue adjusting the screw feet slowly until the pointer rests at the center of the marker plate.

4. Lock the balance. Place a weighing boat or paper on each weighing pan. (If using weighing papers, fold diagonally and then gently flatten.)

5. Unlock the balance by releasing the arrest knob. If the pointer does not rest at the center of the marker plate, then level the balance from left to right to account for weight differences between the weighing boats or papers.

6. Lock the balance and place the required weights in the boat on the right pan. Place the ingredient to be weighed in the boat on the left pan.

7. Unlock the balance and note the shift of the pointer on the marker plate. If the pointer shifts left, too much of the ingredient is on the pan and a portion should be removed. If it shifts right, there is too little ingredient and more should be added. Always arrest the balance when adding or removing ingredients from the left pan.

8. Once you have made an accurate measurement, double check that you have weighed the correct ingredient (check the label) and that you have used the correct weights (internal and external).

VOLUMETRIC EQUIPMENT

In compounding, liquid drugs, solvents, and additives are measured in volumetric glassware or plasticware.

Volumetric means "measures volume." Common volumetric vessels are pipets, cylindrical and conical graduates, burets, syringes, and volumetric flasks. The volume capacity is etched on the vessel wall, and some devices will have graduation marks to measure partial volume.

Volumetric vessels are either "to deliver" (TD) or "to contain" (TC).

"To deliver" means that the vessel must be completely emptied to dispense the needed volume. Single volume pipets, syringes, droppers and some calibrated pipets are TD vessels. "To contain" means that the vessel does not need to be completely emptied to dispense the needed volume. Volumetric flasks and cylindrical and conical graduated cylinders and some calibrated pipets are TC vessels.

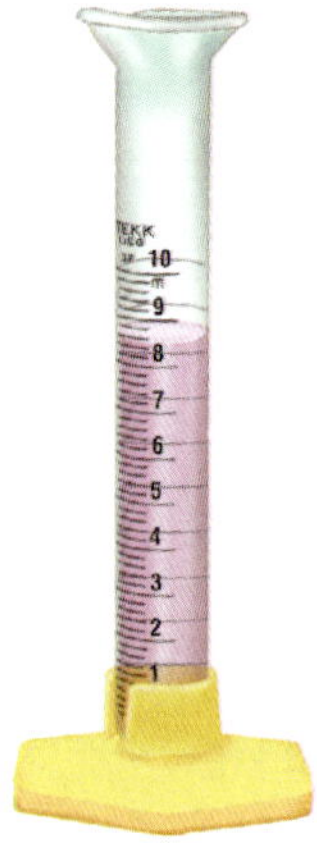

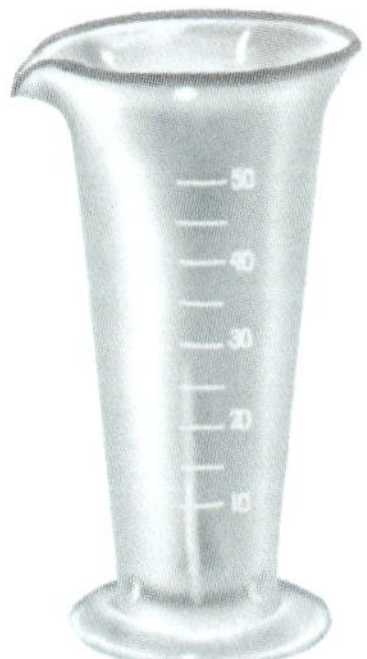

Graduated Cylinders

Graduated cylinders, both cylindrical and cone-shaped, are used for measuring and transferring liquids. Cylindrical graduates are the preferred device because they are more accurate. Graduated cylinders are available in sizes ranging from 5 ml to 4,000 ml. When selecting a graduated cylinder, always choose the smallest one capable of containing the volume to be measured. Avoid measurements of volumes that are below 20% of the capacity of the graduated cylinder because the accuracy is unacceptable. For example, a 100 ml graduated cylinder cannot accurately measure volumes below 20 ml. When measuring small volumes such as 20 ml and less, it is often preferable to use a syringe or pipet.

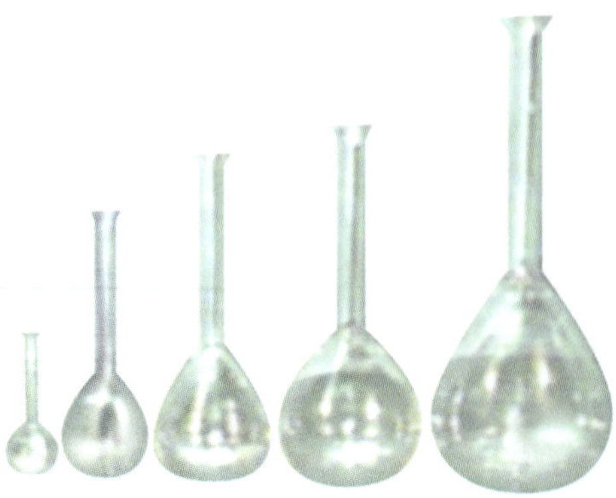

Volumetric Flasks

Volumetric flasks have slender necks and wide, bulb-like bases. Volumetric flasks are single volume glassware and come in sizes ranging from 5 ml to 4,000 ml. There is a calibration mark etched on the neck of the flask. When the flask is filled to that mark, the flask contains that volume. Volumetric flasks are hard to use when dissolving solids in liquid because of the narrowness of the neck. If solids are to be dissolved in the flask, it is best to partially fill the flask with liquid, dissolve the solid, and then fill the flask with more liquid to the calibration mark.

volumetric measures volume. Volumetric vessels are either TD (to deliver) or TC (to contain).

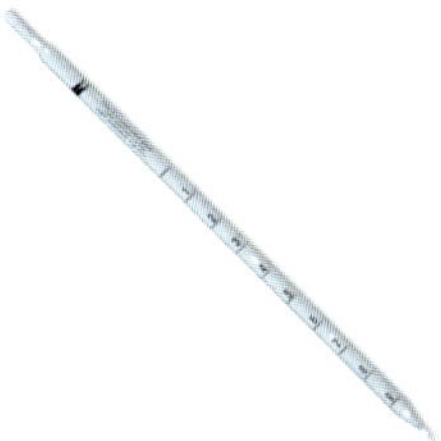

Pipets

Pipets are thin glass tubes recommended for the delivery of all volumes less than 5 ml and required for delivering volumes less than 1 ml (in the absence of an appropriate syringe). A rubber pipet bulb is used to draw liquid into the pipet. There are two basic types of pipets:

- The single volume or transfer pipet is the most accurate and simplest to use, but is limited to the measurement of a single fixed volume. They are normally used for the accurate transfer of 1.0, 2.0, 5.0, 10.0, and 25.0 ml of liquid.
- The calibrated pipet has several calibration marks from a point near the tip to the capacity of the pipet. It can deliver multiple volumes of liquid with good precision.
- A micropipet is a type of pipet with two parts, a hand piece and a disposable tip. The handle section usually has a turn screw that adjusts the volume of liquid drawn into the pipet tip. Each micropipet is calibrated for a range of volumes such as 1–20, 1–100, 1–200 or 1–1000 microliters. When determining which range to use, select the smallest range that will accommodate the volume of liquid to be measured.

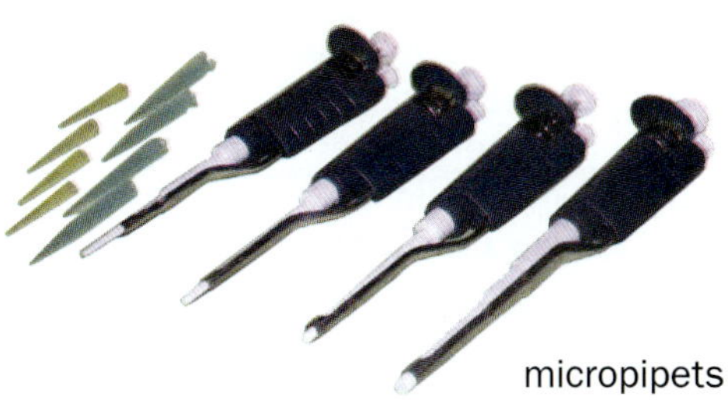

micropipets

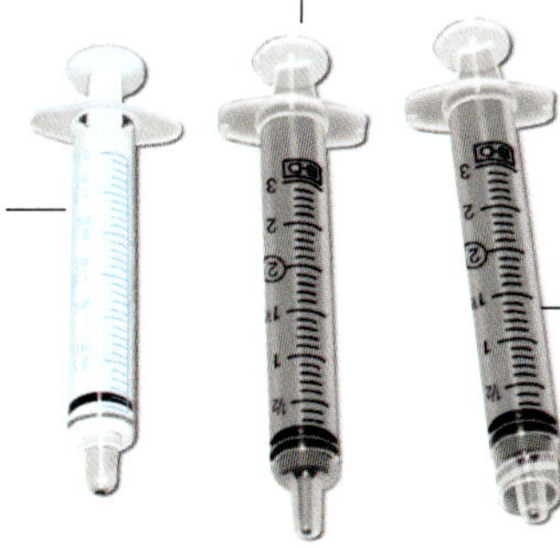

Syringes

Syringes come in sizes from 0.5 ml to 60 ml and in a variety of materials and styles. For most compounding tasks involving small volumes, a disposable hypodermic syringe or an oral syringe made of plastic is used. Syringes have graduation marks on the barrel for measuring partial volumes. As when selecting a graduated cylinder, choose the smallest syringe capable of containing the volume to be measured.

tip

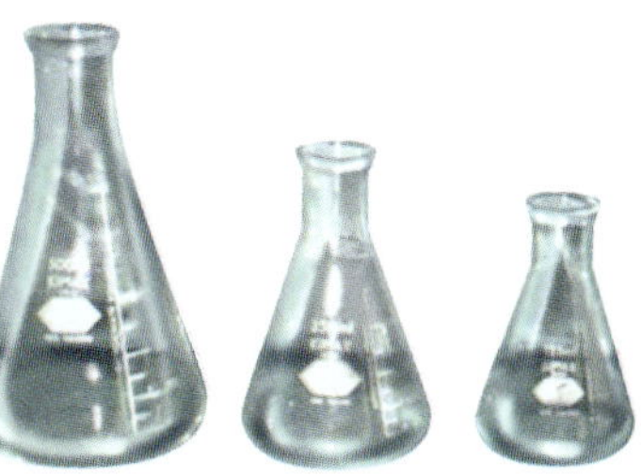

Erlenmeyer flasks (right), beakers, and prescription bottles, regardless of markings, are not volumetric glassware, but are simply containers for storing and mixing liquids. The designated volume is only the approximate capacity of the vessel.

MEASURING LIQUIDS

Selecting a Liquid Measuring Device

- ✔ Always use the smallest device (graduated cylinder, pipet, syringe) that will accommodate the desired volume of liquid. This will minimize the potential for errors in measurement associated with misreading the scale.
- ✔ Use a calibrated pipet, micropipet, or syringe to measure/deliver volumes less than 1 ml.
- ✔ Remember that oily and viscous liquids will be difficult to remove from graduated cylinders and pipets, and at best require long drainage time. Consider using a syringe instead, or measuring by weight rather than volume.
- ✔ Never use prescription bottles, non-volumetric flasks, beakers, or household teaspoons as measurement devices.
- ✔ Liquids have a ***meniscus*** when they are poured into containers. The surface of the liquid curves downward toward the center. If the container is very narrow, the meniscus can be quite large. When reading a volume of a liquid against a graduation mark, hold the measuring device so the meniscus is at eye level and read the mark at the bottom of the meniscus. Viewing the level from above will create the incorrect impression that there is more volume in the measuring device.

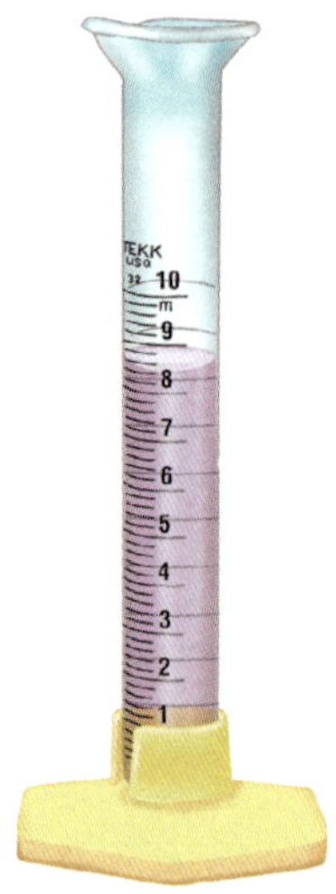

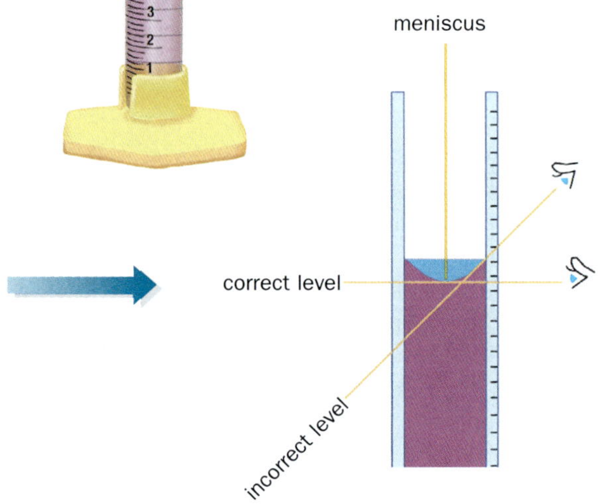

Droppers

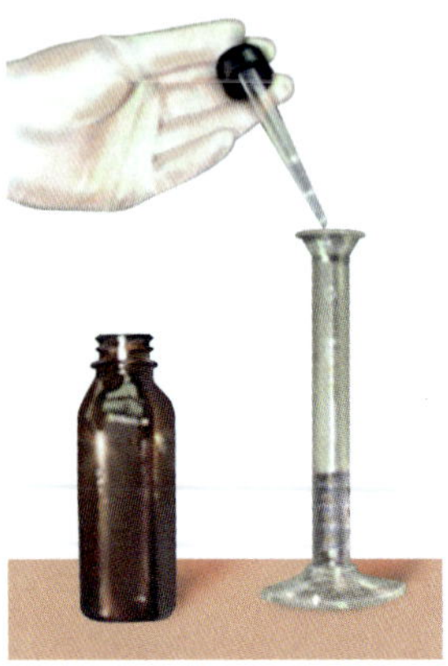

Medicine droppers can be used to deliver small doses of liquid medication. But the medicine dropper must first be calibrated because the drop size will vary from dropper to dropper and from liquid to liquid. Personal factors can also contribute to the inaccuracy of droppers. Two individuals dispensing the same liquid from identical droppers may produce drops of different sizes because of variations in the pressure, speed of dropping, and the angle at which the dropper is held.

To calibrate a medicine dropper, slowly drop the liquid formulation into a small, cylindrical graduate (10 ml), and count the number of drops needed to add several milliliters (ml) to the graduated cylinder. Calculate the average number of drops per ml. Some commercially produced medications are packaged with a marked dropper that has already been calibrated for that preparation.

Graduated Cylinders

Cylindrical graduates are more accurate than conical ones. The following steps will help maximize accuracy when using either a cylindrical or conical graduate.

1. Either place the graduated cylinder on a flat surface that will allow you to view it at eye level or hold the graduated cylinder by the base with the left hand (for a right-handed person) and elevated so that the desired mark is at eye level.
2. Hold the solution container with the right hand and pour the liquid to be measured into the center of the graduated cylinder. This will minimize the liquid adhering to the wall of the graduated cylinder (especially viscous liquids).
3. As the surface of the liquid approaches the desired mark, decrease the pouring rate or use a dropper or pipet to bring the level to final volume. The final volume should be determined by aligning the bottom of the meniscus with the desired graduation mark.
4. Transfer the liquid from the graduated cylinder to the appropriate vessel or container, allowing about 15 seconds for aqueous and hydroalcoholic liquids to drain. Approximately 60 seconds (or more) will be required for more viscous liquids such as syrups, glycerin, propylene glycol, and mineral oil.

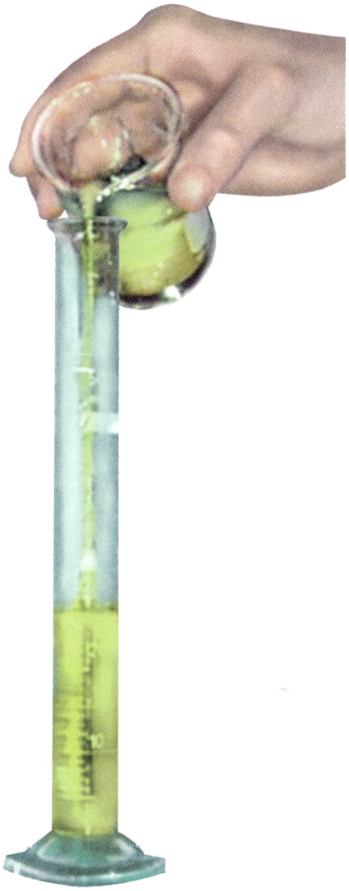

Special Precautions When Using Graduated Cylinders

- ✔ While graduated cylinders are volumetric devices, they are not mixing devices. They should not be used as a container for dissolving solids in liquids. A solution should first be prepared in a beaker or flask, and then placed in the graduated cylinder for final volume adjustments.
- ✔ Do not assume that the final volume of a formulation will be the sum of the individual volumes of liquid ingredients. This is particularly important with the admixture of aqueous and nonaqueous solutions such as alcohol and water. When these solutions are mixed, the total volume is less than the sum of the two volumes.

meniscus the curved surface of a column of liquid.

MEASURING LIQUIDS (cont'd)

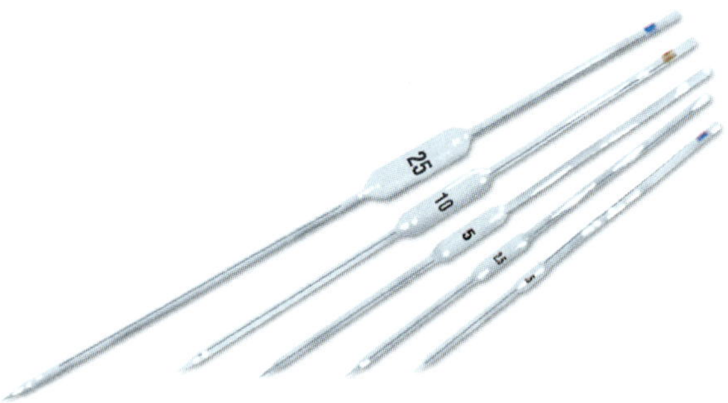

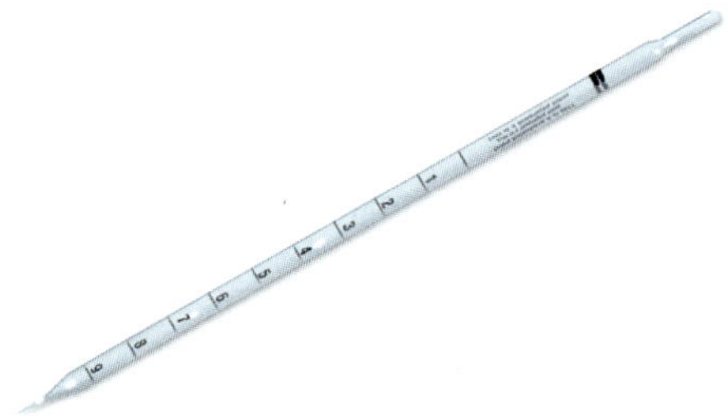

Single Volume Pipets

Single volume pipets have only one graduation mark, and that is the indicated volume of the pipet (e.g., 5 ml, 10 ml). As a result, the pipet is filled, and then emptied. There is no partial filling done with a single volume pipet. The steps in using a single volume pipet are:

1. Using a rubber bulb for suction, draw the liquid into the pipet until it is above the graduation mark.
2. Remove the pipet from the solution.
3. Wipe the end of the pipet with a tissue or Kimwipe®.
4. While holding the pipet in a vertical position, release the pressure inside the bulb and allow the liquid to flow into a waste beaker until the bottom of the meniscus coincides with the graduation mark. Droplets that remain suspended from the tip of the pipet can be removed by touching the pipet to the inside of the waste beaker.
5. Allow the pipet to drain for 30 seconds (or up to 3 minutes for viscous liquids) while touching the tip of the pipet to the inner side of the receiving vessel.

Calibrated Pipets

The calibrated pipet is filled and emptied the same way as a single volume pipet. However, it has multiple graduation marks that allow partial volumes to be transferred by noting the meniscus level before and after delivery. For example, you can deliver 1.50 ml of a liquid by filling the pipet to 8.50 ml and then allowing it to drain until the meniscus reaches 7.00 ml. A second delivery could be made by allowing the meniscus to reach 5.50 ml. The final graduation of the pipet is usually some distance above the pipet tip so that delivery is performed from graduation to graduation and not from graduation to tip as with the single volume pipet.

From a practical standpoint, the calibrated pipet is the preferred pipet for compounding. Just about any prescription requiring small volumes can be compounded with just three basic sizes of pipets: a 1 ml pipet subdivided in 1/100 ml graduations, a 2 ml pipet subdivided in 1/10 ml graduations, and a 5 ml pipet subdivided in 1/10 ml graduations.

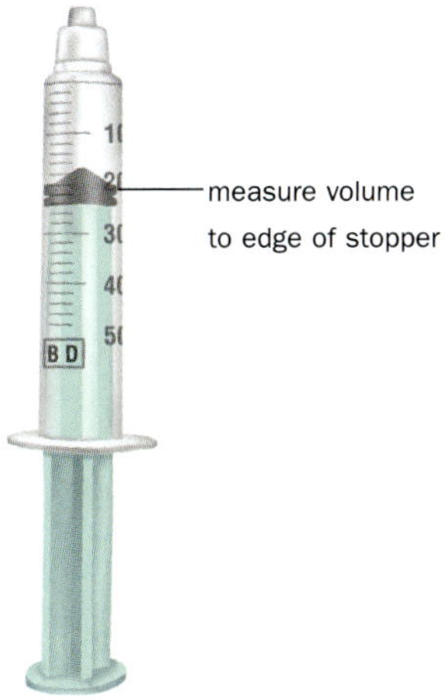

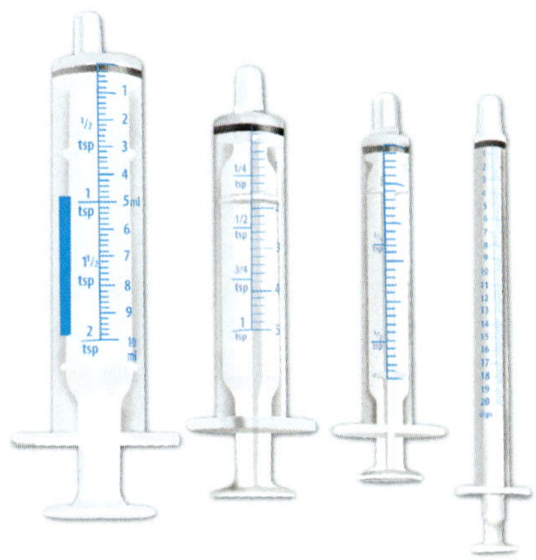

Syringes

Syringes come in a variety of sizes ranging from 0.5 ml (calibrated in 0.01 ml graduations) to 60 ml (calibrated in 2 ml graduations). Syringes may be used to deliver a wide range of liquid volumes with a high degree of accuracy. Measurements made with syringes are more accurate and precise than those made with cylindrical graduates. They are especially useful for measuring and delivering viscous liquids. Besides being easy to use, plastic disposable syringes are unbreakable and economical. As with graduated cylinders and pipets, select a syringe that equals or barely exceeds the volume to be measured.

Liquids are pulled into the syringe by pulling back on the plunger. The tip of the syringe must be fully submerged in the liquid to prevent drawing air into the syringe. Generally, an excess of solution is drawn into the syringe so that any air bubbles may be expelled by holding the syringe tip up, tapping the syringe until the air bubbles rise into the hub, and depressing the plunger to expel the air. This ensures that the hub will be completely filled with solution and the volume of delivery will be accurate.

Oral Syringes

Oral syringes are available for accurately administering liquid medication to the patient. They are especially useful when administering nonstandard doses. Oral syringes have tips that are larger than tips on hypodermic syringes so needles cannot be placed on these syringes. After the dose is drawn into the syringe, a cap is placed on the tip to prevent leakage and prevent contamination.

Oral syringes can be used with a device called an Adapt-a-Cap®. Adapt-a-Caps® do not work with hypodermic syringes (i.e., Slip-Tip® or Luer-Lok®). The cap portion of the Adapt-a-Cap® screws onto the bottle containing the liquid, and the oral syringe is fitted into the other side of the cap. When the bottle is inverted, liquid is withdrawn by pulling back on the syringe plunger. When the required volume has been withdrawn, the bottle is righted, and the syringe is removed from the Adapt-a-Cap®. There are different size caps to fit bottles with different size openings.

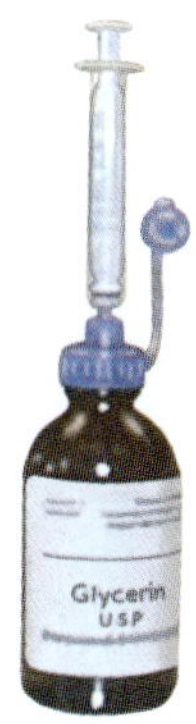

MIXING SOLIDS AND SEMISOLIDS

Mortars and Pestles

Mortars and pestles are commonly used for mixing solids and semisolids. They are made of three types of materials: glass, wedgwood, and porcelain. Wedgwood and porcelain mortars are earthenware, relatively coarse in texture, and are used to grind crystals and large particles into fine powders. The process of grinding powders to reduce the particle size is called ***trituration***. Glass mortars and pestles are preferable for mixing liquids and semisolid dosage forms.

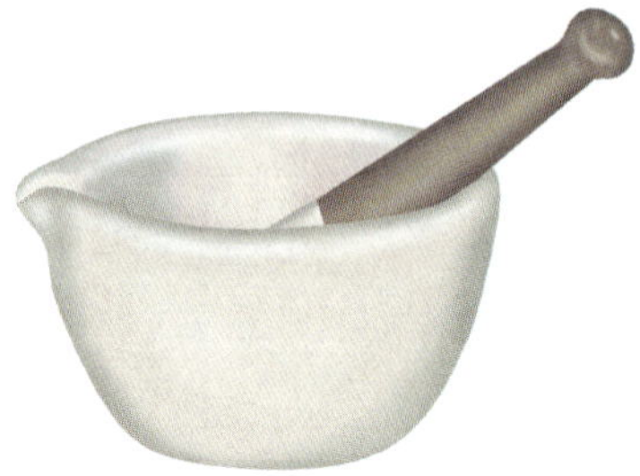

a wedgwood mortar and pestle

Sieves

Compounded powders need to be fine particles. They are then smooth to the touch and nonirritating to the skin. When the size of the particle needs to be reduced, the powder is passed through a sieve. A sieve is a mesh screen that will allow only particles smaller than the mesh openings to pass through it. The size of the mesh opening is expressed as a number indicating the number of openings in the mesh screen per inch. For example, a #40 sieve has 40 openings per inch and particles that can sift through it are said to be "40 mesh" size.

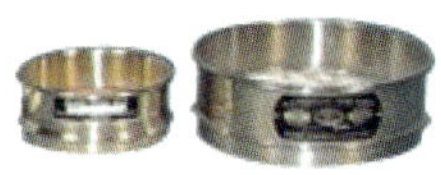

brass sieves

Mixing Powders

When mixing two powders of unequal quantity, a technique called ***geometric dilution*** is used. The smaller amount of powder is diluted in steps by additions of the larger amount of powder. If the two powders are just mixed together without this technique, a homogenous (fully and evenly combined) mixture will not result.

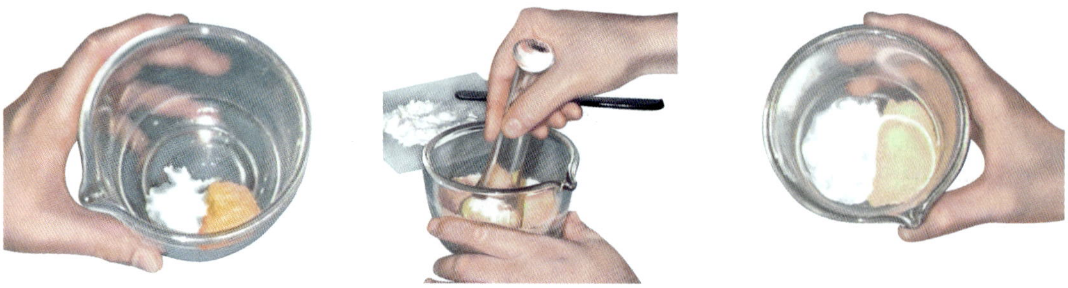

The smaller amount of powder is first triturated with an approximate equal portion of the larger amount of powder in a mortar. This first triturate is then mixed with an approximate equal portion of the larger amount of powder, and these are again triturated in the mortar. This dilution process is continued until all of the two powders have been mixed in the mortar.

Spatulas

Spatulas are used to transfer solid ingredients. They are also used as the mixing instruments in semi-solid dosage forms such as ointments and creams. Spatulas are available in a variety of sizes and are made of stainless steel, hard rubber, or plastic. Stainless steel spatulas can be corroded with certain materials such as iodine, and in these cases, rubber or plastic spatulas should be used. Always clean the spatulas before and after use.

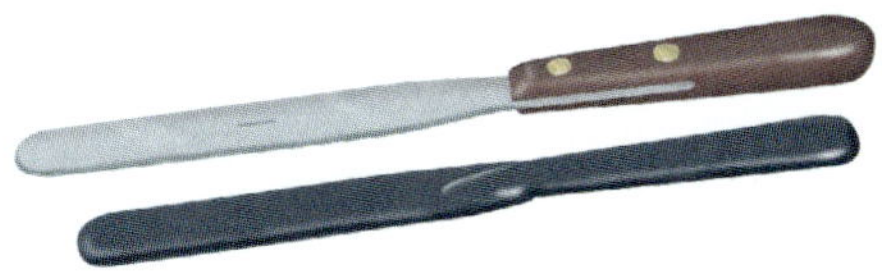

spatulas

Spatulation

Spatulation mixes powders using a spatula. The mixing can be done in a mortar, on an ointment slab, or in a plastic bag.

This method is used when mixing eutectic powders. Eutectic powders partially liquefy when they are brought together. So, the powders are individually mixed with a "carrier" powder (e.g., magnesium oxide, calcium carbonate, starch, lactose) and then blended by spatulation. Some eutectic compounds are aspirin, salicylic acid, camphor, benzocaine, and lidocaine.

When powders are triturated together in a mortar with a pestle, the overall size of the particles is reduced. With spatulation, there is no particle size reduction so the powders must be of fine particle size and of uniform size before the process begins. There is also no pressure applied to the mixture when it is blended so the resulting blend is light and fluffy.

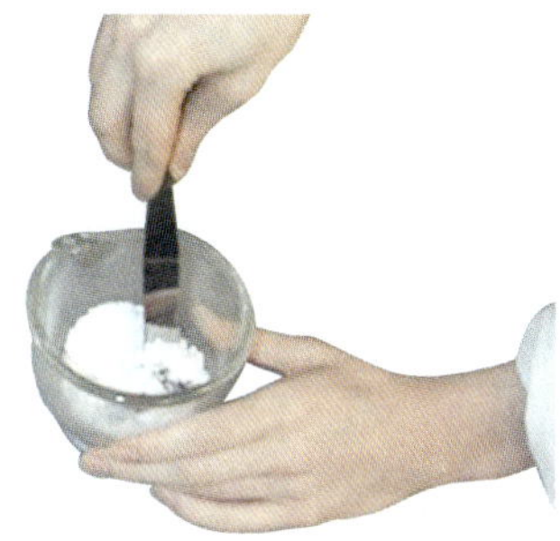

spatulation with a mortar and pestle

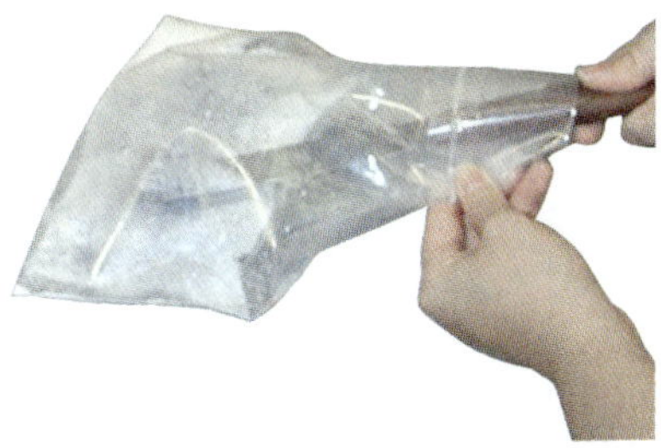

spatulation in a bag

geometric dilution a technique for mixing two powders of unequal quantity.

spatulation mixing powders with a spatula.

trituration the process of grinding powders to reduce particle size.

MIXING SOLIDS AND SEMISOLIDS (cont'd)

Ointment Slabs

Some ointments and creams are prepared on ointment slabs, which are porcelain or ground glass plates. They are often square or rectangular, and provide a hard, nonabsorbable surface for mixing compounds. Spatulas are used to mix the ingredients of the formulation on the slab.

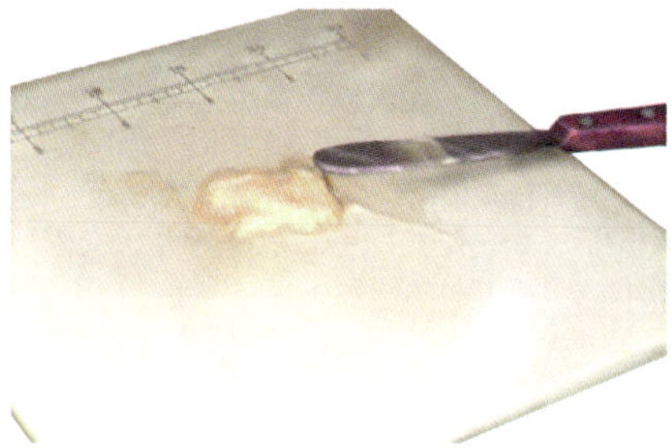

Levigation

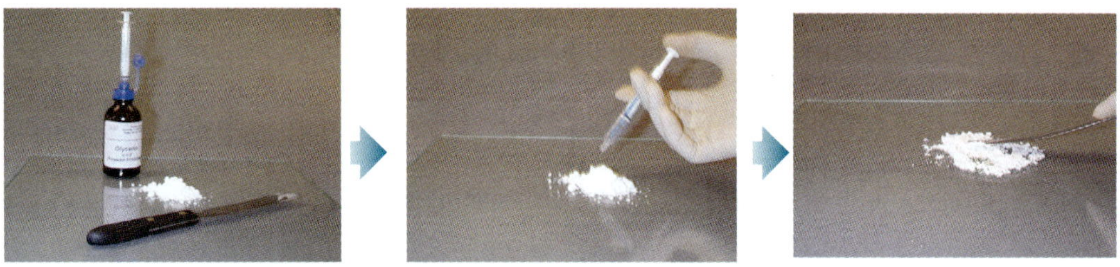

Levigation is a technique used to reduce the particle size of a powder by triturating it with a solvent in which the ingredient is insoluble. This reduces the grittiness of the final formulation. Levigation is generally done before the drug is incorporated into a formulation such as a suspension, ointment, or suppository base.

For example, hydrocortisone (used in ointments) is levigated with glycerin before being incorporated into an ointment base. This reduces the size of the hydrocortisone particles so the resulting ointment will be smooth, not gritty.

Levigation can be done with a mortar and pestle or on an ointment slab.

levigation triturating a powder with a solvent in which it is insoluble to reduce its particle size.

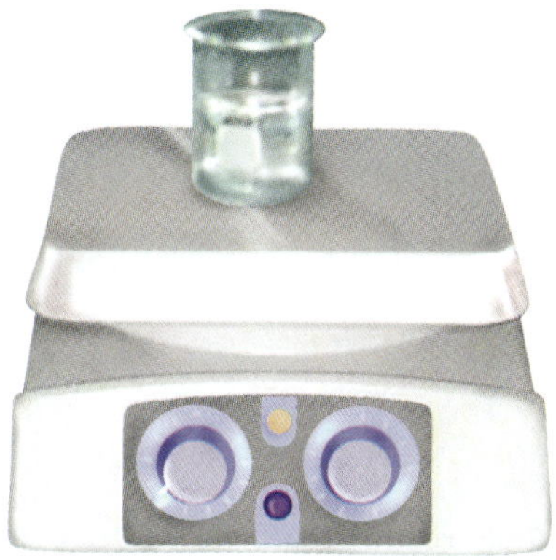

Hot Plates

Sometimes solids and semisolids are mixed by melting them together in a beaker on a hot plate. The hot plate needs to be a special low-temperature (25°C to 120°C) hot plate, and not a standard laboratory type hot plate; those hot plates heat at 125°C to 150°C at their lowest setting. If a low-temperature hot plate is not available, a water bath or steam bath will suffice. Most solids and semisolids used in pharmaceutical compounding will completely melt by 70°C. The melt is removed from the hot plate and allowed to cool to room temperature with constant stirring using a stirring rod, spatula, or magnetic stirring bar. Forced cooling in cold water, ice water, or ice will change the consistency and texture of the final product.

Electric Mortar and Pestles and Ointment Mills

If large quantities of powders need to be blended, or several ingredients in a semisolid need to be mixed, an electric mortar and pestle (EMP) or an ointment mill can be used.

An EMP, such as the Unguator® e/s, Unguator® Q and Unguator® 2100 shown at right, has mixing blades which operates inside a plastic mixing jar. As the EMP operates, the jar moves up-and-down and the mixing blade rotates at moderately high speed inside; this mixes the ingredients in a closed system. The length of the mixing time and speed of the mixing blade can be defined either by programmed presets, or by the operator.

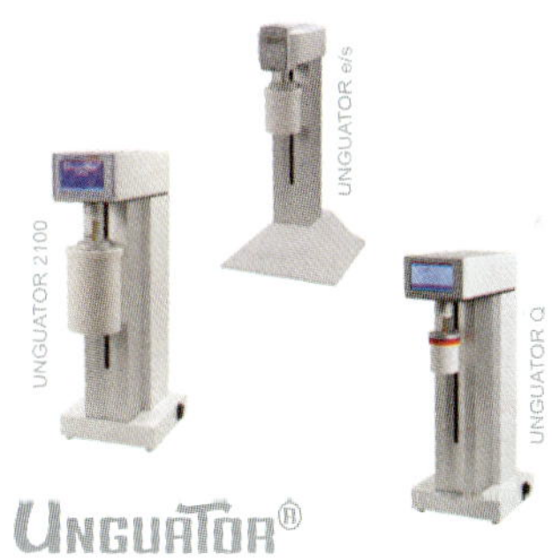

Image courtesy Unguator® Technologies

Ointments mills help achieve very uniform particle sizes in topical, rectal, and oral formulations. The mill has three ceramic rollers that are machined to extremely close tolerance. The degree of uniformity can be controlled by adjusting the spacing between the rollers. The closer the tolerance between the set of rollers, the more the formulation's particle size is reduced, and the more uniform the formulation.

Two side guides on top of the rollers help place the formulation onto the back set of rollers. The formulation then moves through the mill and onto the scraper plate. If the desired smoothness and elegance has been achieved, the formulation can then be dispensed. If more smoothness is needed, the formulation may be scraped off the front plate, and returned to the mill.

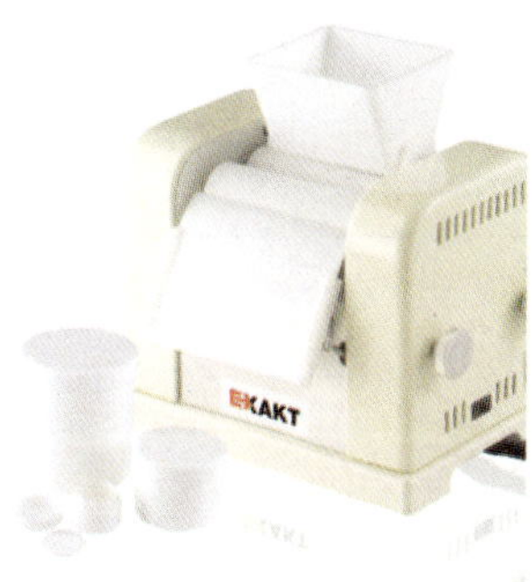

ointment mill
Image courtesy EXAKT Technologies, Inc.

COMPOUNDING SELECT DOSAGE FORMS

Aqueous Solutions

Solutions are probably the most commonly compounded products. Solutions are clear (but not necessarily colorless) liquids in which the drug is completely dissolved. The simplest compounded solution is the addition of a drug in liquid form to a liquid base solution called a "vehicle." This involves the careful measurement of the drug using graduated cylinders or syringes, and then diluting the drug to the final volume with the liquid vehicle. The resulting mixture should be thoroughly shaken or stirred to ensure adequate mixing. Purified water is the most common liquid used in pharmaceutical solutions, but combinations of ethanol, glycerin, propylene glycol, or a variety of syrups may be used, depending on the product requirements.

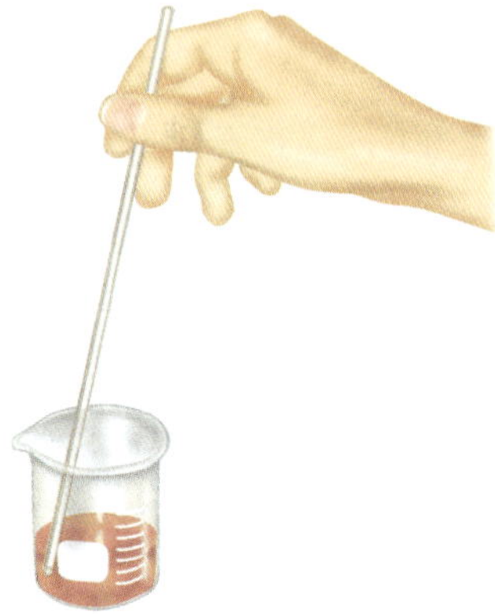

Most solutions require thorough shaking or stirring for adequate mixing.

When solids are to be dissolved in solution, they must be carefully weighed using a prescription balance. Most solids dissolve easily in a solvent. However, some may need to be triturated first to reduce the particle size and increase the dissolution rate. Others require that the solvent be heated (but not overheated, since some drugs decompose at higher temperatures). Some drugs require vigorous shaking, stirring, or ***sonication*** (the application of sound waves using sonic mixing equipment) to affect dissolution.

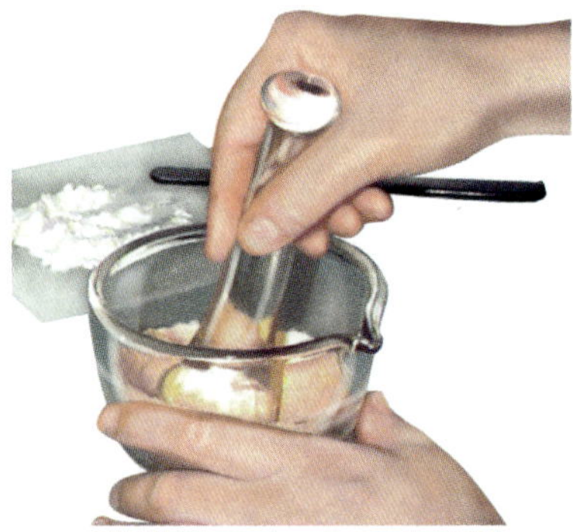

Some solids need to be triturated before mixing in a solution.

The solubility of the drug must be known before attempting to dissolve it in a solution. If a drug is not soluble in a vehicle, then no amount of mixing will help.

The solubility of a drug in a solvent may be described in a variety of ways. References generally express the solubility in terms of the volume of solvent required to dissolve 1 gram of the drug. A small distinction, but an important one, needs to be made about these solubility values. The solubilities are given as grams of solute per milliliter of solvent, not per milliliter of final solution. If the concentration is going to be close to the solubility, this distinction may be relevant. Solubilities may also be expressed in more subjective terms such as those given in the table below from the USP–NF.

Descriptive Terms	Parts of Solvent Needed for 1 Part Solute
Very soluble	< 1
Freely soluble	1–10
Soluble	10–30
Sparingly soluble	30–100
Slightly soluble	100–1,000
Very slightly soluble	1,000–10,000
Practically insoluble or insoluble	> 10,000

sonication exposure to high frequency sound waves.

Syrups

A syrup is a concentrated or nearly saturated solution of sucrose in water. Syrups containing flavoring agents are known as flavoring syrups (e.g., Cherry Syrup, Acacia Syrup); medicinal syrups are those that contain drugs (e.g., Guaifenesin Syrup).

When a reduction in calories or sucrose properties is desired, syrups can be prepared from sugars other than sucrose (e.g., glucose, fructose), non sugar polyols (e.g., sorbitol, glycerin, propylene glycol, mannitol), or other non nutritive artificial sweeteners (e.g., aspartame, saccharin). Non nutritive sweeteners do not produce the same viscosity as with sugars and polyols, so viscosity enhancers such as methylcellulose are often added. Polyols, though less sweet than sucrose, produce good viscosity and have some preservative and solvent qualities. A 70% sorbitol solution is a commercially available syrup vehicle.

Syrups are primarily made by two methods, with or without heat. Using heat is a faster method, but it cannot be used with heat sensitive ingredients. When using heat, the temperature must be carefully controlled to avoid overheating sucrose, which would make the syrup darker in color and more likely to ferment. When making syrups without heat, stirring or shaking generally provides the energy to produce the solution. In this case, a mixing vessel that is about twice as large as the final volume of the product is needed to provide adequate room for mixing.

Syrup	pH	Alcohol Content
Acacia	5.0	0
Aromatic eriodictyon	6.0 - 8.0	6 - 8
Cherry	3.5 - 4.0	1 - 2
Citric acid	—	< 1
Cocoa	—	0
Glycyrrhiza	6.0 - 6.5	5 - 6
Hydriodic acid	—	0
Orange	2.5 - 3.0	2 - 5
Raspberry	3.0	1 - 2
Sarsaparilla		
Syrup USP	6.5 - 7.0	0
Tolu	5.5	2 - 4
Wild cherry	4.5	1 - 2
Coca-Cola™	1.6 - 1.7	0
Syrpalta	4.5	0

Nonaqueous Solutions

Nonaqueous solutions are those that contain solvents other than water, either alone or in addition to water. There are several types of nonaqueous solutions:

- elixirs
- tinctures
- spirits
- fluid extracts
- glycerates
- collodions
- liniments
- oleaginous solutions

Elixirs, collodions, and oleaginous solutions are the most commonly compounded nonaqueous solutions. Elixirs are clear, sweetened, hydroalcoholic liquids intended for oral use. Because elixirs are hydroalcoholic solutions, they can be used to dissolve either alcohol soluble or water soluble drugs. Oleaginous solutions (e.g., corn oil, peanut oil, mineral oil) can be used for oral, topical, or parenteral administration. Collodions are limited to topical application. Collodions and oleaginous solutions would be suitable for more lipophilic (i.e., oil loving) ingredients.

When compounding these formulations, separately dissolve the alcohol soluble ingredients in the alcohol (or oleaginous) portion and the water soluble ingredients in the water portion. Then add the aqueous solution to the alcohol solution, stirring constantly. This will keep the alcohol concentration as high as possible so that the final solution does not become turbid.

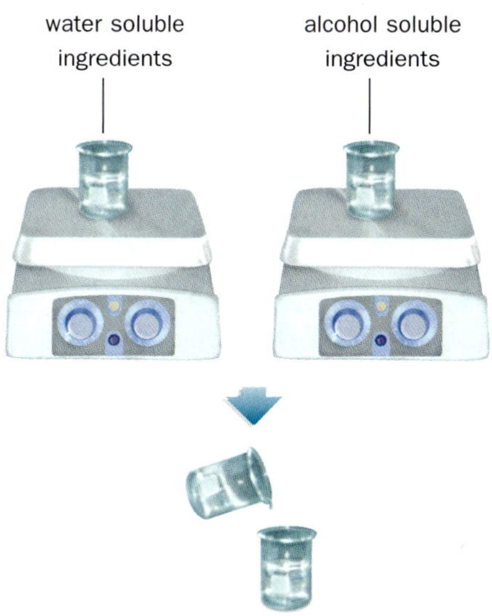

pouring water soluble ingredients into alcohol soluble ingredients

COMPOUNDING SELECT DOSAGE FORMS (cont'd)

Suspensions

The term suspension refers to a two-phase system consisting of a finely divided solid dispersed in a liquid. The solid particles are typically 1 to 50 micrometers in diameter. The primary concern in formulating suspensions is that they tend to settle over time and the dose becomes unevenly dispersed in the liquid. A well-formulated suspension remains dispersed or settles very slowly and can be redispersed easily with shaking. The settling properties of a suspension are controlled by (1) the addition of flocculating agents to enhance particle "dispersibility" and (2) the addition of thickening agents to reduce the settling (sedimentation rate) of the suspension.

- ***Flocculating agents*** are electrolytes that carry an electrical charge. The flocculating agent imparts the electrical charge onto the suspended particle; since all of the particles will have the same charge, there is a slight repulsion between the particles as they settle. What results are clusters of particles, or floccules, which are loosely associated with each other and may be easily redispersed by shaking.
- ***Thickening agents*** are often referred to as viscosity enhancers or suspending agents. They are added to suspensions to thicken the suspending medium, thereby reducing the sedimentation rate of the floccules. Typical thickening agents include carboxymethyl cellulose, methylcellulose, bentonite, and tragacanth.

To begin compounding a suspension, the solid drug to be suspended is levigated in a mortar with a pestle with an appropriate levigating agent. This will reduce the drug's particle size and wet the particles to form a paste. Common levigating agents are mineral oil or glycerin. Then, a portion of the vehicle is added to the mortar, and mixed with the levigated drug until a uniform mixture results. This mixture is then put into the final container or a volumetric measuring device. The mortar and pestle are rinsed with portions of the remaining vehicle, and each rinsing is added to the final container or volumetric measuring device until the final volume is reached.

Some commercially available suspensions require reconstitution with water before they are dispensed. Water is added to the package container and shaken to form the suspension.

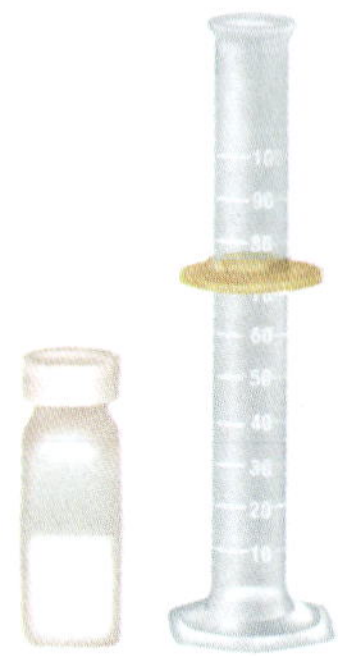

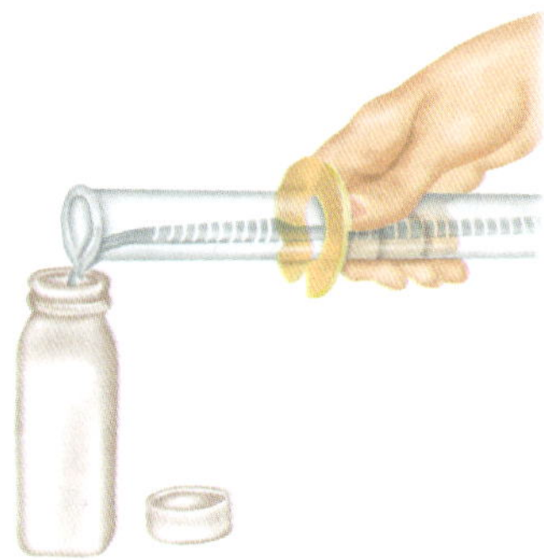

mixing

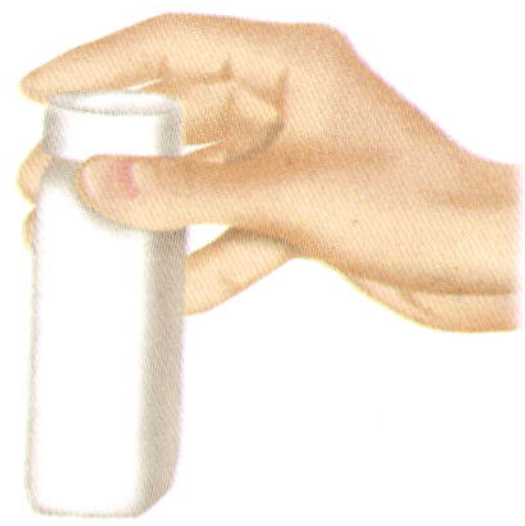

shaking

flocculating agent electrolytes used in the preparation of suspensions to form particles that can be easily redispersed.

thickening agent an ingredient used in the preparation of suspensions to increase the viscosity of the liquid.

tip

Suspensions should be dispensed in bottles with enough air space for adequate shaking and contain the auxiliary label "Shake well."

Flavorings

The human tongue contains about 10,000 taste buds that distinguish salty, bitter, sour, and sweet tastes. The flavor experience is a complex combination of taste, smell, texture, appearance, and temperature. Most patients want:

- immediate flavor recognition;
- rapid full flavor development;
- acceptable mouth feel;
- short after-taste;
- and no undesirable sensations.

Discovering the flavoring agent best suited to masking an unpleasant drug taste is often an empirical matter. It will also be patient dependent. For the basic tastes, several flavors have been found to work well.

Taste	Flavor
Salty	Cinnamon, raspberry, orange, butterscotch
Sweet	Fruit, berry, vanilla
Bitter	Cocoa, chocolate, mint, cherry, walnut
Sour/Acid	Fruit, citrus, cherry
Oily	Wintergreen, peppermint, lemon, anise
Metallic	Mint, marshmallow

Sweeteners

Some desired properties of sweeteners include colorless, odorless, solubility in water at the concentrations needed for sweetening, pleasant tasting with no "after-taste," and stable over a wide pH range. Simple Syrup, 70% sorbitol solution, sodium saccharin (0.05%), aspartame (0.1%), and dextrose have many of these properties.

When increasing the sweetness of a formulation that contains both a sweetening agent and a flavoring agent, increase the sweetener concentration first. All flavoring agents are bitter and need sweetening to make them more pleasing to the taste. If a desirable sweetness cannot be found by changing the sweetener concentration, then experiment with changing the flavoring agent concentration.

Sweetener	Sweetness Compared to Sucrose (Approx.)
Sorbitol	0.5–0.7
Mannitol	0.7
Saccharin	500
Sodium Saccharin	300
Aspartame	180
Stevia	200

Coloring

Coloring agents are not required in every formulation; they are contraindicated in all sterile solutions. However, clear, water-like oral solutions may be perceived to be inert or lack potency. Dark colors such as dark purple, navy, black, and brown may also be rejected because they are often associated with poisons. More pleasant, fruity colors are generally preferred and should be coordinated with flavors and scents (e.g., yellow with lemon, red with cherry). Flesh-toned colors may be added to topical preparations so the product is less visible on the skin.

From a practical standpoint, the pharmacy technician may consider food colorings sold in grocery stores to be safe and appropriate to use. These are red, blue, yellow, or green aqueous solutions and are ideally suited to coloring aqueous solutions. Blends may be used to produce nearly any color.

COMPOUNDING SELECT DOSAGE FORMS (cont'd)

Emulsions and Emulsifiers

An emulsion is an unstable system consisting of at least two ***immiscible*** liquids, one of which is dispersed in the form of small droplets throughout the other, and a stabilizing agent.

Emulsifiers are used as stabilizing agents because emulsions will separate into two distinct phases or layers over time. Some separation can be overcome with shaking. However, some separations result in emulsions that "break" and these cannot be redispersed. Emulsifiers provide a protective barrier around the dispersed droplets. Some commonly used emulsifying agents include tragacanth, sodium lauryl sulfate, sodium dioctyl sulfosuccinate, and polymers known as the Spans® and Tweens®.

When oils, petroleum hydrocarbons, and/or waxes are dispersed into water or another aqueous solution, the system is called an ***oil-in-water (o/w) emulsion***. With o/w emulsions the aqueous solution generally makes up greater than 45% of the total weight. A ***hydrophilic emulsifier*** is used as the stabilizing agent for o/w emulsions

When water or an aqueous solution is dispersed in an oleaginous (oil based) medium, the system is known as a ***water-in-oil (w/o) emulsion***. With w/o emulsions the aqueous solution generally constitutes less than 45% of the total weight. A ***lipophilic emulsifier*** is used as the stabilizing agent for w/o emulsions.

Soy lecithin and a gel containing pluronic 407 can be combined to make pluronic lecithin organogel or "PLO gel." This is really an emulsion and not a true gel. PLO gel is used as a dispersing medium for topical application of active drugs because the pluronic gel dissolves water soluble active drugs and the lecithin dissolves oil soluble drugs, enhancing skin penetration of the active drug(s).

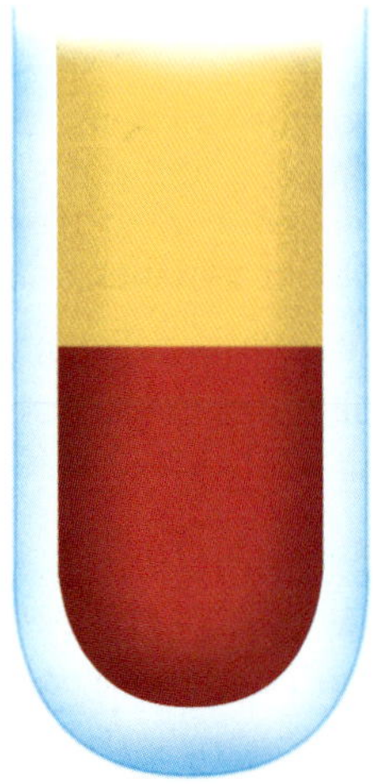

emulsion before mixing

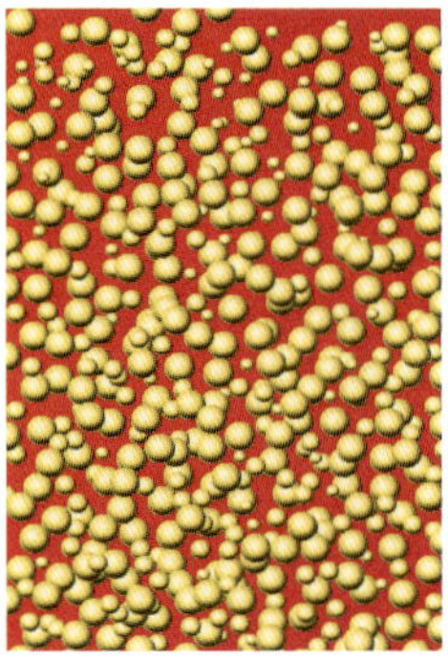

a close-up after mixing

emulsifier a stabilizing agent in emulsions.

hydrophilic emulsifier a stabilizing agent for water based dispersion mediums.

immiscible cannot be mixed.

lipophilic emulsifier a stabilizing agent for oil based dispersion mediums.

mucilage a wet, slimy liquid formed as an initial step in the wet gum method.

oil-in-water emulsion an emulsion in which oil is dispersed in a water base.

primary emulsion the initial emulsion to which ingredients are added to create the final product.

water-in-oil emulsion an emulsion in which water is dispersed in an oil base.

Methods for Preparing Emulsions: Continental (Dry Gum), Wet Gum, and Beaker

There are various methods used to make emulsions. All use energy in the form of shaking, heat, or the action of a mortar and pestle to form the emulsion.

In the Continental method (sometimes also referred to as the Dry Gum method), an initial, or ***primary emulsion***, is formed from 4 parts oil, 2 parts water, and 1 part gum emulsifier such as acacia. In a dry wedgwood or porcelain mortar, the 1 part gum is triturated with the 4 parts oil until the powder is thoroughly levigated. Then the 2 parts water are added, and the mixture is vigorously and continually triturated until the primary emulsion is formed (usually 1–2 minutes). It appears as creamy white and produces a “cracking” sound as it is triturated. Additional ingredients are incorporated after the primary emulsion is formed.

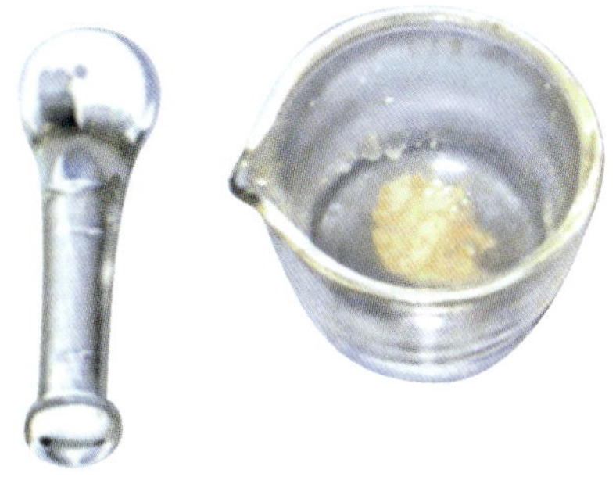

gum and water in preparation for the Wet Gum method

In the Wet Gum method, the primary emulsion is formed by triturating 1 part gum with 2 parts water to form a ***mucilage***, and then slowly adding 4 parts oil, in portions, with trituration after each addition. After all the oil is added, the mixture is triturated for several more minutes to form the primary emulsion. Then other ingredients may be added as in the Continental method.

Some emulsions will have a consistency of a lotion or a cream (i.e., a semisolid). The method of choice in making these types of emulsions is the Beaker method. The ingredients of the formulation are divided into water soluble and oil soluble components. All oil soluble components are dissolved in one beaker and all water soluble components are dissolved in a separate beaker. Both phases are then heated to approximately 70°C using a low-temperature hot plate or steam bath. The two beakers are removed from the heat, and the internal phase is slowly added to the external phase with continual stirring. The product is allowed to cool to room temperature but is constantly stirred with a stirring rod, spatula, or magnetic stirring bar.

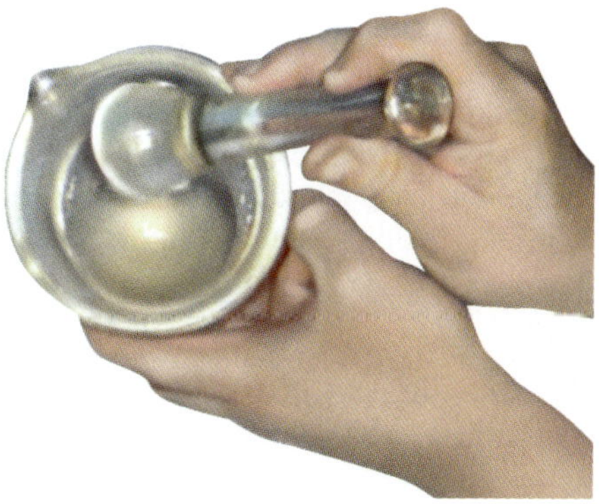

forming the mucilage

℞ **tip**
Stabilizing agents used in emulsions are called emulsifiers, surfactants, or surface active agents.

COMPOUNDING SELECT DOSAGE FORMS (cont'd)

Ointments

Ointments are generally emulsions that have a large portion of un-emulsified solid material. They are used for many different purposes, e.g., as protectants, antiseptics, emollients, and antipruritics.

One major type of compounded ointment is a mixture of an active drug incorporated into an ointment base. There are five types of ointment bases ranging from oleaginous to water ***miscible*** (i.e., capable of being mixed together with water). A particular ointment base is chosen for its fundamental properties or for its potential to serve as a drug delivery vehicle.

If the ointment base will be a drug delivery vehicle, the primary consideration will be its ability to release drug. Oleaginous (oil based) bases generally release substances slowly and unpredictably, since water cannot penetrate them well enough to dissolve the drug and allow for diffusion out of the ointment. Water miscible or aqueous bases tend to release drugs more rapidly.

These types of ointments are generally compounded on an ointment slab. In the simple case of combining two ointments or a drug and an ointment, each component is carefully weighed and placed on an ointment slab. The ingredients are combined by geometric dilution using two spatulas to mix the ointment. One spatula will be used to continually remove ointment from the other spatula. Using a spatula, the ointment is transferred into an ointment jar just big enough for the final volume. When filling the ointment jar, use the spatula to bleed out air pockets. Wipe any excess material from the outside of the jar, including the cap screw threads.

Drugs in powder or crystal form, such as salicylic acid, precipitated sulfur, or hydrocortisone, need to be triturated or levigated in a mortar with a pestle before incorporating them into an ointment base. This will prevent a gritty texture in the final product. Another technique to reduce particle size is to dissolve the drug in a very small amount of solvent and then let the solvent evaporate.

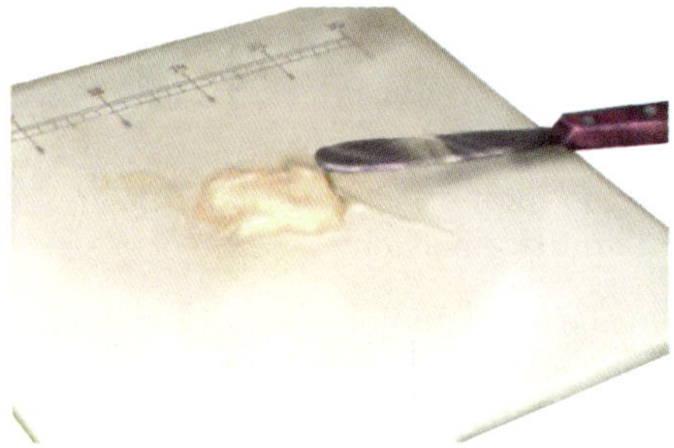

Ointments are generally compounded on an ointment slab.

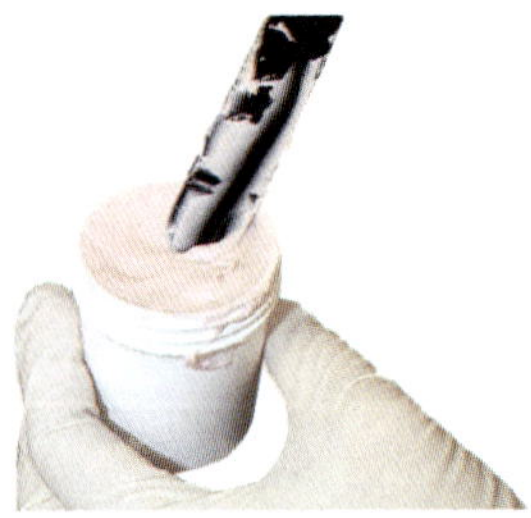

The ointment is then transferred into an ointment jar.

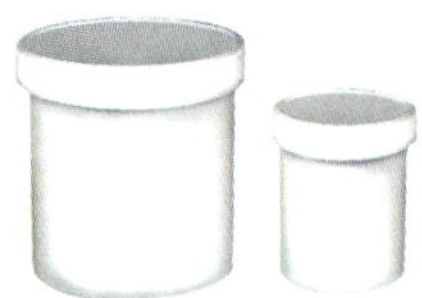

ointment jars

Properties of Ointment Bases

Property	Oleaginous Bases	Absorption Bases	Water/Oil Emulsion Bases	Oil/Water Emulsion Bases	Water Miscible Bases
Water Content	anhydrous	anhydrous	hydrous	hydrous	hydrous
Spreadability	difficult	difficult	moderate to easy	easy	moderate to easy
Washability	nonwashable	nonwashable	non- or poorly washable	washable	washable
Greasiness	greasy	greasy	greasy	nongreasy	nongreasy
Occlusiveness	yes	yes	sometimes	no	no
Examples	White Petrolatum, White Ointment	Hydrophilic Petrolatum, Aquaphor®	Hydrous Lanolin, Eucerin®, Nivea®	Hydrophilic Ointment	PEG Ointment

miscible capable of being mixed together.

Another major type of compounded ointment is one where the base is formed as part of the compounding process. The general scenario is to heat oleaginous soluble ingredients in one beaker and aqueous soluble ingredients in another beaker, and then combine the two phases and let the mixture congeal.

Following are some suggestions for compounding an ointment base:

- When heat is used to melt ingredients, use a water bath or special low-temperature hot plate. Most ingredients used in ointment bases will liquefy around 70°C. Some common substances used in base formulations and their melting points are given in the table below.
- It is helpful to heat the aqueous phase a few degrees higher than the oleaginous phase prior to mixing because the aqueous phase tends to cool faster than the oleaginous phase. However, use the lowest temperature possible and keep the time of heating as short as possible. This will minimize the quantity of water lost through evaporation.
- When melting a number of ingredients, melt the ingredient with the highest melting point first. Then gradually reduce the heat to melt the ingredient with the next highest melting point. Continue this process until all ingredients have been added. This will ensure that the ingredients were exposed to the lowest possible temperature and thus enhance the stability of the final product.

The cooling step in an ointment's preparation is an important part of the compounding process.

- ✔ Do not accelerate the cooling process by putting the melt in water or ice. This can significantly change the consistency of the final product.
- ✔ If adding volatile ingredients such as oils, flavors, or drugs, add them when the product is cool. The melt will still be fluid enough for adequate mixing but not hot enough to evaporate the ingredient.
- ✔ Ointments should be cooled until just a few degrees above solidification before they are poured into tubes or jars. This will minimize "layering" of the ointment in the packaging container.

Mixing Oleaginous and Aqueous Mixtures

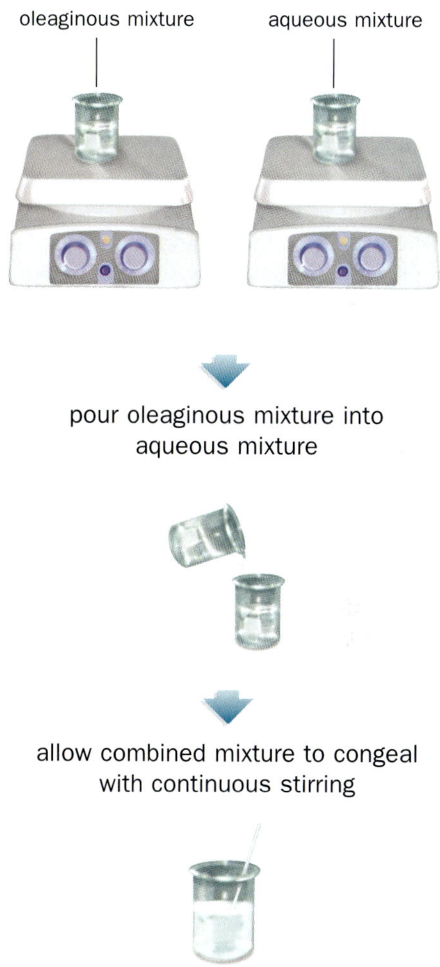

Ingredient	Melting Point (°C)	Ingredient	Melting Point (°C)
Carnauba wax	81–86	Stearic acid	69–70
Cetyl alcohol	45–50	Stearyl alcohol	55–60
Cetyl esters wax	43–47	White wax (Beeswax)	62–65
Cholesterol	147–150	PEG 1500	44–48
Cocoa butter	30–35	PEG 3350	54–58
Glyceryl monostearate	55	PEG 6000	58–63

COMPOUNDING SELECT DOSAGE FORMS (cont'd)

Suppositories

There are three classes of suppository bases defined by their composition and physical properties:

- Oleaginous bases
- Water soluble or miscible bases
- Hydrophilic bases

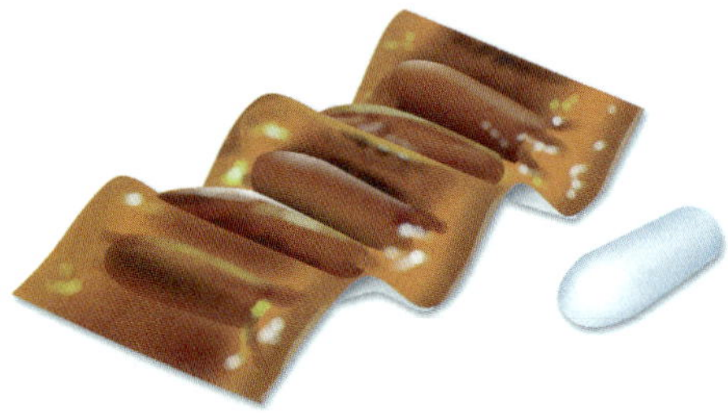

suppositories in plastic shells

Oleaginous Bases

A well-known suppository base is cocoa butter (Theobroma Oil USP). At room temperature, cocoa butter is a solid, but at body temperature, it melts to a bland, nonirritating oil. Cocoa butter is no longer the base of choice because preparing suppositories with it is difficult, and the suppositories require refrigeration. Synthetic triglycerides can be used that do not have the formulation difficulties of cocoa butter, but they are more expensive. There are also newer bases composed of mixtures of fatty acids that do not have the formulation problems or the expense (e.g., FattiBase®, Witepsol®).

Water Soluble or Miscible Bases

Water soluble or miscible bases contain glycerinated gelatin or polyethylene glycol (PEG) polymers. Glycerinated gelatin is a useful suppository base, particularly for vaginal suppositories. Glycerinated gelatin suppositories are gelatinous solids that tend to dissolve slowly to provide prolonged release of active ingredients. Polyethylene glycol (PEGs) polymers are chemically stable, nonirritating, miscible with water and mucous secretions, and can be formulated by molding or compression in a wide range of hardnesses and melting points. Like glycerinated gelatin, they do not melt at body temperature, but dissolve slowly to provide a prolonged release of drugs.

Polyethylene glycols are available in various molecular weight ranges. Those of 200, 400, or 600 molecular weight are liquids. Those with molecular weights over 1,000 are solids. Certain PEGs may be used individually as suppository bases but, more commonly, combinations of two or more molecular weights are mixed in various proportions to give a desired hardness or dissolution time. Since PEGs suppositories dissolve in body fluids and need not be formulated to melt at body temperature, they can be formulated with much higher melting points and can be safely stored at room temperature.

Hydrophilic Bases

Hydrophilic bases are mixtures of oleaginous and water miscible bases. They generally contain a small percentage of cholesterol or lanolin to assist in water absorption.

Some PEG Formulations

Molecular Weight	Percent
PEG 300	60%
PEG 8000	40%
PEG 300	48%
PEG 6000	52%
PEG 1000	95%
PEG 3350	5%
PEG 1000	75%
PEG 3350	25%
PEG 300	10%
PEG 1540	65%
PEG 3350	25%
PEG 8000	50%
PEG 1540	30%
PEG 400	20%
PEG 3350	60%
PEG 1000	30%
PEG 400	10%

compression molding a method of making suppositories in which the ingredients are compressed in a mold.

fusion molding a suppository preparation method in which the active ingredients are dispersed or dissolved in a melted suppository base.

Molding Methods

Suppositories are usually prepared by ***compression molding*** or ***fusion molding***. Compression molding is a method of preparing suppositories by mixing the suppository base and the drug ingredients and forcing the mixture into a special compression mold.

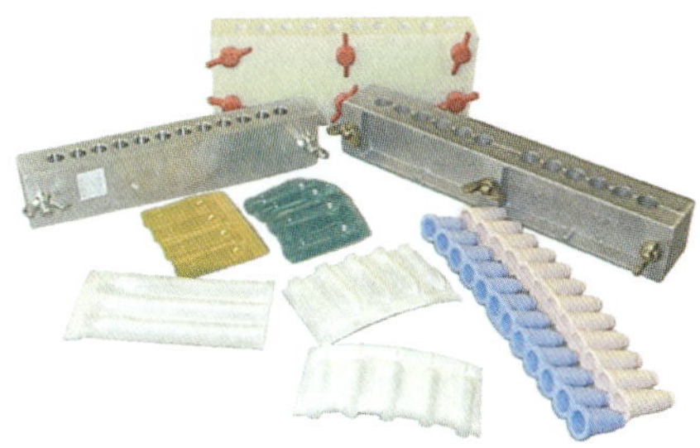

types of suppository molds

Fusion molding is a method in which the drug is dispersed or dissolved in a melted suppository base. The fusion method can be used with all types of suppositories and must be used with most of them. In this method, the suppository base is melted on a low-temperature hot plate, and the drug is dissolved or dispersed in the melted base. The mixture is then removed from the heat and poured into a suppository mold, over filling each cavity. The mixture is allowed to congeal (harden), and the excess material is removed from the top of the mold.

Suppository Molds

There are many types of suppository molds: metal (aluminum or steel) molds, plastic molds, or rubber molds. The metal molds come in a variety of cavity sizes, from 6 to 100. The two halves of the mold are held together with screws. When the suppository mixture has congealed, the excess mass on top of the suppository mold can be removed with a hot spatula or knife scraped flat across the surface of the mold. The screws on the mold are loosened, and the mold is separated. Never open a mold by prying it apart with a knife or spatula. This will damage the matching mold faces which have been accurately machined to make a tight seal. The suppositories are removed from the mold, generally wrapped in foil paper, and put in a suppository box.

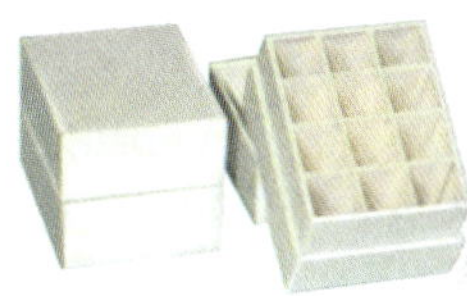

a suppository box

Plastic suppository molds come in long strips and can be torn into any number of cavities. When the suppository has hardened in the cavity, the plastic mold is heat sealed, torn into individual suppository cavities, and put in a suppository box. Rubber molds come in long strips but cannot easily be separated into individual cavities. Suppositories are allowed to remain in the mold (i.e., unwrapped), and the entire mold is put in a dispensing box.

tip

Polyethylene glycol polymers (PEGs) are used in a wide variety of formulations. Low molecular weight PEGs (<1,000) are liquids and impart a softer texture to the formulation. High molecular weight PEGs (>1,000) are solids and add stiffness to the formulation.

COMPOUNDING SELECT DOSAGE FORMS (cont'd)

Capsules

Hard gelatin capsules consist of a body and a cap that fits firmly over the body of the capsule. For human use, eight sizes of capsules are available. Capsules can be filled with liquid or powder formulations. The table below provides capsule sizes and their relative liquid fill capacities.

The total amount of a powder formulation that can be placed in a capsule varies according to the bulk density of the formulation. Several methods have been devised to help select the appropriate size capsule for a particular powder formulation. One method is to compare the density of the formulation being compounded to the density of a known drug. Similar amounts of powder with similar densities will fit in the same size capsule. For example, if a formulation has a density similar to aspirin and 300 mg are needed for each dose, then a #1 capsule would be needed, based on the information in the table on page 241. In general, the smallest capsule that will contain the formulation is used since patients often have difficulty swallowing large capsules.

When filling a small number of capsules, the ***punch method*** is used. The ingredients are triturated to the same particle size and then mixed by geometric dilution. Since some powder will be lost in the punching process, calculations are made for the preparation of at least two extra capsules. The powder is placed on an ointment slab and smoothed with a spatula to a height approximately half the length of the capsule body. The body of the capsule is held vertically and the open end is repeatedly pushed, or "punched," into the powder until the capsule is filled. The cap is then replaced to close the capsule. Each filled capsule is weighed using an empty capsule as a counterweight. Powder is added or removed until the correct weight has been placed in the capsule.

Capsule filling machines are available for filling 100 or 300 capsules at a time. The machines come with a capsule loader that correctly aligns all of the capsules in the machine base. The powder is poured onto the base plate and special spreaders and combs are used to fill the individual capsules. All of the caps are simultaneously returned to the capsule bodies, and the batch is complete. When using a capsule filling machine, it takes practice to ensure that each capsule has the same amount of drug. There is a tendency to overfill the capsules in the center, and under fill the capsules around the edges.

The Punch Method

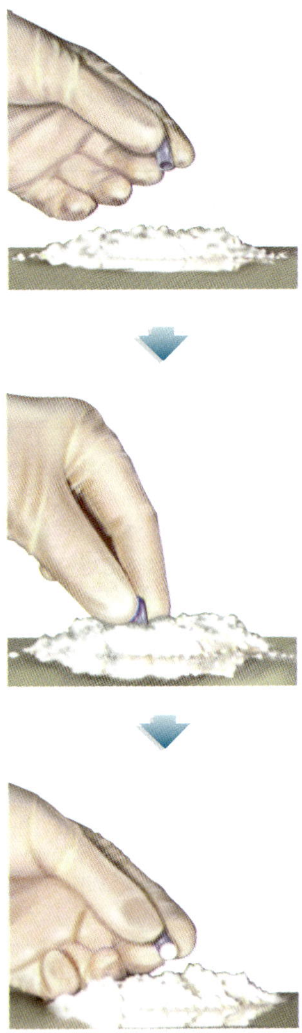

Capsule Size	Liquid Volume (ml)	Capsule Size	Liquid Volume (ml)
000	1.37	2	0.37
00	0.95	3	0.30
0	0.68	4	0.20
1	0.50	5	0.13

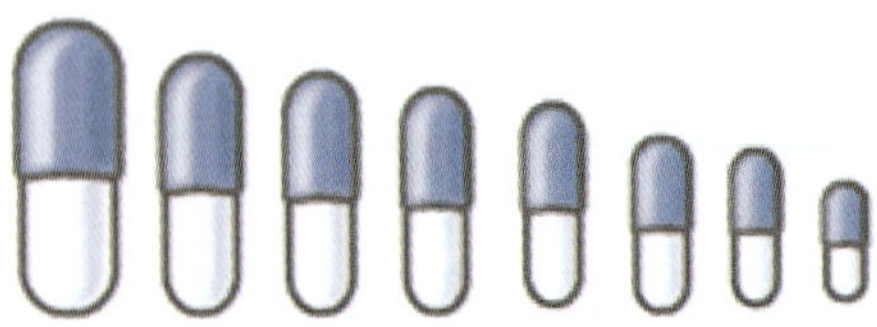

finger cots protective coverings for fingers.

punch method a method for filling capsules by repeatedly pushing, or "punching," the capsule into an amount of drug powder.

Other Tips for Compounding Capsules:

- It is a good practice to have the exact number of empty capsules needed set out before compounding begins. This will avoid preparing the wrong number of capsules and will prevent the contamination of other empty capsules with drug particles that cling to hands.
- The simplest method to keep a capsule free from fingerprints is to use the cap of one capsule as a holder for other capsule bodies during the filling operation. This avoids the capsule bodies coming into contact with the fingers. Another way of protecting the capsules is to wear rubber gloves or protective covering for the fingers called ***finger cots***.
- To remove traces of drug from the outside of the filled capsules, roll them between the folds of clean towel or shake in a towel that has been gathered into the form of a bag.
- Liquids that do not dissolve gelatin, such as alcohol and fixed oils, may be dispensed in capsules. The correct volume of liquid is delivered into the empty capsule body by calibrated dropper or pipet. The size of the capsule should be chosen so that the liquid does not completely fill the body and none of the liquid should touch the outside of the body. The capsule is sealed by moistening the lower portion of the inside of the cap with warm water using a camel's hair brush. The moistened cap is placed on the body and given a half turn. The capsules should be placed on an absorbent paper and inspected for leakage.
- Capsules will absorb moisture and soften in high humidity. In a dry atmosphere, they become brittle and crack. To protect capsules from the extremes of humidity, dispense them in plastic or glass vials, and store in a cool, dry place. A piece of cotton may be added in the top of the vial to keep the capsules from rattling.
- Tablets and smaller capsules can be placed inside capsules. This can be a real convenience to a patient that has many tablets or capsules to take per day.

Capsule Size	mg of lactose	mg of aspirin
000	1250	975
00	850	650
0	600	490
1	460	335
2	350	260
3	280	195
4	210	130
5	140	65

Using a Capsule Filling Machine

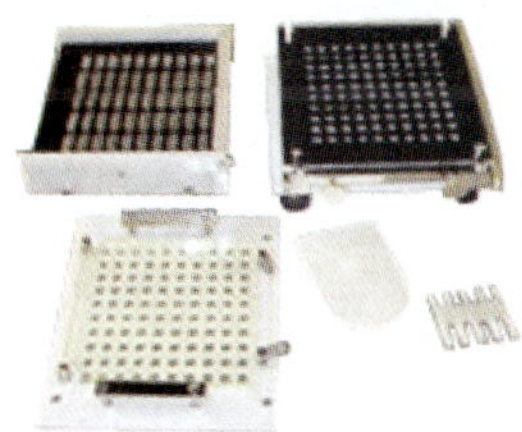

A capsule filling machine consists of a base plate, a capsule loader, a comb, a scraper, and a cap holder.

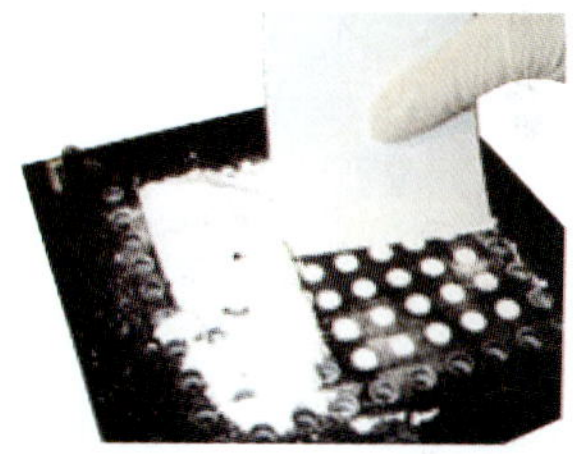

Pour the powder onto the base plate containing the loaded capsule bodies. Spread the powder over the capsules with the scraper.

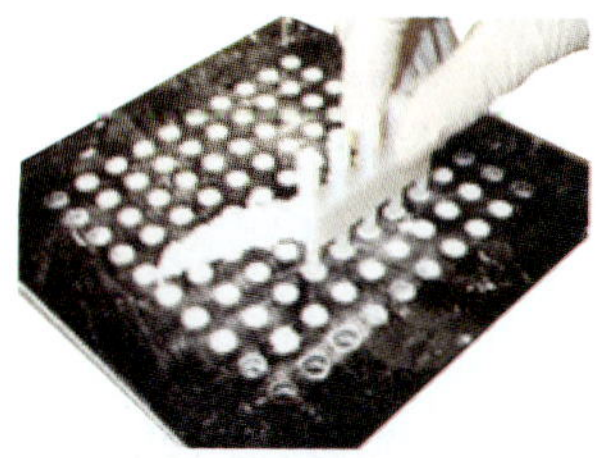

Use the comb to pack the capsules. Continue scraping and packing until the capsules are filled.

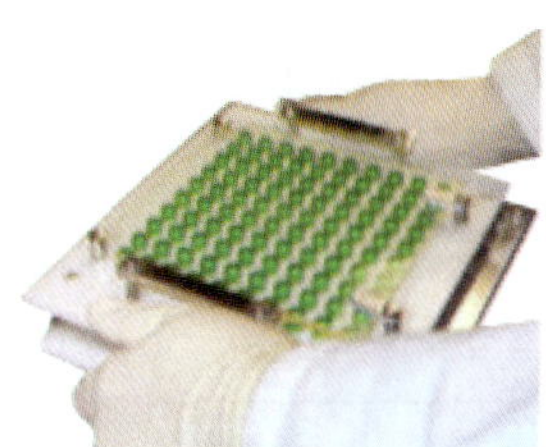

Fit the cap holder onto the base plate, pushing the caps onto the capsule bodies. Then remove the cap holder to remove the capsules.

COMPOUNDING SELECT DOSAGE FORMS (cont'd)

Tablets

Without question, commercially manufactured tablets are the most popular dosage formulation today. Tablets are typically orally administered, but can be used for other routes of administration such as sublingual (under the tongue), buccal (cheek pouch), pellets (subcutaneous implantation), and vaginal inserts. The only limitation of commercially manufactured tablets is that they are available in fixed dosage strengths and combinations. However, pharmacy technicians can extemporaneously compound molded and compressed tablets, providing flexibility and adaptability for their patients.

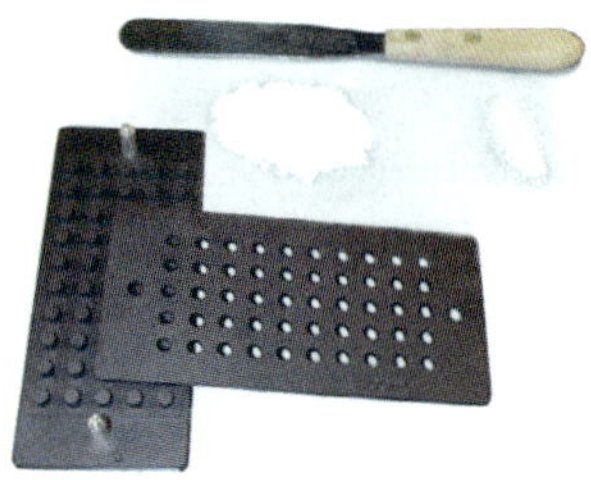

cavity plate, peg plate, powder blend, and spatula

Molded Tablets

Molded tablets are generally prepared by mixing the active drug with a base made of lactose, dextrose, sucrose, mannitol, or some combination of these carbohydrates. These bases are readily water soluble and do not degrade during preparation. Lactose is the preferred base but mannitol adds a pleasant, cooling sensation and additional sweetness in the mouth.

The base ordinarily used for molded tablet triturates is lactose containing 20%–30% sucrose to make a firmer tablet. The mixture of active drug and base is moistened with a solution of alcohol and water (typically about 50–75% alcohol) so the mixture will adhere together while being pressed into the mold cavities. Alcohol will speed up the drying of the tablets and the water will cause the powders to bind together due to its solvent action with sucrose.

Tablet triturate molds are made of metal. There are two plates: the cavity plate that has only holes and the peg plate that has pegs. The mold will indicate the capacity of one cavity (typically 60 mg or 100 mg) but this is only an approximation. The mold must be calibrated with each different formulation since each combination of active drug and base will have a unique density.

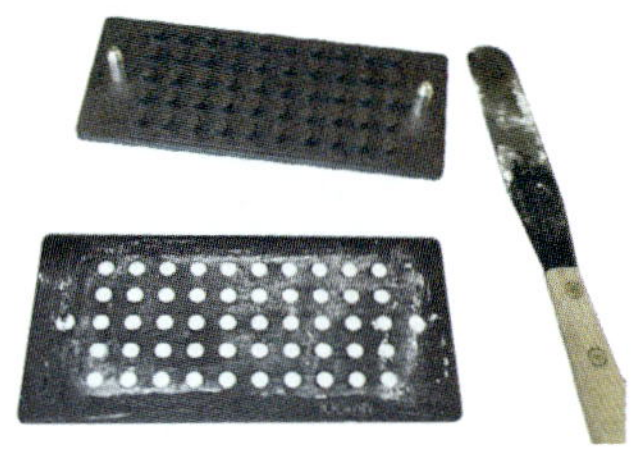

powder pressed firmly into cavity plate

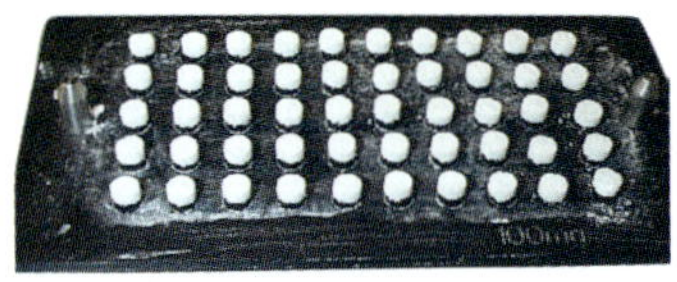

tablets pushed out by lowering cavity plate onto peg plate

Steps for Calibrating Tablet Triturate Molds

1. First make tablets that contain only the base. Weigh the tablets as a batch and calculate the average weight per tablet.
2. Make tablets containing only the active drug. Weigh them as a batch and calculate the average weight per tablet. Usually, just a few tablet cavities are used for this because pure drug is being used.
3. Divide the required quantity of active drug per tablet that will be in the compounded tablets by the value in step 2. This will give a percentage of the cavity volume that the active drug in the compounded tablets will occupy.
4. Subtracting the percentage in step 3 from 100% will give the percentage of the cavity volume that the tablet base will occupy.
5. The percentages of active drug and base in the cavity volume are used to calculate the appropriate amounts of base and drug to weigh. For example, if the mold contains 50 cavities and each will hold approximately 100 mg, then 5,000 mg of mixture will be needed to fill the mold. The amount of base and drug to weigh can be determined by multiplying 5,000 mg by the two different percentages determined in the preceding steps.
6. Prepare a slight excess of powder mixture (5%–10%) to allow for any variance in the approximate and actual capacity of the mold and to allow for powder loss during the compounding procedure.

Single Punch Tablet Machines

Multiple punch tableting machines are commonly used in the pharmaceutical industry and create millions of tablets in a small period of time. When extemporaneously compounding tablets, a single punch tablet machine is used to create compressed tablets. A punch has two pieces of cast metal. The lower piece is a metal plate that has a small cavity in it the size of the tablet to be created; the upper metal piece has one end tapered into a small rod that will just slide into the lower cavity. The upper piece does not go all the way to the bottom of the lower piece, but leaves a small gap. The tablet material is placed into the lower piece, and the upper punch is depressed. The powders are compressed and occupy the size of the gap designed in the punch. Chewable tablets, effervescent tablets, and compressed tablets can all be made using a tablet press.

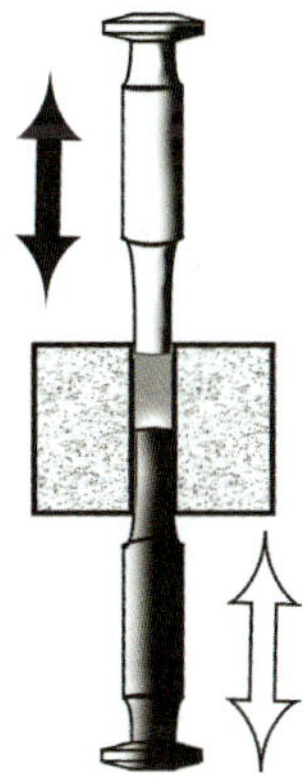

a single-pinch die

Rapid Dissolve Tablets (RDT)

RDTs disintegrate or dissolve within minutes after being placed in the mouth. This is an advantage when administering these dosage forms to children, to elderly, or to anyone who has difficulty swallowing tablets. The tablets liquefy on the tongue, and then the patient swallows the liquid.

RDT tablets contain a number of ingredients in a base formulation. These ingredients are usually extremely water soluble and are used to wick water into the RDT to aid in the dissolution of the tablet. The base ingredients also provide some friability (strength or hardness) to the tablet. The RDT base formulation will also have sweeteners and flavoring agents.

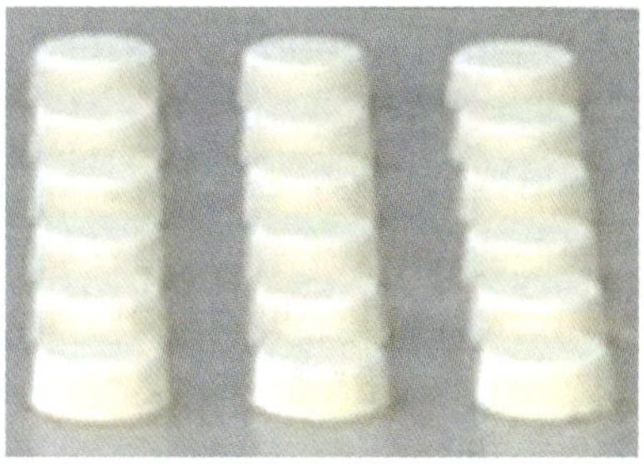

unit-dose rapid dissolve tablets on a card

Typical Ingredients in RDT Formulations

Ingredient	Use
Active drug	Therapeutic effect
Powdered sucrose	Base; hardness
Citric acid, anhydrous	Base; disintegration agent
Sodium bicarbonate	Base; disintegration agent
Mannitol	Base; sweetening agent; flavoring
Polyethylene glycol 3350	Base; stiffening agent
Silica gel	Absorbent; removing bitterness
Stevioside, acesulfame potassium	Sweeteners
Flavors	Flavoring

REVIEW

KEY CONCEPTS

COMPOUNDING

- ✔ Extemporaneous compounding is the on-demand preparation of a drug product according to a physician's prescription, to meet the unique needs of an individual patient.
- ✔ Compounding is regulated by individual state boards of pharmacy. Some states have their own regulations but many accept standards of the United States Pharmacopeia–National Formulary (USP–NF).

REGULATIONS

- ✔ The pharmacist has the responsibility and authority to manage the compounding area.
- ✔ Ingredients of USP–NF purity or better are to be used when compounding formulations.
- ✔ A compounding record and formulation record are required for each compounded formulation.

STABILITY AND BEYOND-USE DATES

- ✔ Beyond-use dates are required on compounded formulations.

COMPOUNDING CONSIDERATIONS

- ✔ There are four areas of considerations when compounding: 1) whether or not to compound; 2) before compounding; 3) during compounding; 4) after compounding.

EQUIPMENT

- ✔ Class A torsion balances can weigh as little as 120 mg of material with a 5% error.
- ✔ When weighing an amount of ingredient that is less than 120 mg, an aliquot or analytical balance can be used.

USING A BALANCE

- ✔ Class A torsion balances and electronic balances need to be leveled before weighing ingredients.
- ✔ Weighing papers or weighing boats should always be placed on the balance pans before weighing ingredients.

VOLUMETRIC EQUIPMENT

- ✔ Liquid drugs, solvents, or additives are measured in volumetric glassware or plasticware such as graduated cylinders, syringes, and pipets.
- ✔ Erlenmeyer flasks, beakers, and prescription bottles, regardless of markings, are not volumetric glassware.

MEASURING LIQUIDS

- ✔ Always use the smallest device that will accommodate the desired volume of liquid.
- ✔ When reading a volume of liquid against a graduation mark, hold the graduated cylinder so the meniscus is at eye level and read the mark at the bottom of the meniscus.

MIXING SOLIDS AND SEMISOLIDS

- ✔ Trituration is the fine grinding of a powder. Levigation is the trituration of a powder drug with a solvent in which the drug is insoluble. Both techniques reduce the drug's particle size.
- ✔ Geometric dilution must be used when mixing powders of unequal quantity.

COMPOUNDING SELECT DOSAGE FORMS

- ✔ Aqueous solutions are clear liquids (but not necessarily colorless) made most commonly with purified water but which may also contain ethanol, glycerin, or propylene glycol.

- ✔ Nonaqueous solutions include elixirs, tinctures, spirits, liniments, and oleaginous solutions.
- ✔ Suspensions are a two-phase system consisting of a finely divided solid dispersed in a liquid.
- ✔ The flavor experience is a complex combination of taste, smell, texture, appearance, and temperature.
- ✔ An emulsion is an unstable system consisting of at least two immiscible (unmixable) liquids, one that is dispersed as small droplets throughout the other, and a stabilizing agent.
- ✔ There are two major methods of compounding ointments: 1) incorporating a drug into an ointment base and 2) forming the base as a part of the compounding process.
- ✔ There are three classes of suppository bases defined by their composition and physical properties: oleaginous bases, water soluble or miscible bases, and hydrophilic bases.
- ✔ When preparing capsules, the smallest capsule capable of containing the final formulation is used since patients often have difficulty swallowing large capsules.
- ✔ Tablets are compounded in either molded, compressed, or rapid dissolve form.

SELF TEST

the answer key begins on page 569

MATCH THE TERMS: I

1. aliquot ____
2. arrest knob ____
3. beyond-use date ____
4. calibrate ____
5. Chapter <795> ____
6. Chapter <797> ____
7. compounding record ____
8. compression molding ____
9. emulsifier ____
10. finger cots ____
11. flocculating agent ____
12. formulation record ____
13. fusion molding ____

a. regulations from USP–NF pertaining to the nonsterile compounding of formulations.
b. the knob on a balance that prevents any movement of the balance pans.
c. a date assigned to a compounded prescription beyond which the formulation should not be used.
d. regulations from USP–NF pertaining to the sterile compounding of formulations.
e. electrolytes used in the preparation of suspensions.
f. formulas and procedures (i.e., recipes) for what should happen when a formulation is compounded.
g. a record of what actually happened when the formulation was compounded.
h. a portion of a mixture.
i. to set or check the graduations of a measuring device.
j. a stabilizing agent in emulsions.
k. method of making suppositories in which the ingredients are compressed in a mold.
l. a suppository preparation method in which the active ingredients are dispersed or dissolved in a melted base.
m. protective coverings for fingers.

REVIEW

MATCH THE TERMS: II

1. geometric dilution ____
2. hydrophilic emulsifier ____
3. immiscible ____
4. levigation ____
5. lipophilic emulsifier ____
6. meniscus ____
7. miscible ____
8. mucilage ____
9. oil-in-water emulsion ____
10. primary emulsion ____
11. punch method ____
12. sensitivity ____
13. sonication ____
14. spatulation ____
15. stability ____
16. thickening agent ____
17. trituration ____
18. volumetric ____
19. water-in-oil emulsion ____

a. a technique for mixing two powders of unequal quantities.
b. wet, slimy liquid formed as an initial step in the Wet Gum method.
c. capable of being mixed together.
d. the curved surface of a volume of liquid.
e. the extent to which a dosage form retains the same properties and characteristics it possessed when it was made.
f. the amount of weight that will move the balance pointer one division mark on the marker plate.
g. measures volume; are either TD (to deliver) or TC (to contain).
h. mixing powders with a spatula.
i. exposure to high frequency sound waves.
j. an ingredient used in the preparation of suspensions to increase the viscosity of the liquid.
k. water dispersed in an oil base.
l. oil dispersed in a water base.
m. the initial emulsion to which ingredients are added to create the final product.
n. the fine grinding of a powder.
o. a method for filling capsules.
p. triturating a powder drug with a solvent in which it is insoluble to reduce its particle size.
q. cannot be mixed.
r. a stabilizing agent for water-based dispersion mediums.
s. a stabilizing agent for oil-based dispersion mediums.

CHOOSE THE BEST ANSWER

1. ____________________ is the on-demand preparation of a drug product according to a physician's prescription.
   a. Manufacturing
   b. Extemporaneous compounding
   c. Trituration
   d. Spatulation

2. Chapter <795> of the USP–NF deals with
   a. compounding sterile products.
   b. compounding nonsterile products.
   c. official compounded formulations and their beyond-use dates.
   d. containers used to package compounded formulations.

3. The documentation that addresses step-by-step written instructions for conducting specific activities in a compounding pharmacy is the
   a. formulation record.
   b. ingredient record.
   c. compounding record.
   d. SOP (standard operating procedure).

4. What factor(s) affect(s) the beyond-use date of a compounded preparation?
   a. whether it is a solid formulation
   b. whether it is an alcohol containing formulation
   c. the length of time therapy is required
   d. all of the above

5. Class A torsion balances have
   a. less than a 5% error when weighing 120 mg.
   b. at least a 6 mg sensitivity.
   c. at least a capacity of 60 grams.
   d. all of the above.

6. Aliquots can be used when a prescription calls for less than _____ of an ingredient.
   a. 120 gm
   b. 500 gm
   c. 500 mg
   d. 120 mg

7. Which is the correct statement when weighing a powder on a Class A torsion balance?
   a. Pour the powder into the pan on the left side of the balance.
   b. Always use the largest possible weigh boat.
   c. Keep the balance unarrested.
   d. Use a clean weigh boat with each new powder.

8. _______ are volumetric vessels and can be used to accurately measure liquids for compounding.
   a. Volumetric flasks, graduated cylinders, pipets, and syringes
   b. Beakers
   c. Prescription bottles
   d. Erlenmeyer flasks

9. A 100 ml graduated cylinder cannot accurately measure volumes less than
   a. 20 ml.
   b. 50 ml.
   c. 30 ml.
   d. 40 ml.

10. If a 5 ml liquid volume needs to be measured, a ___________ should be used.
    a. 10 ml oral syringe
    b. 100 ml cylindrical graduate
    c. 100 microliter micropipet
    d. 25 ml Erlenmeyer flask

11. Adapt-a-Caps® are fitted with
    a. Slip-Tip® syringes.
    b. Luer-Lok® syringes.
    c. oral syringes.
    d. calibrated pipets.

12. Which measuring device would be the most appropriate for dispensing liquid for an infant?
    a. hypodermic syringe
    b. calibrated pipet
    c. oral syringe
    d. volumetric flask

13. _________ is the term for triturating a powder with a solvent in which it is insoluble to reduce its particle size.
    a. suspension
    b. trituration
    c. emulsion
    d. levigation

REVIEW

14. The fine grinding of a powder is called
    a. melting.
    b. trituration.
    c. levigation.
    d. suspension.

15. Which would not be used as a liquid vehicle in a compounded solution?
    a. ethanol
    b. propylene glycol
    c. glycerin
    d. ethylene glycol

16. The USP–NF gives "Relative Terms of Solubility." If a drug is "slightly soluble," how many parts of solvent are required for one part of drug?
    a. 1–10
    b. 10–30
    c. 30–100
    d. 100–1,000

17. Elixirs, tinctures, and liniments are examples of
    a. syrups.
    b. aqueous solutions.
    c. nonaqueous solutions.
    d. emulsions.

18. An aqueous solution of water soluble ingredients is added to an alcoholic solution of alcohol soluble ingredients and the resulting solution turns cloudy or "milky." What is happening?
    a. The alcoholic components are coming out of the solution.
    b. The aqueous components are coming out of the solution.
    c. Nothing; the cloudiness will go away when the solution is stirred.
    d. The small amount of water in the alcohol is separating out.

19. Which characteristics indicate a good suspension?
    a. settles quickly and redisperses slowly
    b. settles quickly and redisperses quickly
    c. settles slowly and redisperses slowly
    d. settles slowly and redisperses quickly

20. Most patients want their flavor experience (i.e., the flavoring in liquid dosage form) to have
    a. slow recognition of the flavor.
    b. a delayed flavor development.
    c. acceptable mouth feel.
    d. extended after-taste.

21. If you need to compound a liquid formulation containing a water-based vehicle and an active drug that is an oil, the appropriate dosage form would be a/an
    a. solution.
    b. elixir.
    c. emulsion.
    d. ointment.

22. The method of choice for making emulsions with the consistency of a lotion or cream is the
    a. Continental method.
    b. Beaker method.
    c. Wet Gum method.
    d. Dry Gum method.

23. When making an ointment in which the base is formed as part of the compounding process,
    a. heat the highest melting point ingredient last.
    b. rapidly cool the mixed water soluble and oil soluble components.
    c. add volatile ingredients when the ointment is almost congealed.
    d. use ingredients that melt only below 55°C.

24. Which suppository base would be preferable for vaginal suppositories?
    a. a combination of low molecular weight PEGs
    b. glycerinated gelatin
    c. cocoa butter
    d. Witepsol®

25. Capsules can contain
    a. other capsules.
    b. bulk powder.
    c. liquids that do not dissolve gelatin.
    d. all of the above.

26. The dose of powder to be placed in a capsule is 525 mg, and the powder has a density similar to lactose. What would be an appropriate hard gelatin shell size to use?
    a. size 3
    b. size 2
    c. size 1
    d. size 0

27. Which carbohydrate is often used to make a firmer molded tablet triturate?
    a. sucrose
    b. lactose
    c. sorbitol
    d. mannitol

CRITICAL THINKING QUESTIONS

1. Why is it important to be able to compound many different dosage forms?
2. Why is it essential that the pharmacy technician know how to use a balance correctly, and how to correctly measure volumes of liquids?
3. Why is geometric dilution used when mixing unequal amounts of powders?
4. Why is it important to know the stability of a compounded product?

THINKING IT THROUGH WRAP-UP

1. The nausea and vomiting could be from an ingredient in the tablets such as lactose (a common tablet filler) or an allergic reaction to a dye and could be prevented in a compounded version using another type of formulation, route of administration, or other ingredients.
2. Other dosage forms to consider would be intravenous solution; sublingual tablet or liquid; oral liquid (syrup, suspension, emulsion); ointment; suppository; or a molded tablet without the filler ingredients (i.e., just the drug).
3. Decisions would need to be made regarding the type of suppository base and suppository mold to use as well as the method for making the suppositories.

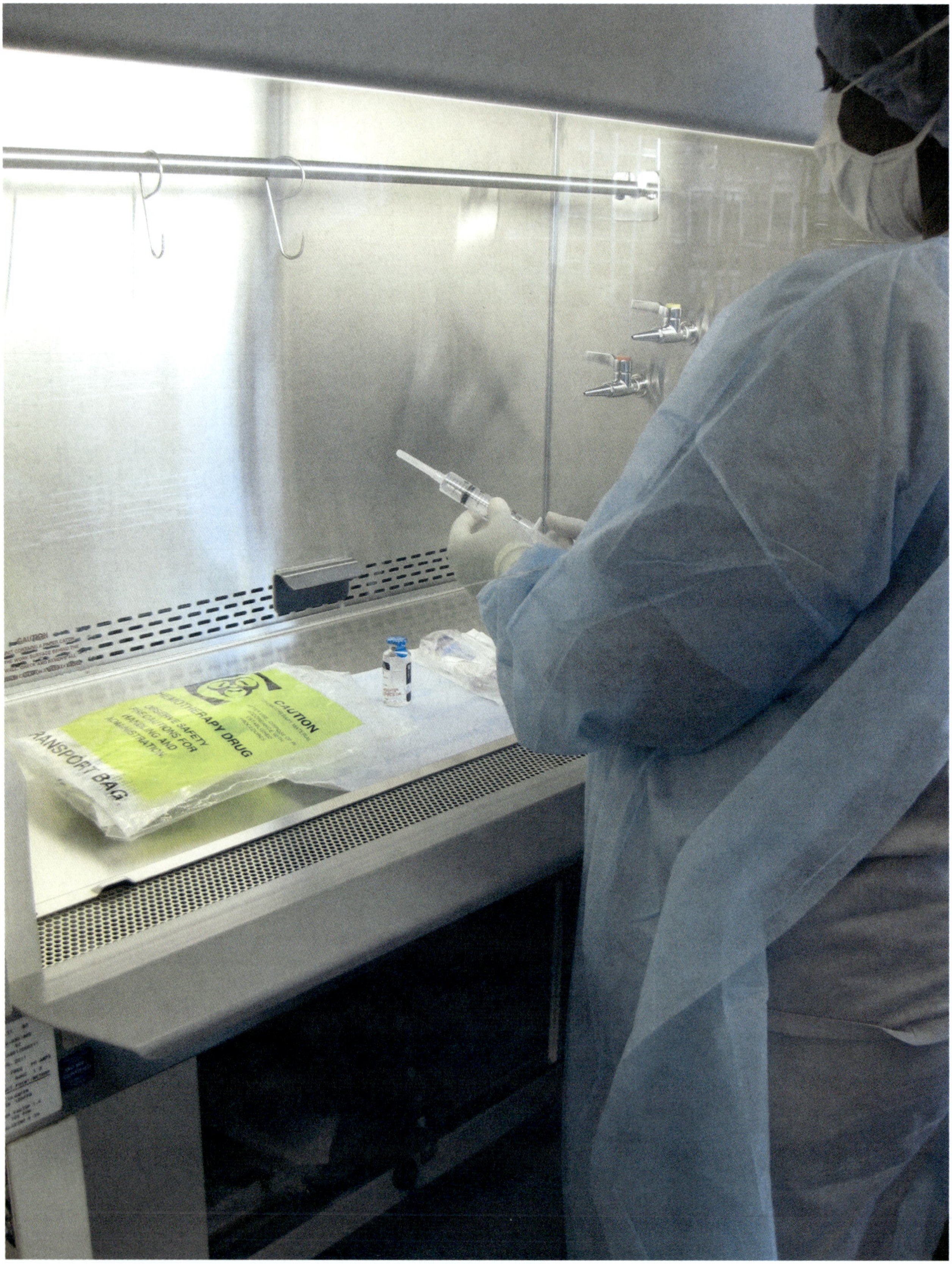
CAUTION

9

PARENTERALS: COMPOUNDING STERILE FORMULATIONS

LEARNING OBJECTIVES

At the completion of study, the student will:

- ✔ understand the requirements of a sterile formulation.
- ✔ describe the differences between LVP and SVP solutions, and explain the purpose of common specialty parenteral solutions.
- ✔ describe the use of administration sets and positive pressure pumps to administer parenteral solutions to patients.
- ✔ explain the importance of using laminar flow hoods and various aseptic techniques in compounding parenteral solutions.
- ✔ list and explain the factors that affect incompatibilities in parenteral solutions.
- ✔ discuss the purposes of the different aspects of a quality assurance program.
- ✔ compare and contrast the units of measurement unique to parenteral solutions.

THINKING IT THROUGH

You are working at a home infusion company as an IV technician responsible for making all the intravenous solutions that are ordered. After turning on the laminar flow hoods and completing the required cleaning of the area, you receive an order for 10 ampicillin 500 mg in 100 ml D5W. You collect the needed supplies and begin preparing the order. Half way through the batch, your supervisor tells you to stop doing the ampicillin and quickly do six vancomycin 1500 mg in 500 ml NS. As you read through this chapter, consider the following questions:

1. Should you stop doing the ampicillin batch and set the supplies outside the hood while you complete the vancomycin order, and then place the ampicillin materials back in the hood to complete the batch? Why or why not?
2. Is there a clean room design that would allow you to set the ampicillin materials outside of the hood for a time to complete the vancomycin order?
3. Ampicillin has D5W as the base IV solution, and vancomycin has NS. Explain why both drugs are not placed in the same base solution.

COMPOUNDING STERILE FORMULATIONS

There are special requirements for how parenteral products are made, packaged, and administered.

Most parenteral formulations are required to be sterile, meaning that the formulation is free from bacteria and other microorganisms. Sterility is not a relative term: the formulation is either sterile or nonsterile. This applies to the injectable formulations given by the intravenous, intramuscular, subcutaneous, and intradermal routes of administration. Dosage forms used for ophthalmic (e.g., intraocular), intranasal, otic, and inhalation administration must also be sterile. Of the other parenteral dosage forms, only dermal and vaginal formulations are not required to be sterile.

These formulations must be sterile because they have rapid access to the circulatory system and can cause a patient great harm if an infection develops or if a mistake in dosage is made.

In addition to being a sterile dosage form, parenteral formulations in most cases must be free from particulate material, pyrogen-free, isotonic, and at physiological pH.

These requirements are met by the manufacturer of a sterile parenteral dosage form.

They produce sterile formulations that are ready for immediate use. However, it is not practical for a manufacturer to supply all of the many different sterile dosage forms used in pharmacy practice. Many manufacturers' formulations are modified in the pharmacy by technicians, under the authorization of a pharmacist. These modified formulations must still remain sterile, pyrogen-free, etc.

This chapter will discuss how many types of sterile solution formulations are compounded in a pharmacy setting.

Sterile parenteral compounding generally occurs in a laminar flow hood or biological safety cabinet, and requires that the operator use ***aseptic techniques***. The most common compounded sterile solutions are large volume parenterals (LVP), small volume parenterals (SVP), total parenteral nutrition (TPN) solutions, dialysis solutions, and irrigation solutions.

SPECIAL REQUIREMENTS

There are a number of special considerations and precautions that must be taken with parenteral dosage forms.

✔ **Solutions must be sterile—i.e., free from bacteria and other microorganisms.**

Techniques that maintain sterile conditions and prevent contamination must be followed. These are called aseptic techniques.

✔ **Solutions must be free of all visible particulate material.**

Examples of such contaminants are glass, rubber cores from vial closures, cloth or cotton fibers, metal, and plastic. Undissolved particles of an active drug will be present in intravenous suspensions, but no contaminants should be present.

✔ **Solutions must be pyrogen-free.**

Intravenous solutions can cause pyretic reactions (fever) if they contain pyrogens. ***Pyrogens*** are chemicals that are produced by microorganisms. They are soluble in water and are not removed by sterilizing or filtering the solution.

✔ **The solution must be stable for its intended use.**

Most admixtures are prepared hours in advance of when they will be administered. So the stability of a particular drug in a particular intravenous solution must be considered in the admixture preparation. This information is generally available in a number of reference sources.

✔ **The pH of an intravenous solution should not vary significantly from physiological pH, about 7.4.**

However, other factors may sometimes be more important, such as when acidic or alkaline solutions are needed to increase drug solubility or used as a therapeutic treatment themselves.

✔ **Intravenous solutions should be formulated to have an osmotic pressure similar to that of blood.**

Osmotic pressure is a characteristic of a solution determined by the number of dissolved particles in it. Osmolarity is a unit of measure of osmotic pressure and is expressed in terms of osmoles (Osmol) or milliosmoles (mOsmol) per liter.

Blood has an osmolarity of approximately 300 mOsmol per liter. Both 0.9% sodium chloride solution and 5% dextrose solution have a similar osmolarity. When a solution has an osmolarity equivalent to that of blood, it is called ***isotonic.***

Intravenous solutions that have greater osmolarity than blood are called ***hypertonic***, and those with lower osmolarity, ***hypotonic.*** Both hypertonic and hypotonic solutions may cause damage to red blood cells, pain, and tissue irritation. However, it is at times necessary to administer such solutions. In these cases, the solutions are usually given slowly through large, free-flowing veins to minimize the reactions.

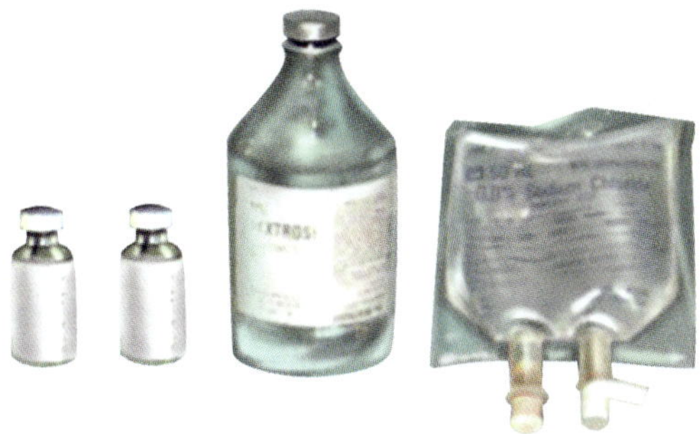

Which parenteral?

Besides meaning any route of administration other than enteral, "parenteral" is commonly used to describe dosage forms administered through syringes or administration sets. It is also used to describe the various bottles, vials, and bags used in preparing and delivering solutions for intravenous administration. It is possible to say that parenterals are prepared and parenterally administered at parenteral sites. As a result, extreme care must be taken when using the word "parenteral" so that the intended meaning is clear to all.

aseptic techniques techniques or methods that maintain the sterile condition of products.

hypertonic when a solution has a greater osmolarity than that of blood.

hypotonic when a solution has a lesser osmolarity than that of blood.

isotonic when a solution has an osmolarity equivalent to that of blood.

osmotic pressure a characteristic of a solution determined by the number of dissolved particles in it.

pyrogens chemicals produced by microorganisms that can cause pyretic reactions (fever) in patients.

LVP SOLUTIONS

Large volume parenteral (LVP) solutions are intravenous solutions packaged in containers holding 100 ml or more.

Common uses of LVP solutions without additives include correction of electrolyte and fluid balance disturbances, nutrition, and vehicles for administering other drugs. The most common sizes are 100, 250, 500, and 1,000 ml. There are three types of containers: glass bottle with an air vent tube, glass bottle without an air vent tube, and plastic bags. The top of the LVP solution container hangs on an administration pole. The other end of the container has two ports of about the same length—one is the administration set port, and the other is the medication port. Graduation marks on the front of the container indicate the volume of solution it can hold. The graduation marks are at 25–100 ml intervals, depending on the overall size of the container.

The administration set port has a plastic cover on it to maintain the sterility of the bag.

The cover is easily removed. A plastic diaphragm inside the port keeps the solution from dripping out of the bag. When the spike of the administration set is inserted into the port, the diaphragm is punctured, and the solution flows out of the bag into the administration set. This inner diaphragm cannot be resealed once punctured.

The medication port is covered by a protective rubber tip.

Drugs are added to the LVP solution through this port using a needle and syringe. There is an inner plastic diaphragm about one-half inch inside the port, just like the administration set port. This inner diaphragm is not self-sealing when punctured by a needle, but the protective rubber tip prevents solutions from leaking from the bag once the diaphragm is punctured.

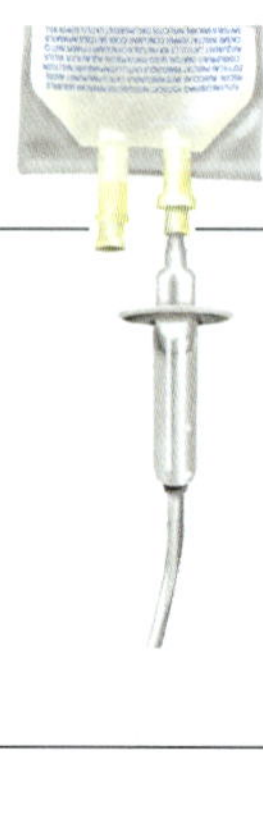

an administration set

REGULATORY REQUIREMENTS FOR PARENTERALS

The United States Pharmacopeia (USP), the Food and Drug Administration (FDA), and state boards of pharmacy set regulations and guidelines for the manufacture, compounding, dispensing, and distribution of parenteral drug products in the United States.

Chapter <797> in the USP–NF titled "Pharmaceutical Compounding—Sterile Preparations" establishes requirements for aseptic preparation of compounded sterile dosage forms. These standards apply to health-care institutions, pharmacies, physician practice facilities, and other facilities that prepare, store, or dispense ***compounded sterile preparations (CSP)***.

A CSP is defined as follows:

- A preparation prepared according to the manufacturer's labeled instructions, or manipulations of a manufactured sterile product that expose the original contents to potential contamination.
- A preparation containing nonsterile ingredients or employing nonsterile components and devices that must be sterilized before administration.
- Biologics, diagnostics, drugs, nutrients, and radiopharmaceuticals which include, but are not limited to, baths and soaks for live organs and tissues, implants, inhalations, injections, powders for injection, irrigations, metered sprays, and ophthalmic and otic preparations.

Plastic bags have advantages not found with glass bottles.

They do not break. They weigh less. They take up less space for both storage and disposal. Because the plastic bag system is not vented to outside air, it collapses as the solution is administered, preventing a vacuum from being created inside.

However, some drugs and solutions may not be used with plastic bags because they interact with the plastic.

Nitroglycerin, amiodarone, and integrelin are examples of solutions dispensed in glass bottles because of this interaction. Glass containers are also required for certain other drugs because polyvinyl chloride (PVC) or di-2-ethylhexylphthalate (DEHP) can leach out of plastic bags into the IV solution and inactivate the drug; however, PVC/DEHP-free plastic bags are now available (VISIV®, Aviva®) that have eliminated the need for glass bottles in theses cases.

When using glass containers, solutions flow from the glass containers to the patient through a special administration set.

Glass containers are packaged with a vacuum and sealed by a solid rubber closure that is held in place by an aluminum band. For solutions to flow out of a glass container, air must be able to enter the container to relieve the vacuum as the solution leaves. Some bottles have air tubes built into the rubber closure for this. Some bottles do not, in which case a special administration set with a filtered airway in the spike must be used.

Common LVP Solutions

Many intravenous solutions are commercially available. Four common solutions used either as LVP solutions or as the primary part of an admixture solution are:

- sodium chloride solution (NS);
- dextrose 5% in water solution (D5W);
- Ringer's solution (Ringer's);
- Lactated Ringer's solution (LR).

Various combinations of different strengths of sodium chloride and dextrose solutions are also available, e.g., 5% dextrose and 0.45% sodium chloride, or 5% dextrose and 0.225% sodium chloride.

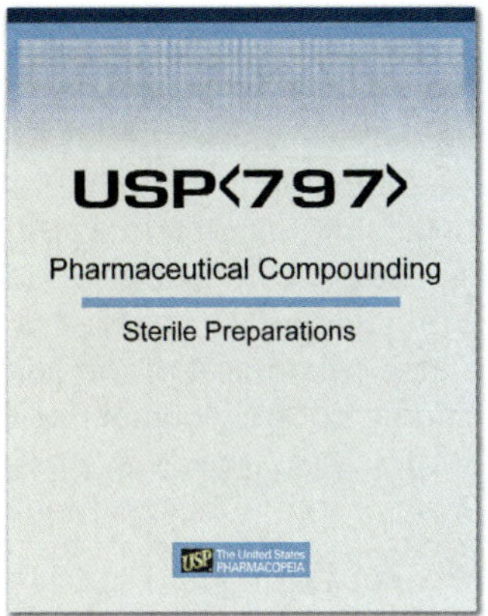

The intent of Chapter <797> is to "prevent harm and fatality that could result from microbial contamination (nonsterility), excessive bacterial endotoxins, large errors in the strength of correct ingredients, and incorrect ingredients in compounded sterile products (CSPs)."

Chapter <797> provides requirements for the development and implementation of essential policies and procedures for the safe preparation of CSPs. Such policies and procedures provide for: cleaner facilities (compared to nonsterile compounding); air quality evaluation and maintenance; and specific training and testing of personnel in aseptic manipulation, sterilization, and solution stability principles and practices.

The level of a pharmacy technician's involvement in developing and implementing these procedures will vary from institution to institution. However, all personnel who prepare CSPs must understand and follow these fundamental practices and precautions.

compounded sterile preparation (CSP) a compounded sterile parenteral dosage form that will be parenterally administered.

SVP SOLUTIONS

Small volume parenteral (SVP) solutions are packaged products that are either directly administered to a patient or added to another parenteral formulation.

SVP solutions are supplied in prefilled syringes, ampules, glass or plastic vials sealed with a rubber closure, or plastic minibags.

When a SVP is added to a parenteral solution, it is referred to as the *additive*, and the final mixture is referred to as the *admixture*.

SVP additives may be either in liquid form or as *lyophilized* (freeze-dried) powders. Powders are supplied in vials and must be reconstituted with a suitable solvent (*diluent*) before being used.

There are two varieties of prefilled syringes.

One, a cartridge-type package, is a single syringe and needle unit that is placed in a special holder before use. Once the syringe and needle unit is used, it is discarded, but the holder can be used again with a new unit. Another type of prefilled syringe consists of a glass tube closed at both ends with rubber stoppers. The prefilled tube is placed into a specially designed syringe that has a needle attached to it. After using this type of prefilled syringe, all of the pieces are discarded.

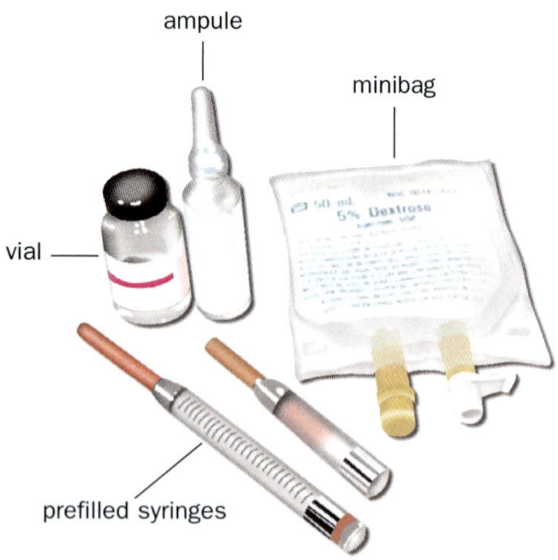

small volume parenterals

ADDING SVPs TO LVPs

Generally the LVP solution is used as a continuous infusion because of its large volume and slow infusion rate. SVP solutions can be introduced into the on-going LVP infusion by injecting the SVP into the medication port of the container or the volume control chamber of the administration set. However, more often the SVP is put into a minibag and used as a piggyback on the LVP.

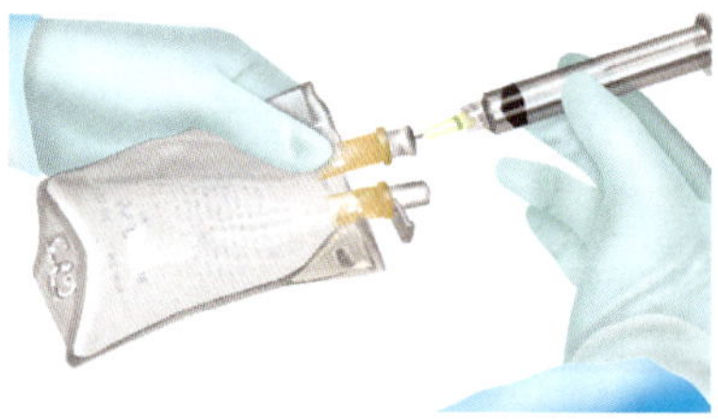

Using a Needle and Syringe to Add a SVP to a LVP

1. Assemble the needle and syringe.
2. If the drug in the SVP is in powder form, reconstitute it with the recommended diluent.
3. Swab the SVP and medication port of the LVP with an alcohol swab.
4. Draw the necessary volume of drug solution into the syringe from the SVP.
5. Insert the needle into the medication port and through the inner diaphragm. The medication port should be fully extended to minimize the chance of going through the side of the port.
6. Inject the SVP solution into the LVP.
7. Remove the needle from the LVP.
8. Shake and inspect the admixture.

Note: This procedure will be done in a laminar flow hood.

READY-TO-MIX SYSTEMS

Ready-to-mix systems consist of a specially designed minibag with an adapter for attaching a drug vial. The admixing takes place just prior to administration. The major advantages of ready-to-mix systems include a significant reduction in waste and lower potential for medication error because the drug vial remains attached to the minibag and can be rechecked if necessary. However, the systems do cost more, and there is the potential that the system will not be properly activated so that the patient receives only the diluent or a partial dose.

Some ready-to-mix systems are: Add-Vantage®, Add-a-Vial®, Mini-Bag Plus®, and CRIS® Controlled Release Infusion System.

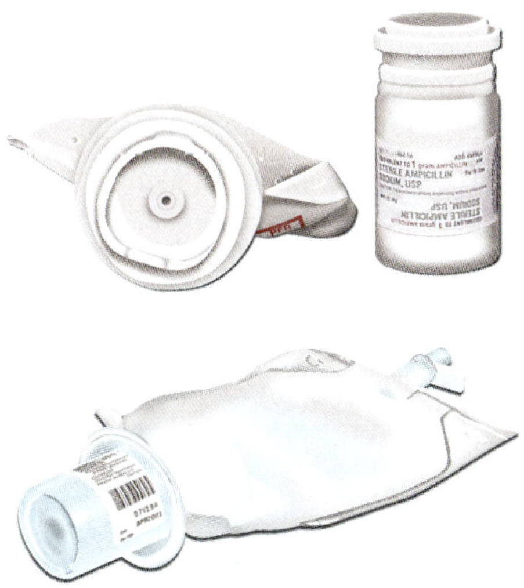

a ready-to-mix system before and after mixing

Ampules are elongated, sealed glass containers with a neck that must be snapped off.

Most ampules are weakened around the base of the neck for easy breaking. These will have a colored band around the base of the neck. Some ampules, however, must first be scored and weakened with a file or the top may shatter. Once an ampule is opened, it becomes an open-system container.

Vials have a rubber stopper through which a needle is inserted to withdraw or add to the contents.

Before withdrawing solution from a vial, an equal volume of air is usually drawn up in the syringe and injected into the vial. This pressurizes the vial and helps in withdrawing solution from the vial. Some medications are packaged under pressure or can produce gas (and pressure) upon reconstitution. In such cases, air is not injected into the vial before withdrawing the solution.

Vials may be prepared for single or multidose use.

Single dose vials do not contain preservatives and should be discarded after one use. Multidose vials contain a preservative to inhibit bacterial contamination once the vial has been used. Also, the rubber closure will reseal on a multidose vial. These vials can be used for a number of doses of variable volume.

Minibags are made of the same plastic materials as LVPs and contain the same types of solutions found in LVPs.

Minibags are just smaller in size since they contain only 50–100 ml of solution.

additive a drug that is added to a parenteral solution.

admixture the resulting solution when a drug is added to a parenteral solution.

diluent a solvent that dissolves a lyophilized powder or dilutes a solution.

lyophilized freeze-dried.

ready-to-mix a specially designed minibag by which a drug is put into the SVP just prior to administration.

SPECIAL SOLUTIONS

TOTAL PARENTERAL NUTRITION SOLUTIONS

Total parenteral nutrition (TPN) solutions are complex admixtures used to provide nutritional support to patients unable to take in adequate nutrients through their digestive tract. These admixtures are composed of dextrose, fat, protein, electrolytes, vitamins, and trace elements. They are hypertonic solutions.

Base parenteral nutrition solutions are available in 2,000 and 3,000 ml sizes. The base solution consists of:

- an amino acid solution (for protein);
- a dextrose solution (for carbohydrates).

These solutions, sometimes referred to as macronutrients, make up most of the volume of a parenteral nutrition solution. Several electrolytes, trace elements, and multiple vitamins (together referred to as micronutrients) may be added to the base solution to meet individual patient requirements. Common electrolyte additives include sodium chloride (or acetate), potassium chloride (or acetate), calcium gluconate, magnesium sulfate, and sodium (or potassium) phosphate. Multiple vitamin preparations containing both water soluble and fat soluble vitamins are usually added on a daily basis. Trace element products contain zinc, copper, manganese, selenium, and chromium.

Intravenous fat (lipid) emulsion can be added as a source of essential fatty acids and a concentrated source of calories. Fat provides 9 calories per gram, compared to 3.4 calories per gram provided by dextrose. Intravenous fat emulsion may be admixed into the total parenteral nutrition solution or piggybacked into the administration line. When intravenous fat emulsion is admixed with a TPN solution, the resulting solution is referred to as a ***total nutrient admixture (TNA)***.

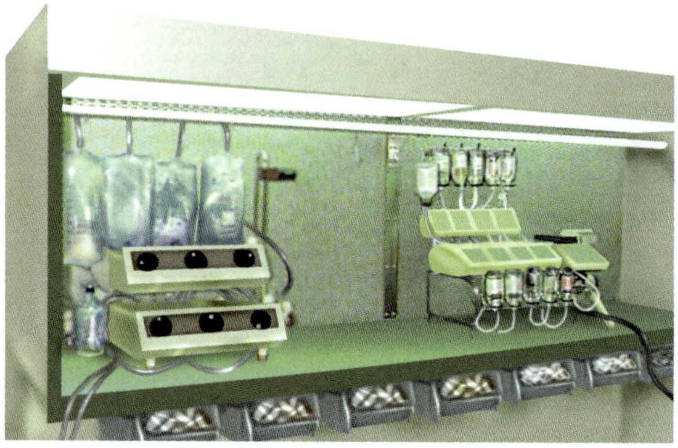

TPN Preparation Systems

Due to the complexity and time needed to prepare TPN solutions, pharmacies use high-speed compounders, automixers, or micromixers. These machines can deliver from 2 to 10 different components safely, accurately, and quickly.

TPN Administration

TPN solutions are usually administered via the subclavian vein under the collar bone over 8 to 24 hours to minimize adverse effects that may occur with a hypertonic solution. The subclavian vein is large and close to the heart, so the solution is diluted rapidly by the large volume of blood in the heart.

To assure their accurate delivery, nutrition solutions are almost always administered with an intravenous infusion pump. Parenteral nutrition solutions are commonly administered through an in-line filter in the administration set positioned as close to the patient as possible. However, intravenous fat emulsion, either alone or as part of a TNA solution, can be administered through an in-line filter only if it has a pore size of 1.2 micron or larger. An alternative is to piggyback the intravenous fat emulsion into the administration set below the in-line filter.

dialysis movement of particles in a solution through permeable membranes.

irrigation solution large volume splash solutions used during surgical or urologic procedures to bathe and moisten body tissues.

osmosis the action in which a drug in a higher concentration solution passes through a permeable membrane to a lower concentration solution.

peritoneal dialysis solution a solution placed in and emptied from the peritoneal cavity to remove toxic substances.

DIALYSIS SOLUTIONS

Dialysis refers to the passage of small particles through membranes. This is caused by ***osmosis***, the action in which a drug in a solution of a higher concentration will move through a permeable membrane to a solution of a lower concentration. This principle is the basis for another type of special parenteral solution.

Peritoneal dialysis solutions are used by patients who have compromised kidney function. The solution is administered directly into the peritoneal cavity (the cavity between the abdominal lining and the internal organs) to remove toxic substances, excess body waste, and serum electrolytes through osmosis. These solutions are hypertonic to blood so the water will not move into the circulatory system. But the toxic substances will move into the dialysis solution.

Peritoneal solutions are administered several times a day. The solution is permitted to flow into the abdominal cavity, and then remains in the cavity for 30 to 90 minutes. It is then drained by a siphon tube into discharge bags. This procedure is repeated many times a day and may use up to 50 liters of solution. For this reason, peritoneal dialysis solutions are supplied in containers that are 2,000 ml or larger in capacity.

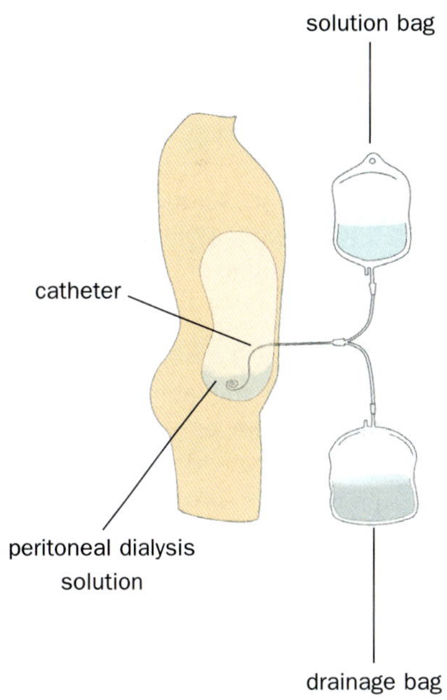

IRRIGATION SOLUTIONS

Irrigation solutions are not administered directly into the venous system but are subject to the same stringent controls as intravenous fluids. They are packaged in containers that are larger than 1,000 ml capacity and are designed to empty rapidly.

Surgical irrigation solutions (splash solutions) are typically Sodium Chloride for Irrigation or Sterile Water for Irrigation. They are used to:

- bathe and moisten body tissues;
- moisten dressings;
- and wash instruments.

Urological irrigation solutions are used during operations to:

- maintain tissue integrity;
- and remove blood to maintain a clear field of vision.

Glycine 1.5% Irrigation and Sorbitol 3% Irrigation solutions are commonly used because they are nonhemolytic (i.e., do not damage blood cells).

total nutrient admixture (TNA) solution a TPN solution that contains intravenous fat emulsion.

total parenteral nutrition (TPN) solution complex solutions with two base solutions (amino acids and dextrose) and additional micronutrients.

ADMINISTRATION DEVICES

ADMINISTRATION SETS

LVP solutions are usually administered with administration sets.

An administration set is a length of flexible plastic tubing with a spike at one end and a needle adapter at the other. The spike fits into the administration set port of the LVP container. The solution flows from the LVP container through the plastic tubing to the needle adapter at the other end. A needle or catheter can be attached to the needle adapter.

The LVP solution will run by gravity flow if no rate-controlling adjustment is on the administration set. The higher the LVP solution is placed above the patient, the faster it will run into the patient. A clamp provides one means of regulating the ***flow rate*** (the rate at which the solution is to be administered to the patient, generally measured in ml/hour). The clamp may be a roll clamp or a slide clamp.

The flow rate can also be determined by counting the number of drops per minute that enter a drip chamber. A drip chamber is a small reservoir in the plastic tubing near the LVP container. Fluid collects in the drip chamber, and then flows continuously through the remainder of the tubing without mixing with air. Drip chambers may be a regular drip chamber (e.g., 10 drops/ml), or a minidrip chamber (e.g., 60 drops/ml).

An administration set can have many variations. The spike may have an air vent built into it. A drip chamber or a volume control chamber may or may not be present. The length of the tubing varies as well as the lumen size (i.e., regular or micro size). There may also be a filter incorporated into the tubing.

Some administration sets have a flexible rubber bulb located near the needle adapter called a ***Flashball***. The Flashball can be squeezed before starting the administration to see if the needle is correctly located in the patient's vein. If blood comes up into the Flashball, the needle is properly placed.

A controller may also be used to regulate the flow rate. Most controllers use a photoelectric sensor to compare the actual gravity flow rate to a programmed (desired) flow rate and relax or constrict the administration set tubing to increase or decrease the flow rate.

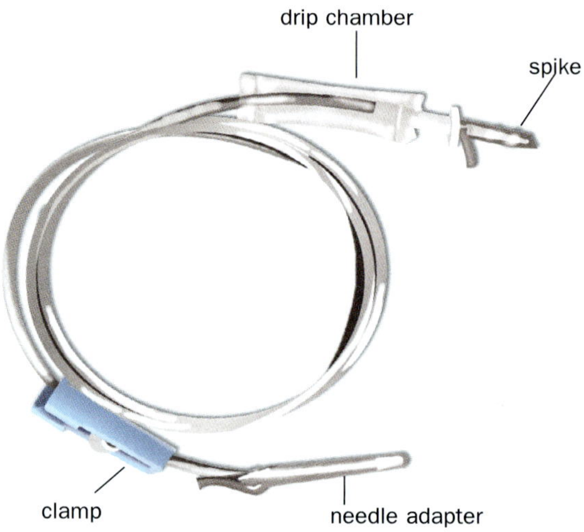

an administration set

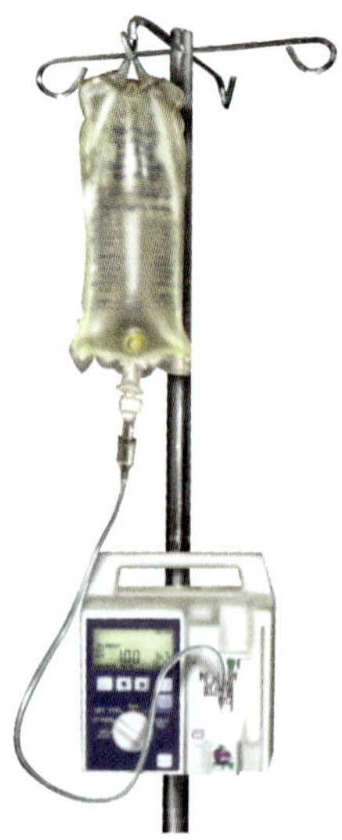

an LVP connected to an administration set with a controller

Flashball flexible rubber bulb near the needle adapter on an administration set; used to determine if the needle is properly placed in the vein.

flow rate the rate (in ml/hour or ml/minute) at which solution is administered to the patient.

Combination controllers/pumps provide both the safety of low infusion pressures from the controller part of the device and the availability of a positive pressure pump in the other part of the device. The user selects whether to use the device as a controller or a pump.

"Smart" pumps are a technological innovation in positive pressure pumps. They have drug administration rate libraries and decision support as part of their programming. This software provides an additional medication safety check at the point of care by reducing administration rate errors.

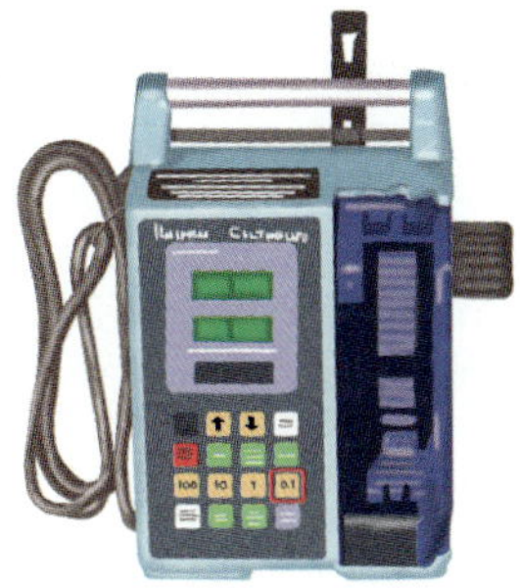

a controller/pump

VOLUME CONTROL CHAMBERS

A volume control chamber is often used with a clamp to control the flow rate. A volume control chamber is a plastic cylindrical device with graduation marks along the sides for measuring the volume of solution. As the IV solution flows from the LVP container, the chamber is filled to a measured volume. A clamp immediately above the chamber is closed when the desired volume of solution has been added. In this manner, the volume control chamber serves as a mini reservoir from which the solution is allowed to flow when a clamp below the chamber on the administration set is opened. It also is a safety precaution that will limit the volume of fluid that may be infused accidentally. These chambers are generally recommended only for pediatric patients.

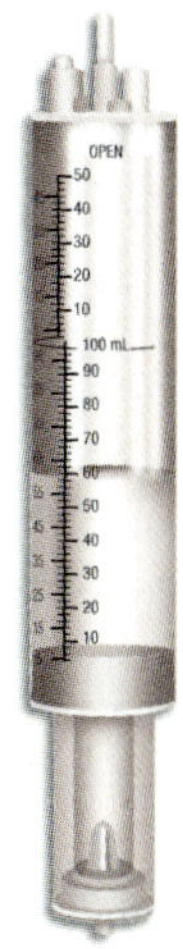

a volume control chamber

IV CATHETERS

An IV catheter is a 1- to 5-inch piece of fine, flexible plastic tubing connected to a plastic hub that is in turn attached to a syringe or to an administration set. The catheter has a needle to allow for insertion but it is pulled out after insertion. IV catheters are sometimes used instead of needles because they are more flexible and therefore can be less irritating to the patient. It is important to remember, however, that the risk of inflammation increases the longer any foreign material is left inserted in a vein.

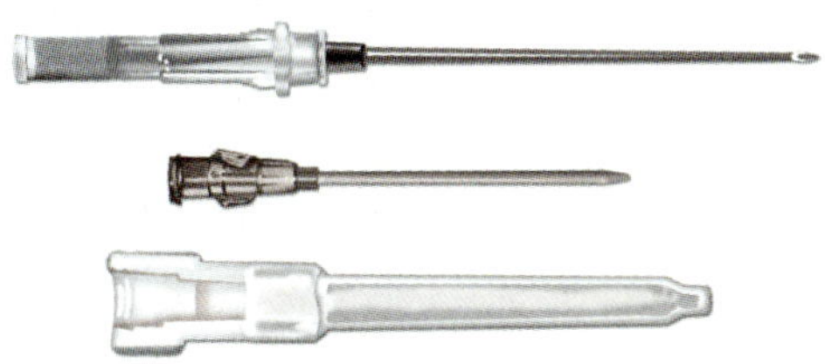

ADMINISTRATION DEVICES (cont'd)

POSITIVE PRESSURE PUMPS

Positive pressure infusion devices (pumps) generate a pressure that will cause fluid to flow through the administration set into the patient's vascular system. These devices overcome minor occlusions and resistance associated with an intravenous system, viscous solutions, and vascular back pressure. Most pumps have operating pressures in the 2–12 pounds per square inch (PSI) range. Pressures around 2 PSI are used to keep the vascular access open (called "keep open"), whereas arterial access requires pressures about 10–12 PSI.

Cassette Pumps

Cassette pumps are often used as ambulatory pumps since many are about the size of a hand, allowing the patient to have freedom of movement.

In this type of pump, a cassette acts as a reservoir and fits into the pump housing. Tubing connects the cassette to the patient. The pump makes the cassette fill and then empty in two separate, sequential cycles to deliver a measured volume of fluid.

Syringe type cassette pumps move a motor-driven plunger into and out of a fluid filled chamber. In a piston-activated diaphragm cassette pump, a flexible diaphragm is mounted near a moving piston. Each inward stroke of the piston compresses the diaphragm, directing solution to the patient. Each outward stroke allows the diaphragm to relax and refills the chamber.

Multiple chamber pumps allow one chamber to refill while the other directs fluid to the patient.

Elastomeric Reservoirs

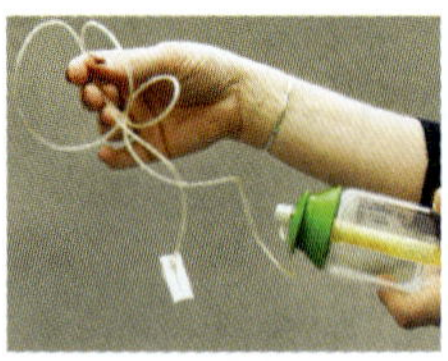

These are tennis ball sized pumps with a balloon-like reservoir surrounded by a rigid, protective outer shell. The elastic reservoir is filled with a solution that exerts a constant positive pressure, forcing the solution through the tubing into the patient. The combination of the pressure and dimensions of the tubing determine the flow rate of the pump.

Syringe Pumps

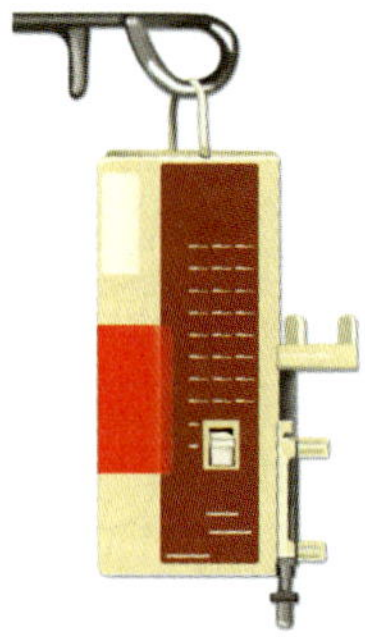

In this type of pump, a syringe attached to a pump expels solution from the syringe by advancing either the plunger or the barrel at a predetermined rate. Syringe pumps are commonly used for infusion of intermittent medications such as antibiotics. They are also used to administer antineoplastic drugs, analgesics, and anesthetics. Because they can deliver solutions at very low and precisely controlled flow rates, they are especially useful for neonatal, infant, and critical care applications where small volumes need to be given over extended periods of time.

Peristaltic Pumps

Peristaltic pumps infuse solutions in "micro-pulses" produced by a massaging action on the IV tubing. Special infusion sets are used because the tubing has been reinforced with a silastic insert at the point of contact with the peristaltic mechanism. This reinforcement keeps the tubing from stretching and deforming which would lead to variations in the flow rate. A linear peristaltic pump has finger-like projections that occlude the tubing in a successive manner in a rippling, wave-like motion. Rotary peristaltic pumps compress the tubing against a rotor housing with rollers mounted on it. As the rotor turns, the rollers occlude the tubing and force the fluid to flow toward the patient while drawing new fluid from the IV bag.

heparin lock an administration device used when a primary LVP solution is not available.

piggybacks small volume solutions connected to an LVP.

PIGGYBACKS

Intermittent intravenous medications are often administered using ***piggybacks***. This involves infusing medications in a small volume of solution at regular intervals, typically 30 to 60 minutes. The intermittent IV solution flows into the patient's vein through the same administration set as the LVP, and at the same time. When the intermittent infusion is not being administered, the LVP infusion continues to keep the vein open.

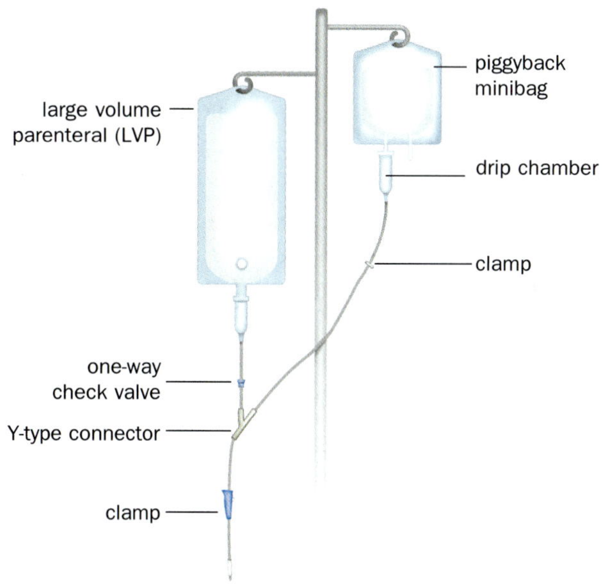

The LVP solution container and the piggyback solution container are connected at a Y-type connector in the administration set. The minibag container is placed higher than the LVP container so its greater pressure will ensure the minibag solution will enter the administration set. At the appropriate time, the clamp to the piggyback container is opened. The minibag solution is prevented from flowing into the LVP container by a one-way check valve in the LVP administration set. The two solutions are not mixed together except in the administration set tubing below the Y-connector.

Piggyback containers are usually made of the same material as the plastic LVP bags and hold 50–100 ml of 5% Dextrose Injection or 0.9% Sodium Chloride Injection.

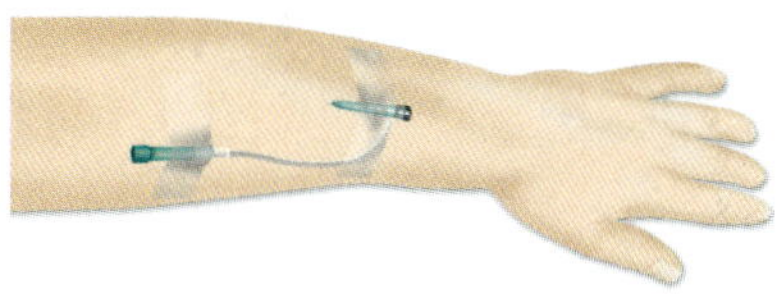

HEPARIN LOCKS

In some instances, a patient may not have a primary LVP solution, yet must receive minibag medications. This is done through a ***heparin lock*** which is a short piece of tubing attached to a needle or intravenous catheter. When the tubing is not being used for the minibag, heparin is used to fill the tubing. Heparin prevents blood from clotting in the tubing.

LAMINAR FLOW HOODS

Microorganisms invisible to the eye are present on dust and particulate matter in the air as well as on most surfaces, even those that appear clean.

Microorganisms are also present in a person's exhaled air and on their skin, which sheds approximately 15–20 million cells per hour. Because of these enormous contamination risk factors, environmental protection and aseptic techniques must be used when preparing parenteral solutions.

The best way to reduce the environmental risk is to use a laminar flow hood, which establishes and maintains an ultraclean work area.

Room air is drawn into a laminar hood and passed through a prefilter to remove relatively large contaminants such as dust and lint. The air is then channeled through a high-efficiency particulate air *(HEPA) filter* that removes ≥ 99.97% of particles larger than 0.3 μm (microns).

According to USP–NF Chapter <797> regulations, laminar flow hoods must maintain an ISO Class 5 environment when used to prepare sterile parenteral preparations.

An ISO Class 5 environment has no more than 3,520 particles ≥ 0.5 μm per cubic meter of air. This purified air flows over the work surface at a uniform velocity (i.e., *laminar flow*) of 80–100 ft./min. The constant flow of air from the hood prevents room air from entering the work area and removes contaminants introduced into the work area by material or personnel. However, they do not protect personnel or the environment from the hazards of drug products.

The surfaces of the hood's work area are clean, but they are not sterile.

Therefore, it is necessary to use aseptic techniques that maintain the sterility of all sterile items. These techniques apply to the technician, the laminar flow hood, and all substances and materials involved in the procedure.

TYPES OF LAMINAR FLOW HOODS

Laminar flow hoods are designed as either "horizontal" or "vertical" flow hoods. ***Horizontal flow hoods*** take up room air and channel it through the HEPA filter. The air crosses the work area in a horizontal direction and exits the hood. The illustration below shows a design where room air enters the hood through the bottom. Other models have room air entering from the back or top of the hood.

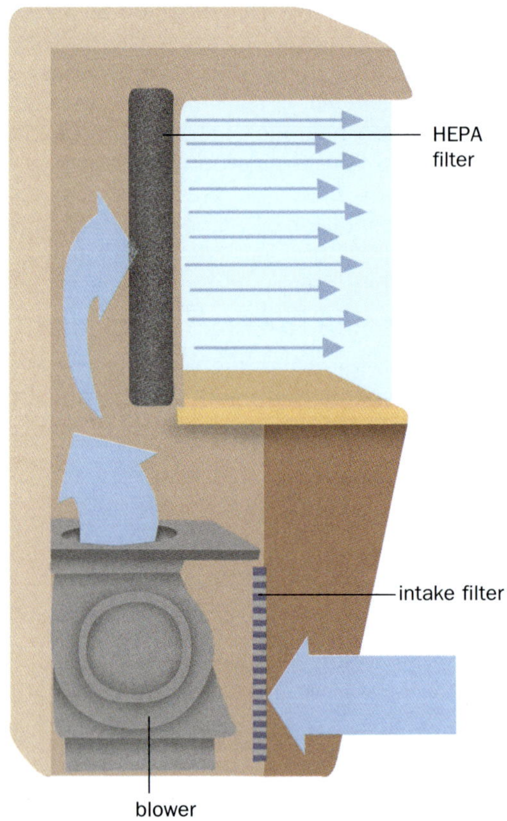

a horizontal flow hood

HEPA filter a high efficiency particulate air filter.

horizontal flow hood a laminar flow hood with horizontal air flow across the work area.

laminar flow continuous movement at a uniform rate in one direction.

vertical flow hood a laminar flow hood with vertical air flow across the work area.

zone of turbulence an area of blocked air flow in a laminar flow hood.

safety you should know

Laminar flow hoods do not provide a sterile environment. They provide an ultraclean work area.

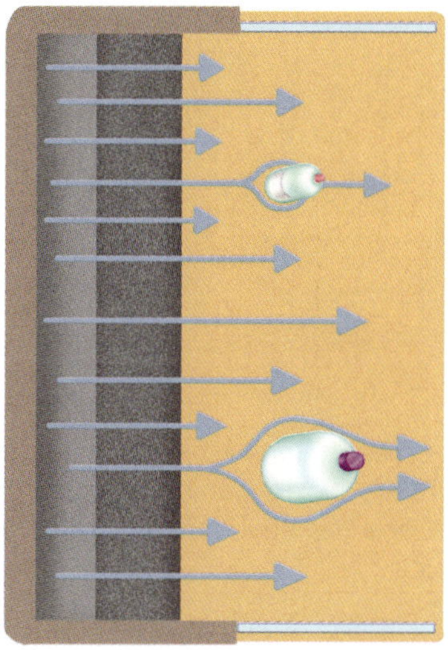

view from above
a horizontal hood

The illustration above shows how air is channeled around objects in the work area of a horizontal hood. Note that there is a "dead" area (sometimes called the ***zone of turbulence***) in front of the large container. Because of the air flow pattern, smaller items should be placed close to the HEPA filter and larger items closer to the opening of the hood.

Whenever possible, hand movements should not disturb the air flow pattern. For example, moving hands between the HEPA filter and the materials placed on the hood will disrupt or block the air flow, which will decrease the efficiency of the hood in that area. This can happen with an act as simple as wrapping a hand around an item. It is best to approach materials from the open side of the hood, and avoid the tendency to grasp the item with a full hand.

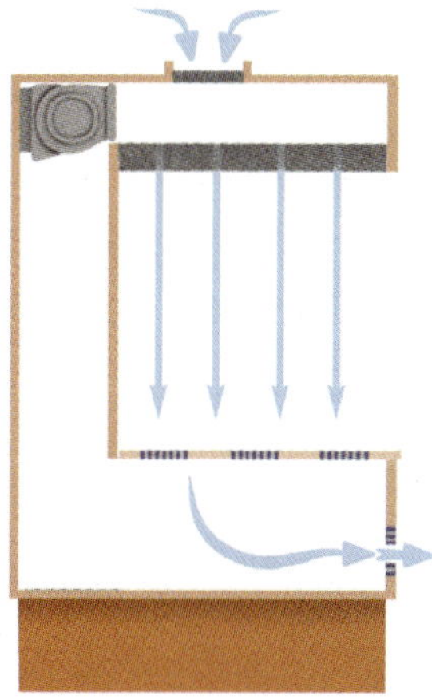

a vertical flow hood

With ***vertical flow hoods***, filtered air enters at the top of the work area, and moves downward. In some models the air moves downward all the way through the work area before it is returned to the room air.

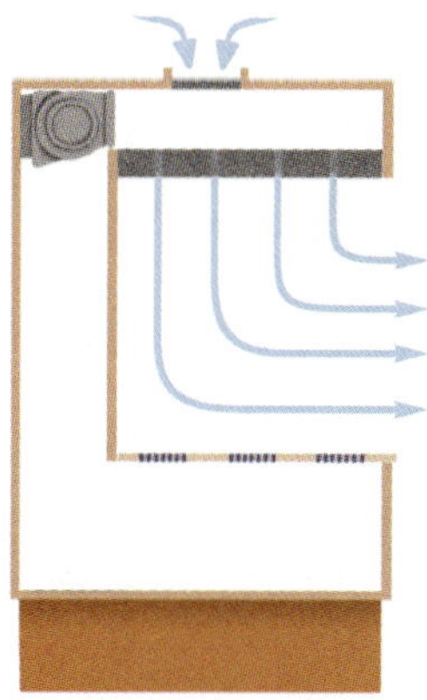

In other vertical models the air moves downward initially but then turns inside the work area and exits from the hood through the opening in the front.

Moving hands above items placed in either type of vertical hood will block air flow, decreasing the hood's efficiency in that area.

BIOLOGICAL SAFETY CABINETS

Biological safety cabinets are designed differently than laminar flow hoods.

They take air into the cabinet through the work surface vents and recirculate it through a HEPA filter located in the top of the cabinet. The air is channeled so that a major portion is recirculated back into the cabinet, and a minor portion is passed through another HEPA filter before being exhausted into the room. Once the air is filtered, it is directed downward toward the work surface, just as with a vertical laminar flow hood. However, as the air approaches the work surface, it is pulled through vents at the front, back, and sides of the work surface and again recirculated back into the cabinet.

There are several types of biological safety cabinets.

A Class II, Type A1 cabinet, which was just described, represents the minimum recommended environment for preparing chemotherapy agents. But they are not suitable for work with volatile toxic chemicals and radionucleotides which require a different type of cabinet.

Biological safety cabinets protect both personnel and the environment from contamination.

Laminar flow hoods should not be used to prepare chemotherapy agents because they blow air across the work surface toward the operator and into the work environment.

Institutions will have policies and procedures for personnel working with cytotoxic and hazardous drugs.

In addition to working in biological safety cabinets, these policies will cover areas such as personnel training in the identification, containment, collection, segregation, and disposal of these agents. The procedures should also describe the use of equipment, protective clothing to be worn, and procedures to be followed in case of exposure.

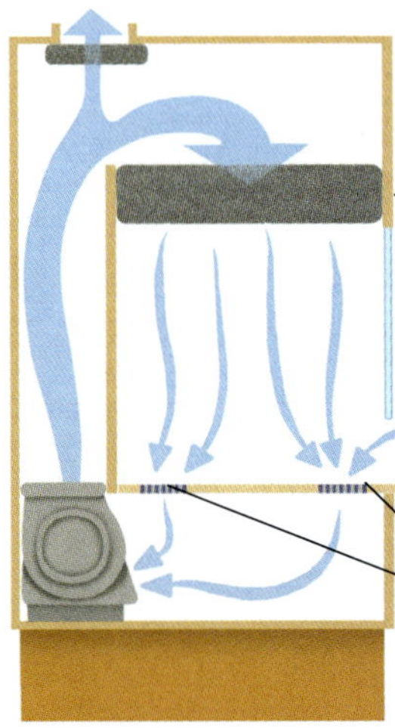

This is a Class II, Type A1 biological safety cabinet. These safety cabinets protect both personnel and the environment from contamination.

Common Chemotherapy Drugs

Route	Drug(s)
Oral	Capecitabine
Intravenous	Doxorubicin
Intraarterial (into the arteries)	Floxuridine Fluorouracil Mitomycin-C Cisplatin Streptomycin
Intralesional (directly into a tumor)	Vinblastine Vincristine
Intraperitoneal (into the cavity surrounding the abdominal organs)	Paclitaxel Mitoxantrone Carboplatin Alpha interferon
Intrathecal (into the spinal fluid)	Methotrexate Cytarabine

9

CLEAN ROOMS

Laminar flow hoods and biological safety cabinets must be housed in an area isolated from the pharmacy's main traffic.

These areas are commonly referred to as "clean rooms." In the past, clean room facilities varied significantly from pharmacy to pharmacy, but USP–NF Chapter <797> regulations now have mandated standard requirements for such facilities.

USP–NF <797> regulations state that clean room facilities must be an ISO Class 7 environment.

ISO Class 7 means that the environment has no more than 352,000 particles ≥ 0.5 µm per cubic meter of air. In addition, the clean room must be in a designated area with limited traffic and have unrestricted air flow. Further, only designated personnel should enter the space, and only for the purpose of preparing sterile preparations. The room should be large enough to accommodate all the necessary equipment needed for aseptic compounding, and provide for the proper storage of drugs and supplies. There should be an additional room adjacent to the clean room (the anteroom) where gowning and hand washing take place.

The regulations also state that the air quality, temperature, and humidity in clean rooms must be tightly controlled in order to greatly reduce the risk of contamination.

The air in a clean room must be repeatedly filtered to remove dust particles, particulates, and other impurities. The clean room usually has only one door, which should remain closed when not in use. It should have positive pressure, which means that when the door is open, the air will flow out of the clean room.

In some facilities, the entire clean room is an ISO Class 5 environment.

These rooms will not have laminar flow hoods or biological safety cabinets since the air in the room is the same as in laminar flow hoods. In these clean rooms, the anteroom is typically an ISO Class 7 environment.

PREPARING FLOW HOODS AND SAFETY CABINETS FOR USE

Turning on the Hood or Cabinet

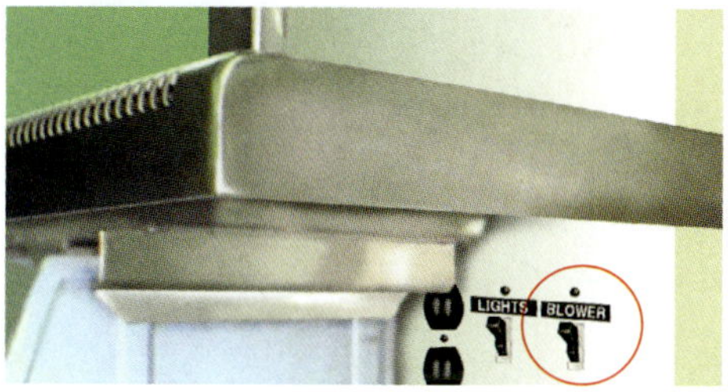

- ✔ In order to produce an ultraclean environment turn on the hood at least 30 minutes before use.
- ✔ Maintain a designated clean area around the hood.

Cleaning the Hood or Cabinet

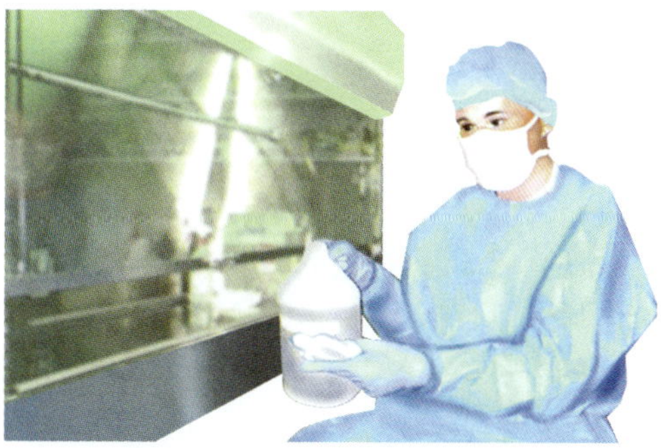

Follow these steps to clean the inside of the hood with a suitable disinfectant.

- ✔ If using a cleaner in a spray bottle, be sure not to spray the HEPA filter.
- ✔ Clean the metal pole used to hang the containers.
- ✔ Next clean the sides of the hood using up and down motions and moving from the back of the hood toward the front.
- ✔ Finally clean the bottom of the hood using side-to-side motions, again moving from the back of the hood toward the front.

ASEPTIC TECHNIQUES IN HOODS & CABINETS

Personnel involved with admixing parenteral solutions must use good aseptic techniques.

Aseptic techniques are the sum total of methods and manipulations required to minimize the contamination of sterile products. Contamination can be from microorganisms and/or particulate material. Working in a laminar flow hood does not, by itself, guarantee a sterile formulation.

Positioning of material and aseptically working inside hoods and cabinets requires training, practice, and attention to details.

Following are some general aseptic techniques for working in a laminar flow hood or biological safety cabinet:

- ✔ Never sneeze, cough, or talk directly into a hood.
- ✔ Close doors or windows. Breezes can disrupt the air flow enough to contaminate the work area.
- ✔ Perform all work at least 6 inches inside the hood to derive the benefits of the laminar air flow. Laminar flow air begins to mix with outside air near the edge of the hood.
- ✔ Maintain a direct, open path between the HEPA filter and the area inside the hood.
- ✔ Place nonsterile objects, such as solution containers or your hands, downstream from sterile ones. Particles blown off these objects can contaminate anything downstream from them.
- ✔ Do not put large objects at the back of the work area next to the filter. They will disrupt air flow.

The additional guidelines on these pages must also be followed, along with any applicable facility and manufacturer guidelines.

safety you should know

Sterile supplies often have expiration dates as well as instructions for use. Always follow these instructions.

Clothing and Barriers

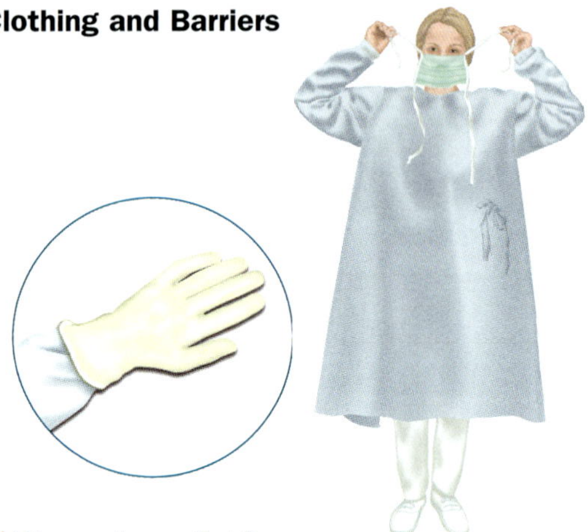

- ✔ Wear clean lint-free garments or barrier clothing, including shoe covers, gowns, hair covers, and a mask.
- ✔ Wear sterile gloves.
- ✔ Follow facility or manufacturer guidelines for putting on and removing barrier clothing. Unless barriers are put on properly, they can easily become contaminated.

Collect Supplies

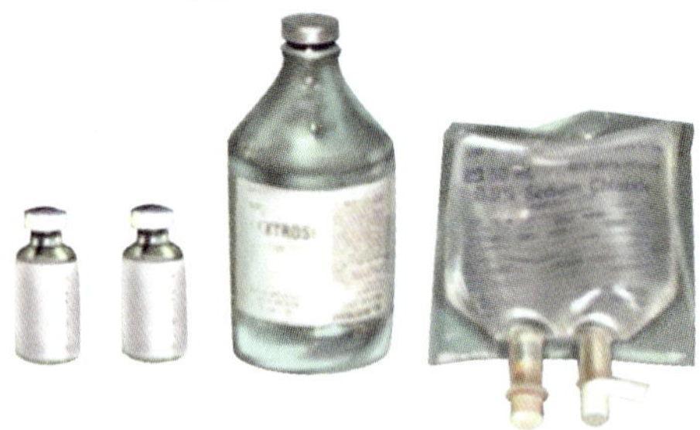

- ✔ Assemble all necessary supplies, checking each for expiration dates and particulate material.
- ✔ Plastic solution containers should be squeezed to check for leaks.
- ✔ Use only pre-sterilized needles, syringes, and filters. Check the protective covering of each to verify they are intact.
- ✔ Remove dust coverings before placing supplies in the hood.

safety you should know

Contamination comes from the environment and from personnel. Flow hoods, safety cabinets and clean rooms control the environment, and personnel using aseptic techniques control contamination from personnel.

Wash Hands

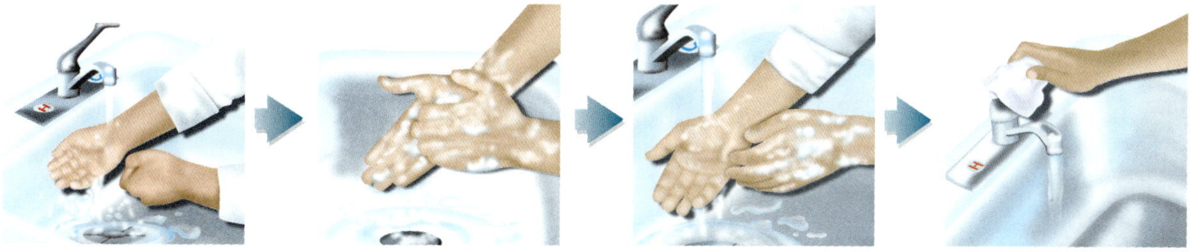

- ✔ Remove all jewelry.
- ✔ Stand far enough away from the sink so clothing does not come in contact with it.
- ✔ Turn on water. Wet hands and forearms thoroughly. Keep hands pointed downward.
- ✔ Scrub hands vigorously with an antibacterial soap.
- ✔ Work soap under fingernails by rubbing them against the palm of the other hand.
- ✔ Interlace the fingers and scrub the spaces between the fingers.
- ✔ Wash wrists and arms up to the elbows.
- ✔ Thoroughly rinse the soap from hands and arms.
- ✔ Dry hands and forearms thoroughly using a nonshedding paper towel.
- ✔ Use a dry paper towel to turn off the water faucet.
- ✔ After hands are washed, avoid touching clothes, face, hair, or any other potentially contaminated object in the area.

Position Supplies in Hood

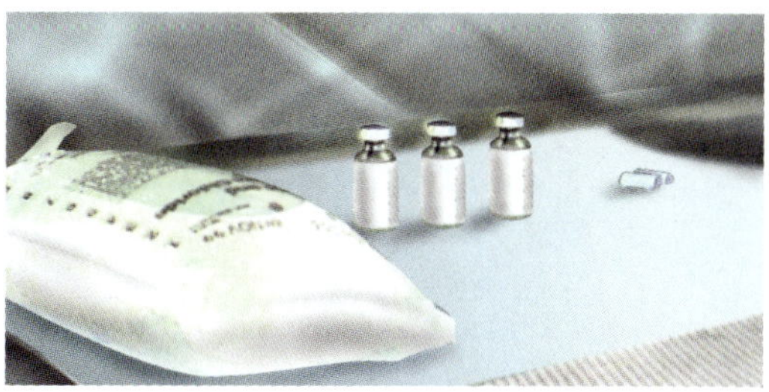

- ✔ Place supplies in the hood with smaller supplies closer to the HEPA filter and larger supplies further away from the filter.
- ✔ Space supplies to maximize laminar flow.
- ✔ Plan for the work area to be at least three inches from the back of the hood, and six inches inside the front of the hood.

Sterilize Puncture Surfaces

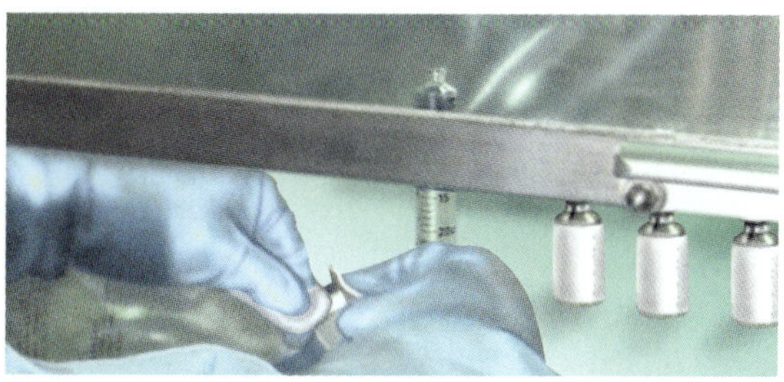

- ✔ Swab all surfaces that require entry (puncture) with an alcohol wipe. Avoid excess alcohol or lint that might be carried into the solution.
- ✔ Use a new alcohol wipe with each surface.

WORKING WITH VIALS

There are two types of parenteral vials that are used in making admixtures.

One contains the drug already in the solution. The other contains a powder that must be dissolved in a diluent to make a solution. In either case, a needle will be used to penetrate the closure in the vial.

VIALS CONTAINING SOLUTIONS

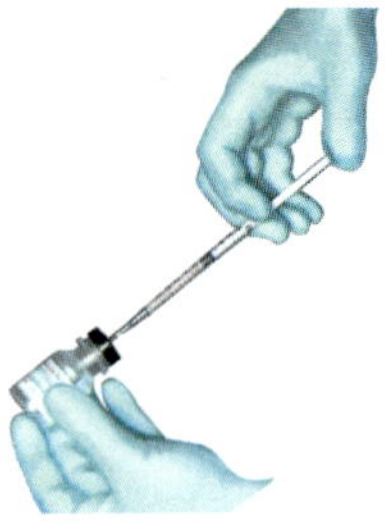

- ✔ Draw into the syringe a volume of air equal to the volume of solution to be withdrawn from the vial.
- ✔ Penetrate the vial without coring and inject the air. This will pressurize the vial and help in withdrawing the solution.

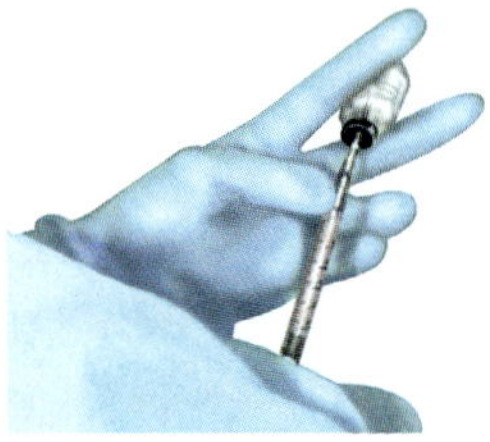

- ✔ Turn the vial upside down. Using one hand to hold the vial and the barrel of the syringe, pull back on the plunger with the other hand to fill the syringe. Fill the syringe with a slight excess of solution.

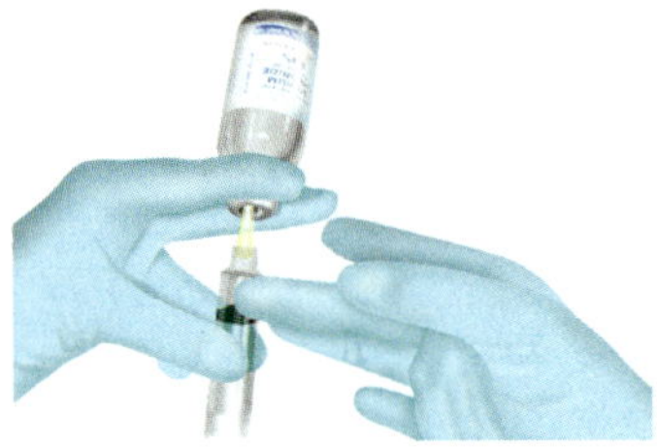

- ✔ Tap the syringe to allow air bubbles to come to the top of the syringe. Press the plunger to push air and excess solution into the vial.
- ✔ Transfer the solution into the final container, again minimizing coring.

VIALS CONTAINING LYOPHILIZED POWDER

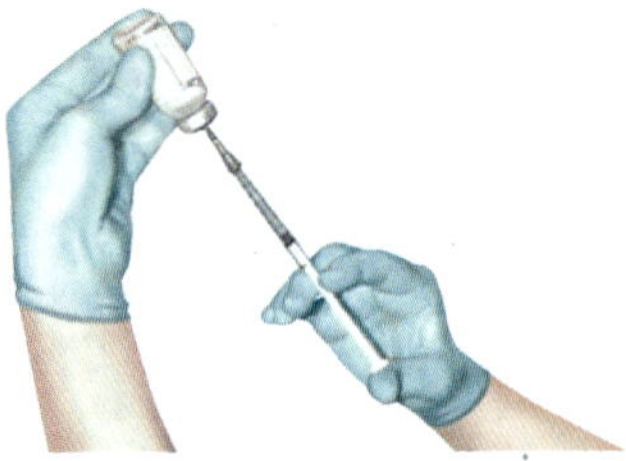

- ✔ Follow the above steps to withdraw the correct volume of diluent from its vial.
- ✔ Transfer the diluent into the vial containing the powder.
- ✔ Remove a volume of air from the vial into the syringe that is slightly greater than the volume of diluent. This creates a slight negative pressure in the vial, lowering chances that aerosol droplets will spray out when withdrawing the needle.

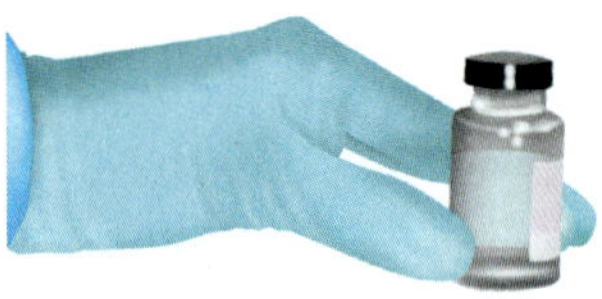

- ✔ After withdrawing the needle, swirl the vial until the drug is dissolved.

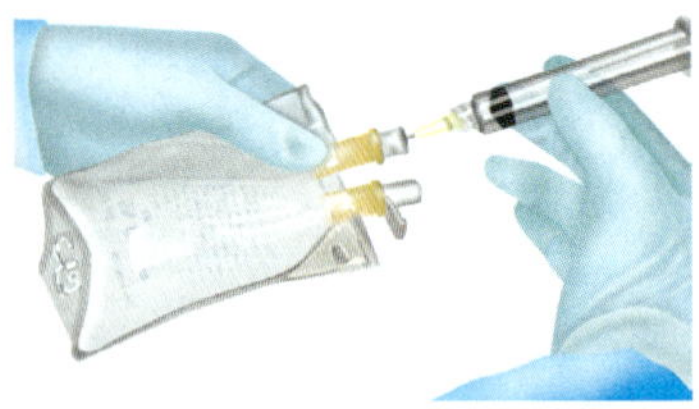

- ✔ Using a new needle and syringe, use the steps outlined above for vials containing solutions to withdraw the correct volume of reconstituted drug solution into the syringe.
- ✔ Transfer the reconstituted solution to the final container, again making sure to minimize coring.

coring when a needle damages the rubber closure of a parenteral container, causing fragments of the closure to fall into the container and contaminate its contents.

PREVENTING CORING

Coring happens when a needle damages the rubber closure of a parenteral container, causing fragments of the closure to fall into the container and contaminate its contents. To prevent coring, follow these steps:

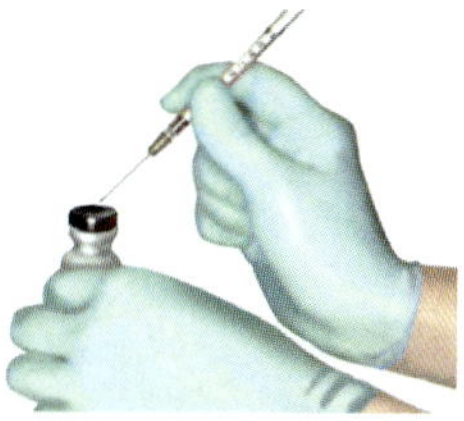

✔ Place the vial on a flat surface and position the needle point so that the bevel is facing upward and the needle is at about a 45° to 60° angle to the closure surface.

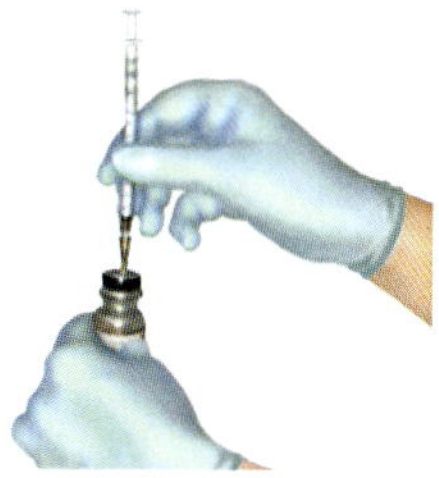

✔ Press downward on the needle while gradually bringing it to an upright position. Just before penetration is complete, the needle should be at a vertical (90°) angle.

MULTIPLE DOSE VIALS AND OVERFLOW VOLUMES

Multiple dose vials usually contain about 10 doses of the drug and have a rubber closure that can be punctured multiple times. When a needle is removed from the vial, the closure reseals and protects the vial contents from airborne contamination.

Since it is impossible to get the exact number of doses from a multiple dose vial unless it contains a slight excess of solution (overfill), the USP–NF recommends the following overages for multiple dose vials.

Labeled size (ml)	Excess volume for mobile liquids (ml, unless noted)	Excess volume for viscous liquids (ml, unless noted)
0.5	0.10	0.12
1.0	0.10	0.15
2.0	0.15	0.25
5.0	0.30	0.50
10.0	0.50	0.70
20.0	0.60	0.90
30.0	0.80	1.20
50.0 or more	2.00%	3.00%

WORKING WITH AMPULES

Glass ampules are always broken open at the neck.

Pre-scored *ampules* have a colored stripe around the neck to indicate it has been weakened by the manufacturer to facilitate opening. Some ampules are not pre-scored by the manufacturer, and the neck must first be weakened (scored) with a fine file.

OPENING AN AMPULE

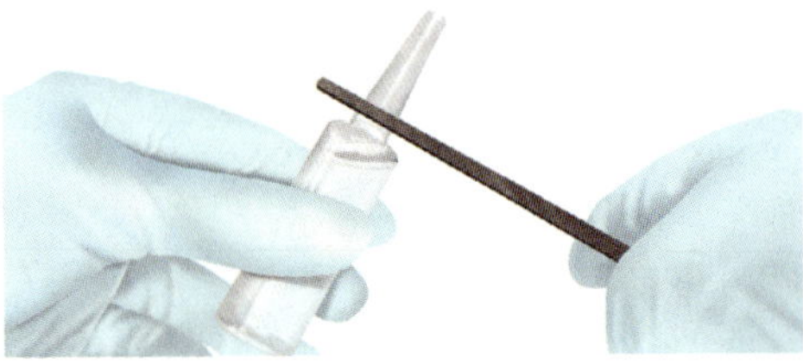

- ✔ If the ampule is not pre-scored, use a fine file to lightly score the neck at its narrowest point. Do not file all the way through the glass.
- ✔ Hold the ampule upright and tap the top to settle the solution into the bottom of the ampule.
- ✔ Swab the neck of the ampule with an alcohol swab.

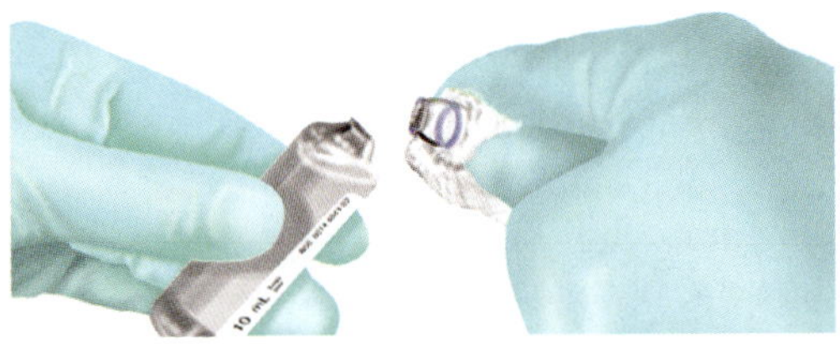

- ✔ Wrap a gauze pad around the neck of the ampule. This will help protect fingers if the ampule shatters and will reduce the possibility of splinters becoming airborne.
- ✔ Grasp the top of the ampule with the thumb and index finger of one hand. Grasp the bottom of the ampule with the other hand.
- ✔ Quickly snap the ampule moving your hands outward and away. Do not open the ampule toward the HEPA filter or any other sterile supplies in the hood. If the ampule does not snap easily, rotate it slightly and try again.
- ✔ Inspect the opened ampule for glass particles that may have fallen inside, and use a filter needle when withdrawing the solution.

ampules sealed glass containers with an elongated neck that must be snapped off.

TRANSFERRING SOLUTION

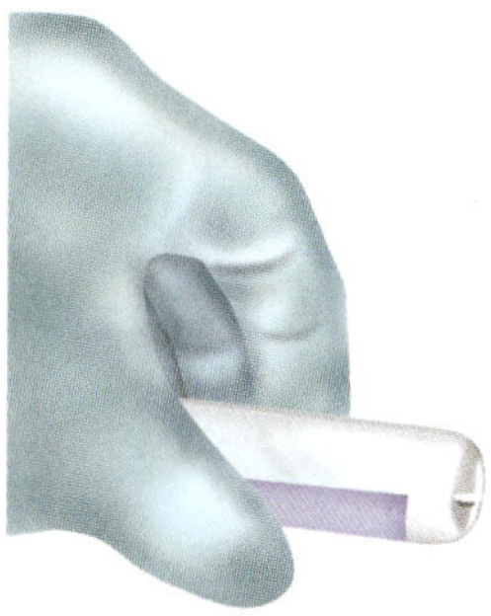

- ✔ Hold the ampule down at about a 20° angle.
- ✔ Attach a 5 micron filter needle to a syringe.
- ✔ Insert the filter needle into the ampule. Avoid touching the opening of the ampule with the needle point.

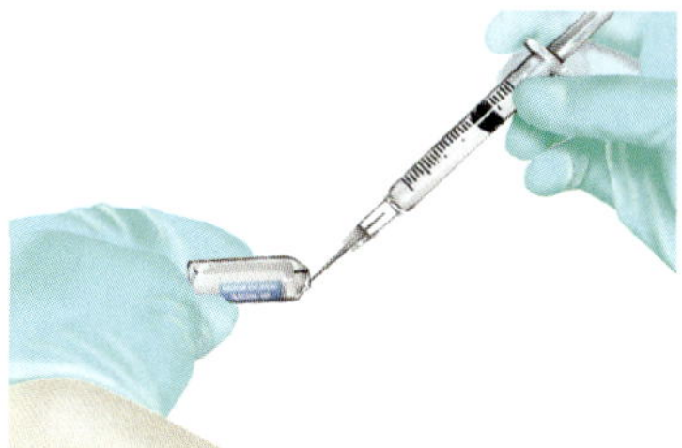

- ✔ Position the needle on the shoulder area of the ampule. Place its beveled edge against the side of the ampule to avoid pulling glass particles into the syringe.
- ✔ Withdraw solution into the syringe but keep needle submerged to avoid drawing air into the syringe.

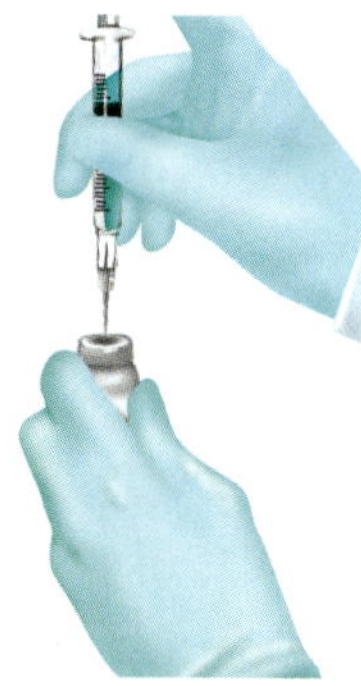

- ✔ Withdraw needle from ampule and remove all air bubbles from the syringe.
- ✔ Exchange the filter needle for a new filter needle or membrane filter and transfer the solution into the final container.

List of Drugs Commonly Packaged in Glass Ampules

Drug	Common Ampule Size
Epinephrine Injection 1:1000	1 ml
Lidocaine HCl Injection 2%	2 ml
Propranolol HCl Injection 1 mg/ml	1 ml
Naloxone HCl Injection 0.4 mg/ml	1 ml
Magnesium Sulfate Injection 50%	2 ml
Digoxin Injection 250 mcg/ml	2 ml
Isoproterenol HCl Injection 1:5000	5 ml
Calcium Gluconate Injection 10%	10 ml
Fentanyl Citrate Injection 50 mcg/ml	20 ml
Hydromorphone HCl Injection 1 mg/ml	1 ml

Some Disadvantages of Ampules

- ✔ A major disadvantage of ampules is that the solution can be contaminated by glass shards when the ampule is opened.
- ✔ Another disadvantage is that the solution in the ampule must be transferred out of the ampule with a syringe and filter needle.
- ✔ Finally, an ampule cannot be resealed once it has been opened and any remaining solution must be discarded.

SYRINGES & NEEDLES

Many of the manipulations performed with aseptic techniques require the use of syringes, needles, and filters.

The basic parts of a syringe are the barrel, plunger, and tip. The barrel is a tube that is open at one end and tapers into a hollow tip at the other end. The plunger is a piston-type rod with a slightly cone-shaped stopper that passes inside the barrel of the syringe. The tip of the syringe provides the point of attachment for a needle. The volume of solution inside a syringe is indicated by graduation lines on the barrel. Graduation lines may be in milliliters or fractions of a milliliter, depending on the capacity of the syringe. The larger the capacity, the larger the interval between graduation lines.

There are several common types of syringe tips. *Slip-Tip®* tips use friction to hold the needle on the syringe; the needle is reasonably secure, but it may slip off if not properly attached or if considerable pressure is used. *Luer-Lok®* tips have a collar with grooves that lock the needle in place. *Eccentric* tips, which are off-center, are used when the needle must be parallel to the plane of injection such as in an intradermal injection. *Oral syringes* have tips larger than a Slip-Tip® and are used to administer liquids by routes other than parenteral administration; needles will not fit on oral syringes.

Syringes come in sizes ranging from 1 to 60 ml. As a rule, the correct syringe size is the next size larger than the volume to be measured. For example, a 3 ml syringe should be selected to measure 2.3 ml, or a 5 ml syringe to measure 3.8 ml. In this way, the graduation marks on the syringe will be in the smallest possible increments for the volume measured. Syringes should not be filled to capacity because the plunger can be easily dislodged.

Measuring Volume

The volume of solution in a syringe is measured to the edge of the plunger's stopper while the syringe is held upright and all the air has been removed from the syringe.

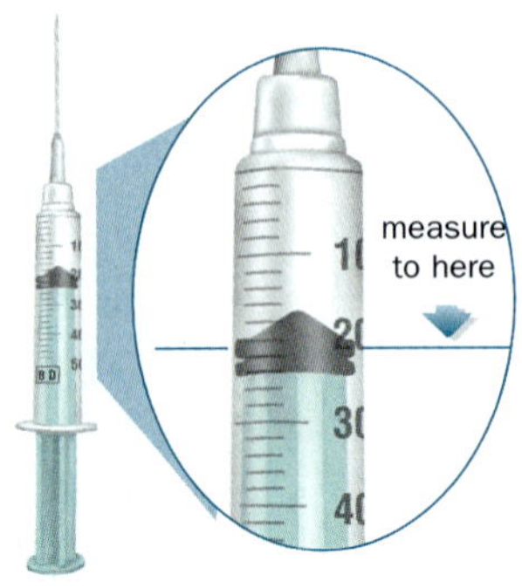

SYRINGES

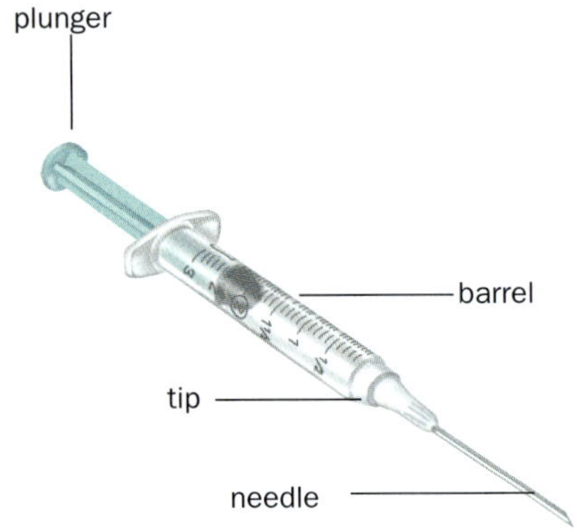

a syringe with graduation marks

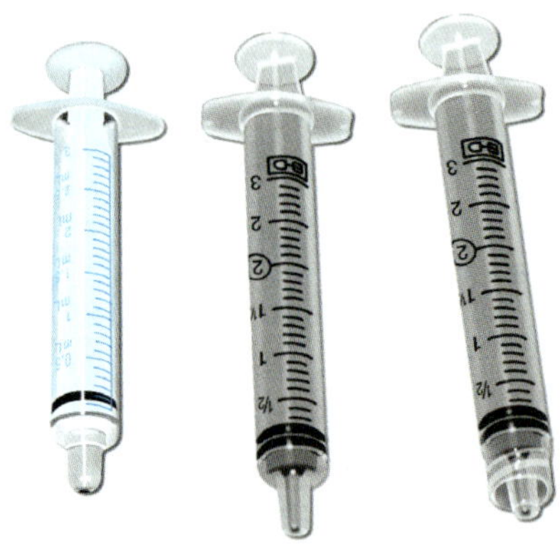

different syringe tips: oral (left); Slip-Tip® (center); and Luer-Lok® (right)

Drawing Liquids into the Syringe

Liquids are drawn into the syringe by pulling back on the plunger. The tip of the syringe must be fully submerged in the liquid to prevent air from being drawn into the syringe. Generally, an excess of solution is drawn into the syringe so that any air bubbles may be expelled by holding the syringe tip up, tapping the syringe until the air bubbles rise into the hub, and depressing the plunger to expel the air. This ensures that the hub will be completely filled with solution and the volume of delivery will be accurate.

safety you should know
Disposable needles should always be used when preparing admixtures because they are pre-sterilized and individually wrapped to maintain sterility.

NEEDLES

Parts

A needle has three parts: the ***hub***, the ***shaft***, and the ***bevel***. The hub is at one end of the needle and attaches to the syringe. It is designed for quick and easy attachment and removal. The shaft is the long, slender stem of the needle that is angled at one end to form a point called the "bevel." The hollow bore of the needle shaft is known as the **lumen**.

A transfer needle has shafts on both ends of the hub, allowing the solution in one container to be transferred to another without using a syringe.

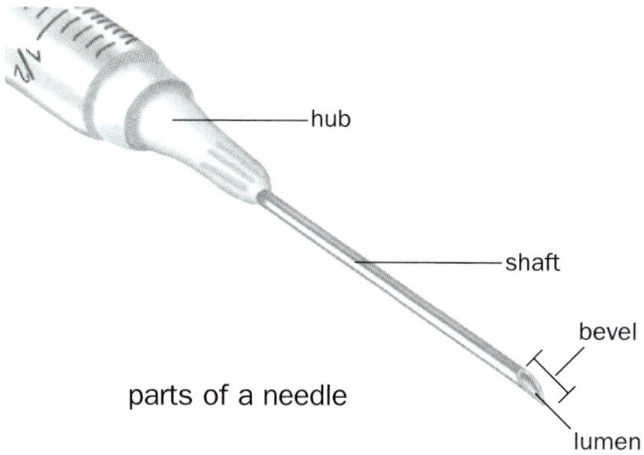

parts of a needle

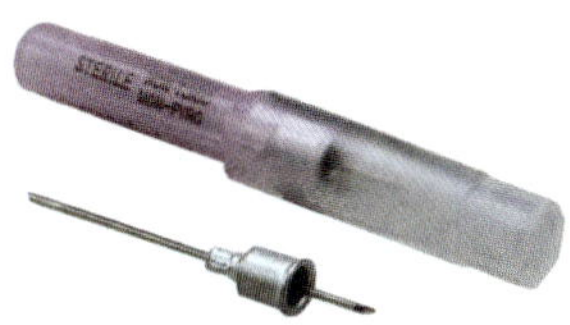
a transfer needle

Sizes

Needle sizes are indicated by length and ***gauge***. The length of a needle is measured in inches from where the shaft meets the hub to the tip of the bevel. Needle lengths range from 3/8 inch to three and a half inches. Some special-use needles are even longer. The gauge of a needle, used to designate the size of the lumen, ranges from 27 (the smallest) to 13 (the largest). In other words, the higher the gauge number, the smaller the lumen. The hubs are color coded for each gauge size.

Needle sizes are chosen based on both the viscosity (thickness) of the parenteral solution and the type of rubber closure in the container. Needles with relatively small lumens can be used for most dosage forms. However, some viscous solutions require needles with larger lumens. One problem is that larger needles are more likely to cause coring. Therefore, small gauge needles are used if the rubber closure can be easily cored, regardless of the solution viscosity.

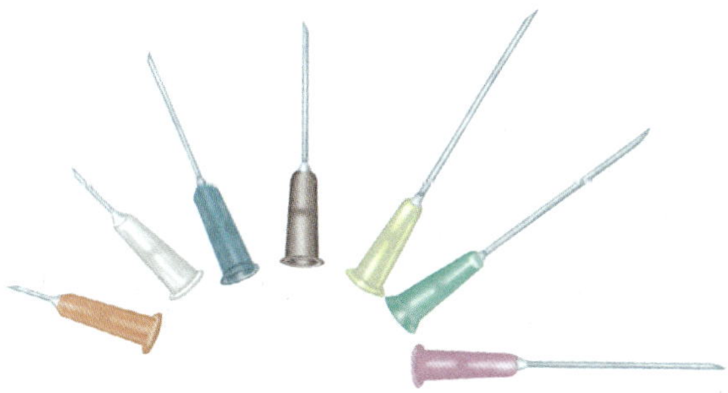
different needle sizes

bevel an angled surface at the tip of a needle.

gauge a measurement with needles: the higher the gauge, the smaller the lumen.

hub the part of the needle that attaches to the syringe.

lumen the hollow center of a needle.

shaft the stem of the needle that provides the overall length of the needle.

Slip-Tip®, Luer-Lok®, eccentric, oral different types of syringe tips.

FILTERS

Filters are used to remove particulate materials or microorganisms from solutions.

They are divided into two basic groups: depth filters and membrane filters. ***Depth filters*** work by trapping particles as solution moves through twisting channels. A ***membrane filter*** consists of many small pores of a uniform size that retain particles larger than the pores. Filters have a wide range of pore sizes. Common ones are 0.22, 0.45, 1.2, 5, or 10 microns.

Filters can be found in a variety of packaging.

Filters often are packaged in a round plastic holder that can be attached easily to the end of a syringe. Some filters are attached to administration sets and serve as ***final filters***, filtering the solution immediately before it enters the patient's vein. Some administration sets have filters that are already built into the set.

Filters also can be placed inside of needles; these are called filter needles.

Filter needles can have just one shaft with the filter inside the hub. They can also be transfer-type needles with the filter between the two shafts.

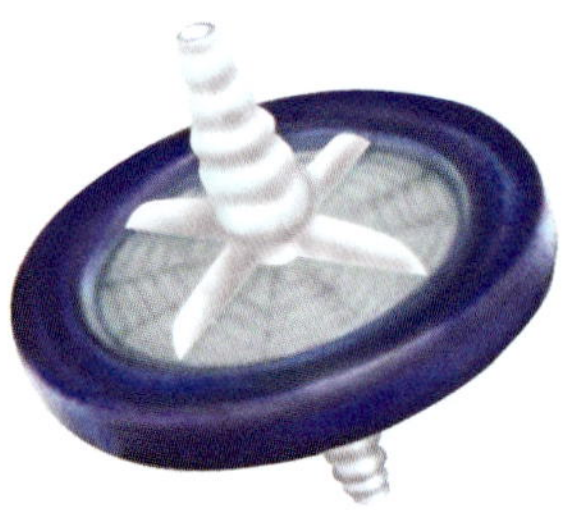

Membrane Filters

A membrane filter similar to the one above is often placed between the syringe and needle before the medication is introduced into a LVP or SVP container.

MEMBRANE FILTERS

Membrane filters are intended to filter a solution only as it is expelled from a syringe. A common scenario would be to transfer a reconstituted powder drug solution into a LVP or SVP following these steps:

1. Attach a needle to the syringe.
2. Pull the reconstituted powder drug solution into the syringe.
3. Remove air bubbles from the syringe.
4. Remove the needle from the syringe.
5. Attach a membrane filter to the syringe.
6. Place another needle on the end of the filter.
7. Eliminate air from the filter chamber by holding the syringe in a vertical position so that the needle is pointing upward. The air in the filter chamber is then expelled by slowly pushing in the plunger. Air must be expelled before the filter becomes wet or the air will not pass through the filter.
8. Once air has been expelled, introduce the needle into the final LVP or SVP container; slowly and continuously apply pressure to push the solution through the filter into the container.
9. Do not pull back on the plunger when the membrane filter is in use because the filter may rupture.

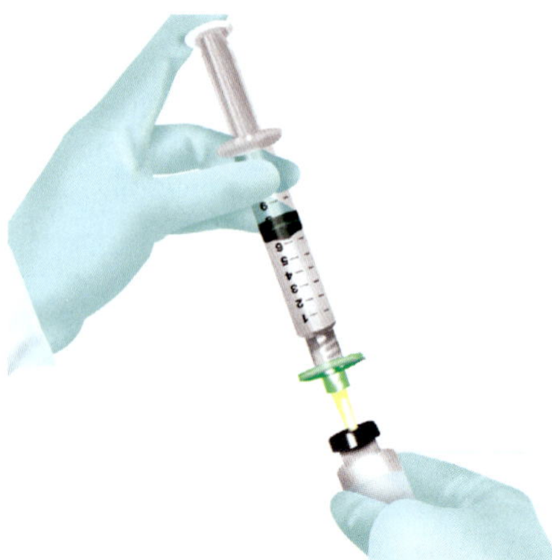

a membrane filter attached to a syringe and needle

DEPTH FILTERS

Depth filters are constructed of randomly oriented fibers or particles (e.g., diatomaceous earth, porcelain, asbestos) that have been pressed, wound, or otherwise bonded together to form a tortuous pathway for solution flow.

The depth filter is rigid enough to filter the solution either as it is pulled into or expelled from the syringe, but not both ways in the same procedure. If a drug solution is to be filtered as it is pulled into a syringe, use the following steps:

1. Attach the filter needle to the syringe.
2. Pull the solution into the syringe.
3. Remove the filter needle.
4. Attach a new needle to the syringe.
5. Expel the solution from the syringe.

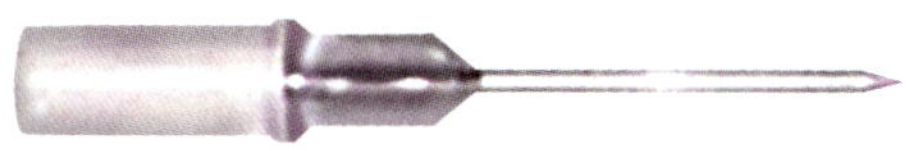

The depth filter is inside the hub of this filter needle.

FINAL FILTERS

A filter that filters a solution immediately before it enters the patient's vein is called a final filter. Some administration sets contain final filters as part of the set. Some filters are designed to be attached to administration sets and serve as final filters.

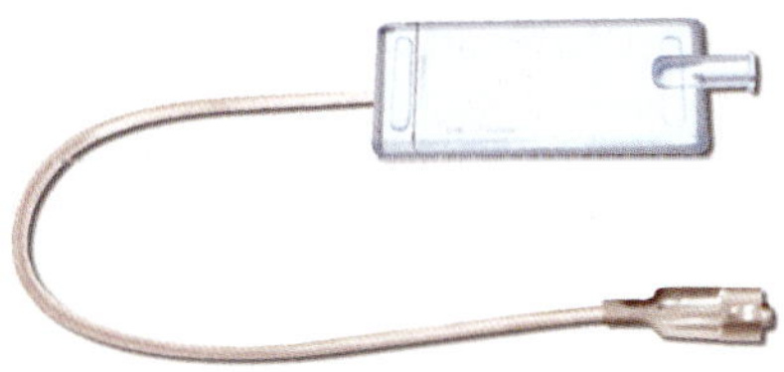

a final filter

depth filter a filter that can filter solutions being drawn into or expelled from a syringe, but not both ways in the same procedure.

final filter a filter placed immediately before a solution enters a patient's vein.

membrane filter a filter that filters solution as the solution is expelled from the syringe.

QUALITY ASSURANCE & INFECTION CONTROL

The USP–NF <797> regulations require every parenteral compounding facility to have a quality assurance program.

Quality assurance (QA) is a series of activities ensuring that a compounded formulation will be safe, stable, and of the proper identity, strength, purity, and quality. Another goal is to provide for product uniformity since a given formulation may be compounded by different pharmacy personnel at different times.

A major component of a quality assurance program is a written environmental quality and infection control plan.

These plans provide for:

- ✔ semiannual testing and certification of ISO classified work areas;
- ✔ routine monitoring of environmental airborne particulates and microbiologicals;
- ✔ routine monitoring of operating temperatures and humidity;
- ✔ maintaining continuous positive pressure and pressure differentials or gradients between clean areas;
- ✔ continuous HEPA filtered air;
- ✔ maintaining environmentally zoned areas based on critical activities (i.e., ISO Class 5 or 7);
- ✔ and limiting access to environmentally controlled areas.

Inspection

Formulated or admixed solutions should be inspected after compounding.

Visual inspection can check only for particulate material and stability.

Special equipment and skilled personnel are needed to check for sterility, pH, osmolarity, presence of pyrogens, and chemical degradation of the drug.

Final Check

The final check by the pharmacy technician of compounded parenteral formulations should verify that:

- ✔ the label is complete and error free;
- ✔ the correct base parenteral ingredients (quantity, strength) have been used;
- ✔ the correct drug additive (strength, quantity) has been added to the base parenteral ingredient;
- ✔ admixtures for IV solutions are clear and free from particulate matter; this part of the inspection can be aided by holding the admixture in front of both a black and white background;
- ✔ the correct beyond-use date is stated.

Sharps Disposal

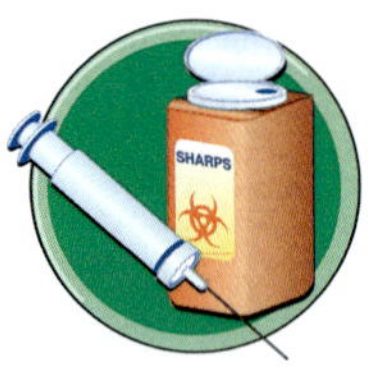

Once a parenteral solution has been prepared and inspected, any used syringes, bottles, vials, or other supplies should be disposed of properly in a container labeled sharps. A ***sharp*** is any object that might puncture or cut the skin of anyone who handles them. Sharps containers should be easily identified, leak proof, puncture proof, and able to be sealed permanently.

Following are procedures for preparing materials for disposal into a sharps container:

- ✔ Excess solutions should be returned to their original vial, an empty vial, or some other closed container before disposal.
- ✔ Needles should be left on syringes to prevent possible injuries.
- ✔ To prevent aerosolization of any remaining solution, needles should not be clipped.
- ✔ Used needles should never be recapped; they should be discarded as an intact unit, along with IV catheters or other sharp objects.
- ✔ Sharps containers should be disposed of when three-quarters full or at least daily.

Environmental quality and infection control plans also specify the methods for and frequency of cleaning and sanitizing parenteral compounding areas.

Cleaning and sanitizing are the responsibility of pharmacy personnel since these areas are off limits to housekeeping personnel.

Recommended standard operating procedures for cleaning sterile compounding facilities, including all anteroom carts, equipment, work benches, work surfaces, and floors, are to:

- ✔ clean and sanitize the direct and contiguous compounding area at the beginning of each shift;
- ✔ clean and sanitize work surfaces in the anteroom daily;
- ✔ mop floors daily (when no aseptic operations are in progress);
- ✔ empty storage shelving in the anteroom of all supplies and clean and sanitize at least weekly;
- ✔ clean and sanitize the walls and ceilings in the work space at least monthly.

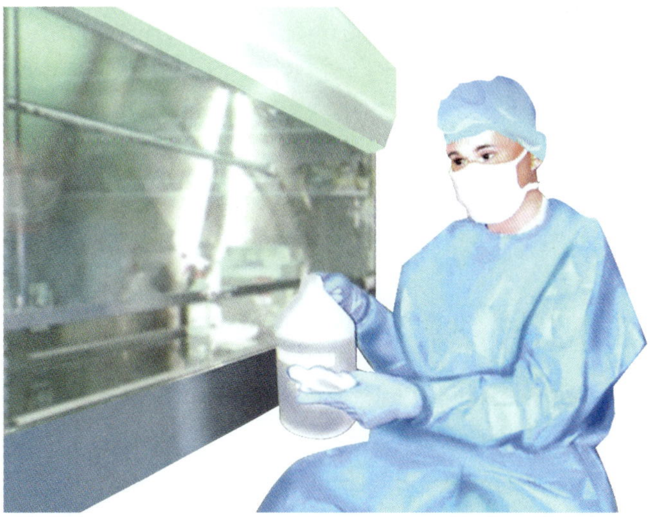

Hazardous Waste Regulations

The Resource Conservation and Recovery Act gives the EPA authority to regulate the handling of hazardous wastes from their generation to their disposal. These regulations apply to drugs and chemicals discarded by pharmacies, hospitals, clinics, and other entities.

Hazardous materials are divided into two lists. "P-list" wastes include epinephrine, nitroglycerin, and physostigmine. "U-list" wastes are toxic, flammable, corrosive, or reactive and include cyclophosphamide; these materials are considered hazardous even in trace amounts of no more than 3% of the capacity of a container.

Hazardous waste must be collected and stored according to specific EPA and Department of Transportation (DOT) requirements. Sharps containers and other properly labeled, leak proof, and spill proof containers of nonreactive plastic are required where hazardous waste is generated. Hazardous drug waste may be initially contained in thick, sealable plastic bags before placing in approved containers.

Transport of waste containers from satellite accumulation areas to storage sites must be done by individuals who meet OSHA-mandated hazardous waste training. Hazardous waste must be properly manifested and transported by a federally permitted transporter to a federally permitted storage, treatment, or disposal facility.

sharps needles, jagged glass or metal objects, or any items that might puncture or cut the skin.

PARENTERAL INCOMPATIBILITIES

Not all drugs are compatible with each other: an incompatibility may exist between two or more drugs or between a drug and a base IV solution.

The number of unexpected or undesired combinations is relatively low compared to the number of IV admixtures prepared. But incompatibilities can lead to a patient not receiving the full dose of the medication or to an adverse reaction.

Some incompatibilities, such as a color change or hazy appearance, can be seen.

Precipitates form in the solution, or an evolution of gas may even be smelled. For example, variations in color can occur for imipenem-cilastatin or dobutamine. When ceftazidime is reconstituted, carbon dioxide gas is released. The precipitate that forms when paclitaxel is refrigerated dissolves at room temperature. Reading the package insert or checking with the pharmacist can confirm the reason for these changes in appearance.

But other incompatibilities are not indicated by color changes, precipitation, or gas formation.

If two or more drugs react that are incompatible with each other, one drug can cause the degradation of the other drug(s). These types of incompatibilities are only confirmed by analytical methods.

Incompatibility Information References

The most often used reference for incompatibility information is the manufacturers' package insert. There are also incompatibility charts that list drugs horizontally across the top and vertically down one side. Where the column and row intersect, there is a code relating information about the incompatibility of the two drugs.

Other sources of information include articles in professional journals, reference books such as Trissel's *Handbook on Injectable Drugs*, and the *American Hospital Formulary Service: Drug Information*. There is computer software available based on these references.

MINIMIZING INCOMPATIBILITIES

The following guidelines can help minimize incompatibilities.

- ✔ Use solutions promptly after preparation. Drugs in solutions tend to degrade in a relatively short time. If an admixture is not immediately used, it should be placed in the refrigerator (if appropriate).
- ✔ Minimize the number of drugs that will be added to a solution at one time. As the number of added drugs increase, so does the likelihood of an incompatibility.
- ✔ Check incompatibility references when an additive drug will produce a very high or very low pH solution. Some drugs will precipitate out of solution if the pH isn't favorable.
- ✔ Check incompatibility references when an additive drug contains a calcium, magnesium, or phosphate salt. These salt forms can precipitate many drugs and each other.
- ✔ Check incompatibility references when an additive drug contains an acetate or lactate salt. These solutions tend to have increased buffer capacities and are resistant to changes in pH.

tip
Make use of information references if you have any questions about a possible incompatibility. See Chapter 12, *Information*, for more on information resources.

FACTORS AFFECTING COMPATIBILITY & STERILITY

Following are some common factors that can affect the compatibility and/or stability of drugs in IV solutions.

pH

Combining two drugs that require different pH values for their final solution can cause one or both drugs to either degrade or precipitate.

Light

Some drugs will start to break down and lose their therapeutic effect if exposed to light.

- Example: Amphotericin B, cisplatin, and metronidazole must be protected from light to maintain their potency.

Temperature

Storing and maintaining IV solutions at the appropriate temperature are important factors in keeping admixtures stable. Because heat increases the rate of most chemical reactions (including degradation), most drugs are more stable when refrigerated than at room temperature.

- Example: Cefazolin IV is stable for only 24 hours at room temperature, but for 96 hours under refrigeration.

However, some drugs should not be refrigerated because a precipitate will form.

Dilution

The concentration of a drug in a solution may be a factor in its compatibility with other drugs. A common problem is mixing electrolytes for parenteral nutrition solutions. Make sure that a drug is properly diluted before combining it with another drug.

- Example: Up to 15 mEq of calcium can be added to a liter of solution containing up to 30 mEq of phosphate but higher concentrations of either drug will cause precipitation.

Buffer Capacity

This is the ability of a solution to resist a change in pH when another drug is added. In general, IV solutions do not have high buffer capacities so when a drug with a high buffer capacity is added, the resulting solution will have a pH that results from the drug added.

Time

Many drugs start to degrade shortly after being added to an IV solution. Others may require a longer period of time before degradation is evident.

Filters

Filters, especially final filters, can reduce the concentration of a drug if it becomes trapped by the filter.

- Example: An in-line filter can cause up to a 90% reduction in the delivered concentration of nitroglycerin.

Solutions

Some drugs require a specific solution or diluent to be used with them. Choosing the wrong solution can make the drug break down more quickly or cause a precipitate to form.

- Example: amphotericin B is not compatible with normal saline.
- Example: Trastuzumab (Herceptin®) is packaged with a specific diluent for reconstitution.

Chemical Complexation

Complexation occurs when two drugs combine together and a new chemical combination is formed. Often, the therapeutic effect of one of the drugs changes.

- Example: The combination of tetracycline and calcium reduces the activity of tetracycline.
- Example: Cisplatin-AQ should not be used with needles, administration sets, or filters that contain aluminum.

Plastics

Some drugs are incompatible with the plastics in containers or certain administration sets. This is especially true of polyvinyl chloride (PVC) plastics. The drug can bind to the plastic material, making it unavailable for therapeutic activity. Albumin is sometimes added to solutions because it preferentially binds to the plastic surfaces. Also, plasticizers can leach out of the plastic bag or from the administration set into the IV solution, and might bind with the drug, inactivating it.

UNITS OF MEASUREMENT

There are different ways to express the concentration of a drug in a parenteral solution.

Each method of expressing the concentration is related to a particular property of the solution. The common concentrations and their units are listed on these pages.

MOLARITY

Molarity is an expression of the number of moles of a drug in a volume of solution. A mole is the number of grams numerically equal to the ***molecular weight*** of the drug. The molecular weight is the sum of the atomic weights of all the atoms that make up the drug molecule. Potassium chloride (KCl) has a molecular weight of 74.6. So, one mole of potassium chloride is 74.6 grams.

Molarity concentrations are expressed as mole/liter (written as mol/L, or M). A 1M solution of potassium chloride contains 74.6 grams of the drug in 1,000 ml (1 liter) of solution.

Some molarity concentrations are expressed as millimoles per liter (written as mM/L). A millimole is one-thousandth of a mole.

Salt Forms

Drugs come in different salt forms for a variety of reasons, and the salt form and ***waters of hydration*** must be factored into determining the molecular weight of a drug. For example, chloride is available as sodium salt, potassium salt, and calcium salt.

Waters of hydration are water molecules that can attach to drug molecules. Calcium chloride ($CaCl_2$) exists in three different forms, ***anhydrous*** (no waters), dihydrate (two associated waters), and hexahydrate (six waters of hydration). The dihydrate form is the one used in making parenteral solutions.

OSMOLES

Another expression for an amount of drug is the osmole (Osmol). An osmole is equal to the molecular weight of the drug divided by the number of ***ions*** formed when a drug dissolves in solution.

$$\textbf{osmole} = \frac{\textbf{molecular weight}}{\textbf{\# of ions}}$$

For example, potassium chloride forms two ions when it dissolves in solutions. Therefore, 1 Osmol of potassium chloride would be its molecular weight (74.6 grams) divided by two: 37.3 grams. Anhydrous calcium chloride forms three ions when it dissolves in solution: one calcium ion and two chloride ions. 1 Osmol would be its molecular weight (111.0 grams) divided by three: 37.0 grams.

Most drug solution concentrations are expressed as Osmol/liter (written as Osmol/L). Some concentrations are expressed as mOsmol/L. A milliosmole is one-thousandth of an osmole.

anhydrous without water molecules.

equivalent weight a drug's molecular weight divided by its valence, a common measure of electrolyte concentration.

ions molecular particles that carry electric charges.

molecular weight the sum of the atomic weights of a molecule.

valence the number of positive or negative charges on an ion.

waters of hydration water molecules that attach to drug molecules.

EQUIVALENTS

Another expression for an amount of drug is the ***equivalent weight (Eq)***. It is used to describe concentrations of electrolytes such as potassium chloride, sodium chloride, sodium acetate, etc.

When an electrolyte dissolves in solution, it divides into ions, particles that carry electric charges that can be positive or negative. The number of positive or negative charges (but not both added together) is called the ***valence*** of the ions. It indicates the ions' ability to combine with other atoms or molecules.

An equivalent weight is equal to the molecular weight of the drug divided by the valence of the ions that form when the drug is dissolved.

$$\textbf{equivalent weight} = \frac{\textbf{molecular weight}}{\textbf{valence}}$$

Equivalent concentrations are expressed as an equivalent weight per liter (written as Eq/L). Equivalent concentrations are also expressed as milliequivalents per liter (written as mEq/L). A milliequivalent is one-thousandth of an equivalent weight.

EXAMPLE

Potassium chloride (KCl) splits into one potassium ion (K^+) and one chloride ion (Cl^-).

- KCl's valence is 1 since there is either one positive charge on the potassium ion or one negative charge on the chloride ion.
- The equivalent weight of KCl is 74.6 grams divided by one: 74.6 grams.

EXAMPLE

Anhydrous calcium chloride ($CaCl_2$, 111.0 grams) splits into one calcium ion having two positive charges (++) and two chloride ions, each having one negative charge (-). Its valence is 2.

- The equivalent weight of $CaCl_2$ is 111.0 grams divided by two: 55.5 grams.

PERCENTAGE WEIGHT BY VOLUME

Percentage concentrations refer to the drug's weight per 100 ml if the drug is a solid, or the drug's volume per 100 ml if the drug is a liquid.

$$\textbf{solid: \%} = \frac{\textbf{weight (gm)}}{\textbf{100 ml}}$$

$$\textbf{liquid: \%} = \frac{\textbf{volume (ml)}}{\textbf{100 ml}}$$

For example, a 5% dextrose solution contains 5 grams of dextrose (a solid) in 100 ml of solution. A 5% acetic acid solution (common household vinegar) contains 5 ml of acetic acid (a liquid) per 100 ml of solution.

Percentage concentrations are applied to other formulations besides parenteral solutions. A 10% zinc oxide ointment would have 10 grams of zinc oxide (a solid) in 100 grams of ointment.

INTERNATIONAL UNITS

Because the potency and purity of drugs from biological sources vary depending on the source, they are measured by units of activity rather than by weight. Units may be abbreviated as IU, or U, and are expressed for example as 2,000 U, 1,000,000 U, etc. However, most institutions do not recommend the "IU" or "U" abbreviation because it can be misinterpreted. It is suggested that international units be spelled out.

Drugs commonly measured in international units include penicillin, insulin, heparin, and some vitamins.

REVIEW

KEY CONCEPTS

COMPOUNDING STERILE FORMULATIONS

- ✔ Parenteral solutions must be sterile, free of all visible particulate material, pyrogen-free, stable for their intended time of use, be isotonic, and in most cases (but not all) have a pH around 7.4.

LVP SOLUTIONS

- ✔ Large volume parenterals (LVP) are 100 ml or more and come in plastic bags or glass bottles.

SVP SOLUTIONS

- ✔ When a drug is added to a parenteral solution, the drug is referred to as the additive, and the final mixture is referred to as the admixture.

SPECIAL SOLUTIONS

- ✔ Parenteral nutrition solutions are complex admixtures composed of dextrose, fat, protein, electrolytes, vitamins, and trace elements used to meet a patient's nutritional needs.

ADMINISTRATION DEVICES

- ✔ LVP solutions are usually administered with an administration set. In addition to the basic components (tubing, spikes, clamps, needle adapters), administration sets may have drip chambers, volume control chambers, and Flashballs.
- ✔ Parenteral administration devices use either gravity or a pump to push the solution into the patient.

LAMINAR FLOW HOODS

- ✔ A laminar flow hood establishes and maintains an ultraclean work area for preparing parenteral solutions.

BIOLOGICAL SAFETY CABINETS AND CLEAN ROOMS

- ✔ Chemotherapy agents are to be made in a biological safety cabinet, not a laminar flow hood.
- ✔ Clean rooms are isolated rooms that house laminar flow hoods and biological safety cabinets; however, clean rooms that meet ISO Class 5 standards do not need a hood or cabinet.

ASEPTIC TECHNIQUES FOR HOODS AND CABINETS

- ✔ Aseptic techniques maintain the sterility of all sterile items and are used in preparing admixtures.

WORKING WITH VIALS

- ✔ There is the potential of coring the rubber stopper of a vial when inserting a needle.

WORKING WITH AMPULES

- ✔ Ampules may be pre-scored by the manufacturer or need to be scored with a file.

SYRINGES AND NEEDLES

- ✔ Syringes come in sizes ranging from 1 to 60 ml.
- ✔ Needle sizes are indicated by length and gauge. Large needle lumens may be needed for highly viscous solutions but are more likely to cause coring.

FILTERS

- ✔ Syringe filters are used to remove particulate materials or microorganisms from parenteral solutions.

QUALITY ASSURANCE AND INFECTION CONTROL

- ✔ A significant part of preparing parenteral solutions is to have and follow an environmental quality and infection control plan.
- ✔ Drugs and supplies used in making parenteral solutions should be disposed of properly. This may involve using a sharps container, or following procedures prescribed by the EPA and local landfill requirements.

PARENTERAL INCOMPATIBILITIES

- ✔ An incompatibility can exist between the drugs in an admixture or between a drug and the base IV solution.

UNITS OF MEASUREMENT

- ✔ Equivalent (Eq/L) or milliequivalent (mEq/L) concentrations are commonly used to describe concentrations of electrolytes in parenteral solutions.
- ✔ Percentage concentrations refer to the drug's weight per 100 ml if the drug is a solid, or the drug's volume per 100 ml if the drug is a liquid.

SELF TEST

the answer key begins on page 569

MATCH THE TERMS: I

1. additive _____
2. admixture _____
3. ampules _____
4. anhydrous _____
5. aseptic techniques _____
6. bevel _____
7. compounded sterile preparation (CSP) _____
8. coring _____
9. depth filter _____
10. dialysis _____
11. diluent _____
12. equivalent weight _____
13. final filter _____

a. sealed glass containers with an elongated neck.
b. a filter placed immediately before a solution enters a patient's vein.
c. a solvent that dissolves a lyophilized powder or dilutes a solution.
d. an angled surface, at the tip of a needle.
e. movement of particles in a solution through permeable membranes.
f. methods that maintain sterility of sterile products.
g. the resulting solution when a drug is added to a parenteral solution.
h. a compounded sterile parenteral dosage form that will be parenterally administered.
i. a drug that is added to a parenteral solution.
j. without water molecules.
k. a filter that can filter solutions being drawn into or out of a syringe, but not both ways in the same procedure.
l. a drug's molecular weight divided by its valence, a common measure of electrolyte concentration.
m. when needle damage to the rubber closure of a vial causes fragments to fall into the vial.

REVIEW

MATCH THE TERMS: II

1. Flashball _____
2. flow rate _____
3. gauge _____
4. HEPA filter _____
5. heparin lock _____
6. horizontal flow hood ____
7. hub _____
8. hypertonic _____
9. hypotonic _____
10. ions _____
11. irrigation solution _____
12. isotonic _____
13. laminar flow _____
14. lumen _____
15. lyophilized _____
16. membrane filter _____
17. molecular weight _____
18. osmosis _____
19. osmotic pressure _____
20. peritoneal dialysis solution ____
21. piggybacks _____
22. pyrogens _____
23. ready-to-mix _____

a. the sum of the atomic weights of a molecule.
b. a specially designed minibag by which a drug is put into the SVP fluid just prior to administration.
c. a laminar flow hood where the air crosses the work area in a horizontal direction.
d. a high efficiency particulate air filter.
e. chemicals produced by microorganisms that can cause fever reactions in patients.
f. molecular particles that carry electric charges.
g. when a solution has an osmolarity equivalent to blood.
h. when a solution has an osmolarity less than blood.
i. when a solution has an osmolarity greater than blood.
j. the rate (in ml/hour or ml/minute) at which the solution is administered to the patient.
k. freeze dried.
l. the action in which a drug in a higher concentration solution will pass through a permeable membrane to a lower concentration solution.
m. a solution placed in and emptied from the peritoneal cavity to remove toxic substances.
n. large volume splash solutions used during surgical or urologic procedures to bathe and moisten body tissues.
o. continuous movement at a uniform rate in one direction.
p. flexible rubber bulb near the needle adapter of an administration set used to determine if the needle is properly placed in the vein.
q. the part of the needle that attaches to the syringe.
r. a needle size measurement.
s. the hollow center of a needle.
t. a filter that filters solution expelled from the syringe.
u. a characteristic of a solution determined by the number of dissolved particles in it.
v. small volume solutions connected to an LVP.
w. an injection device used when a primary LVP solution is not available.

MATCH THE TERMS: III

1. shaft ____
2. sharps ____
3. Slip-Tip®, Luer-Lok®, eccentric, oral ____
4. total nutrient admixture (TNA) solution ____
5. total parenteral nutrition (TPN) solution ____
6. valence ____
7. vertical flow hood ____
8. waters of hydration ____
9. zone of turbulence _____

a. water molecules that attach to drug molecules.
b. the number of positive or negative charges on an ion.
c. a laminar flow hood where the air crosses the work area in a vertical direction.
d. any object that can puncture or cut the skin of anyone who handles them.
e. different types of syringe tips.
f. complex solutions with two base solutions (amino acids and dextrose) and additional micronutrients.
g. a TPN solution that contains intravenous fat emulsion.
h. the stem of the needle that provides the overall length of the needle.
i. an area of blocked air flow in a laminar flow hood.

CHOOSE THE BEST ANSWER

1. What does "sterile" mean with regard to an intravenous solution?
   a. It is free from bacteria.
   b. It is free from particulate material.
   c. It is free from pyrogens.
   d. all of the above

2. The purpose of USP–NF <797> is to prevent harm and fatality to patients that can result from
   a. nonsterile formulations.
   b. excessive bacterial endotoxins.
   c. large errors in the strength of correct ingredients.
   d. all of the above

3. Which of the following is not a small volume parenteral (SVP)?
   a. multivitamins, two 5 ml vials
   b. glycine 1.5% irrigation solution
   c. folic acid, 5 mg/ml, 10 ml vial
   d. magnesium sulfate, 4 g in 100 ml D5W

4. Irrigation solutions are administered
   a. through a filter needle.
   b. through a special administration set.
   c. orally.
   d. by pouring them out of the bottle.

5. Which part of an administration set is used to set the flow rate?
   a. spike
   b. volume control chamber
   c. Flashball
   d. needle adapter

6. Peristaltic, cassette, and elastomeric pumps are examples of
   a. automixers.
   b. positive pressure pumps.
   c. controllers.
   d. administration sets.

REVIEW

7. In horizontal laminar flow hoods, air blows
   a. down toward the work area.
   b. away from the operator.
   c. toward the operator.
   d. up toward the HEPA filter.

8. Which is an incorrect statement regarding clean rooms?
   a. must be a designated area of the pharmacy
   b. must have restricted air flow
   c. must accommodate most of the equipment for aseptic compounding
   d. must have proper storage of supplies

9. Which must be used to create and maintain a sterile environment?
   a. ISO Class 5 laminar flow hood
   b. aseptic technique
   c. positive pressure clean room
   d. none of the above

10. When using the laminar flow hood, a technician should work at least __________ inside the hood.
    a. two inches
    b. four inches
    c. six inches
    d. eight inches

11. A LVP plastic bag has a protective covering to keep __________ from the bag.
    a. pyrogens
    b. bacteria
    c. dust
    d. humidity

12. Why is air generally injected into a vial before a volume of solution is removed?
    a. keeps the drug dissolved in the solution
    b. provides a negative pressure in the vial so the solution will not spray when the needle is removed
    c. helps withdraw the solution by pressurizing the vial
    d. prevents the vial closure from coring

13. Which is the correct procedure of adding a lyophilized drug packaged in a vial to a LVP solution?
    a. Draw the lyophilized drug into a syringe, and add to the LVP.
    b. Draw the lyophilized drug into a syringe, add to the LVP, then reconstitute.
    c. Reconstitute the lyophilized drug in the vial and attach to the LVP.
    d. Reconstitute the lyophilized drug in the vial and add to the LVP.

14. Lyophilized powder in a vial
    a. can be drawn directly into a syringe.
    b. requires a diluent to solubilize the powder before withdrawing from the vial.
    c. forms aerosol droplets when withdrawn from the vial.
    d. cannot be added to any other LVP or SVP.

15. Which is a false statement about ampules?
    a. If an ampule is not pre-scored, it cannot be used.
    b. The ampule should be opened by breaking the neck away from the operator.
    c. The contents of an ampule should be withdrawn through a filter needle.
    d. Ampules should be disposed of in sharps containers.

16. You are to use 2.4 ml of diluent to reconstitute a vial of medication. What size of syringe should be used?
    a. 20 ml
    b. 10 ml
    c. 5 ml
    d. 3 ml

17. _______ is the part of the needle that attaches to the syringe.
    a. The lumen
    b. The bevel
    c. The core
    d. The hub

18. Visual inspection of parenteral solutions can show the presence of ________ and ________.
    a. particle contamination, precipitation
    b. pH, precipitation
    c. chemical degradation of a drug, osmolarity
    d. pyrogens, precipitation

19. USP–NF Chapter <797> recommends that the contiguous compounding area be cleaned and sanitized
    a. every shift.
    b. daily
    c. weekly
    d. monthly

20. Which concentration term used with parenteral solutions does not use the drug's molecular weight to determine its value?
    a. molarity
    b. osmoles
    c. equivalents
    d. percentage weight per volume

CRITICAL THINKING QUESTIONS

1. When working in a laminar flow hood, a technician should work at least 6 inches inside the hood. Why?
2. Why is it necessary to use a filter with a 1.2 micron or larger pore size as a final filter for a TNA parenteral solution?
3. Why should a filter needle be used when withdrawing drug solution from an opened ampule?

THINKING IT THROUGH WRAP-UP

1. No. Once you remove the opened materials from the hood, they will be contaminated by the air and lose their sterility. You will need to complete the ampicillin batch completely, and then begin the vancomycin order.
2. Hoods are required to be class ISO 5, and clean rooms are to be class ISO 7. If you were actually in a clean room that was class ISO 5, it would be permissible to set the ampicillin aside while you do the vancomycin order. That is because the air quality in the clean room would be the same as in the hood.
3. There is an incompatibility of ampicillin in NS or vancomycin in D5W. Resources would need to be consulted to understand the mechanism of the incompatibility since there are many different factors that could be involved.

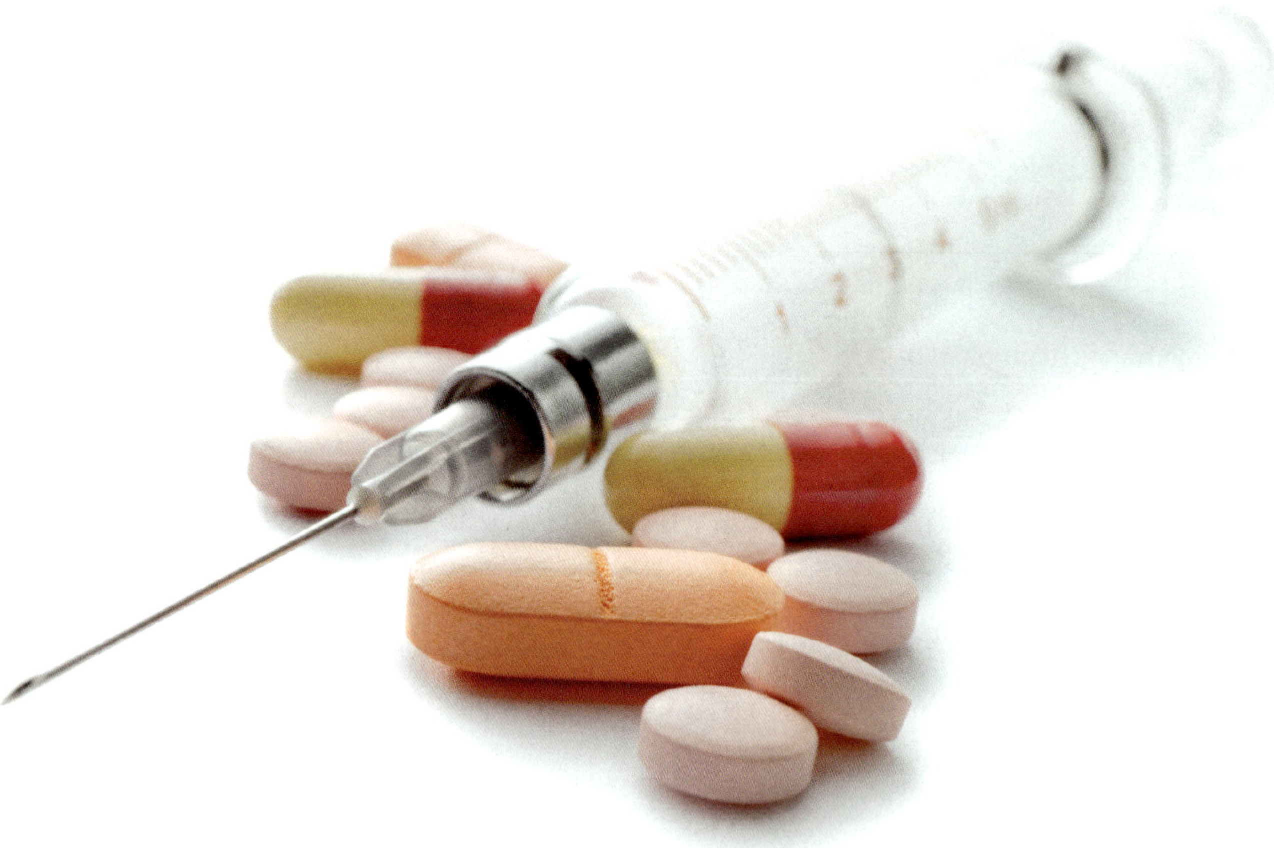

10

BASIC BIOPHARMACEUTICS

LEARNING OBJECTIVES

At the completion of study, the student will be able to:

- ✔ explain how a drug produces a pharmacological effect.
- ✔ explain why a blood concentration–time profile is an accepted method of indirectly determining the concentration of a drug at the site of action.
- ✔ identify and explain the influence of ADME processes on a blood concentration–time curve.
- ✔ identify and explain the influence of three factors on the processes of absorption, distribution, metabolism, and excretion.
- ✔ define bioavailability and explain the difference between absolute and relative bioavailability.
- ✔ define bioequivalency and explain how the FDA uses this information.
- ✔ explain how to determine a drug's half-life.

THINKING IT THROUGH

Levothyroxine is a drug that can be given by rapid intravenous administration to patients who need it administered in that fashion. Typically, however, it is administered in a tablet dosage form because of its convenience and lower cost. A patient is switching from 50 mcg of levothyroxine IV to the tablet form. Your pharmacists asks you look up the bioavailability of levothyroxine tablets and you find it has an absolute bioavailability of 50%.

As you read this chapter, consider the following questions:

1. What are some of the potential problems you might encounter in changing from an IV solution to an oral tablet form of a drug in terms of its absorption, distribution, metabolism, and elimination?
2. What does an absolute bioavailability of 50% mean?
3. If the patient was receiving 50 mcg of intravenous levothyroxine, can you estimate what the equivalent oral tablet dose would be?

HOW DRUGS WORK

Drugs produce either desired or undesired effects in the body.

Once they are in the blood, drugs are circulated throughout the body. The properties of both the drug and the body influence where the drug will go, and what concentration it will have at each place. The place where a drug causes an effect to occur is called the ***site of action***. The objective of drug therapy is to deliver the right drug, in the right concentration, to the right site of action, and at the right time to produce the desired effect.

When most drugs produce an effect, they are interacting at a molecular level with cellular material.

The cellular material directly involved in the action of a drug is called a ***receptor***. The receptor is often described as a lock into which the drug molecule fits as a key, and only those drugs able to interact with the receptors at a particular site of action can produce effects at that site. This is why specific cells respond only to certain drugs, even though their receptors are exposed to any drug molecules that are present in the body. This is also why drugs are ***selective*** in their action: that is, they act only on specific targeted receptors and tissues.

Receptors are located on the surfaces of cell membranes and inside cells.

There are many different types of receptors, each type having a different influence on the body's processes. Most receptors can be found throughout the body, though some occur in only a few places.

agonists drugs that activate receptors to accelerate or slow normal cellular function.

antagonists drugs that bind with receptors but do not activate them. They block receptor action by preventing other drugs or substances from activating them.

receptor the cellular material located at the site of action that interacts with the drug.

selective (action) the characteristic of a drug that makes its action specific to certain receptors and tissues.

site of action the location where an administered drug produces an effect.

DRUG ACTION AT THE SITE OF ACTION

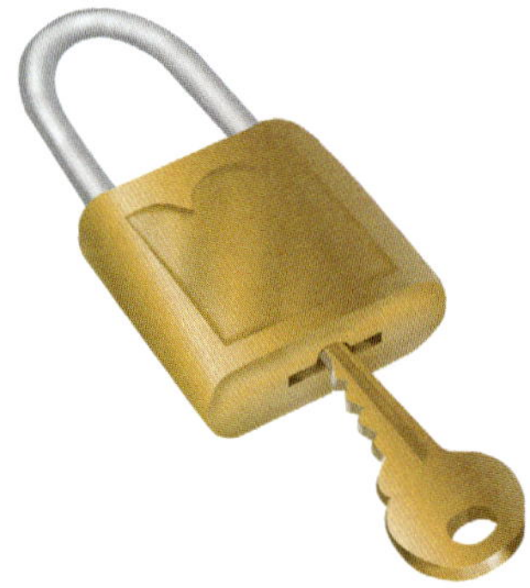

Like a lock and key, only certain drugs are able to interact with certain receptors.

Types of Action

When drugs interact with the site of action, they can:

- act through physical action, such as the protective effects of ointments upon topical application;
- react chemically, such as antacids that reduce excess gastric acidity;
- modify the metabolic activity of pathogens, such as antibiotics;
- change the osmolarity of blood and draw water out of tissues and into the blood;
- incorporate into cellular material to interfere with normal cell function;
- join with other chemicals to form a complex that is more easily excreted;
- modify the biochemical or metabolic process of the body's cells or enzyme systems.

When drug molecules bind with a receptor, they can cause a reaction that stimulates or inhibits cellular functions.

The pharmacological effects of these interactions are termed agonism or antagonism. ***Agonists*** are drugs that activate receptors and produce a response that may either accelerate or slow normal cellular processes, depending on the type of receptor involved. For example, epinephrine-like drugs act on the heart to increase the heart rate while acetylcholine-like drugs act on the heart to slow the heart rate. Both are agonists. ***Antagonists*** are drugs that bind to receptors but do not activate them. Instead, antagonists block the receptors' action by preventing other drugs or substances from interacting with them.

The number of receptors available to interact with a drug will also directly influence the effect.

A minimum number of receptors have to be occupied by drug molecules to produce an effect. If there are too few drug molecules to occupy the necessary number of receptors, there will be little or no effect. In this case, increasing the dosage will cause more receptors to be occupied. On the other hand, once all the receptors are occupied, further increasing the dosage will not increase the effect.

Receptors can be changed by drug use.

For example, extended stimulation of cells with an agonist can reduce the number or sensitivity of the receptors, and the effect of the drug is reduced. Extended inhibition of cell functions with an antagonist can increase the number or sensitivity of receptors. If the antagonist is stopped abruptly, the cells can have an extreme reaction to an agonist. To avoid such withdrawal symptoms, some drugs must be gradually discontinued.

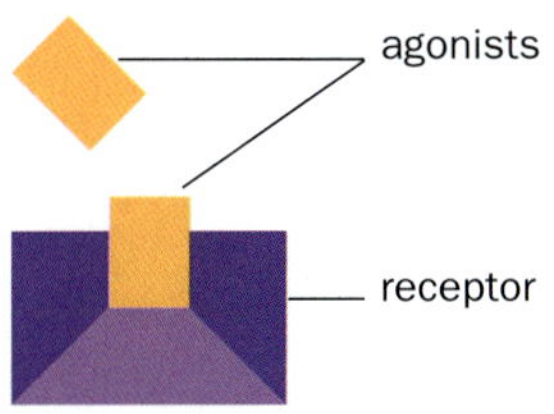

agonists activate receptors

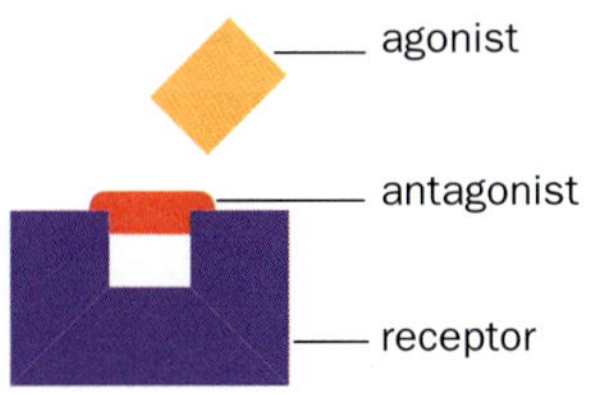

antagonists block receptors

Other Drug Actions

- Some drugs work by changing the ability of ions to move into or out of cells. For example, sodium or calcium ion channels can open and allow movement of the ions into nerve cells, stimulating their function. With potassium channels, the opposite can happen. The channels can open and allow the movement of potassium ions out of nerve cells, obstructing their function.
- Some drugs modify the creation, release, or control of hormones that regulate different physiological processes.

Rx tip

The objective of drug therapy is to deliver the right drug, in the right concentration, to the right site of action, and at the right time to produce the desired effect.

CONCENTRATION & EFFECT

It is difficult to measure the amount of drug at the site of action and therefore to predict an effect based upon that measurement.

One problem is that many factors influence a drug's movement from the site of administration to the site of action (absorption, elimination, membrane permeability, etc.). It can also be physically impossible to measure the drug at the site of action either because of its unknown location or small size.

One way to monitor the amount of a drug in the body and its effect at the site of action is to use a dose–response curve.

A dose–response curve shows an increase in response to a drug as its dosage is increased. However, when a series of drug doses is given to a variety of people, the results show that some people respond to low doses while others require a larger dose to produce an equal response. This is due to human variability: different people have different characteristics that affect how a drug product performs in them and how a drug moves from the site of administration to the site of action. For these reasons, dose–response curves are not ideal for correlating the amount of drug in the body to its actual effect in individuals.

A better way to relate the amount of a drug in the body to its effect is to determine drug concentrations in the body's fluids.

Of the body's fluids, blood is generally used because of its rapid equilibrium between the site of administration and the site of action. As a result, knowing a drug's concentration in the blood can be directly related to its effect. This is the most common way to analyze the potential effect of a drug.

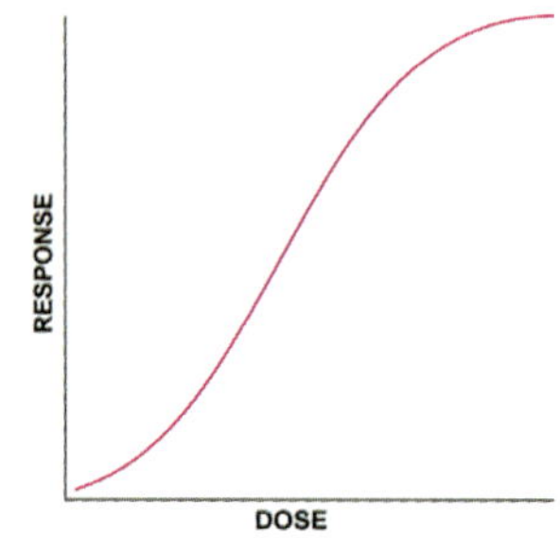

An expected dose–response curve shows that a response increases as the dose is increased.

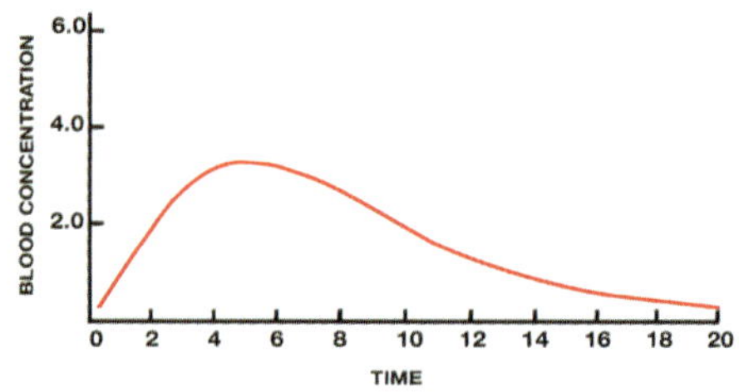

a blood concentration–time profile

duration of action the time drug concentration is above the MEC.

minimum effective concentration (MEC) the blood concentration needed for a drug to produce a response.

minimum toxic concentration (MTC) the upper limit of the therapeutic window. Drug concentrations above the MTC increase the risk of undesired effects.

onset of action the time MEC is reached and the response occurs.

therapeutic window a drug's blood concentration range between its MEC and MTC.

An advantage of using blood concentrations to measure the amount of drug in the body is that blood can be repeatedly sampled.

When sampling covers several hours or more, a blood concentration–time profile can be developed. Plasma or serum concentrations can be used instead of blood concentrations, and the same type of profile will result.

For many drugs, changes in the blood concentration–time profile reflect changes in concentration at the site of action and therefore changes in effect.

These drugs are typically monitored by determining the blood concentration peak and trough at the beginning and end of a dosing interval. Drugs usually monitored include vancomycin, phenytoin, gentamycin, digoxin, and valproic acid.

There are exceptions to when a blood concentration–time profile reflects the site of action concentration.

The concentration of some drugs at the site of action produces an action hours or days later after the drug is given. Other drugs show no relationship between blood concentrations and concentrations in the site of action. Still others don't depend on blood concentrations to produce an effect.

A Sample Blood Concentration–Time Profile

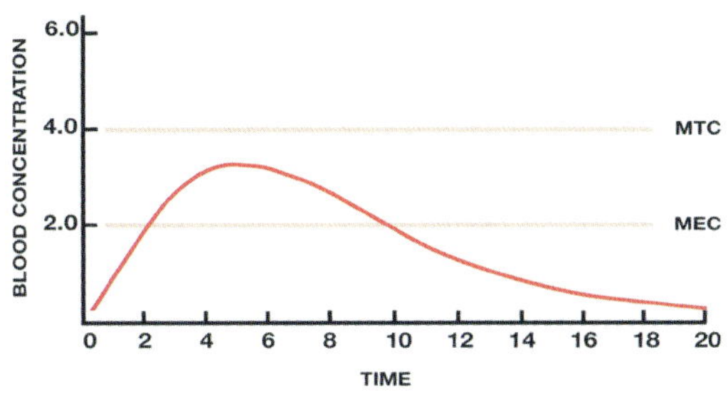

This illustration shows a typical blood concentration–time profile for a drug given orally. The blood concentration begins at zero at the time the drug is administered (before it has been absorbed into the blood). With time, the drug leaves the formulation and enters the blood, causing concentrations to rise.

To produce an effect, the concentrations must achieve a ***minimum effective concentration (MEC)***. This is when there is enough drug at the site of action to produce a response. The time this occurs is called the ***onset of action***. With most drugs, when blood concentrations increase, so does the intensity of the effect, since blood concentrations reflect the concentrations at the site of action that produce the response.

Some drugs have an upper blood concentration limit beyond which there are undesired or toxic effects. This limit is called the ***minimum toxic concentration (MTC)***. The range between the minimum effective concentration and the minimum toxic concentration is called the ***therapeutic window***. When concentrations are in this range, most patients receive the maximum benefit from their drug therapy with a minimum of risk.

The last part of the curve shows the blood concentrations declining as absorption is ending and elimination is proceeding. The time between the onset of action and the time when the minimum effective concentration is reached by the declining blood concentrations is called the ***duration of action***. The duration of action is the period of time during which the drug should produce the desired effect.

Applications of Blood Concentration–Time Profiles

- Manufacturers use the data to evaluate their drug products.
- Pharmacy professionals use them to visualize the consequences of incorrectly compounding a formulation or of using the wrong route of administration.
- Researchers and clinicians use them to measure human variability (e.g., influence of age, gender, nationality, or disease) in drug product performance.
- Physicians and pharmacists use them to monitor the drug therapy of patients.

ADME PROCESSES & DIFFUSION

Blood concentrations are the result of four simultaneously occurring processes: absorption, distribution, metabolism, and excretion. These four processes are referred to as the ADME processes, but may also be called *disposition*. Metabolism and excretion combined are called *elimination*.

The transfer of drug into the blood from an administered drug product is called absorption.

When a drug product is first administered, absorption is the primary process whereby the drug is released from the product and moves into the blood. Distribution, metabolism, and excretion will also occur, but the amount of drug available for them is much less than the amount of drug available for absorption, so these processes have little effect. As more of the drug is absorbed into the blood, it is available to undergo these other processes and their roles increase.

A drug's distribution will be affected by physiological functions and its own properties.

Though blood may deliver the drug to a body tissue, if the drug cannot penetrate the tissue's membranes, it will not interact with the receptors. The opposite situation can also occur. A drug may be able to penetrate to the tissue's membranes, but if there is not enough blood flow to the tissue, little of the drug will be available. Distribution is also influenced by drug binding to proteins in the blood or in tissues.

The ADME processes are all illustrated by blood concentration–time curves.

Concentrations rise during absorption, but as absorption nears completion, metabolism and elimination become the primary processes, and they cause the blood concentration to decline.

ADME Processes and Blood Concentration-Time Curves

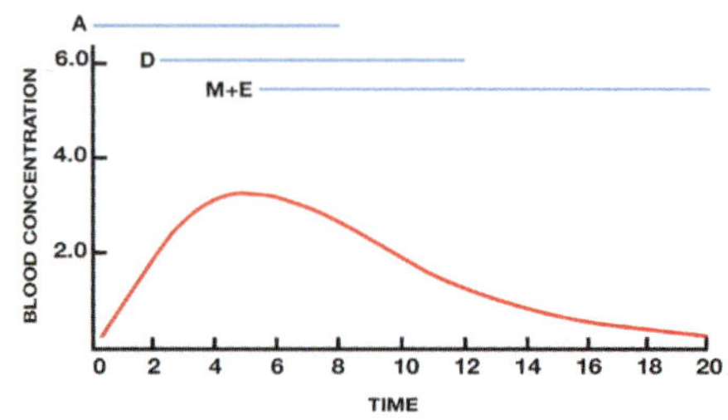

In the first part of a blood concentration–time curve, absorption is the primary process and concentrations rise. As absorption nears completion, metabolism and excretion become the primary processes, causing the concentration to decline. Distribution occurs throughout. The blue lines show the parts of the profile most influenced by the various ADME processes.

Half-life

Half-life is the amount of time it takes for the blood concentration of a drug to decline to one-half an initial value. For example, if at 6 hours a drug's blood concentration was 30 mcg/ml, and at 15 hours it was 15 mcg/ml, then the half-life would be 9 hours (15 hours minus 6 hours). To estimate how long it takes to essentially remove the drug from the body via the process of elimination, five times the half-life is used. So, in the preceding example, that would be 5 x the half-life of 9 hours, or 45 hours.

active transport the movement of drugs from an area of lower concentration to an area of higher concentration; cellular energy is required.

disposition a term sometimes used to refer to all of the ADME processes together.

elimination the processes of metabolism and excretion.

hydrophilic capable of associating with or absorbing water.

hydrophobic water repelling; cannot associate with water.

lipoidal fat-like substance.

passive diffusion the movement of drugs from an area of higher concentration to lower concentration.

Besides the four ADME processes, a critical factor of drug concentration and effect is how drugs move through biological membranes.

Before an effective concentration of a drug can reach its site of action, it must overcome many barriers, most of which are biological membranes.

Biological membranes are complex structures composed of lipids (fats) and proteins.

They are generally classified in three types: those made up of several layers of cells, such as the skin; those made up of a single layer of cells, as in the intestinal lining; and those of less than one cell in thickness, as in the membrane of a single cell.

Most drugs penetrate biological membranes by passive diffusion.

Drugs in the body's fluids will generally move from an area of higher concentration to an area of lower concentration until the concentrations in each area are balanced, or in a state of equilibrium. This process is called *passive diffusion*. It is the most common way a drug penetrates biological membranes and is a primary factor in the distribution process. This movement from higher to lower concentration causes most orally administered drugs to move from the intestine to the blood and from the blood to the site of action.

Drug concentration is not the only factor influencing diffusion.

Membranes are *lipoidal* (fat-like); drugs that are more lipid-soluble will penetrate membranes better than drugs that are not. These lipid-soluble drugs are called *hydrophobic* drugs. They hate or repel water and are attracted to lipids. *Hydrophilic* drugs are attracted to water and can also penetrate membranes. It is thought that they move through water-filled passages called aqueous pores which allow water (and any drug contained in it) to move through the membrane.

In addition to passive diffusion, some drugs may be carried across membranes by specialized transport mechanisms.

This type of *active transport* (as opposed to passive diffusion) is thought to explain how certain substances that do not penetrate membranes by passive diffusion nevertheless succeed in entering a cell.

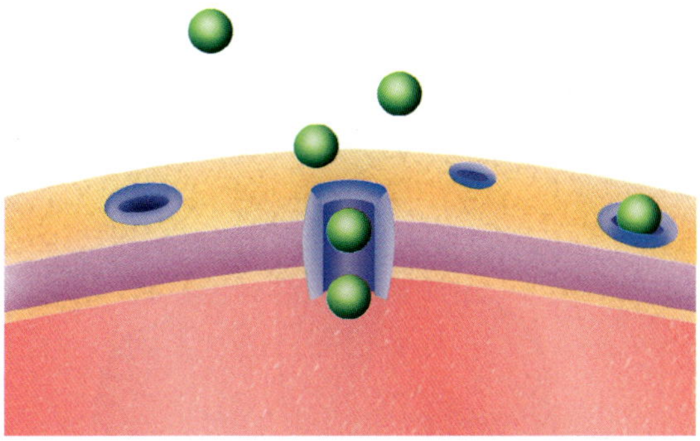

drug molecules penetrating a cell membrane

Ionization and Unionization

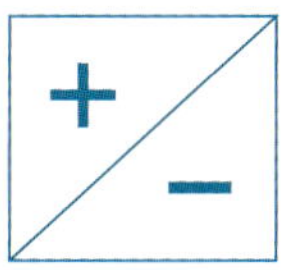

Because they are weak organic acids and bases, most drugs will dissociate (come apart) and associate (attach to other chemicals) in solutions. When acids dissociate, they become ionized. When bases dissociate, they become unionized.

Unionized drugs penetrate biological membranes more easily than ionized drugs for these reasons:

- unionized drugs are more lipid soluble;
- charges on biological membranes bind or repel ionized drug;
- ionized drugs associate with water molecules, creating larger particles with reduced penetrating capability.

Rx tip

Even though the ADME processes occur simultaneously, they are studied separately to understand the critical factors responsible for each process.

ABSORPTION

Once a drug is released from its dosage formulation, the process that transfers it into the blood is called *absorption*.

Absorption occurs to some extent with any route of administration. For example, even a drug in an intravenous suspension or emulsion must first be released from the dosage form to be absorbed into the blood. However, since many drugs are given orally, we will look at the ADME processes from the perspective of oral administration.

One of the primary factors affecting oral drug absorption is the *gastric emptying time*.

This is the time a drug will stay in the stomach before it is emptied into the small intestine. Since stomach acid can degrade many drugs and since most absorption occurs in the intestine, gastric emptying time can significantly affect a drug's action. If a drug remains in the stomach too long, it can be degraded or destroyed, and its effect decreased. Gastric emptying time can be affected by various conditions, including the amount and type of food in the stomach, the presence of other drugs, the person's body position, and their emotional condition. Some factors increase the gastric emptying time, but most slow it.

Once a drug leaves the stomach, its rate of movement through the intestines affects its absorption.

Slower than normal intestinal movement can lead to increased drug absorption because the drug is in contact with the intestinal membrane longer. Faster than normal intestinal movement can produce the opposite result since the drug moves through the intestinal tract too rapidly to be fully absorbed.

Bile salts and enzymes from the intestinal tract also affect absorption.

Bile salts improve the absorption of certain hydrophobic drugs. Enzymes added to the intestinal tract's contents from pancreatic secretions destroy certain drugs and consequently decrease their absorption. Enzymes are also present in the intestinal wall and can destroy drugs as they pass from the gut into the blood, decreasing their absorption.

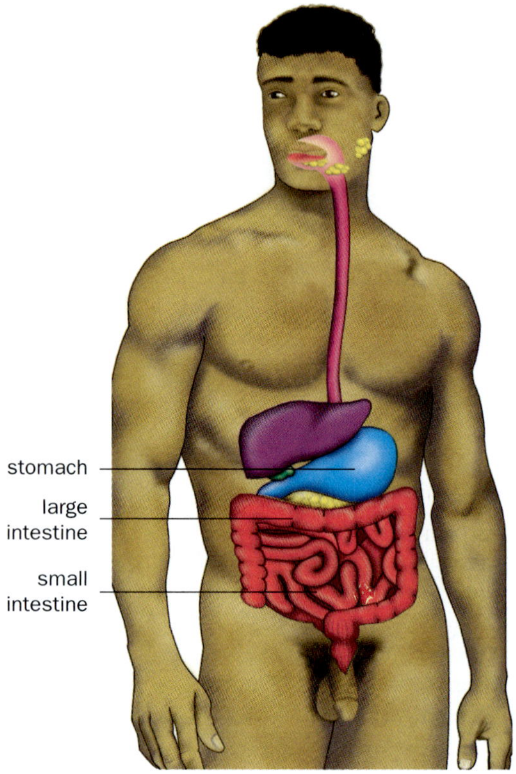

gastrointestinal organs

Most drugs are given orally and absorbed into the blood from the small intestine. The small intestine's large surface area benefits drug absorption. However, there are many conditions in the stomach that can affect absorption positively or negatively before the drug even reaches the small intestine. Once in the intestines, many additional factors can affect a drug's absorption.

absorption the movement of a drug from the dosage formulation to the blood.

gastric emptying time the time a drug will stay in the stomach before it is emptied into the small intestine.

DISTRIBUTION

Distribution involves the movement of a drug within the body once the drug has reached the blood.

Blood carries the drug throughout the body and to its sites of action, as well as to the organs responsible for the metabolism and excretion of the drug.

The blood flow rates to certain organs have a significant effect on distribution.

Drugs are rapidly distributed to organs having high blood flow rates such as the heart, liver, and kidneys. Distribution to areas such as muscle, fat, and skin is usually slower because they have lower blood flow rates.

The permeability of tissue membranes to a drug is also important.

Most tissue membranes are easily penetrated by most drugs. Small drug molecules (those having a low molecular weight) and drugs that are hydrophobic will generally diffuse through tissue membranes with ease. Some tissue membranes have specialized transport mechanisms that assist penetration. A few tissue membranes are highly selective in allowing drug penetration: The blood-brain barrier, for example, limits drug access to the brain and the cerebral spinal fluid.

Protein binding can also affect distribution.

Many drugs will bind to proteins in blood plasma, forming a *complex*. The large size of such complexes prevents the bound drug from entering its sites of action, metabolism, and excretion—essentially making the drug inactive. Only free, or unbound, drug can move through tissue membranes and cellular openings. Another drug with a stronger binding capacity can displace or unbind a more weakly bound drug from a protein, making it available for pharmacological activity. This has been the basis for a well-known drug interaction between aspirin and coumadin.

complexation when different molecules associate or attach to each other.

protein binding the attachment of a drug molecule to a plasma or tissue protein, effectively making the drug inactive, but also keeping it within the body.

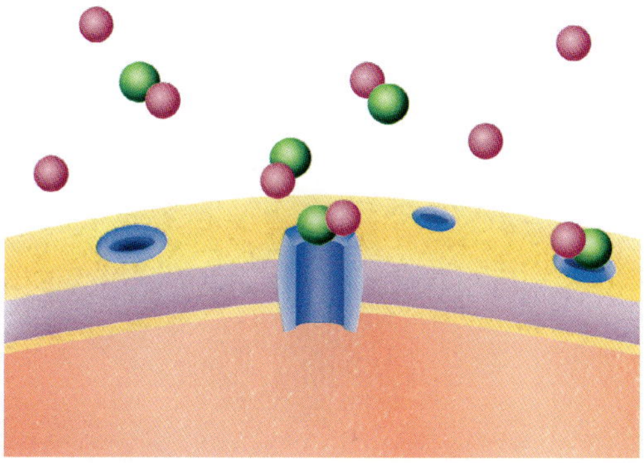

Protein Binding

Many drugs bind to proteins in blood plasma to form a complex that is too large to penetrate biological membranes. So the drug remains inactive.

Protein binding can be considered a type of drug storage or "depot" within the body. Some drugs bind extensively to proteins in fat and muscle, and are gradually released as the blood concentration of the drug falls. These drugs remain in the body a long time, and therefore have a long duration of action.

Selective Action

Though drugs are widely distributed throughout the body once they reach the bloodstream, they will have action that is selective to certain tissues or organs. This is due both to the specific nature of the receptor in the tissue and the various factors that affect the distribution of the drug (e.g., blood flow) to the tissue. This is why drugs can be targeted for specific therapeutic effects.

However, since most receptors can be found in multiple tissues throughout the body, most drugs have multiple effects. This is why a drug may be used for different therapies. For example, terbutaline is used for bronchodilation but it will also delay labor in pregnant women. It is also one reason drugs have side effects.

METABOLISM

Drug metabolism refers to the body's process of transforming drugs.

The transformed drug is called a *metabolite*. Most metabolites are inactive molecules that are excreted. However, the metabolites of some drugs are active, and they will produce effects in the patient until they are further metabolized or excreted.

The primary site of drug metabolism in the body is the liver.

Enzymes are complex proteins that catalyze chemical reactions. Enzymes found in the liver interact with drugs and transform them into metabolites.

In response to the chronic administration of certain drugs, the liver will increase its enzyme activity.

This is called *enzyme induction*, and it results in greater metabolism of a drug. As a result, larger doses of the drug must be administered to produce the same therapeutic effects. Some drugs decrease enzyme activity, a process called *enzyme inhibition*. In this case, smaller doses of the drug will be needed to avoid toxicity from drug accumulation.

The liver may secrete drugs or their metabolites into bile that is stored in the gallbladder.

The gallbladder empties the bile (and any drugs or metabolites in it) into the intestine in response to food entering the intestinal tract. Any drugs or metabolites contained in the bile may be reabsorbed or simply eliminated within the feces. If the drugs or metabolites are reabsorbed back into the blood circulation, this is called *enterohepatic cycling*.

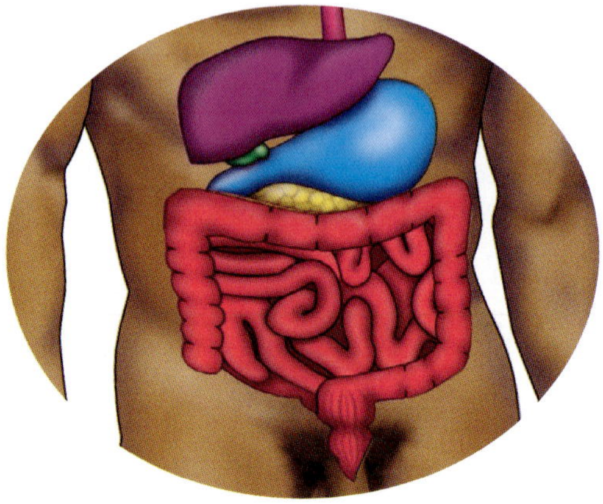

First-Pass Metabolism

With oral administration, once a drug is absorbed from the gastrointestinal tract, it is immediately delivered to the liver. It will then be transferred into the general systemic circulation.

However, before it reaches the circulatory system, the drug can be substantially degraded or destroyed by the liver's enzymes. This is called ***first-pass metabolism*** and is an important factor with orally administered drugs. Because of it, certain drugs must be administered by other routes. Any route of administration other than the oral route either partially or completely bypasses first-pass metabolism.

enterohepatic cycling the transfer of drugs and their metabolites from the liver to the bile in the gallbladder, then into the intestine, and then back into circulation.

enzyme a complex protein that catalyzes chemical reactions.

enzyme induction the increase in hepatic enzyme activity that results in greater metabolism of drugs.

enzyme inhibition the decrease in hepatic enzyme activity that results in reduced metabolism of drugs.

first-pass metabolism the substantial degradation of an orally administered drug caused by enzyme metabolism in the liver before the drug reaches the systemic circulation.

metabolite the substance resulting from the body's transformation of an administered drug.

EXCRETION

Most drugs and their metabolites are excreted in the urine by the kidneys.

Some orally administered drugs are not easily absorbed from the gastrointestinal tract and as a result are significantly excreted in the feces. Excretion can also occur through the bile (if enterohepatic cycling does not occur) and certain drugs are removed through the lungs in the expired breath.

The kidneys filter the blood and remove waste materials (including drugs and metabolites) from it.

As blood flows through a kidney, some of the plasma water is filtered from it into the ***nephron*** (the functional unit of the kidney) tubule in a process called ***glomerular filtration***. This filtered plasma water may contain waste materials and drugs from other parts of the body. As the water moves along the tubule, additional waste substances and drugs can be secreted into the fluid. Some drugs can be reabsorbed back into the blood during a process called urinary reabsorption. After glomerular filtration, renal secretion, and urinary reabsorption are completed, the remaining fluid is excreted from the body as urine.

The rate of urinary excretion is much faster than that of fecal excretion.

Drugs that will be excreted through the feces generally take a day or two to be excreted, whereas drugs may be excreted through the urine within hours of administration.

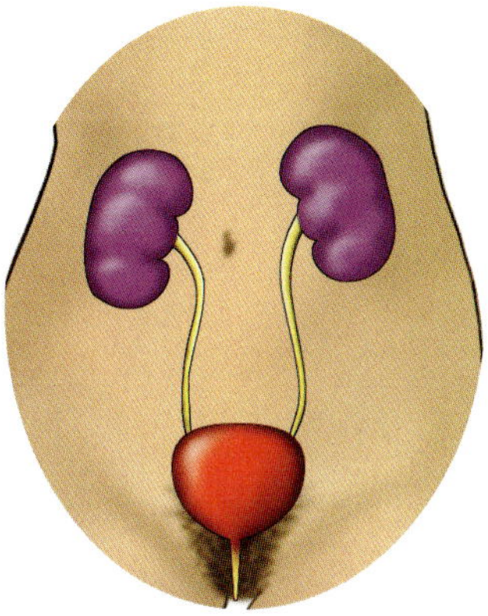

Factors Affecting Urinary Excretion

- If the kidney's process of excretion becomes impaired, excretion will be reduced and some drugs will accumulate in the blood. In such cases, the dosage of these drugs must be decreased or the dosing interval lengthened. Drugs such as vancomycin and gentamicin are monitored for this reason.
- Some drugs affect the excretion of others. In such cases, the affected drug will accumulate in the blood, and its dosage must be decreased or the dosing interval lengthened.
- Some drugs are actively transported into the urine (i.e., renal secretion). These active transport sites can be the location of important drug interactions that affect excretion.
- The pH of urine can affect the reabsorption of some drugs. A high pH can increase excretion of weak acids such as salicylates and phenobarbital. However, a high pH will decrease the excretion (i.e., increase reabsorption) of weak bases.
- The amount of drug excreted in urine is the amount filtered + the amount secreted - the amount reabsorbed.

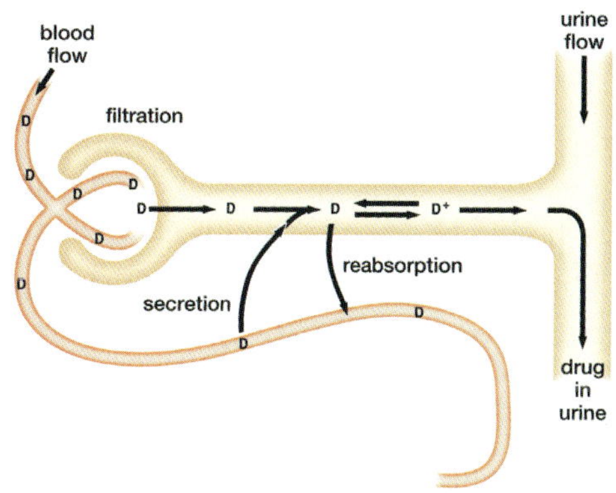

glomerular filtration the blood filtering process of the nephron.

nephron the functional unit of the kidneys.

BIOAVAILABILITY

The amount of a drug delivered to the site of action and the rate at which it becomes available is referred to as its *bioavailability*. By FDA definition, bioavailability is measured by determining the fraction of an administered dose of a drug that reaches the general systemic circulation and the rate at which this occurs.

The bioavailability of a drug is measured using the data from a blood concentration–time profile.

From this graphical representation, it is possible to calculate the rate at which the drug is absorbed, the duration of action of the drug, and the relationship between blood concentrations and the effect of the drug. What cannot be measured from a single profile is the amount or proportion of the drug that is absorbed from a drug product (i.e., the extent of absorption).

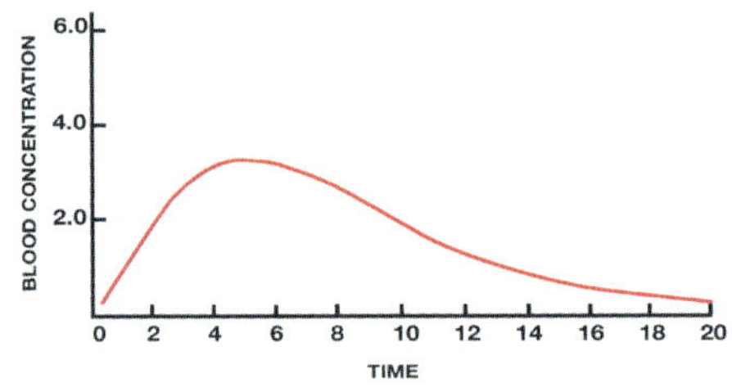

blood concentration–time profile

To determine the extent of absorption, the blood concentration–time profile from the drug product must be compared to a profile of a drug product that is used as a standard and for which the extent of absorption is already known.

The blood concentration–time profile of a rapidly administered intravenous solution is often used as the standard. Its extent of absorption is 100% since it does not have an absorption process but is immediately available in the blood circulation. When a rapidly administered IV solution is used as the standard, the comparison of the two profiles is termed *absolute bioavailability*.

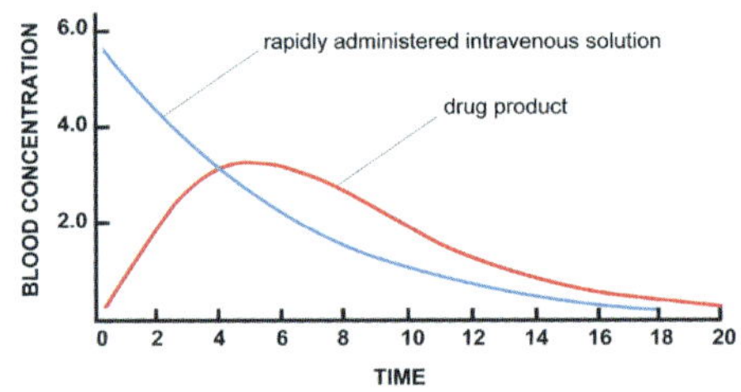

absolute bioavailability

If a blood concentration–time profile from a drug administered by any other means is used as a standard, it is termed *relative bioavailability*.

Any drug product other than a rapidly administered intravenous solution will have an absorption process that will affect the extent of absorption. This is obvious for rectal, oral, and topical routes, but it is also true for slowly administered intravenous solutions and other intravenous products such as suspensions or emulsions.

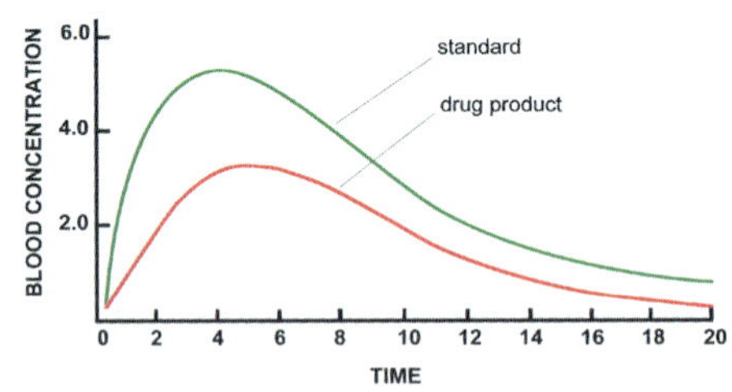

relative bioavailability

absolute bioavailability the bioavailability of a drug product compared to the same drug in a rapidly administered IV solution.

bioavailability the amount of an administered dose that reaches the general circulation and the rate at which this occurs.

relative bioavailability the bioavailability of a drug product compared to the same drug in any other dosage form than a rapidly administered IV solution.

DETERMINING A DRUG PRODUCT'S EXTENT OF ABSORPTION

The numeric value for the extent of absorption of a drug product is determined by comparing its area-under-curve (AUC) to the AUC of a standard product. If F represents the extent of absorption, then the ratio of the two AUCs will give the extent of absorption:

$$F = \frac{\text{drug product AUC}}{\text{standard product AUC}}$$

For example, if the absolute bioavailability of a drug in a tablet formulation is 50%, that means one-half of the dose is not absorbed from the site of administration when compared to the same drug in the form of a rapidly administered intravenous solution. This becomes an important factor when switching between IV and oral routes of administration.

Bioavailabilities of Commonly Prescribed Drugs Given by Oral Administration

Drug Name	Bioavailability %	Drug Name	Bioavailability %	Drug Name	Bioavailability %
Acyclovir	20	Diphenhydramine	72	Olanzapine	60
Albuterol (R)	30	Enalapril	41	Ondansetron	62
Albuterol (S)	71	Enoxaparin	92 (SC)	Oxycodone	42
Alprazolam	88	Felodipine	15	Phenytoin	90
Amiodarone	46	Furosemide	71	Prednisone	80
Amlodipine	74	Gabapentin	60	Quetiapine	9
Atenolol	58	Gemfibrozil	98	Ranitidine	52
Atorvastatin	12	Haloperidol	60	Ropinirole	55
Carvedilol	25	Hydrochlorothiazide	71	Sildenafil	38
Ceftazidime	91 (IM)	Ibuprofen	80	Sumatriptan	14
Chlorthalidone	64	Lisinopril	25	Tramadol	70
Ciprofloxacin	60	Losartan	36	Trazadone	81
Citalopram	80	Metformin	52	Warfarin	93
Clonazepam	98	Metoprolol	38	Zolpidem	72
Digoxin	70	Moxifloxacin	86		
Diltiazem	38	Nifedipine	50		

* The percentages are absolute bioavailabilities.

Rx **tip**

Rapidly administered intravenous solutions (i.e., bolus) do not have an absorption process.

BIOEQUIVALENCE

Comparing the bioavailabilities of one drug product to another drug product determines their *bioequivalency*.

Bioequivalent drug products are pharmaceutical equivalents or alternatives that have essentially the same rate and extent of absorption when administered using the same dose of the active ingredient under similar conditions. The FDA requires drug manufacturers to perform bioequivalency studies on their products before they are approved for marketing. In such studies, the bioavailability of the active ingredient in the manufacturer's drug product is compared to the bioavailability of the innovator's product. Bioequivalency studies are also used to compare bioavailability between different dosage forms (tablets, capsules, etc.), different manufacturers, and different production lots.

Bioequivalency can be graphically illustrated by placing the blood concentration–time profiles of the manufacturer's product and the innovator's product on the same plot.

In the illustration below, the same dose is contained in both the manufacturer's and the innovator's drug product, but the two curves are not the same. The innovator product (blue line) has a faster rate of absorption than the manufacturer's product (red line) but the manufacturer's product has a longer duration of action.

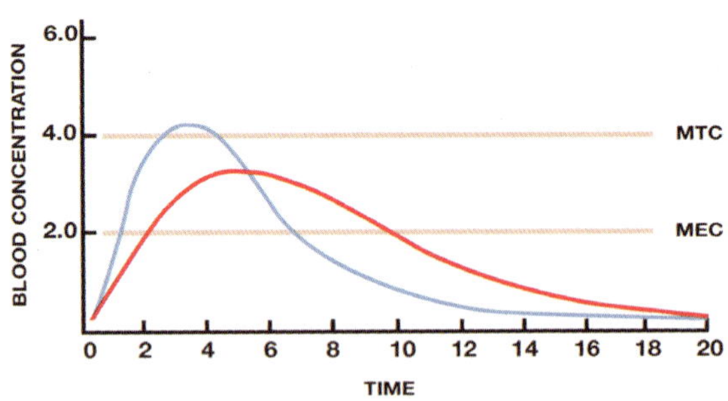

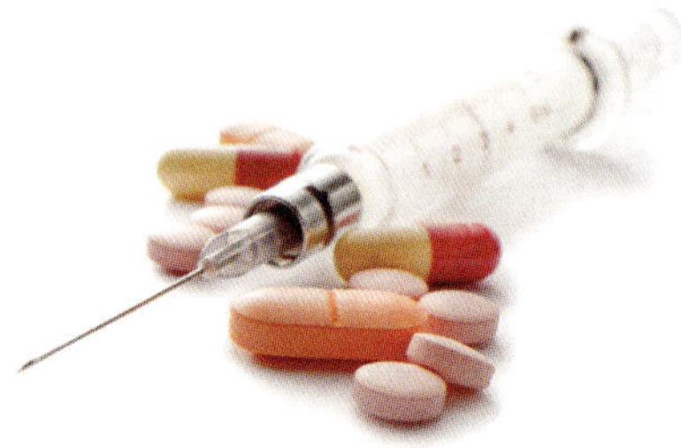

Differences Between Bioavailabilities

Exact bioequivalency between drug products (where blood concentration–time profiles for each product are identical) does not occur, and is not expected. There are simply too many variables that can contribute to differences between products. In tablets, for example, there can be different amounts or types of fillers, binders, lubricants, and other components. The particle size of the active drug itself may be slightly different. The manufacturing process may also produce different results in size, hardness, or other characteristics (especially for different manufacturers, but also for the same manufacturer at different times or different manufacturing facilities). Changes in these or various other factors can affect the bioavailability of a drug. Though there can be differences in the bioavailability of different products, when the differences are not significant the products are bioequivalent.

bioequivalency the comparison of bioavailability between two dosage forms.

pharmaceutical alternative drug products that contain the same active ingredient, but not necessarily in the same salt form, amount, or dosage form.

pharmaceutical equivalent drug products that contain identical amounts of the same active ingredient in the same dosage form.

therapeutic equivalent pharmaceutical equivalents that produce the same effects in patients.

The following terms are used by the FDA to define types of drug products used in bioequivalency studies.

Pharmaceutical equivalents are drug products that contain identical amounts of the same active ingredient in the same dosage form, and are identical in strength, concentration, and route of administration. They do not have to contain the same inactive ingredients, or have the same physical shape, release mechanisms, packaging, or expiration time. Since pharmaceutical equivalents may have different inactive ingredients, different pharmaceutically equivalent products may not be equally suitable for a given patient. One drug formulation may perform differently enough to change the overall effect.

- same active ingredient (same salt form)
- same amount of active ingredient
- same dosage form
- inactive ingredients can be different

Pharmaceutical alternatives are drug products that contain the identical active ingredient, but not necessarily the same salt form or amount or dosage form. An example is tetracycline hydrochloride 250 mg capsules versus tetracycline phosphate complex 250 mg capsules, or quinidine sulfate 200 mg tablets versus quinidine sulfate 200 mg capsules. They do not have to contain the same inactive ingredients, or have the same physical shape, release mechanisms, packaging, or expiration time.

- same active ingredient (but different salt form)
- amount of active ingredient can be different
- dosage form can be different
- inactive ingredients can be different

Therapeutic equivalents are pharmaceutical equivalents that produce the same therapeutic effect in patients.

- pharmaceutical equivalents that produce the same effects in patients

Rx tip

The FDA annually publishes *Approved Drug Products With Therapeutic Equivalence Evaluations* (the "Orange Book"). It is available online at www.accessdata.fda.gov/scripts/cder/ob/default.cfm. For further discussion, see Chapter Three of *The Pharmacy Technician Workbook and Certification Review, Fifth Edition.*

REVIEW

KEY CONCEPTS

HOW DRUGS WORK

- ✔ The objective of drug therapy is to deliver the right drug, in the right concentration, to the right site of action, and at the right time to produce the desired effect.
- ✔ Only those drugs able to interact with the receptors in a particular site of action can produce effects in that site. This is why specific cells respond only to certain drugs.

CONCENTRATION & EFFECT

- ✔ To produce an effect, a drug must achieve a minimum effective concentration (MEC). This is when there is enough drug at the site of action to produce a response.
- ✔ The range between the minimum effective concentration and the minimum toxic concentration is called the therapeutic window. When concentrations are in this range, most patients receive the maximum benefit from their drug therapy with a minimum of risk.
- ✔ Therapeutic drug monitoring can be useful when the blood concentration of the drug reflects the concentration at the site of action.

ADME PROCESSES & DIFFUSION

- ✔ Blood concentrations are the result of four simultaneously occurring processes: absorption, distribution, metabolism, and excretion (the ADME processes).
- ✔ Besides the four ADME processes, a critical factor in drug concentration and effect is how drugs move through biological membranes. Most drugs penetrate biological membranes by passive diffusion.

ABSORPTION

- ✔ One of the primary factors affecting oral drug absorption is the gastric emptying time.

DISTRIBUTION

- ✔ Many drugs bind to proteins in blood plasma to form a complex that is too large to penetrate biological membranes, essentially making the drug inactive.

METABOLISM

- ✔ Enzymes catalyze the transformation of drugs to metabolites. Most metabolites are inactive molecules that are excreted.

EXCRETION

- ✔ The kidneys filter blood and remove wastes, drugs, and metabolites from the body.
- ✔ Urinary excretion = glomerular filtration + renal secretion - urinary reabsorption.

BIOAVAILABILITY

- ✔ The amount of a drug that is delivered to the site of action and the rate at which it becomes available is called the bioavailability of the drug.

BIOEQUIVALENCE

- ✔ Bioequivalent drug products are pharmaceutical equivalents or alternatives that have essentially the same bioavailabilities (i.e., rate and extent of absorption) when administered in the same dose of the active ingredient under similar conditions.
- ✔ Pharmaceutical equivalents are drug products that contain identical amounts of the same active ingredient in the same dosage form, but may contain different inactive ingredients.
- ✔ Pharmaceutical alternatives are drug products that contain the identical active ingredient, but not necessarily in the same salt form, same amount, or dosage form.

SELF TEST

the answer key begins on page 569

MATCH THE TERMS: I

1. absolute bioavailability ____
2. absorption ____
3. active transport ____
4. agonists ____
5. antagonists ____
6. bioavailability ____
7. bioequivalency ____
8. complexation ____
9. disposition ____
10. duration of action ____
11. elimination ____
12. enterohepatic cycling ____
13. enzyme ____
14. enzyme induction ____
15. enzyme inhibition ____
16. first-pass metabolism ____
17. gastric emptying time ____
18. glomerular filtration ____
19. hydrophilic ____
20. hydrophobic ____
21. lipoidal ____

a. the substantial degradation of an orally administered drug caused by enzyme metabolism in the liver before the drug reaches the systemic circulation.
b. the increase in hepatic enzyme activity that results in greater metabolism of drugs.
c. the comparison of bioavailability between two dosage forms.
d. the amount of an administered dose that reaches the general circulation and the rate at which this occurs.
e. water repelling; cannot associate with water.
f. capable of associating with or absorbing water.
g. the blood filtering process of the nephron.
h. the time a drug will stay in the stomach before it is emptied into the small intestine.
i. the decrease in hepatic enzyme activity that results in reduced metabolism of drugs.
j. a complex protein that catalyzes chemical reactions.
k. the transfer of drugs and their metabolites from the liver to the bile in the gall bladder, then into the intestine, and then back into circulation.
l. the process of metabolism and excretion.
m. the time the drug concentration is above the MEC.
n. a term sometimes used to refer to all the ADME processes together.
o. when different molecules associate or attach to each other.
p. the movement of drugs from an area of lower concentration to an area of higher concentration; requires cellular energy.
q. the movement of a drug from the dosage formulation to the blood.
r. drugs that activate receptors to accelerate or slow normal cellular function.
s. drugs that bind with receptors but do not activate them.
t. fat-like substance.
u. the bioavailability a drug product compared to the same drug in a rapidly administered IV solution.

REVIEW

MATCH THE TERMS: II

1. metabolite ____
2. minimum effective concentration (MEC) ____
3. minimum toxic concentration (MTC) _____
4. nephron ____
5. onset of action _____
6. passive diffusion ____
7. pharmaceutical alternative ____
8. pharmaceutical equivalent ____
9. protein binding ____
10. receptor ____
11. relative bioavailability _____
12. selective (action) _____
13. site of action ____
14. therapeutic equivalent ____
15. therapeutic window ____

a. the attachment of a drug molecule to a protein, effectively making the drug inactive.
b. the cellular material that interacts with a drug.
c. the movement of drugs from an area of higher concentration to lower concentration.
d. the characteristic of a drug that makes its action specific to certain receptors.
e. the location where an administered drug produces an effect.
f. the blood concentration needed for a drug to produce a response.
g. the time MEC is reached and the response occurs.
h. a drug's blood concentration range between its MEC and MTC.
i. the upper limit of the therapeutic window.
j. the substance resulting from the body's transformation of an administered drug.
k. the functional unit of the kidney.
l. drug products that contain identical amounts of the same active ingredient in the same dosage form.
m. pharmaceutical equivalents that produce the same effects in patients.
n. drug products that contain the same active ingredient but not necessarily in the same salt form, amount, or dosage form.
o. the bioavailability of a drug product compared to the same drug in any other dosage form than a rapidly administered IV solution.

CHOOSE THE BEST ANSWER

1. The place where a drug causes an effect to occur is called the
   a. site of action.
   b. site of administration.
   c. therapeutic window.
   d. minimum toxic concentration (MTC).

2. When a drug produces an effect, it is acting at a/an ________________ level.
   a. tissue
   b. atomic
   c. cellular
   d. organ

3. Drug action can be determined by the
   a. number of receptors occupied.
   b. number of receptors present.
   c. sensitivity of the receptors.
   d. all of the above.

4. An agonist will
   a. not bind to a receptor.
   b. accelerate a normal body process.
   c. prevent other drugs from binding to a receptor.
   d. increase the number of stimulated receptors.

5. Blood concentrations are the result of ____ simultaneously occurring processes.
   a. two
   b. four
   c. three
   d. five

6. Blood concentration–time profiles can be used to predict the amount of drug at the site of action because
   a. blood is in rapid equilibrium with the site of administration and the site of action.
   b. blood is in rapid equilibrium with the site of action.
   c. blood is in rapid equilibrium with the receptor.
   d. blood can be repeatedly sampled.

7. In a blood concentration–time curve, the range between the minimum toxic concentration (MTC) and the minimum effective concentration (MEC) is called the
   a. onset of action.
   b. concentration at site of action.
   c. duration of action.
   d. therapeutic window.

8. If the blood concentration–time profile reflects the amount of drug at the site of action, the maximum therapeutic response would occur
   a. at the onset of action.
   b. at the MEC.
   c. at the peak blood concentration.
   d. when elimination is the predominant process.

9. Which drug would not typically be monitored with peak and trough blood concentrations?
   a. vancomycin
   b. valproic acid
   c. promethazine
   d. phenytoin

10. For elimination of a drug to be essentially complete, ____ times the half-life must elapse.
    a. two
    b. three
    c. five
    d. seven

11. Unionized drugs are
    a. actively transported.
    b. hydrophobic drugs.
    c. passively diffused through membranes.
    d. hydrophilic drugs.

12. The transfer of a drug out of a dosage form and into the blood is called
    a. absorption.
    b. dissolution.
    c. metabolism.
    d. elimination.

REVIEW

13. Which processes can influence the absorption of drugs given orally?
    a. first-pass metabolism
    b. intestinal transit time
    c. gastric emptying
    d. all of the above

14. Which formulation does not have an absorption step?
    a. rapidly administered intravenous solution
    b. intramuscular emulsion
    c. topical cream
    d. vaginal suppository

15. Why is a plasma protein bound drug essentially "inactive"?
    a. bound drug cannot enter the site of action
    b. bound drug can enter the site of metabolism
    c. bound drug can move through tissue membranes and cellular openings.
    d. bound drug can be displaced by a drug with a stronger binding capacity.

16. First-pass metabolism refers to the substantial degradation of the drug following
    a. passage through the small intestine.
    b. oral absorption.
    c. distribution to the liver.
    d. interaction with liver enzymes.

17. When some drugs are chronically administered, the liver will decrease its enzyme activity. This is called
    a. enzyme induction.
    b. enzyme inhibition.
    c. enzyme secretion.
    d. first pass metabolism.

18. Enterohepatic recycling occurs when
    a. a drug is metabolized to a metabolite.
    b. drug is secreted into the intestines along with the bile
    c. drug is secreted into the intestines along with the bile and reabsorbed back into the blood circulation.
    d. all of the above.

19. Elimination is
    a. absorption and metabolism.
    b. metabolism and excretion.
    c. distribution and excretion.
    d. distribution and metabolism.

20. Which set of circumstances will result in a drug undergoing urinary reabsorption?
    a. basic drug in high urine pH
    b. basic drug in low urine pH
    c. acidic drug in high urine pH
    d. none of the above

21. The amount of drug excreted in the urine is the amount
    a. filtered + secreted + reabsorbed.
    b. filtered + secreted - reabsorbed.
    c. filtered - secreted + reabsorbed.
    d. filtered - secreted - reabsorbed.

22. The amount of drug that is delivered to the site of action and the rate at which it becomes available is the drug's
    a. bioequivalence.
    b. bioavailability.
    c. biotransformation.
    d. biopharmaceutics.

23. To determine the bioavailability of a drug product, it must be compared to another product containing the same drug. If the second product is a rapidly administered intravenous solution, the bioavailability is termed ________ availability.
    a. relative
    b. bioequivalent
    c. redundant
    d. absolute

24. The _____ requires drug manufacturers to perform bioequivalency studies on their products before they are approved for marketing.
    a. DEA
    b. AMA
    c. FDA
    d. USP

CRITICAL THINKING QUESTIONS

1. Blood concentration–time data is used for many purposes, one of which is to monitor the blood levels of certain drugs such as vancomycin, phenytoin, digoxin, and valproic acid. Why is it necessary or desirable to measure the blood concentration–time data for these drugs?
2. An antagonist has been given for an extended period of time. When the patient quits taking the drug, they quit all at one time without tapering the dose down. Then an agonist was given that same day, and the patient had a very severe reaction. How would you explain this severe reaction?
3. The amount of drug excreted in the urine equals the amount filtered + the amount secreted – the amount reabsorbed. Explain how each process contributed to the overall amount of drug excreted.

THINKING IT THROUGH WRAP-UP

1. The major consideration would be the absorption step from the tablets. Once a drug gets into the general circulation, the distribution, metabolism, and elimination processes are the same regardless of which route of administration was used. But absorption may be greatly influenced by factors such as gastric emptying, first-pass metabolism, and disintegration and dissolution.
2. A study was done using levothyroxine solution administered by rapid intravenous administration, and the AUC of that blood concentration–time curve was compared to a similar curve obtained when levothyroxine was given in the tablet dosage form. The 50% means that one-half as much drug reached the systemic circulation after the oral tablet administration compared to the rapid intravenous administration.
3. Since the absolute bioavailability data shows that only one-half as much drug reached the systemic circulation using the tablets, then a 100 mcg tablet dose would give the same amount of drug in the systemic circulation as the 50 mcg of intravenous solution dose.

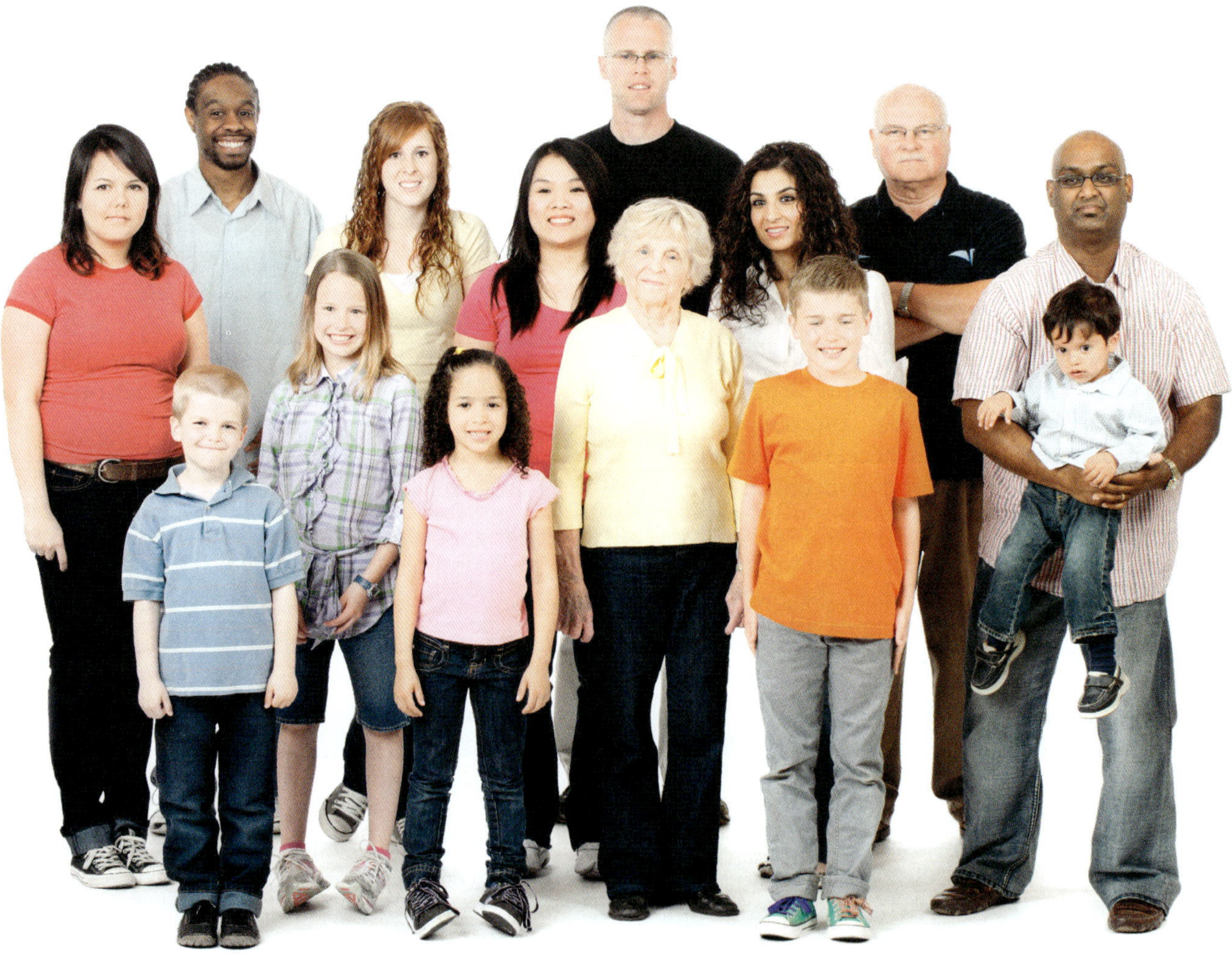

11

FACTORS AFFECTING DRUG ACTIVITY

LEARNING OBJECTIVES

At the completion of study, the student will:

- ✔ enumerate physiological factors that influence drug disposition and lead to variation in drug response.
- ✔ describe how common disease states can lead to altered drug response.
- ✔ understand common adverse drug reactions and that such reactions can occur in one patient but not another.
- ✔ describe the mechanisms of drug–drug interactions that affect the disposition of one or both drugs and result in either increases or decreases in therapeutic or side effects.
- ✔ explain the types of drug–drug interactions that do not alter the drugs' disposition but interact at the site of action.
- ✔ describe drug–diet interactions that alter drug disposition.

THINKING IT THROUGH

You decide to ask your family members how they react to a single 325 mg dose of aspirin when they get a headache. You know you don't have any problems taking aspirin, but it doesn't always get rid of your headache, and you end up taking some other drug like ibuprofen.

Your mom says aspirin gives her terrible nausea so she just doesn't take it. Your older uncle says he "almost died" when he took a dose of aspirin—he couldn't breathe and it felt like his chest was going to explode. Your dad says three aspirins seem to be the best dose for him, and that it works better with a cup of coffee. Your aunt is on warfarin therapy; her doctor told her to take only the 81 mg size of aspirin, but not for headaches—he said to take Tylenol® for headache.

As you read this chapter, identify which factors might be affecting each family member's experience with aspirin.

HUMAN VARIABILITY

Human variability can significantly alter blood concentration–time profiles and drug efficacy.

Differences in age, weight, genetics, and gender are among the variables that influence the differences in disposition and response to medications.

Age

Human life is a continuous process but it is usually characterized as having stages. The distinctions between the stages are open to individual interpretation, but they are often based on physiological characteristics. The stages are generally considered as:

- Neonate, up to one month after birth
- Infant, between the ages of one month and two years
- Child, between the ages of two and 12 years
- Adolescent, between the ages of 13 and 19 years
- Adult, between 20 and 70 years
- Elder, older than 70 years

Neonates and Infants

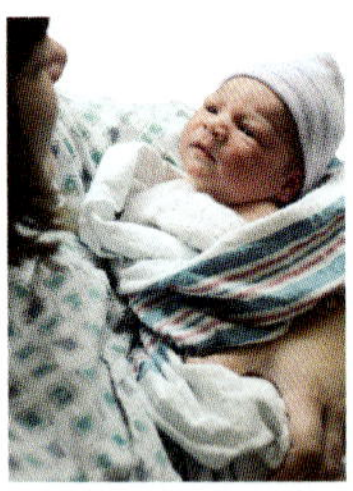

Drug distribution, metabolism, and excretion are quite different in the neonate and infant than in adults because their organ systems are not fully developed. They are not able to eliminate drugs as efficiently as adults. Older infants reach approximately adult levels of protein binding and kidney function, but liver function and the blood-brain barrier are still immature.

Children

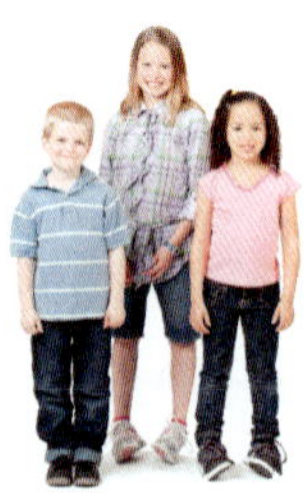

Children metabolize certain drugs more rapidly than adults. Their rate of metabolism increases between ages 1 and 12, depending on the child and the drug. Afterward, metabolism rates decline with age to normal adult levels. Some of the drugs eliminated faster in children include clindamycin, valproic acid, ethosuximide, and theophylline.

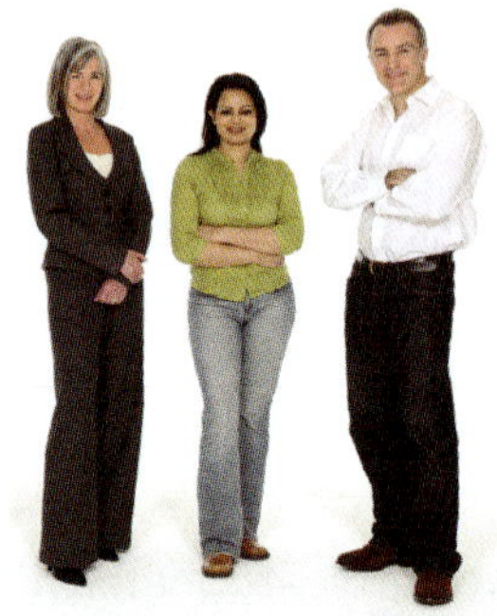

Adults

Adults experience a decrease in many physiological functions between ages 30 to 70, but such decreases and their effects on drug activity are gradual.

The Elderly

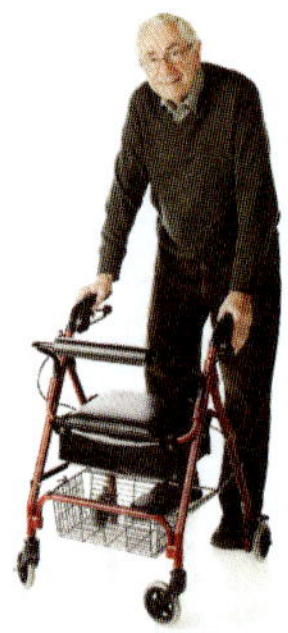

The elderly typically consume more drugs than any other age group. Because they have a greater incidence of chronic illnesses and multiple disease states, they take multiple medications, which leads to a higher incidence of drug interactions.

They also experience more physiological changes that significantly affect drug action:

- Changes in gastric pH, gastric emptying time, intestinal motility, and gastrointestinal blood flow all tend to slow the rate of absorption.
- Changes in the cardiovascular system (including lower cardiac output) tend to slow distribution of drug molecules to their sites of action, metabolism, and excretion.
- Though there is probably a decrease in the liver's production of metabolizing enzymes, the metabolism of most drugs does not appear to decrease.
- A decline in kidney function (including glomerular filtration and secretion) occurs, which in turn tends to slow urinary excretion of drugs.

pharmacogenomics a field of study that defines the hereditary basis of individual differences in absorption, distribution, metabolism, and excretion (the ADME processes).

Gender

For many years women were excluded from clinical drug investigations. One reason for this was to avoid exposing a fetus or potential fetus to unknown risks. This resulted in an inappropriate application of data collected from male subjects or patients to women. Now women are included in clinical drug investigations unless there is a clear and compelling reason not to do so.

Many studies have been completed in both genders that show differences in drug disposition, depending on the drug. For example, males and females have similar elimination for cimetidine and lorazepam, but women eliminate propranolol, isosorbide dinitrate, diazepam, and temazepam more slowly than men. Acetaminophen and clofibric acid are eliminated more rapidly in women than men.

Some gender-based differences in drug response appear to be related to hormonal fluctuations in women during their menstrual cycle. Women with clinical depression, for example, may need higher dosages of antidepressant medication when menstrual symptoms are worse.

Drug distribution may also be somewhat different between men and women simply as a result of differences in body composition (males have more muscle, women more fat).

Pregnancy

A number of physiological changes, including delayed gastric emptying and decreased gastrointestinal tract motility, occur in women in the later stages of pregnancy. These changes tend to reduce the rate of absorption.

Drug plasma protein binding may be reduced and metabolism increased in pregnant women for a number of drugs. The rate of urinary excretion for a number of drugs is much greater in pregnant women than in nonpregnant women.

Drugs can also readily transport from the maternal to the fetal circulation. Because the fetus has underdeveloped mechanisms to handle drug exposure, drug concentrations may be greater in the fetus than in the mother.

Genetics

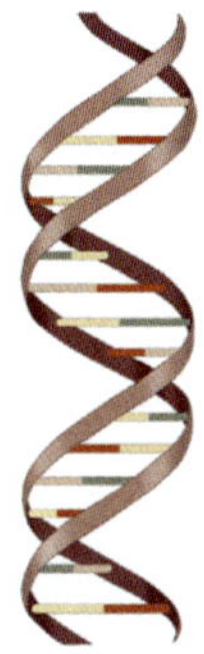

Genes determine the types and amounts of proteins produced in the body, with each person being somewhat different. Since drugs interact with proteins in plasma, tissues, receptor sites, and elsewhere, genetic differences can result in differences in drug action. It has been estimated that 20–50% of human variability is due to genetics alone.

Pharmacogenomics is a field of study that defines the hereditary basis of individual differences in absorption, distribution, metabolism, and excretion (the ADME processes). The largest contributing factor to inherited variability is metabolism. For example, people with certain genetic characteristics will not metabolize a drug that most people do, or will metabolize it at an abnormal rate. In such cases, the individual may experience no therapeutic effect at all, or perhaps even an adverse or toxic effect instead.

Body Weight

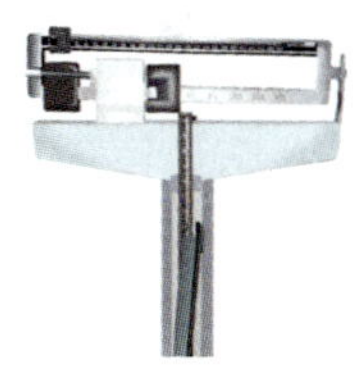

Dosage adjustments based on weight are generally not made for adults who are slightly overweight. However, weight is often considered in infants, children, or unusually small, emaciated, or obese patients. Adults who are obese (i.e., body fat content greater than 30% of total body weight) will have significant changes in the distribution and renal excretion of a number of drugs.

Psychological Factors

Though the specific reasons are unknown, it is clear that psychological factors can influence individual responses to drug administration. For example, in clinical trials in which placebos are used, patients receiving them often report both therapeutic and adverse effects. This may account for some variability in patient responses to an administered non-placebo drug. At a fundamental level, it is a factor in patient willingness to follow prescribed dosage regimens.

DISEASE STATES

Numerous studies have shown that the presence of disease can alter the disposition and effect of some drugs in some people. This is because disease can disrupt the normal functioning of organs involved in a drug's absorption, distribution, metabolism and/or excretion, which in turn alters the drug's effect. However, it is not always possible to predict the outcome.

HEPATIC

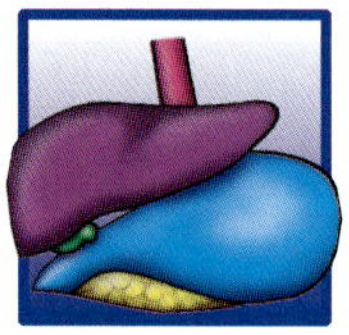

Patients with ***cirrhosis***, ***obstructive jaundice***, and ***acute viral hepatitis*** must be monitored when receiving certain drugs.

Cirrhosis is a chronic and potentially fatal liver disease that can lead to a loss of hepatic function. Obstructive jaundice occurs when the bile duct is blocked and hepatic waste products accumulate inside the liver. Both of these diseases appear to decrease hepatic metabolism and thereby diminish the first-pass metabolism of some drugs. When this happens, the bioavailability of the drug that would otherwise be degraded by the first-pass metabolism rises substantially.

Cirrhosis can also develop a condition in which a significant amount of blood coming from the intestine by-passes the liver and enters the circulation directly. When this happens, the bioavailability of some drugs also increases. Examples of drugs affected by this condition include verapamil, chlormethiazole, morphine, nifedipine, and midazolam.

The effects of acute viral hepatitis on liver function are less than those seen with cirrhosis. However, long term exposure to hepatitis can progress into a condition similar to cirrhosis.

Selected Drugs with Decreased Elimination in Cirrhosis and Obstructive Jaundice

- Caffeine
- Diazepam
- Encainide
- Erythromycin
- Lidocaine
- Meperidine
- Metronidazole
- Metoprolol
- Theophylline
- Verapamil

RENAL

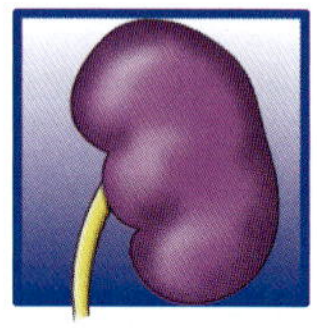

Reduced renal function, especially in end-stage renal disease, can affect the elimination and plasma protein binding of many drugs.

As renal function decreases, the dosage of a drug that is eliminated by the kidneys should be reduced to avoid accumulation of the drug in the body.

The plasma protein binding of acidic drugs is markedly reduced in severe renal insufficiency. Albumin is the major plasma and tissue protein that is responsible for acidic drug binding. Normally, the kidneys do not allow the elimination of albumin, but in chronic renal disease excessive protein filtration may occur which leads to a loss of albumin from the body.

Orosomucoid is a plasma protein that is rapidly produced when the body is injured. It also is a protein that many basic drugs bind to in the body. In chronic renal disease, orosomucoid blood concentrations are higher than normal and this results in increased basic drug binding.

Decreases in renal function can be measured by monitoring the amount of creatinine excreted in the urine. Creatinine is produced by muscles in the body and excreted at a constant rate primarily by glomerular filtration. In diseased kidneys, the rate of creatinine excretion decreases.

Selected Drugs with Decreased Elimination in Renal Disease

- Atenolol
- Digoxin
- Gentamicin
- Lithium
- Piperacillin
- Ranitidine
- Vancomycin

CIRCULATORY

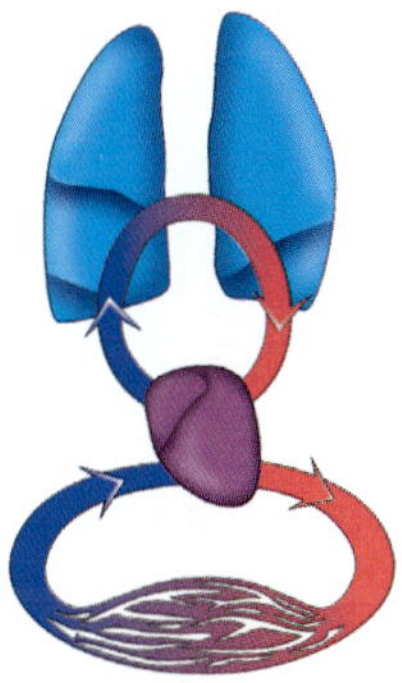

Circulatory disorders generally cause a diminished blood flow to one or more organs of the body. The decreased blood flow affects drug absorption, distribution, and elimination and therefore potentially also influences a drug's effect.

Effects on absorption include delayed gastric emptying, decreased intestinal motility, and/or changes in gastrointestinal pH. These changes lead to delayed or erratic drug absorption.

Decreased blood flow can also affect how drugs are metabolized by the liver. A diminished blood flow can affect the ability of certain drugs to move from the blood into hepatic cells that contain metabolizing enzymes. Decreased blood flow can also decrease the clearance of drugs that are eliminated in proportion to hepatic blood flow.

Changes in blood flow usually have less effect on the renal elimination of drugs since only 20% of the cardiac output flows to the kidney. However, there are high renal clearance drugs such as penicillin, lithium, and allopurinal that have decreased elimination when renal blood flow is markedly decreased.

THYROID

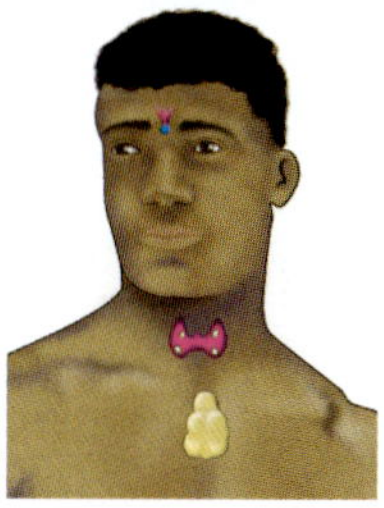

Changes in thyroid function can affect many of the aspects of absorption, excretion, and metabolism.

In ***hypothyroidism*** (a condition in which the thyroid is underactive), the bioavailability of a few drugs (e.g., riboflavin, digoxin) is increased. In ***hyperthyroidism*** (an overactive thyroid condition) their bioavailability is decreased because of changes in gastrointestinal motility.

Some other changes affected by thyroid conditions are:

- Renal blood flow is decreased in hypothyroidism and increased in hyperthyroidism.
- The activity of metabolizing enzymes in the liver is reduced in hypothyroidism and increased in hyperthyroidism.
- The metabolism of theophylline, propranolol, propylthiouracil, and methimazole is increased by hyperthyroidism.

acute viral hepatitis an inflammatory condition of the liver caused by viruses.

cirrhosis a chronic liver disease causing loss of function.

hyperthyroidism a condition in which thyroid hormone secretions are above normal, often referred to as an overactive thyroid.

hypothyroidism a condition in which thyroid hormone secretions are below normal, often referred to as an underactive thyroid.

obstructive jaundice an obstruction of the bile duct that causes hepatic waste products and bile to accumulate in the liver.

ADVERSE DRUG REACTIONS

Because of human variability, adverse drug reactions can occur in one person but not another.

An *adverse drug reaction* can be any undesired symptom and can involve any organ. It may be common or rare, localized or widespread, mild or severe, depending on the drug and the patient. Some adverse drug reactions occur with usual doses of drugs (often called side effects). Others are more likely to occur only at higher than normal dosages. Following are some common adverse drug reactions.

Central Nervous System Effects

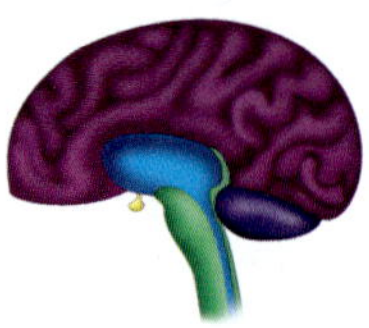

CNS effects may result from CNS stimulation (e.g., agitation, confusion, delirium, disorientation, hallucinations) or CNS depression (e.g., dizziness, drowsiness, sedation, coma, impaired respiration and circulation). Some examples are efavirenz, antimalarial drugs such as chloroquine and amodiaquine, and amantadine.

Hepatotoxicity

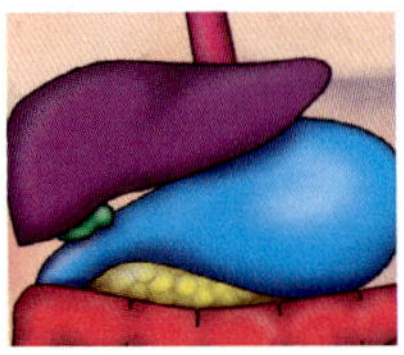

Hepatotoxicities (liver toxicities) include hepatitis, hepatic necrosis, and biliary tract inflammation or obstruction. These are relatively rare but potentially life threatening. Commonly used hepatotoxic drugs include acetaminophen, halothane, isoniazid, chlorpromazine, methotrexate, nitrofurantoin, phenytoin, and aspirin.

Nephrotoxicity

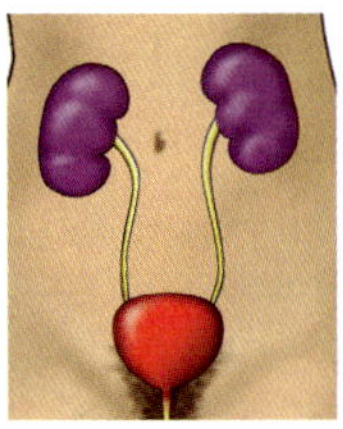

Renal toxicity can occur with gentamicin and other aminoglycosides, with ibuprofen and other nonsteroidal anti-inflammatory drugs, and with many other drugs such as celecoxib, omeprazole, and acyclovir.

Hematological Effects

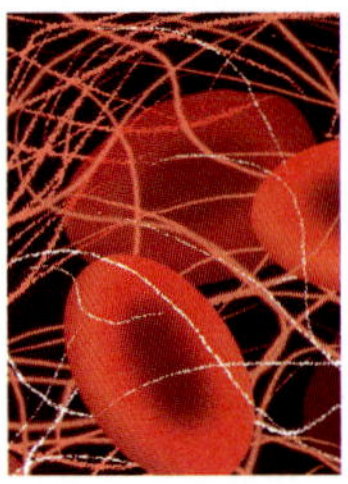

Blood coagulation, bleeding, and bone marrow disorders are potentially life threatening and can be caused by various drugs. Anticoagulants can cause excessive bleeding, so patients taking aspirin and warfarin must be carefully monitored. Vitamin K (phytonadione) can be given if bleeding becomes severe. Antineoplastic drugs such as busulfan, capecitabine, and chlorambucil may cause bone marrow depression.

Gastrointestinal Effects

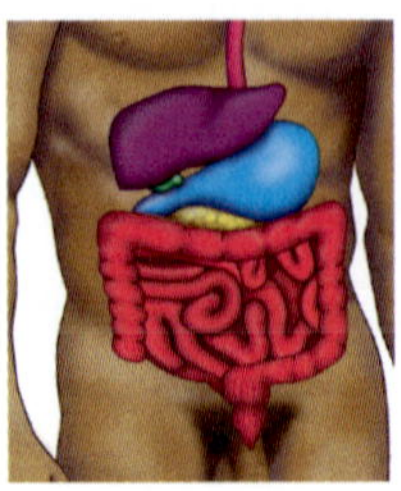

Anorexia, nausea, vomiting, constipation, pain, heartburn, and diarrhea are among the most common adverse reactions to drugs. More serious effects include ulcerations and colitis (e.g., irritable bowel disease).

Drug	Some Common Adverse Gastrointestinal Effects
aspirin, potassium chloride	➡ esophageal ulcer
NSAIDs, theophylline	➡ esophageal reflux
NSAIDs	➡ gastritis
aluminum containing antacids	➡ constipation
clindamycin, amoxicillin	➡ diarrhea

safety you should know

Pharmaceutical manufacturers are legally required to report any serious unlabeled (i.e., unexpected) adverse drug reactions through the FDA MedWatch Program. If the product presents a significant threat to consumer safety, that product can be recalled. A numerical classification (Class I, II, or III) indicates the potential hazard of the product. Adverse reactions to vaccines are reported through the Vaccine Adverse Event Reporting System (VAERS) maintained by the Centers for Disease Control (CDC).

Teratogenicity

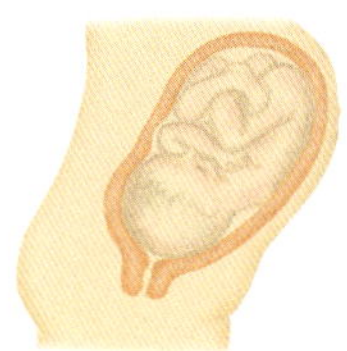

This is the ability of a substance to cause abnormal fetal development when given to pregnant women. Drug groups considered teratogenic include analgesics, diuretics, antihistamines, antibiotics, and antiemetics.

Carcinogenicity

Carcinogenicity is the ability of a substance to cause cancer. Several drugs are carcinogens, including some hormones and anticancer drugs. Some lifestyle choices such as using tobacco and alcohol have also been implicated in causing cancer.

Drug Dependence

Chronic usage of narcotic analgesics, sedative-hypnotic agents, antianxiety agents, and amphetamines can result in physiological or psychological dependence. Physiological dependence is accompanied by unpleasant physical symptoms when the drug is discontinued or the dose reduced. Psychological dependence involves an emotional or mental fixation on drug usage.

Idiosyncrasy

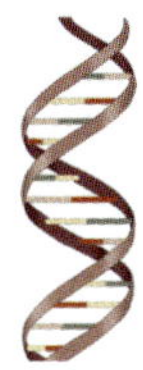

Idiosyncrasy is the unexpected reaction to a drug the first time it is given to a patient. Such reactions are thought to be caused by genetic characteristics that alter the patient's drug metabolizing enzymes.

Hypersensitivity or Allergy

Almost any drug, in almost any dose, can produce an allergic or ***hypersensitive*** reaction in a patient. This generally happens because a patient developed antibodies while previously taking the drug or a drug with a similar chemical structure. The drug will interact with the antibodies, releasing histamine and other substances that produce reactions that can range from mild rashes to potentially fatal ***anaphylactic shock***.

Allergic reactions can occur within minutes or weeks of drug administration. Anaphylactic shock occurs within minutes. It is a hypersensitivity reaction that can lead to cardiovascular collapse and death if untreated. Its symptoms include severe respiratory distress and convulsions. Immediate emergency treatment with epinephrine, antihistamines, or bronchodilator drugs is required.

adverse drug reaction an unintended side effect of a medication that is negative or in some way injurious to a patient's health.

anaphylactic shock a potentially fatal hypersensitivity reaction producing severe respiratory distress and cardiovascular collapse.

carcinogenicity the ability of a substance to cause cancer.

hypersensitivity an abnormal sensitivity generally resulting in an allergic reaction.

idiosyncrasy an unexpected reaction the first time a drug is taken, generally due to genetic causes.

DRUG–DRUG INTERACTIONS

A drug's effect can be altered by a drug–drug interaction.

The probability of a drug–drug interaction increases with the number of drugs a patient takes and in certain disease states. Many drug–drug interactions can affect how another drug is absorbed, distributed, metabolized, or excreted. Following are examples of some of the more common types of drug–drug interactions. It should be remembered that herbal supplements can also be involved in these types of interactions.

ABSORPTION

There are several means by which one drug may affect another's gastrointestinal absorption.

Complexation

Some drugs can form nonabsorbable complexes by binding to other drugs, resulting in decreased absorption. For example, iron salts bind to and decrease the absorption of several tetracyclines, methlydopa, and levodopa. Antacids and sucralfate bind to norfloxacin and ciprofloxacin, decreasing their absorption.

Gastric Emptying

Certain drugs will affect gastric emptying and therefore the absorption of other drugs. For example, propantheline will delay acetaminophen absorption by slowing the rate of gastric emptying. On the other hand, metoclopramide will increase acetaminophen absorption, since metoclopramide increases the rate of gastric emptying. Another problem with reducing gastric emptying time is that drugs that are degraded by gastric acid have a longer time to degrade, resulting in a decreased amount of drug available for absorption from the intestine.

Gastric pH

Drugs that alter gastrointestinal pH can have varied effects on the absorption of other drugs. Some factors affected by pH are the amount of unionized drug available for absorption, the rate of dissolution, intestinal motility, and degradation.

Intestinal Metabolism

Alterations in metabolism are involved in the interaction between oral contraceptives and oral antibiotic therapy. The antibiotic kills the normal bacterial flora in the GI tract, which disrupts the enterohepatic recycling of the oral contraceptive's estrogens.

DISTRIBUTION

Displacement

One drug can displace another from a plasma protein binding site and so increase the amount of the free drug available for distribution. This will increase its pharmacological effect. The displaced drug will also have faster elimination since more of the free drug is available for metabolism and excretion.

Such ***displacement*** interactions generally occur within the first week or two of administration. When they do occur, many turn out to be self-correcting after a few days, at which point the concentration of displaced drug often returns to pre-interaction levels, even if the patient continues to take both drugs.

The biggest consequence of displacement interactions is the change in pharmacological effect. If drugs are highly protein bound, displacement tends to have a greater effect than with drugs that are not highly bound. For example, warfarin is 98% plasma protein bound, with only 2% free or unbound. If a drug interaction displaces only 2% of the bound warfarin, then 96% will be bound, but 4% will now be free. That is a 100% increase in the free concentration of warfarin, and it might double its pharmacological effect. By comparison, for a drug that is only 60% bound, displacing 2% will cause only a 5% increase in the concentration.

complexation when two different molecules associate or attach to each other.

displacement a drug that is bound to a plasma protein is removed when another drug of greater binding potential binds to the same protein.

enzyme induction the increase in hepatic enzyme activity that results in greater metabolism of drugs.

enzyme inhibition the decrease in hepatic enzyme activity that results in reduced metabolism of drugs.

METABOLISM

Enzyme Induction

Some drugs are capable of increasing the concentration of metabolizing enzymes in the liver. This process is called ***enzyme induction***. It increases the metabolism of drugs that use the same enzyme system and usually results in a reduction in pharmacological effect. Examples of enzyme inducers include phenobarbital, carbamazepine, phenytoin, and rifampin. Cigarette smoking and chronic alcohol use may also induce metabolism.

The time course of drug interactions from enzyme induction is slower than for many other types of interactions. Though enzyme induction may be dose related, it can also be influenced by age, genetics, or liver disease. As a result, it is a difficult type of interaction to predict.

Enzyme Inhibition

Another alteration in metabolism is called ***enzyme inhibition***. This usually occurs when two drugs compete for binding sites on the same metabolizing enzyme. This generally increases the plasma concentration (and consequently the pharmacological effect) of at least one of the drugs. Enzyme inhibition is one of the most common drug interactions. In fact, if a drug is known to be metabolized by the liver, manufacturers often study its potential for enzyme inhibition early in the drug development process. Examples of enzyme inhibitors include allopurinol, cimetidine, erythromycin, disulfiram, isoniazid, ketoconazole, and verapamil.

Unlike enzyme induction, which has a much slower time course, enzyme inhibition has a rapid onset, generally within 24 hours, and tends to disappear quickly once the inhibitor is discontinued. Enzyme inhibition is also easier to predict since it appears to be dose related. It is also true that drugs that share a similar chemical structure often share the potential for enzyme inhibition.

EXCRETION

Glomerular Filtration

Drug interactions that actually change the filtration rate itself are rare. Changes in the filtration rate are more likely to occur in response to specific drugs, such as those that change the systemic blood pressure, for example. Whatever the cause, changes in the filtration rate will also change the rate of drug excretion.

Renal Secretion

There are different secretory systems in the kidneys for basic drugs and acidic drugs. Basic drugs do not seem to compete for the acidic drug transport system, or vice versa. However, two basic drugs or two acidic drugs may compete for the same transport system and this can cause one or both of the drugs to accumulate in the blood. For example, probenecid competes with penicillin and reduces penicillin's secretion. Probenecid also inhibits the secretion of cephalosporins. The interaction between NSAIDs and methotrexate is another example. Some of these interactions can increase methotrexate concentrations two- to threefold. An example of such a competition involving basic drugs is quinidine and digoxin. Quinidine reduces digoxin excretion by 30% to 50%.

Urinary Reabsorption

Urinary reabsorption, a passive transport process, is influenced by the pH of the urine and the extent of ionization of the drug. In acidic urine, acidic drugs tend to be reabsorbed while basic drugs are not. As a result, basic drugs are excreted in the urine. In alkaline urine, acidic drugs will not be reabsorbed but will instead be excreted in the urine, while basic drugs will be reabsorbed. An example of these interactions is quinidine, which is a base. The excretion of quinidine is reduced nearly 90% when the urine pH is increased from less than 6.0 to over 7.5.

DRUG–DRUG INTERACTIONS (cont'd)

Some drug–drug interactions do not alter the drugs' disposition but interact at the site of action.

Sometimes, interacting drugs directly compete for the same receptor. Other times, the interaction is more indirect and involves interfering with normal physiological processes. These interactions are commonly called "additive," "synergistic," or "potentiation." But most often it is difficult to quantify the extent of altered drug activity.

- ***Additive effects*** occur when two drugs with similar pharmacological actions result in an effect equal to the sum of the individual effects.

  Example: trimethoprim + sulfamethoxazole for antibiotic effect.

  Sulfamethoxazole and trimethoprim are commonly used in combination to treat *Pneumocystis carinii* pneumonia, an opportunistic infection in AIDS patients.

  Example: amiodarone + dofetilide for prolongation of heart's QT interval.

  Many drugs affect the electrical activity of the heart. Amiodarone and dofetlide prolong repolarization as part of their therapeutic effect. But phenothiazines (tranquilizers) and some antibiotics slow repolarization as an undesired effect. If these drugs are used together, repolarization may be delayed too long, and arrhythmias may occur.

- ***Synergism*** occurs when two drugs with similar pharmacological actions produce greater effects than the sum of individual effects.

  Example: aspirin + warfarin = increased anticoagulation.

  Aspirin increases the risk of bleeding in anticoagulated patients because it inhibits platelet function and causes gastric erosions. Large doses of aspirin (3 g/day or more) can increase the entire anticoagulation response. However, low doses of aspirin appear to primarily increase minor bleeding, and so the combination of aspirin and warfarin is used intentionally in many patients.

  Example: vancomycin + gentamicin = increased antibacterial effects of gentamicin.

  Enterococcus fecalis is a gram-negative microorganism that is not susceptible to gentamicin. But if another antibiotic (e.g., vancomycin) is given that inhibits the synthesis of the microorganism's cell walls, the effect of gentamicin is increased.

Time Course of Drug Interactions

The time it takes for drug–drug interactions to occur can vary substantially. Some interactions occur almost immediately while others may take weeks. Knowing the time course of an interaction allows quick identification and treatment of potential interactions. It also allows clinicians to evaluate the relative importance of an interaction from two drugs compared to their therapeutic effects. For example, if an interaction requires one to two weeks to occur, short-term administration over a few days will not cause a significant adverse effect.

additive effects the summation in effect when two drugs with similar pharmacological actions are taken.

antidote a drug that antagonizes the toxic effect of another.

potentiation when one drug with no inherent activity of its own increases the activity of another drug that produces an effect.

synergism when two drugs with similar pharmacological actions produce greater effects than the sum of individual effects.

- ***Potentiation*** occurs when one drug with no inherent activity of its own increases the activity of another drug that produces an effect.

  Example: amoxicillin + clavulanic acid = increased duration of amoxicillin's antibiotic effect.

  Clavulanic acid inhibits the enzyme that degrades amoxicillin, and thereby allows amoxicillin to be more potent than if used alone.

  Example: penicillin + probenecid = increased duration of penicillin's antibiotic effect.

  Probenecid competes with penicillin for the renal secretory site that is responsible for the rapid secretion of penicillin when used alone. With probenecid, penicillin is removed more slowly, and therefore has a longer effect.

- An ***antidote*** to a particular drug is given to block or reduce its toxic effects.

  Example: naloxone + morphine = relief of morphine induced respiratory depression.

  Naloxone displaces morphine from their receptor sites, preventing morphine from causing further depressive effects.

  Example: vitamin K + warfarin = opposition of the anticoagulant effect of warfarin and a return to normal blood clotting time.

  The anticoagulation effects of warfarin can be reduced or abolished by the concurrent use of vitamin K. Vitamin K can be given as a drug, but can also be consumed by the patient in some green vegetables such as spinach, brussel sprouts, or broccoli. Some liquid dietary supplements (e.g., Ensure-Plus, Nutrilite 330) contain vitamin K and can also cause the interaction.

  Example: Protamine sulfate is given as an antidote to heparin overdose. Protamine combines with heparin to form a stable complex, which leads to the decrease in the anticoagulant activity of both drugs.

  Example: Flumazenil is a benzodiazepine antagonist that reverses the sedative effects of diazepam, midazolam, and zolpidem. Flumazenil competes for the same receptors as the benzodiazepines and displaces them.

DRUG–DIET INTERACTIONS

Dietary intakes and patterns vary widely and can contribute to variability in the disposition and effects of drugs.

Drug–diet interactions may be attributed to various factors including food preferences and availability, weight loss or gain diets, and variations for seasonal, religious, and/or therapeutic reasons.

ABSORPTION

The physical presence of food in the gastrointestinal tract can alter absorption in several ways. It can:

- interact chemically (e.g., tetracycline and iron);
- improve the solubility of some drugs by increasing bile secretion;
- affect the performance of the dosage form (e.g., altering the release characteristics of polymer coated tablets);
- alter gastric emptying;
- alter intestinal motility;
- alter liver blood flow.

As a result, some drugs have increased bioavailability and some have decreased bioavailability in the presence of food. For example, the bioavailability of propranolol, metoprolol, hydralazine, cefuroxime, erythromycin, and phenytoin is enhanced by the presence of food. It appears that food enhances the dissolution of these drugs.

The bioavailability of a drug is generally decreased when the presence of food slows absorption. For example, when tablets or capsules are taken with food, they dissolve more slowly, and have decreased absorption as a result. The absorption of alendronate is decreased 60% with coffee or juice; there is no absorption at all when taken with within two hours of a meal.

Food may also combine with a drug to form an insoluble drug–food complex. This is how tetracycline interacts with dairy products, such as milk and cheese. It combines with the calcium in milk products to form an insoluble, nonabsorbable compound that is excreted in the feces. The same interaction occurs with ciprofloxacin and dairy products. In general, dietary fiber decreases the absorption of drugs.

DISTRIBUTION

The presence of food can also influence drug distribution. For example, high fat meals can increase fatty acid levels in the blood that bind to the same plasma protein binding sites as many drugs. This displaces the bound drug and increases the free concentration of that drug, leading to an increased effect.

There are also differences in the plasma protein binding of certain drugs between well-nourished and undernourished people. Undernourished people with low albumin levels have fewer binding sites available for highly bound drugs such as phenytoin (90% bound) and warfarin (96% bound); these drugs would potentially have a greater effect in this population.

ADMINISTRATION TIMES

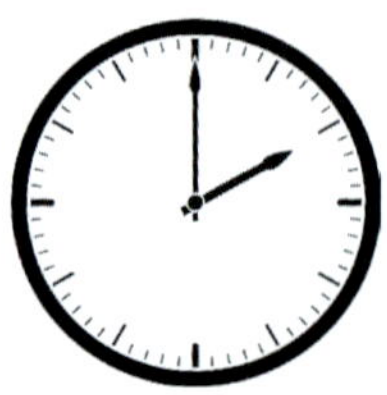

Interactions that alter drug absorption can be minimized by separating the administration of drugs and food intake by about 2 hours.

drug–diet interactions when elements of ingested nutrients interact with a drug and this affects the disposition of the drug.

METABOLISM

Most foods are complex mixtures of carbohydrate, fat, and protein. Research studies designed to determine the influence of diet on drug metabolism use diets in which one of these nutrients is increased, another decreased, and the third nutrient and total caloric intake are kept constant. In general, high protein (low carbohydrate) diets are associated with accelerated metabolism while high carbohydrate (low protein) diets appear to decrease metabolism. The substitution of fat calories for carbohydrate seems not to affect drug metabolism rates.

In general, mildly or moderately undernourished adults have normal or enhanced metabolism of drugs while severely malnourished adults have decreased drug metabolism. However, there are many variables in malnourishment that can produce an effect on metabolism.

EXCRETION

Increasing protein in the diet appears to increase glomerular filtration, decrease reabsorption, and decrease secretion in the kidneys. The total effect of restricted protein intake will depend on the urinary excretion characteristics of the specific drug.

High sodium diets tend to increase the excretion of sodium and they also increase the excretion of lithium because it shares the same reabsorption site in the nephron as sodium.

Effects of Dietary Factors on Metabolism

Change in Food Composition	Effect on Metabolism
increased protein	increased metabolism
increased carbohydrate	decreased metabolism
increased fat	no effect
decreased calories	decreased metabolism

SPECIFIC FOODS

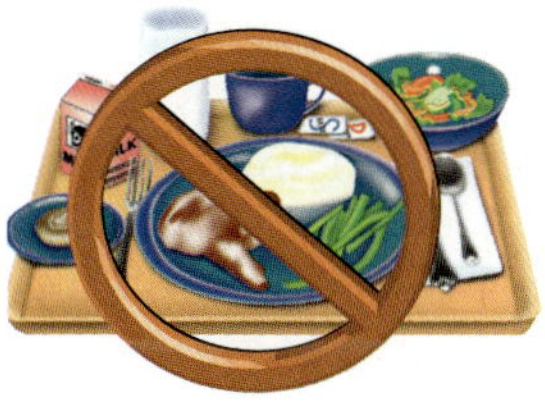

Some foods contain substances that react with certain drugs. For example, eating foods containing tyramine while using monoamine oxidase (MAO) inhibitors may produce severe hypertension or intracranial hemorrhage. MAO inhibitors include isocarboxazid, phenelzine, and procarbazine. Foods containing tyramine include beer, red wine, aged cheeses, yeast products, chicken livers, and pickled herring.

Certain cruciferous vegetables (e.g., brussels sprouts, cabbage) stimulate the metabolism of a few drugs. Other foods that might also have a similar effect are alfalfa, turnips, broccoli, cauliflower, or spinach. Some of the same foods are also involved with an interaction with oral anticoagulants such as warfarin. Spinach and other greens contain vitamin K, and vitamin K inhibits the action of oral anticoagulants. A patient ingesting foods containing vitamin K while taking an anticoagulant would not receive the full therapeutic effect from warfarin.

REVIEW

KEY CONCEPTS

HUMAN VARIABILITY

- ✔ Differences in age, weight, genetics, and gender are among the significant factors that influence the differences in medication responses among people.
- ✔ Drug distribution, metabolism, and excretion are quite different in the neonate and infant than in adults because their organ systems are not fully developed.
- ✔ Children metabolize certain drugs more rapidly than adults.
- ✔ The elderly typically consume more drugs and have a higher incidence of drug interactions than other age groups. They also experience more physiological changes that significantly affect drug action.
- ✔ Genetics can cause differences in the types and amounts of proteins produced in the body, which can result in different responses to the same drug at the same dose.

DISEASE STATES

- ✔ The disposition and effect of some drugs may be altered in one patient but not another by the presence of diseases. Such changes are well-documented in cardiovascular, hepatic, renal, and thyroid diseases.

ADVERSE DRUG REACTIONS

- ✔ Almost any drug, in almost any dose, can produce an allergic or hypersensitive reaction in a patient. Anaphylactic shock is a potentially fatal hypersensitivity reaction.
- ✔ Anorexia, nausea, vomiting, constipation, and diarrhea are among the most common adverse reactions to drugs in the GI tract.

DRUG–DRUG INTERACTIONS

- ✔ Many drug–drug interactions affect the disposition of one drug and result in either an increased or decreased effect.
- ✔ Decreased intestinal absorption of oral drugs occurs when drugs complex to produce nonabsorbable compounds.
- ✔ Displacement of one drug from protein binding sites by a second drug increases the effects of the displaced drug.
- ✔ Drugs that induce liver metabolism may also increase metabolism of other drugs that use the same metabolizing enzymes.
- ✔ Some drugs increase excretion by altering urinary pH and lessening renal reabsorption.
- ✔ Some drug–drug interactions do not alter a drug's disposition but interact at the site of action.
- ✔ Additive effects occur when two drugs with similar pharmacological actions result in an effect equal to the sum of the individual effects.
- ✔ Synergism occurs when two drugs with similar pharmacological actions produce greater effects than the sum of the individual effects.
- ✔ Potentiation occurs when one drug with no inherent activity of its own increases the activity of another drug that produces an effect.

DRUG–DIET INTERACTIONS

- ✔ Dietary intake can influence drug action by altering one or all of the ADME processes.
- ✔ Some foods contain substances that react with certain drugs, e.g., foods containing tyramine can react with monoamine oxidase (MAO) inhibitors.

SELF TEST

the answer key begins on page 569

MATCH THE TERMS

1. acute viral hepatitis ____
2. additive effects ____
3. adverse drug reaction ____
4. anaphylactic shock ____
5. antidote ____
6. carcinogenicity ____
7. cirrhosis ____
8. complexation ____
9. displacement ____
10. drug–diet interactions ____
11. enzyme induction ____
12. enzyme inhibition ____
13. hypersensitivity ____
14. hyperthyroidism ____
15. hypothyroidism ____
16. idiosyncrasy ____
17. obstructive jaundice ____
18. pharmacogenomics ____
19. potentiation ____
20. synergism ____

a. when two different molecules associate or attach to each other.
b. an abnormal sensitivity resulting in an allergic reaction.
c. a potentially fatal hypersensitivity reaction producing severe respiratory distress and cardiovascular collapse.
d. an unexpected reaction the first time a drug is taken, generally due to genetic causes.
e. the ability of a substance to cause cancer.
f. when two drugs with similar pharmacological actions produce an effect equal to the sum of their individual effects.
g. when two drugs with similar pharmacological actions produce an effect greater than the sum of their individual effects.
h. a drug that antagonizes the toxic effect of another drug.
i. a chronic and potentially fatal liver disease causing loss of function and increased resistance to blood flow through the liver.
j. an inflammatory liver condition caused by viruses.
k. when elements of ingested nutrients interact with a drug and this affects the disposition of the drug.
l. an obstruction of the bile duct that causes hepatic waste products and bile to accumulate in the liver.
m. a condition in which thyroid hormone secretions are above normal; having an overactive thyroid.
n. a condition in which thyroid secretions are below normal, often referred to as an underactive thyroid.
o. a field of study that defines the hereditary basis of individual differences in the ADME processes.
p. an unintended side effect of a medication that is negative or in some way injurious to the patient's health.
q. an effect produced when one drug with no inherent activity of its own increases the activity of another drug.
r. a drug bound to a plasma protein is removed when another drug of greater binding potential binds to the same protein.
s. the decrease in hepatic enzyme activity that results in reduced metabolism of drugs.
t. the increase in hepatic enzyme activity that results in greater metabolism of drugs.

REVIEW

CHOOSE THE BEST ANSWER

1. What criteria is commonly used to define the elderly?
   a. age greater than 55
   b. age greater than 65
   c. age greater than 70
   d. age greater than 80

2. Children between the ages of _______ metabolize certain drugs more rapidly than adults.
   a. 0 and 6 months
   b. 6 and 18 months
   c. 1 and 2 years
   d. 1 and 12 years

3. Some drugs given to children require a higher than normal adult dose. Why?
   a. Children have a more rapid renal excretion than adults.
   b. Children metabolize some drugs faster than adults.
   c. Children have a more immature renal function than adults.
   d. Children have a higher cardiac output than adults.

4. The distribution of drugs may be different between men and women due to
   a. normal fluctuations.
   b. age.
   c. body composition.
   d. activity.

5. The placebo effect is a
   a. psychological variable.
   b. gender variable.
   c. hypersensitive reaction.
   d. drug dependence variable.

6. Adults have a gradual decline in many physiological functions between the ages of
   a. 12–20 years.
   b. 20–40 years.
   c. 30–70 years.
   d. 40–75 years.

7. Adults that have greater than _____ body fat have significant changes in drug distribution and renal excretion.
   a. 10%
   b. 20%
   c. 30%
   d. 40%

8. Decreased blood circulation can affect drug metabolism by
   a. shunting blood away from functioning hepatic cells.
   b. changing the rate at which drugs move from the blood into hepatic cells.
   c. reducing drug clearance.
   d. all of the above

9. In end-stage renal disease, _________ levels increase and _________ levels decrease.
   a. albumin, orosomucoid
   b. orosomucoid, albumin
   c. anastomoses, orosomucoid
   d. albumin, thyroid

10. Which endogenous compound is used to monitor renal function?
    a. cortisol
    b. creatinine
    c. cholesterol
    d. calcium

11. When hepatic function is decreased by a hepatic disease, it is expected that
    a. first-pass metabolism will increase.
    b. urinary excretion will decrease.
    c. first-pass metabolism will decrease.
    d. hepatic blood flow will increase.

12. Acute viral hepatitis is an inflammatory condition caused by
    a. chronic alcohol abuse.
    b. obstructive jaundice.
    c. decreased hepatic blood flow.
    d. viruses.

13. Which set of conditions is required for an adverse drug reaction to occur?
    a. normal drug dosage, affects only the organ being treated, occurs in most patients taking the drug
    b. normal drug dosage, affects all of the organs, occurs in most patients taking the drug
    c. elevated drug dosage, affects only the organ being treated, occurs in a few patients
    d. none of the above

14. Hypersensitivity generally happens because a patient develops
    a. anaphylaxis.
    b. anorexia.
    c. antibodies.
    d. hepatotoxicity.

15. The ability of a substance to cause abnormal fetal development when given to pregnant women is called
    a. hematological effects.
    b. idiosyncrasy.
    c. nephrotoxicity.
    d. teratogenicity.

16. Anaphylactic shock usually occurs within
    a. minutes.
    b. hours.
    c. days.
    d. weeks.

17. Ciprofloxacin bioavailability can be reduced when given with calcium, magnesium, and aluminum ion containing drugs. What type of drug–drug interaction is this?
    a. additive
    b. potentiation
    c. induction
    d. complexation

18. Induction and inhibition involve enzymes in the ______ system.
    a. gastric
    b. circulatory
    c. hepatic
    d. renal

19. If a drug is _____ plasma protein bound, a displacement interaction will probably be significant.
    a. 10%
    b. 30%
    c. 60%
    d. 90%

20. The renal excretion of a drug is a combination of
    a. glomerular filtration plus renal secretion.
    b. glomerular filtration plus urinary reabsorption minus renal secretion.
    c. glomerular filtration plus renal secretion minus urinary reabsorption.
    d. glomerular filtration plus renal secretion plus urinary reabsorption.

REVIEW

21. In acidic urine, acidic drugs are reabsorbed and basic drugs are not. This occurs because
    a. acidic drugs are more unionized in acidic urine.
    b. acidic drugs are more ionized in acidic urine.
    c. basic drugs are more unionized in acidic urine.
    d. basic drugs are more ionized in basic urine.

22. When two drugs with similar pharmacological actions produce an effect equal to the sum of the individual effects, the interaction is called
    a. an additive effect.
    b. a complexation effect.
    c. an induction effect.
    d. a displacement effect.

23. A/an ______________ is a drug that antagonizes the toxic effects of another drug.
    a. agonist
    b. synergist
    c. antidote
    d. inducer

24. Which effect will the presence of food in the gastrointestinal tract have on drug absorption?
    a. react chemically with the drug and decrease absorption
    b. alter the solubility of a drug by increasing bile secretion
    c. alter the gastric emptying time
    d. all of the above

25. Drug–diet interactions that alter drug absorption can be minimized by separating the administration of the drug and food intake by
    a. 15 minutes.
    b. 30 minutes.
    c. 2 hours.
    d. 4 hours.

26. A high carbohydrate (low protein) diet would be expected to ______________ the metabolism of many drugs.
    a. decrease
    b. have no effect
    c. increase

27. What do these foods have in common: beer, red wine, yeast products, chicken livers, and aged cheeses?
    a. They inhibit hepatic metabolism.
    b. They contain tyramine.
    c. They contain monoamine oxidase inhibitors.
    d. They contain an inherent anticoagulant activity.

CRITICAL THINKING QUESTIONS

1. Why is it important to know something about the physical characteristics of a patient?
2. How can you easily distinguish between an adverse drug reaction and a drug–drug interaction?
3. Not all drug–drug interactions occur immediately. Some require days or weeks to develop. Why?

THINKING IT THROUGH WRAP-UP

Your mom says she doesn't take aspirin because of the nausea. Nausea when taking aspirin is a very common adverse effect. For almost all drugs that cause gastrointestinal adverse effects, nausea, vomiting, and diarrhea are the three most common reactions.

Since your uncle said he "almost died," either literally or figuratively, he might have been describing an anaphylactic reaction to the aspirin. If you wanted to confirm your suspicion, you could ask him how quickly the reaction came on and how long it lasted.

Your dad says coffee makes the aspirin work better. The most likely explanation is that the caffeine is adding to the pain relieving effect of aspirin through a potentiation drug–drug interaction. But the caffeine may also provide either an additive or synergistic effect. Coffee has been shown to decrease the absorption of alendronate, so a complexation interaction may also be occurring, which would explain why your dad takes three aspirins, instead of the normal two tablet dose.

Your aunt's doctor is advising her to take only small doses of aspirin because it has a synergistic effect with warfarin's effect of thinning blood. Tylenol® does not contain aspirin and so does not have that effect.

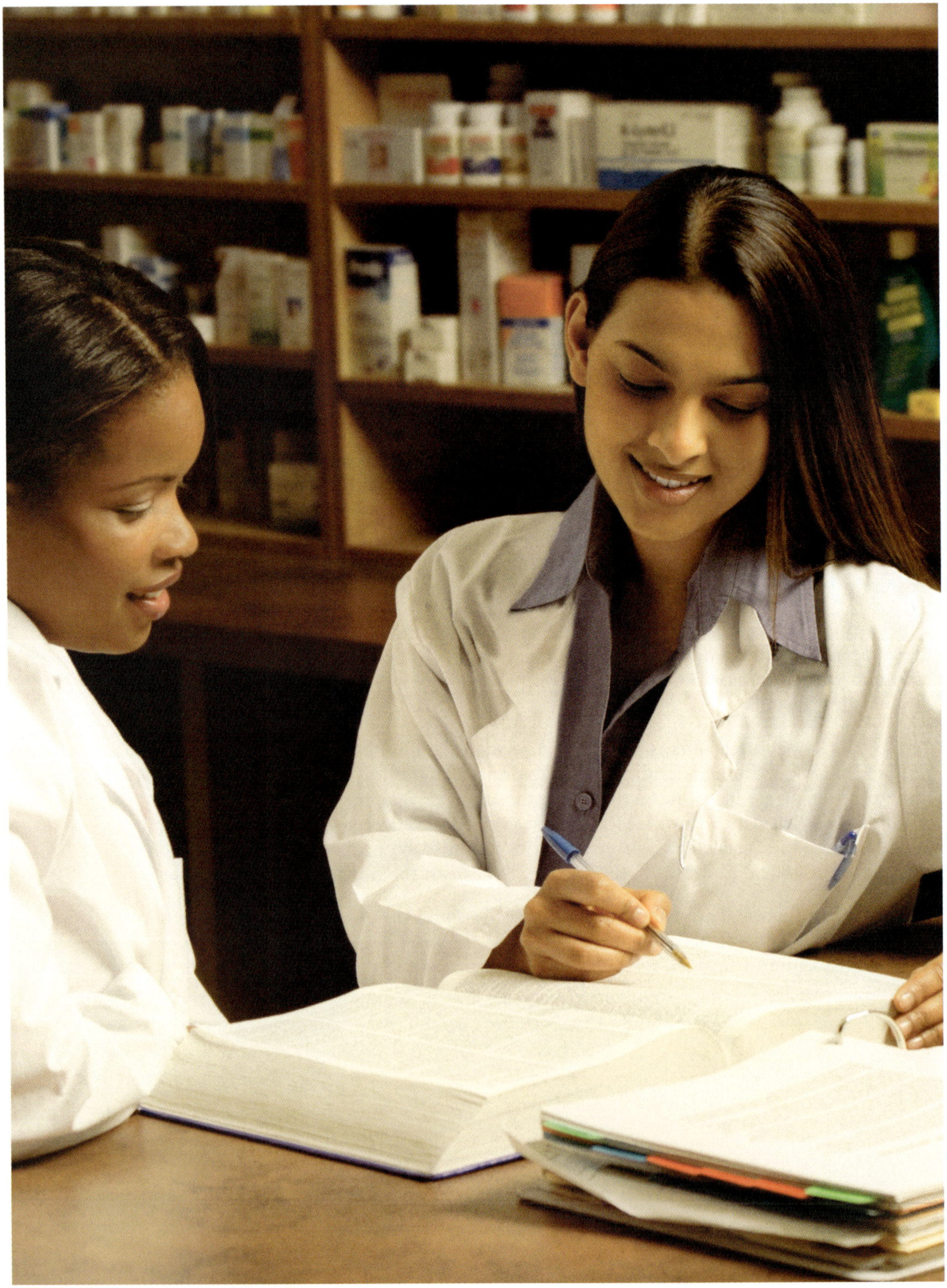

Photo courtesy Hanson Ng/Design Pics/Getty Images

12

INFORMATION

LEARNING OBJECTIVES

At the completion of study, the student will:

- ✔ understand the three types of pharmacy literature.
- ✔ become familiar with pharmacy references and understand how to use them.
- ✔ know key pharmacy websites.
- ✔ be familiar with references on the pharmacy technician profession.

THINKING IT THROUGH

You are a pharmacy technician working the evening shift in a hospital pharmacy that also fills a limited number of outpatient prescriptions. As you read this chapter, consider what you would do in the following situations:

1. A nurse calls the pharmacy stating a stock bottle of Lugol's® solution fell off a shelf and broke.
2. An elderly patient comes to the pharmacy with a baggie containing different tablets and wonders if you could identify them.
3. The ER calls and asks if they can run Cephazolin® and Heparin® together through the same IV line.

INFORMATION

The tremendous amount of drug research done each year results in the appearance of many new drugs on pharmacy shelves.

As a pharmacy technician, you may find it difficult to absorb and keep up with pharmaceutical information. Becoming familiar with the various pharmaceutical information sources will allow you to keep current with the information necessary to perform your job on an ongoing basis.

Pharmacy literature can be thought of as a pyramid divided into three sections.

Primary literature sits at the base. It is original research rather than a synthesis of information from other sources. It provides the foundation for the development of *secondary* and *tertiary literature*, which are syntheses and interpretations of primary literature.

Of the three types of reference materials, pharmacists and technicians usually find the tertiary sources the easiest and most convenient to use.

However, no single tertiary reference source contains all the information that will be needed by the pharmacy department. Also, view tertiary references carefully, since authors may misinterpret or misquote the original literature. Finally, keep in mind that tertiary references are usually published one or more years after the original literature and therefore may no longer be current.

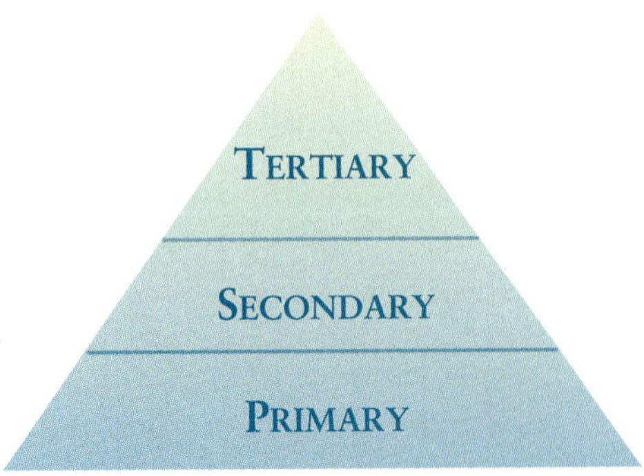

primary literature original reports of clinical trials, research, and case studies; use for the most up-to-date information.

secondary literature general reference works based upon primary literature sources; use to find primary literature.

tertiary literature condensed works based on primary literature (e.g., textbooks); use to find background information or a summary of information.

PHARMACY LITERATURE

Primary Literature

Primary literature provides direct access to the largest amount of and most current information from contemporary research. It includes original reports of scientific, clinical, technological, and administrative research and is found in professional and scientific journals such as the *journal of Pharmacy Technology* (www.jpharmtechnol.com). Specific information in primary literature can be found with database searches on PubMed (www.ncbi.nlm.nin.gov/pubmed), a service of the U.S. National Library of Medicine, using topics, authors, or journals. The need for large storage spaces and the varying quality of journal articles constitute the greatest disadvantages of this type of literature.

Secondary Literature

Secondary literature references are used to identify and locate primary literature and consist of indexing or ***abstracting services***.

Abstracting services (e.g., *PubMed*) summarize information contained in some professional and scientific journals. Indexing services (e.g., *Medline*) provide more comprehensive listings of current articles in worldwide professional and scientific journals. You can usually find these indexing services online. There is a lag time in-between the publication of primary sources and their reference in secondary sources.

Tertiary Literature

Tertiary literature sources contain condensed and compact information based on established knowledge in primary literature. This type of literature includes textbooks, monographs, standard reference books, and review articles.

abstracting services services that summarize information from various primary sources for quick reference.

Health Insurance Portability and Accountability Act (HIPAA) a federal law created to protect the privacy of patient health records.

LEGAL ASPECTS

Federal

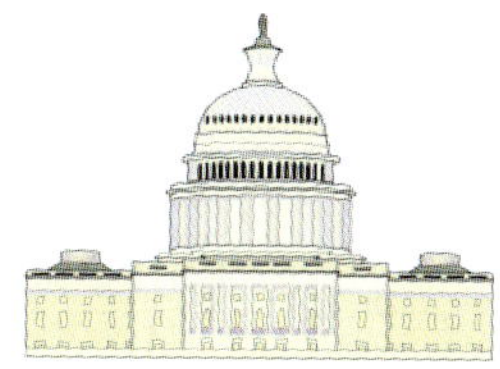

At present, no federal law mandates that pharmacies maintain professional drug information literature. The Occupational Safety and Health Administration (OSHA) does however require pharmacies to have a Material Safety Data Sheet (MSDS) for each hazardous chemical they stock. A pharmacy can obtain MSDSs from the manufacturers or the local OSHA area office. A MSDS provides information you need to ensure the implementation of proper protective measures for exposure to hazardous chemicals. The National Institute for Occupational Safety and Health (NIOSH) develops recommendations for occupational safety and health standards (www.cdc.gov/niosh).

For drugs manufactured and marketed in the United States, the U.S. Food, Drug and Cosmetic Act recognizes the USP-NF general chapters <1> to <999> as enforceable by the Food and Drug Administration. The USP-NF is available in print, on CD, and online at www.usp.org.

The Health Insurance Portability and Accountability Act (HIPAA) of 1996 affects many of the daily activities that take place in the pharmacy. The act's privacy regulation, *HIPAA Privacy Standards: A Compliance Manual for Pharmacies,* was created to protect the privacy of patient health records and requires pharmacies to set boundaries on the use and disclosure of patients' protected health information (PHI).

State

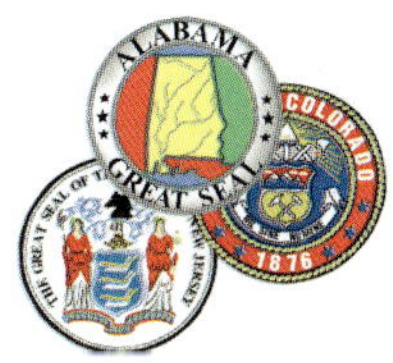

Most states have Pharmacy Statutes and State Board of Pharmacy Rules and Regulations that require pharmacies to maintain specific professional literature references. Pharmacy technicians should know which are mandated by their state regulatory agencies. Examples might include the current edition of *21 Code of Federal Regulations (CFR) Part 1300 to End* contained in the *DEA Pharmacist Manual* (www.deadiversion.usdoj.gov/pubs/manuals/pharm2/index.html) or a state's *Uniform Controlled Substances Act.*

Legal References

An awareness of the legal aspects of pharmacy protects both the pharmacy technician and the patients. The pharmacy law references described below provide information about laws concerning controlled substances, drug control, and other laws critical to the practice of pharmacy.

- *Pharmacy Law Desk Reference* provides information about legal aspects of pharmaceutical practice such as professional liability insurance, support personnel, law and ethics, HIPAA, compounding, and medication error reporting.
- *Legal Handbook for Pharmacy Technicians* by Dione Davey, PharmD, JD, teaches technicians the essentials on how pharmacy is regulated.

COMMON REFERENCES

The tertiary literature sources described below are the most commonly available references in pharmacies and drug information centers in the United States.

Some of these references focus on specific areas, while others seek to be very comprehensive. As such, there is overlap in the kinds of information these references provide. You may be able to find what you are looking for in more than one source. At the same time, it is helpful to know if one reference will be particularly useful for certain kinds of information, which we have noted in *blue-green italics* in the following descriptions.

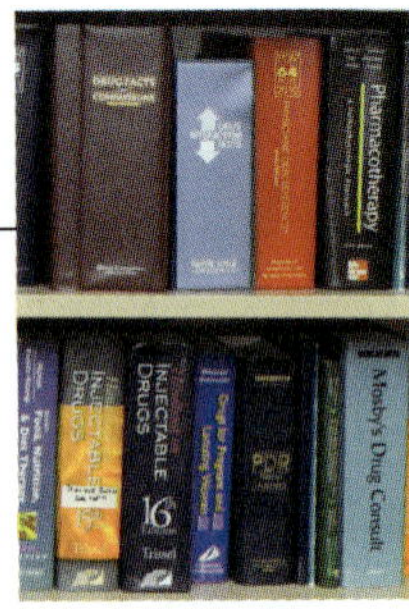

***AHFS Drug Information* (www.ahfsdruginformation.com)**

The *American Hospital Formulary Service (AHFS)* is accepted as the source of comparative, unbiased, and evidence-based drug information. It groups drugs by therapeutic use and is updated electronically and in an annual print update. *Use AHFS when investigating* ***off-label medication indications*** (i.e., an indication not approved by the FDA). *PDA* and *Desktop* formats are available.

Martindale, *The Complete Drug Reference*

Formerly known as Martindale, *The Extra Pharmacopoeia,* this reference contains international drug monographs with drug names, manufacturers, country of origin, active constituents, and licensed indications. *Use Martindale to research foreign drugs.*

***The Merck Index* (www.merckmanuals.com)**

Provides information on chemicals, drugs, and biologicals via monographs, supplemental tables, and organic name reactions. It includes chemical, common, and generic names; chemical structures; molecular formula; physical and toxicity data; therapeutic and commercial uses; and caution and hazard information. *Use* The Merck Index *when information on chemical attributes of drugs is needed.* The printed edition includes a companion CD and a free one-year subscription to *The Merck Index Internet Edition*.

***Physicians' Desk Reference* (PDR) (www.pdr.net)**

The PDR provides FDA regulation information on prescription drugs. *The information is similar to pharmaceutical manufacturers' drug package inserts since manufacturers prepare the essential drug information found in the PDR.* It contains drug usage information and warnings, drug interactions, and full-size color photos of drugs. PDR.net® is the online version of the PDR® and the mobile PDR® provides complete access to the PDR® from any mobile device.

***Drug Facts and Comparisons* (DFC) (www.factsandcomparisons.com/)**

The DFC, a preferred reference for comprehensive and timely drug information, contains information about prescription and OTC products presented in easy-to-use comparative tables of therapeutic groups. *It is used to compare medications in the same therapeutic class.* A loose-leaf edition provides the most up-to-date drug reference through monthly updates. The drug information is also available online and on monthly and annual CDs.

off-label indication a use of a medication for an indication not approved by the FDA.

"Orange Book" the common name for the FDA's *Approved Drug Products with Therapeutic Equivalence.*

American Drug Index

This bound index published by Facts and Comparisons provides quick access to a comprehensive list of drugs and drug products. Drug names are cross-referenced with monographs that provide generic pronunciations, manufacturer, strength, composition, package size, dosage forms, uses, and common abbreviations. *Use this reference to find trade and generic names.*

***Handbook on Injectable Drugs* (www.ashp.org/)**

This is a collection of monographs on commercially available parenteral drugs. *It includes information on preparation, storage, administration, compatibility, and stability of injectable drugs.* It is available through ASHP's online marketplace (www.ahfsdruginformation.com/products_services/hid.aspx).

***King's Guide to Parenteral Admixtures* (www.kingguide.com)**

This reference provides information on injectable drug compatibility and stability, updated quarterly. It is available in print, online, and in PDA and wall chart formats.

***Red Book: Pharmacy's Fundamental Reference* (www.redbook.com)**

The *Red Book* is the guide to accurate product information and prices on prescription drugs, OTCs, nutraceuticals, and bulk chemicals. *It provides the latest pricing information, including nationally recognized AWP's and suggested retail prices for OTC products.* The *Red Book* is utilized for: drug utilization review, market analysis and research, prescription pricing and order entry, establishing and validating reimbursement, claims adjustment, forecasting, drug-pricing research, generic substitutions, therapeutic interchange, purchasing, formulary development, and as a source for AWP and WAC. *Red Book* online is now available.

"Orange Book" (www.accessdata.fda.gov/scripts/cder/ob/default.cfm)

"Orange Book" is the common name for the FDA's *Approved Drug Products with Therapeutic Equivalence Evaluations. Use the Orange Book to determine the therapeutic equivalence of a brand and generic drug.* Drugs with Code A are considered equivalent while drugs with Code B are documented as nonequivalent.

***OSHA Technical Manual* (OTM) Section VI: Chapter 2, Controlling Occupational Exposure to Hazardous Drugs (www.osha.gov/dts/osta/otm/otm_vi/otm_vi_2.html)**

***ASHP Technical Assistance Bulletin on Handling Cytotoxic and Hazardous Drugs* (www.baxa.com/resources/docs/technicalpapers/ASHPTechbulltn.pdf)**

These references are needed if a pharmacy compounds cytotoxic products.

OTHER REFERENCES

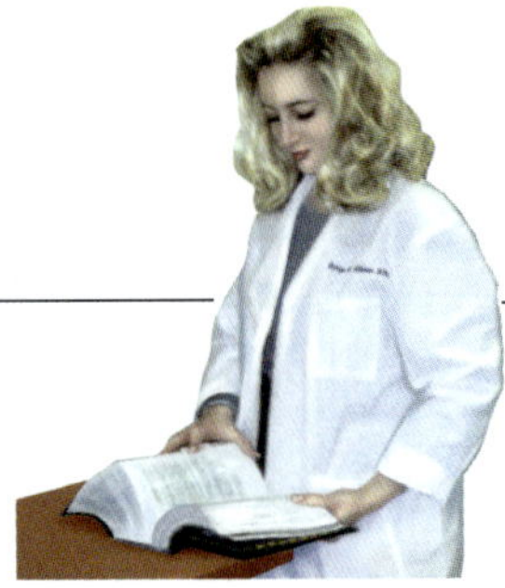

Professional Practice Journals

These journals are official publications of pharmacy organizations and can reflect the political views or policies of these groups. They also reflect changes in standards of practice and indicate trends in the profession. They may publish some original research studies. Examples are *Today's Technician (NPTA)*, *America's Pharmacist* (NCPA), *American Journal of Health-System Pharmacy* (ASHP) and the *Journal of the American Pharmacists Association* (APhA).

Trade Journals

Trade journals are published commercially but are not produced by any professional association. They tend to contain large amounts of advertising material. Examples are: *Pharmacy Times* (www.pharmacytimes.com) and *US Pharmacist* (www.uspharmacist.com).

Indexes of Primary Literature

Primary literature can be accessed by online database searching. The continuing development of online databases has increased the efficiency of the access, retrieval, and storage of information. *PubMed* (www.ncbi.nlm.nih.gov/pubmed) contributes the most comprehensive index of international medical literature and clinical trials. In addition, the *Cochrane Library* consists of systematic reviews of primary research in human health care and health policy that is recognized as the highest standard of evidence-based health care (www.thecochranelibrary.com).

Newsletters

Newsletters are published rapidly and frequently and provide a useful source of current information.

- *The Medical Letter on Drugs and Therapeutics* (www.medicalletter.org) contains short abstracts from journal articles. It also provides information on clinical trials and profiles on products recently granted New Drug Application (NDA) status.
- *The Pharmacists Letter* (pharmacistsletter.therapeuticresearch.com) provides unbiased evidence and recommendations on new developments in drug therapy.
- *Natural Medicines Comprehensive Database* (naturaldatabase.therapeuticresearch.com) contains unbiased scientific clinical information on complementary, alternative, and integrative therapies.

Textbooks

Textbooks can provide basic information on a particular topic or a range of topics. As with any publication, there is a wide range in the quality, level, and usefulness of textbooks. It is important to not accept the information in them as the last word on a subject. However, textbooks are very useful for explaining basic concepts and in refreshing your understanding of a topic. The texts below are noted for their authoritativeness and reliability in providing pharmaceutical information.

- *Handbook of Nonprescription Drugs: An Interactive Approach to Self Care* (www.pharmacylibrary.com/otchandbook).

  The *Handbook* provides a quick access to OTC drug information, complementary therapies, nondrug measures, treatment algorithms, assessment and triage techniques, and patient counseling tips. It serves both as a textbook for the pharmacy student and an information source for the practicing pharmacist. A searchable e-book in PDF format can be downloaded.

- Remington, *The Science and Practice of Pharmacy*

  Published every five years since 1885, Remington is the most comprehensive work in the pharmaceutical sciences. It covers all aspects of pharmacy for students, practitioners, and researchers, including ethical principles, technology and automation, professional communication, specializations in pharmacy practice, and medication errors. Drug monographs are categorized by drug class. The companion CD is essentially a scanned version of the entire book.

Mobile Devices

Health care providers utilize mobile devices to consult formularies and other reference materials such as drug and medical information. There are a variety of brands and operating systems, including smart phones, iPADs, and e-readers.

TECHNICIAN REFERENCES

There are many references that provide valuable information about the pharmacy technician profession.

They are useful for those interested in entering the field, technicians wishing to improve their skills and professionalism, and instructors.

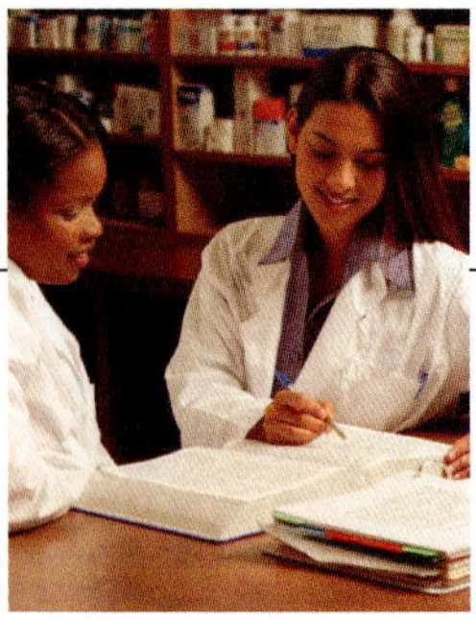

Photo courtesy Hanson Ng/ Design Pics/Getty Images

Occupational Information

A good first step to find job descriptions and overall job outlooks is the *Occupational Outlook Handbook* (Washington, D.C.: Bureau of Labor Statistics) and/or the Occupational Outlook Handbook website at www.bls.gov/ooh. You can also visit www.rxinsider.com to find jobs and salaries for pharmacy technicians in the United States and Canada.

Another good way to look up job descriptions, training programs, and opportunities is to use an Internet search engine. Just enter "pharmacy technician" and start exploring! A considerable amount of information is available about the responsibilities of a pharmacy technician, required training, salary ranges, and job opportunities.

Training Programs

Many pharmacy technicians receive informal, on-the-job training, but formal training programs are becoming more widespread. These programs differ in many respects, from credentials to program length. A directory of ASHP-accredited training programs can be found at www.ashp.org/directories/technicians. The Pharmacy Technician Educators Council (PTEC) guidance for training pharmacy technicians can be found at www.pharmacytecheducators.com.

Pharmacy Technician Organizations and Publications

- American Association of Pharmacy Technicians (www.pharmacytechnician.com)
- National Pharmacy Technician Association (www.pharmacytechnician.org)
- Canadian Association of Pharmacy Technicians (www.capt.ca)
- The Association of Pharmacy Technicians, UK (www.aptuk.org)
- Pharmacy Technician's Letter (pharmacytechniciansletter.therapeuticresearch.com)
- *journal of Pharmacy Technology* (www.jpharmtechnol.com)*:* provides information about the entire body of pharmacy practice and includes continuing education articles.
- *Today's Technician* (www.pharmacytechnician.org/en/cms459): published six times a year specifically for pharmacy technicians; includes a minimum of two hours of ACPE-accredited continuing education for CPhTs.

Rx tip

Whether you are considering becoming a pharmacy technician, receiving certification or recertification, or simply maintaining your competency and skills, it's always a good idea to research and read about your job. There's a lot you can learn on your own, if you make the effort.

Certification Examination Preparation

In 1995 the Pharmacy Technician Certification Board (PTCB) began administering the national Pharmacy Technician Certification Examination (PTCE). The PTCB website at www.ptcb.org offers information, a practice exam, and a guidebook to help individuals prepare for the PTCE. Other preparation texts include:

- *Pharmacy Technician Certification Review and Practice Exam, 3rd Edition*. Bethesda, MD: American Society of Health-System Pharmacists, 2010.
- *The Pharmacy Technician Workbook and Certification Review, 5th edition*. Englewood, CO: Morton Publishing, 2013.
- *Certification Review for Pharmacy Technicians, 9th Edition*. Bloomington, IN: Author House, 2012.
- *Pharmacy Calculations, 4th Edition*, Englewood, CO: Morton Publishing, 2013.
- *Medication Workbook for Pharmacy Technicians: A Pharmacology Primer*. Englewood, CO: Morton Publishing, 2012.

Continuing Education Information

Once certified, the PTCB requires you to obtain 20 hours of continuing education credit every two years to maintain your certification. At least one contact hour in pharmacy law is required. Resources for continuing education include:

- www.pharmacytechnician.org: free continuing education for NPTA members
- www.rxtechschool.com: training and education of pharmacy technicians
- www.techlectures.com: continuing education that meets PTCB requirements
- www.pharmacist.com: APhA online continuing education center for members
- www.powerpak.com: a source of continuing education for health-care professionals

Professional Liability

Since the pharmacy technician is a recognized professional, companies offer pharmacy technician liability policies that meets the needs of today's pharmacy technician.

- Pharmacists Mutual (www.phmic.com)
- HealthCare Providers Service Organization (HPSO) (www.hpso.com)

THE INTERNET

A computer network is a series of computers connected by a communication line, allowing the computers to exchange information.

The Internet is a supernetwork, with many networks from around the world all connected to each other and all using a common "language" (software and rules for communication) that enables them to communicate with each other.

The Internet is the world's largest network.

It has grown from a skeletal experimental network used by scientists to a gigantic commercial information superhighway used daily by millions of people. It also contains the world's largest source of information, the *World Wide Web* or web.

The web is a virtual library in which electronic information existing on hundreds of thousands of websites is accessible to Internet users.

Among this information is a growing amount of pharmacy literature and reference. Patients are also increasingly using the web to find pharmaceutical and health information.

What It Costs

There is a fee for an ISP. Most heavy Internet users set up their Internet service using high speed access via DSL, cable or satellite.

browser a software program that allows users to view websites on the World Wide Web (e.g., Safari, Internet Explorer).

Internet service provider (ISP) a company that provides access to the Internet.

search engine software that searches the web for information related to criteria entered by the user (e.g., Google, Bing, Yahoo!).

uniform resource locator (URL) a web address.

World Wide Web (WWW) a collection of electronic documents at addresses called websites.

GETTING CONNECTED

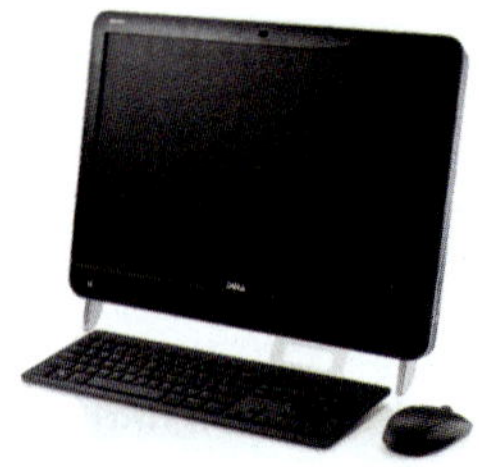

Image courtesy Dell, Inc.

A computer user can connect to the Internet and explore the web if they have the following:

- an Internet-ready computer that can use ethernet, wi-fi, or bluetooth to connect them to the Internet;
- an ***Internet service provider (ISP)***, such as Verizon, Comcast or CenturyLink, that provides Internet access;
- a wired or wireless connection to an ISP;
- and Internet ***browser*** software, such as Internet Explorer, Safari, or Mozilla Firefox. Browsers have many functions that allow you to move around the web, view websites, print their contents, save information, and so on. They generally include an e-mail function that allows you to send messages to anyone on the Internet who has an e-mail address.

℞ tip
Web addresses can and do change. If one of the addresses on this page doesn't work, try looking up the address in a search engine.

FINDING WHAT YOU WANT

Connecting to the Internet is only a starting point. To find information, you must have specific addresses of websites you want to visit. Web addresses are referred to as ***URLs—uniform resource locators***. For example, to go to the USP site, you would enter www.usp.org in the address line of your browser.

If you don't know the address you want, you can use a ***search engine*** to look for specific information. Search engines have different rules for entering a query, but they are very easy to use, and most Internet users rely on them heavily. Here are addresses for a few:

- Google: www.google.com
- Bing: www.bing.com
- Yahoo! www.yahoo.com

It is a good idea to check the quality of a site's information. The Health on the Net (HON) Foundation (www.hon.ch/home.html) is a nonprofit organization that helps guide web users to reliable information.

SOME KEY PLACES TO VISIT

Pharmacy Education and Related Information

- www.medscape.com/pharmacists
  integrated medical information and educational tools
- www.rxlist.com
  list of the top 200 drugs, pill identifier, and medical dictionary
- www.ismp.org
  The Institute for Safe Medication Practices —medication safety alerts, error reporting, and self-assessment guidelines
- www.ptcb.org
  Pharmacy Technician Certification Board —certification exam information
- www.pharmacist.com
  American Pharmacists Association —professional/career development resources
- www.ashp.org
  American Society of Health-System Pharmacists —pharmacy technician membership and continuing education
- www.nabp.net
  National Association of Boards of Pharmacy —links to Verified Internet Pharmacy Practice Sites (VIPPS)

Drug Information

- www.clinicalpharmacology.com
  Elsevier / Gold Standard
- www.lexi.com
  Walters Kluwer Health
- www.micromedex.com
  Truven Health Analytics
- www.epocrates.com
  Epocrates, Inc.

Government Sites

- www.justice.gov/dea/index.shtml
  U.S. Drug Enforcement Administration
- www.fda.gov
  U.S. Food and Drug Administration
- www.osha.gov
  Occupational Safety & Health Administration
- www.hhs.gov/ocr/privacy
  information on how to handle HIPAA
- www.hhs.gov
  U.S. Department of Health and Human Services

REVIEW

KEY CONCEPTS

INFORMATION

- ✔ Primary literature provides direct access to the most current contemporary research. Secondary literature primarily consists of general reference works based upon primary literature sources. Tertiary literature sources contain condensed information based on primary literature.
- ✔ OSHA requires pharmacies to have Material Safety Data Sheets (MSDS) for all their hazardous chemicals.
- ✔ The USP-NF Chapters <1> through <999> are enforced by the FDA.
- ✔ State laws and State Board of Pharmacy rules and regulations require pharmacies to maintain specific professional literature references.

COMMON REFERENCES

- ✔ *Drug Facts and Comparisons* (DFC) is a preferred reference for comprehensive and timely drug information, containing information about prescription and OTC products.
- ✔ Martindale, *The Complete Drug Reference* provides the best source of information about drugs in clinical use internationally.
- ✔ *AHFS* is accepted as the authority for drug information questions. It groups drug monographs by therapeutic use and provides off-label medication uses.
- ✔ The "Orange Book" is the common name for the FDA publication titled *Approved Drug Products with Therapeutic Equivalence Evaluations*.
- ✔ The *Handbook on Injectable Drugs* is a collection of monographs on commercially available parenteral drugs that include concentration, stability, dosage, and compatibility information.
- ✔ The *Red Book: Pharmacy's Fundamental Reference* is the pharmacist's guide to products and prices and provides annual price lists of drug products, as well as manufacturer, package size, strength, and wholesale and retail prices.
- ✔ *PDR* provides FDA regulation information about prescription drugs similar to the manufacturer's drug package inserts.

OTHER REFERENCES

- ✔ *Today's Technician*, a professional practice journal, is the official publication of the NPTA.
- ✔ *The Pharmacist's Letter* provides recommendations on new developments in drug therapy.

TECHNICIAN REFERENCES

- ✔ The Pharmacy Technician Certification Board (PTCB) administers the National Pharmacy Technician Certification Exam (PTCE). The PTCB website at www.ptcb.org provides information regarding exam application and preparation.
- ✔ Once certified as a pharmacy technician, the PTCB requires you to obtain 20 hours of continuing education credit every two years to maintain your certification. At least one of the 20 hours must be in pharmacy law.

THE INTERNET

- ✔ The Internet is a super network, with many networks from around the world all connected to each other and all using a common language.
- ✔ A search engine such as Google will search the web for specific information you enter.
- ✔ A browser, such as Internet Explorer, allows you to view websites.

SELF TEST

the answer key begins on page 569

MATCH THE TERMS

1. abstracting services ____
2. browser ____
3. HIPAA ____
4. Internet service provider (ISP) ____
5. off-label indication ____
6. "Orange Book" ____
7. primary literature ____
8. search engine ____
9. secondary literature ____
10. tertiary literature ____
11. uniform resource locator (URL) ____
12. World Wide Web ____

a. original reports of clinical and other types of research projects and studies.

b. condensed works based on primary literature, such as textbooks, monographs, etc.

c. services that summarize information from various primary sources for quick reference.

d. regulation created to protect the privacy of patient health records.

e. a collection of electronic documents at an Internet address.

f. a company that provides access to the Internet.

g. software that searches the web for information related to criteria entered by the user.

h. general reference works based upon primary literature sources.

i. the common name for the FDA's Approved Drug Products publication.

j. a software program that allows users to view websites on the World Wide Web.

k. a web address.

l. a use of a medication for an indication not approved by the FDA.

REVIEW

CHOOSE THE BEST ANSWER

1. ______________________ summarizes information in professional and scientific literature.
   a. Primary literature
   b. Abstracting services
   c. Secondary literature
   d. AHFS Drug Information

2. Pharmacy technicians find ___________ literature the easiest and most convenient to use.
   a. Primary
   b. Tertiary
   c. Secondary
   d. Abstract

3. The Occupational Safety and Health Administration (OSHA) requires pharmacies to have this literature on hand:
   a. Material Safety Data Sheets
   b. *The Merck Index*
   c. policy and procedure manuals
   d. Remington, *The Science and Practice of Pharmacy*

4. A pharmacy can obtain MSDSs from the local area __________ office.
   a. FDA
   b. DEA
   c. NIOSH
   d. OSHA

5. The general chapters <1> through <999> of the USP–NF are enforced by (the)
   a. DEA.
   b. FDA.
   c. OSHA
   d. HIPAA.

6. Which common reference would a pharmacy technician search to compare medications in the same therapeutic class for a patient on a restricted formulary?
   a. *American Hospital Formulary Service*
   b. *Drug Facts and Comparisons*
   c. *Physicians' Desk Reference*
   d. *USP DI*

7. Which reference would you use to identify a drug that a patient purchased in England?
   a. *Drug Facts and Comparisons*
   b. Martindale, *The Complete Drug Reference*
   c. *The Merck Index*
   d. *USP-NF*

8. To what pharmacy reference would you direct a physician who is looking for prescription information on major pharmaceuticals similar to drug package inserts?
   a. *The Merck Index*
   b. *Drug Facts and Comparisons*
   c. *Physicians' Desk Reference*
   d. *USP-NF*

9. Which pharmacy drug reference would you search for an indication for an off-label medication?
   a. *Drug Facts and Comparisons*
   b. *Physicians' Desk Reference*
   c. *AHFS Drug Information*
   d. Martindale, *The Complete Drug Reference*

10. Where would a pharmacy technician look for nationally recognized AWPs and NDCs for FDA approved drugs?
   a. *AHFS*
   b. "Orange Book"
   c. *Red Book*
   d. *USP-NF*

11. *The Medical Letter on Drugs and Therapeutics* is an example of a
   a. pink sheet.
   b. trade journal.
   c. professional practice journal.
   d. newsletter.

12. The common name for the FDA's *Approved Drug Products with Therapeutic Equivalent Evaluations* is the
   a. "Medical Book."
   b. "Orange Book."
   c. "Red Book."
   d. "USP-NF."

13. A patient would like to order their medications online. To which website would a pharmacy technician direct them?
   a. ashp.org
   b. nabp.org
   c. osha.gov
   d. ptcb.org

14. The most comprehensive text covering pharmaceutical sciences is
   a. Remington, *The Science and Practice of Pharmacy.*
   b. *Goodman and Gilman's The Pharmacological Basis of Therapeutics.*
   c. the "Orange Book."
   d. the *American Drug Index.*

15. The Bureau of Labor Statistics provides information about pharmacy careers on the Internet in the
   a. *Occupational Outlook Handbook.*
   b. "Orange Book."
   c. *Red Book.*
   d. *Pink Sheet.*

16. The directory of accredited technician training programs can be found at the website for
   a. TJC.
   b. ASHP.
   c. APhA.
   d. NABP.

17. A pharmacy technician searching for PTCE information, a practice exam, and a guidebook to help prepare for the PTCE should contact which organization?
   a. ASHP
   b. AAPT
   c. NPTA
   d. PTCB

18. As a member of NPTA, a pharmacy technician will receive which bimonthly journal that provides information and continuing education specifically for pharmacy technicians?
   a. *journal of Pharmacy Technology*
   b. *Today's Technician*
   c. *Pharmacy Times*
   d. *The Pink Sheet*

REVIEW

19. How many contact hours of continuing education in pharmacy law is required every two years to maintain your certification?
    a. one
    b. three
    c. five
    d. ten

20. Which reference would a pharmacy technician choose to research the compatibility of IV cefazolin and heparin running through the same IV line?
    a. *Drug Facts and Comparisons*
    b. *King's Guide to Parenteral Admixtures*
    c. Martindale, *The Complete Drug Reference*
    d. PDR

21. Which pharmacy reference would a pharmacy technician compounding a product consult to find the solubility properties of a chemical in water?
    a. *American Drug Index*
    b. Martindale, *The Complete Drug Reference*
    c. *The Merck Index*
    d. *Red Book*

22. Safari and Internet Explorer are examples of a
    a. browser.
    b. DSL.
    c. ISP.
    d. URL.

23. A company that provides access to the Internet is a/an
    a. browser.
    b. ISP.
    c. search engine.
    d. URL.

24. Google is an example of a
    a. modem.
    b. browser.
    c. search engine.
    d. uniform resource locator.

25. A collection of electronic documents at addresses called websites:
    a. WWW
    b. ISP
    c. DSL
    d. URL

CRITICAL THINKING QUESTIONS

1. A drug company sales rep requests a list of patients on one of their medications being reviewed by the FDA. What should you do and why?
2. You receive an order for Dilantin® and the patient asks for the generic equivalent phenytoin. Can phenytion be substituted for Dilantin®? Where would you find this information?
3. While training a new pharmacy technician you are asked for how long narcotic records need to be kept on file. What do you tell the technician and where do you direct him/her to find this information?
4. A patient asks if you can order empty gelatin capsules and approximately how much they will cost? What pharmacy reference can you search for this information?
5. A friend asks you about your job as a pharmacy technician and would like more information about the job outlook, training, and certification. Where do you send them?

THINKING IT THROUGH WRAP-UP

1. First, determine if Lugol's® is a toxic agent by reviewing its MSDS. Then follow your facility's hazardous spill policies.
2. Use a medication identifier such as www.rxlist.com or www.clinicalpharmacology.com to identify the medication; then provide this information to the pharmacist to discuss with the patient.
3. Check the *Handbook on Injectable Drugs* for compatibility information. Give this information to the pharmacist so they can discuss it with the nurse.

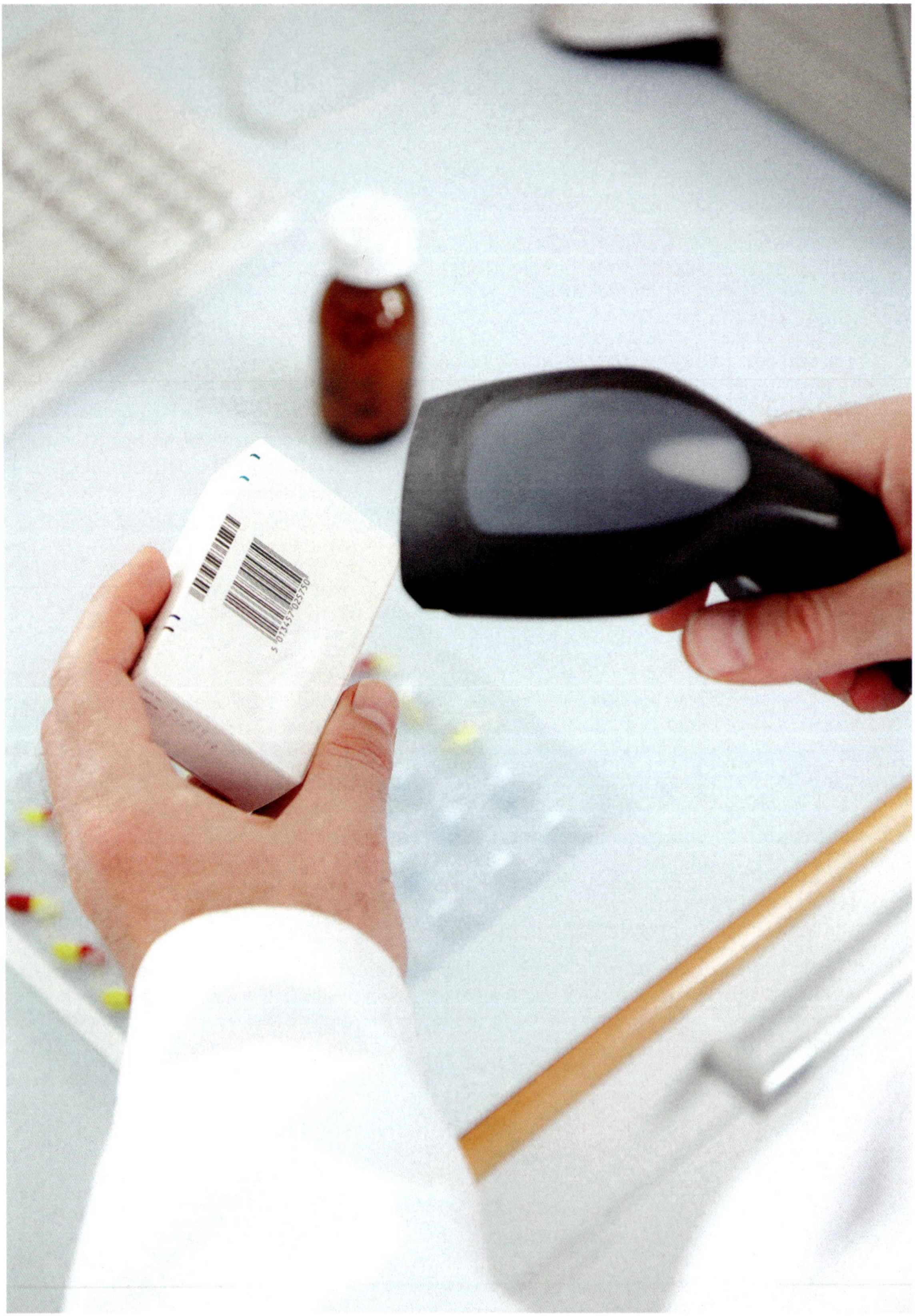

Photo courtesy Adie Bush/Cultura/Getty Images

13

INVENTORY MANAGEMENT

LEARNING OBJECTIVES

At the completion of study, the student will:

- ✔ understand the goal of inventory management.
- ✔ understand the use of wholesalers and a formulary.
- ✔ become familiar with inventory systems for maintaining adequate inventory.
- ✔ be knowledgeable of the technology used in inventory systems.
- ✔ know the ordering and receiving process related to inventory management.
- ✔ be familiar with the forms used during inventory and ordering.
- ✔ understand the procedures for stocking and storing pharmacy inventory.

THINKING IT THROUGH

You are a pharmacy technician who has been assigned buyer duties for the day. This means you are responsible for stocking and ordering drugs. You start your shift with boxes or totes full of drugs from an order that was placed with the wholesaler the night before. As you read this chapter, consider the following:

1. You are stocking the order that was placed yesterday when you discover that several medications listed on the invoice are not in the tote boxes, and that some items included in the shipment were not ordered. What is the process for checking in the order and dealing with wrong stock?
2. What should be reviewed during the process of stocking the shelves?
3. How would you determine if the correct amount of stock is on hand/if additional stock should be ordered?
4. What process would you use to place an order for additional stock?

INVENTORY MANAGEMENT

An *inventory* is a listing of the goods or items that a business will use in its normal operation.

Pharmacies generally develop an inventory of medications based upon what they expect to need. Rarely used medications might not be kept in inventory but instead ordered as needed.

Because medication needs are often urgent, pharmacies must maintain good control of their stock or inventory.

This means that all drugs that are likely to be needed are both on hand and usable—that is, they have not expired or been damaged, contaminated, or otherwise made unfit for use.

Inventory management is an integral part of the technician's job responsibility.

Each technician is required to master the specific inventory system in use at their workplace. In some cases, inventory management may be the technician's primary responsibility, and the technician has the opportunity to become a "pharmaceutical buyer." At hospitals and other institutions, for example, a purchasing/inventory technician is often responsible for obtaining and maintaining the institution's medication and device supply.

safety you should know

It is important to deal only with well-known or established wholesalers and suppliers that can document the pedigree or path of a drug from manufacturer to consumer. Unscrupulous manufacturers have made counterfeit medications, which may look like an established drug but that have little or no active ingredients, and then sell them to lesser known wholesalers or suppliers.

FORMULARIES

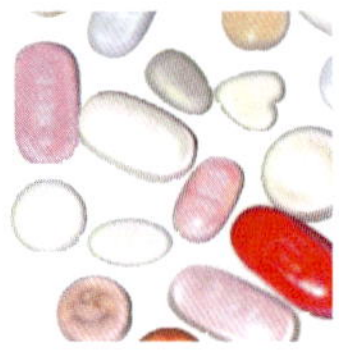

Many hospitals, HMOs, insurers, and other health-care systems maintain a list of medications called a ***formulary***. These are the medications that are approved for use in the system.

- An ***open formulary*** is one that allows purchase of any medication that is prescribed.
- A ***closed formulary*** is a limited list of approved medications. A physician must receive permission to use a medication that is not on the list. Closed formularies are generally used as a cost savings tool, in which less expensive substitutes are stocked. Though these substitutes are mainly generic equivalents, in some hospitals a drug on the formulary that is ***therapeutically equivalent*** (chemically different but with similar actions and effects) may be substituted for a drug not on the formulary.
- Formulary medications are routinely reviewed when new information is available about side effects or contraindications. In addition, look-Alike and soundalike medications may be stored, labeled, or marked separately to prevent mix-ups. Medications may be removed from the formulary or from public access if significant side effects are found.

closed formulary a limited list of approved medications.

formulary a list of medications approved for use.

inventory a list of goods or items a business uses in its normal operations.

open formulary a system that allows a pharmacy to use any prescribed medication.

therapeutic equivalent pharmaceutical equivalents that produce the same effects in patients.

THE INVENTORY ENVIRONMENT

There are many participants in the inventory process—the pharmacy, the institution, the wholesaler, the manufacturer, the government, insurers, and other third parties.

The Pharmacy

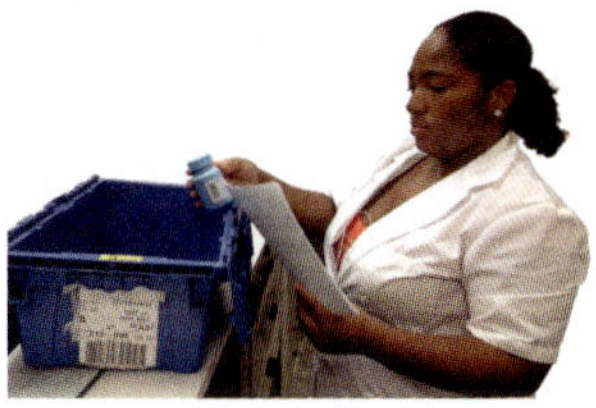

Pharmacies usually buy drugs from wholesalers, but sometimes they buy directly from manufacturers. Pharmacies also sometimes participate in large purchasing groups called GPOs (group purchasing organizations) that negotiate contracts to buy in bulk at a discount.

Wholesalers

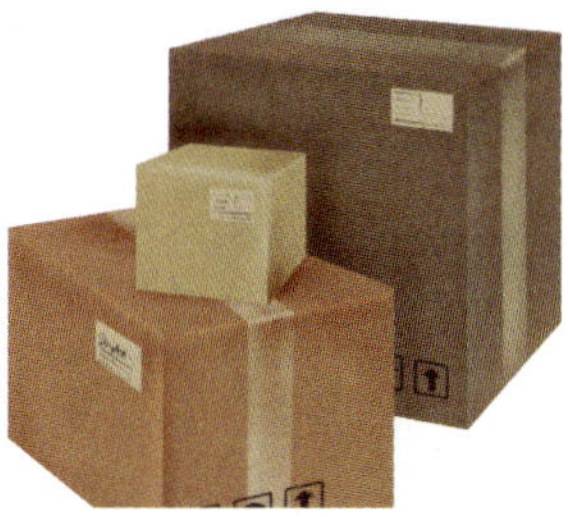

More than three-quarters of pharmaceutical manufacturers' sales are directly to drug wholesalers,* which in turn resell their inventory to hospitals, pharmacies, and other pharmaceutical dispensers.

Wholesalers are government-licensed and regulated. They stock tens of thousands of items from hundreds of manufacturers, everything from disposable razors to life-saving, emergency-use drugs. Wholesalers also obtain less-used medications as they are needed, often making daily deliveries. In addition, they can provide generic substitution options, private label products, and automated purchasing and inventory systems.

Because they offer pharmacies dependable one-stop shopping for most of their medication needs, using wholesalers greatly simplifies the drug purchasing process, saving time, effort, and money: there are fewer purchase orders, invoices, and payments; fewer procedures to learn regarding placing orders, shipping, and returns; and fewer employees needed to manage the inventory.

**Source: National Wholesale Drug Association*

Drug Manufacturers

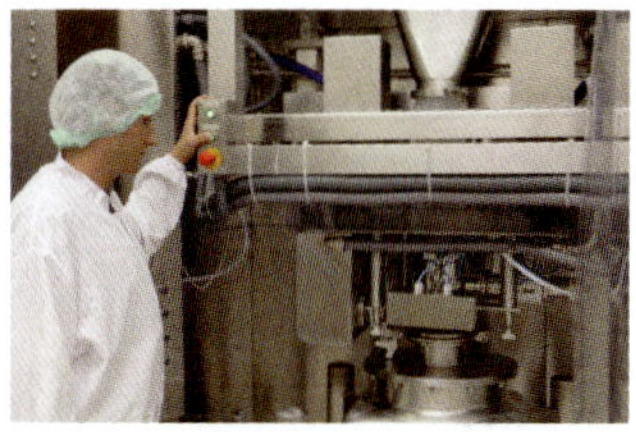

When drugs are not available from wholesalers due to expense, storage requirements, or other reasons, they can be obtained directly from the manufacturer. In this case, a purchasing account for the pharmacy must be set up with the manufacturer.

The Government

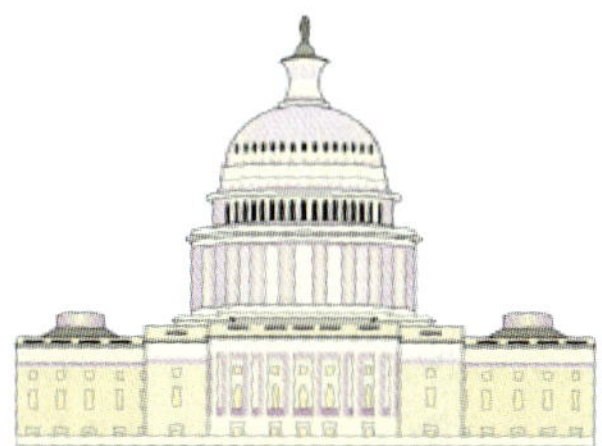

A major role the government plays is in regulating controlled substances. In the United States, the Drug Enforcement Administration (DEA) regulates the distribution, storage, record keeping, and ordering requirements for controlled substances. See the following pages on ordering and stocking and storing drugs for more specific information.

The government can also pass laws to help reduce the cost of drugs. The 340B Drug Pricing Program resulted from the Veterans Health Care Act and limits the cost of covered outpatient drugs to safety-net providers such as federal grantees, federally qualified health center look-alikes, and qualified hospitals. The program saves these providers 20–50% on the cost of pharmaceuticals. Manufacturers are willing to participate in order to have their drugs included in these government sponsored programs. Strict record-keeping regulations must be followed; more information can be obtained from the Health Resources and Services Administration (HRSA) Office of Pharmacy Affairs (OPA) at www.hrsa.gov/opa/index.html.

INVENTORY SYSTEMS

A pharmaceutical inventory system tracks inventory, forecasts needs, and generates reorders to maintain adequate inventory.

The goal of a good inventory system is to have the right amount of stock at the right price available at all times. Too many drugs on hand involves unnecessary cost and maintenance and may result in spoilage. Too few drugs means that medications won't be available when needed.

In order to maintain an adequate supply of medications, pharmacies use a *perpetual inventory system*.

A perpetual inventory system maintains a continuous record of every item in inventory so that it always shows the stock on hand. This is a requirement for Schedule II substances, but it is also important for many medications since their availability has health consequences.

Spoilage

Time or storage conditions may cause the chemical compounds in medications to break down, resulting in either lost potency or changed function. This is called inventory spoilage. Use of such medications may be dangerous. Medications carry expiration dates and storage requirements that must be honored. It is an important task of the pharmacy technician to constantly check all stock for drugs going out of date.

✔ **Note:** As an expiration date approaches, it may already be too late to dispense the medication, since it must be used before the date passes. If an expiration date for a medication has passed, or the medication cannot be completely used before that date, the medication must be appropriately disposed of or returned to the supplier for credit. In some cases, wholesalers will not accept expired drugs, but the drug manufacturer will. When returned, packages must generally be unopened.

Disposal of Nonreturnable Medications

Federal legislation such as in the Safe Water Drinking Act requires safe disposal of medications. Companies such as Stericylce (www.stericycle.com) can assist with complying with OSHA, EPA, and DOT regulations for disposing of nonreturnable medications.

INVENTORY CONCEPTS

Turnover

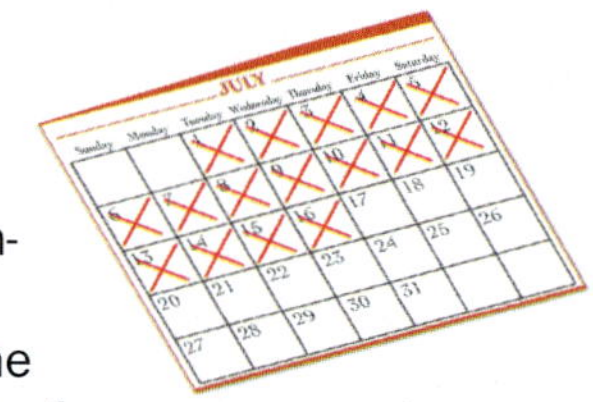

The ***turnover*** rate is the number of days it takes to use the complete stock of an item. Besides quality and spoilage issues, there is also a financial consideration. If a supplier's payment terms are "30 days net" and stock turnover averages less than 30 days, the stock will be sold before the supplier must be paid, which lowers the cost of the stock.

Fast Movers and Slow Movers

A general rule is that 20% of the stock will account for 80% of the orders or prescriptions. To keep inventory dollars low, pharmacies keep a 1–2 week supply of fast moving drugs and a month's supply of slower moving drugs.

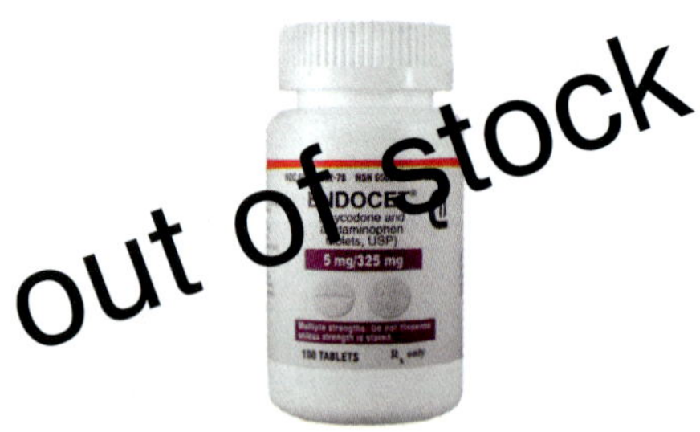

Availability

Besides monitoring stock on hand, it is important to monitor the market availability of medications. A particular drug may be unavailable due to manufacturing difficulties, raw material unavailability, recalls, etc. This can increase market demand for substitutes for the unavailable drug, sometimes causing shortages in the substitutes as well.

TOOLS FOR PERPETUAL INVENTORY

Point-of-Sale (POS) System

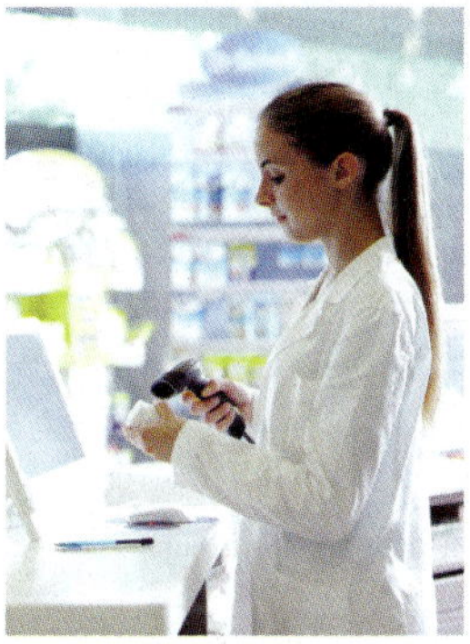

Pharmacy operations generally use a ***point-of-sale system***, which deducts items from inventory as they are sold or dispensed. The transaction is often triggered by scanning a bar code on the medication packaging, though it can also be keyed into the system. Pharmacies may use their own inventory system, one provided by a corporate parent if they are part of a chain, or one provided by a third party such as a wholesaler.

Order Entry Devices

Portable hand-held devices are widely used to enter ordering data. When inspection of stock shows that a drug is approaching the minimum inventory level, the reorder can be made using one of these devices. The drug's ID number is entered by hand or scanned into the device using a bar-coded shelf tag and the wand attached to the device. A desired quantity, generally enough to reach the maximum inventory level, is then entered to complete the order. The data is sent to the institution's ordering computer. Confirmation is received to verify stock will be sent.

perpetual inventory a system that maintains a continuous record of every item in inventory so that it always shows the current amount of stock on hand.

point of sale (POS) system an inventory system in which the item is deducted from inventory as it is sold or dispensed.

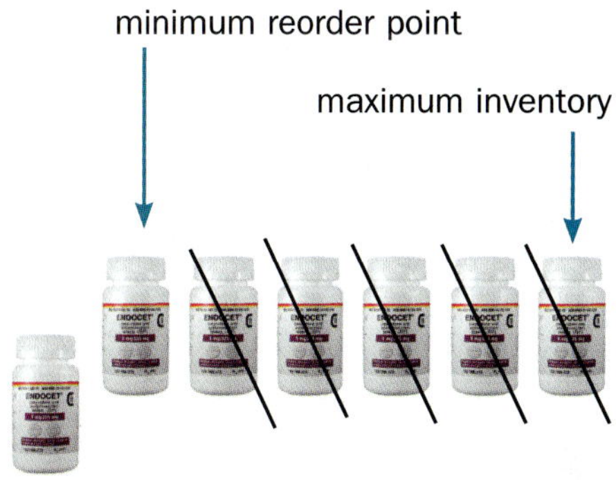

Reorder Points

In order to maintain adequate inventory for their needs, community and institutional pharmacies maintain computer databases of their inventory using drug ***reorder points***. These are maximum and minimum inventory levels for each drug. As the minimum reorder point of a medication is reached, most computer systems will generate an automatic purchase order for more of it. What medications should be ordered (and how much) is automatically identified on a daily basis. The order amount will be calculated to reach the maximum reorder point. Reorder points for any item can generally be set according to the needs of the facility.

Automated Reports

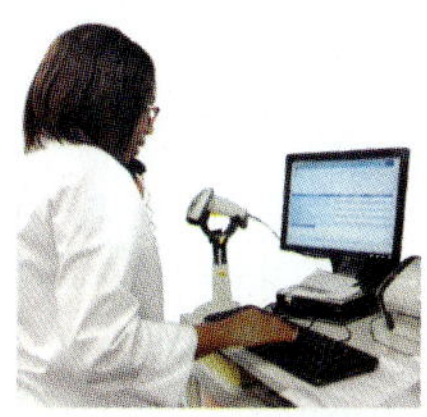

Computerized inventory systems provide a continuous picture of the inventory situation through automated reports that allow users to analyze and monitor their inventory in a variety of ways. They automatically update stock amounts, track turnover, produce purchase orders based on reorder points, and forecast future needs.

reorder points minimum and maximum stock levels that determine when a reorder is placed and for how much.

turnover the rate at which inventory is used, generally expressed in number of days.

COMPUTERS & INVENTORY

There are many different kinds of computer systems in retail and hospital pharmacy.

Among the many available options, these systems can automate label printing, coordinate billing and pricing with insurance, use bar codes to check medication identification, check for allergies and possible drug interactions, print medication information for the patient, provide drug information for the pharmacists and nurses, automate filling prescriptions and medication orders, manage inventory. and, in some hospital systems, also calculate weight-based dosing and provide disease-specific alerts based on lab values.

Computerized inventory systems automatically adjust inventory and generate orders based on maintaining set inventory levels.

The inventory system is often a component of a comprehensive pharmacy management system that includes elements like patient profiling, management reporting, and so on. In many cases, the drug wholesaler provides the system to its customers as part of the wholesaler service. The customer's system interacts with the wholesaler's so that various types of information (pricing, order information, etc.) can be exchanged automatically between the two systems.

Entering correct information is essential to any computer system.

Computerized systems can automatically create and maintain records based on each inventory transaction. However, because many of these transactions are manually entered into the system there is always a possibility of error. For this reason, each system produces reports that cover virtually every aspect of the inventory process from stock to turnover to reorders. These reports can be read on screen or printed so that errors can be detected.

To protect against possible abuses, users are given passwords to access different features of the system.

This not only protects the employer, but the employee as well. It prevents unauthorized activities and also documents who did what and when.

KEY COMPUTER CONSIDERATIONS

System Care and Maintenance

Computer systems have become very durable, but they need care and maintenance. It is important to know and follow the operating instructions for any system. Some factors that can cause damage to computers are temperature, dust, moisture, movement, vibrations, and power surges.

System Backup

Each system's ***database*** of information is a critical component of the pharmacy or institution in which it functions. These files must be regularly backed up or copied to an appropriate storage media. There are many types of such media but whatever the media, it is important to know its reliability. Depending on the operation, back up may need to be performed daily.

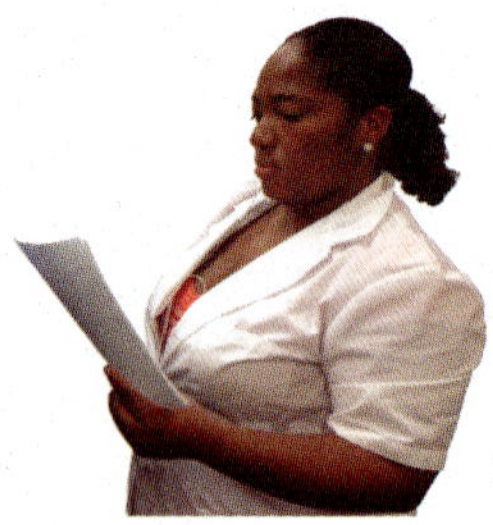

Manual Checking

Checking reports manually is an important step in ensuring that records are correct. Simple data entry errors can result in serious mistakes affecting orders, stock availability, prices, and other issues. For example: If a box containing 150 u/d tablets of Tylenol® is set up in the system as one unit, but is incorrectly keyed into the system as 150 units, the system's information will be grossly incorrect.

automated dispensing machine a device that dispenses medications at point-of-use upon confirmation of an order that has been communicated from a centralized computer system.

database a collection of information structured so that specific information within it can easily be retrieved and used.

AUTOMATED DISPENSING SYSTEMS

There are many types of automated dispensing systems whose functions may vary somewhat. Some are designed for retail prescriptions while others are designed for hospitals using unit doses.

Retail Automation

Parata Max® is an automated counting system. Unique, bar-coded cells hold different drugs. When a prescription is received at the pharmacy drop-off and entered into the host system, it is sent to Max, which labels, fills, caps, sorts and stores the prescription. Technicians replenish the cells. To ensure accuracy, Max prompts the technician to scan the barcodes on the stock bottle and the Max cell to ensure drugs are loaded into the correct cells.

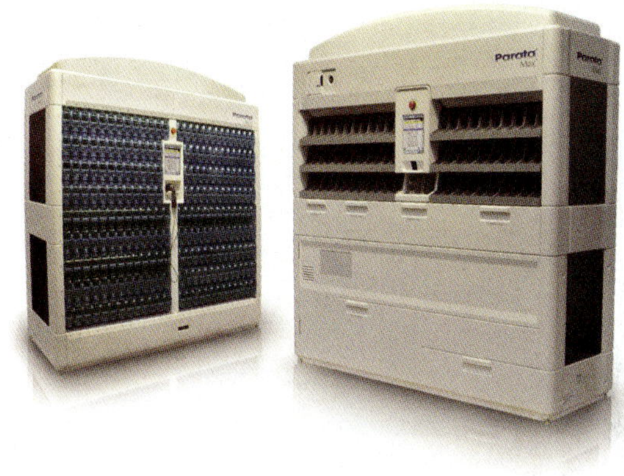

Parata Max®
Photo courtesy of Parata Systems, LLC

Hospital Automation

The Pyxis Med/Supply Station® is like an ATM for medications used in hospitals. This type of device is generally known as an ***automated dispensing machine (ADM)***. A network of storage stations are located throughout a facility and are connected to a Pyxis® server, which in turn links to the hospital's ADT, billing, and materials management information systems. The system tracks inventory and keeps a record of which drugs/supplies were taken by which nurse for which patient. There are several such devices available (e.g., AcuDose Rx®, OmniCell®, and MedSelect®Flex).

Homerus® is an example of a centralized robotic unit-dose dispensing device. It can individually package and store large amounts of medications from bulk supplies, deliver bar-coded medications to 24-hour patient-specific medication bins, and return medications to storage after a patient is discharged.

Some hospitals have mobile robots that travel throughout a facility delivering drugs to various nursing units and departments.

Carousels are used to efficiently store bulk or unit dose medications. They use bar codes to track medications placed in the machine. This system allows quick removal and returning of medications through computerized access panels.

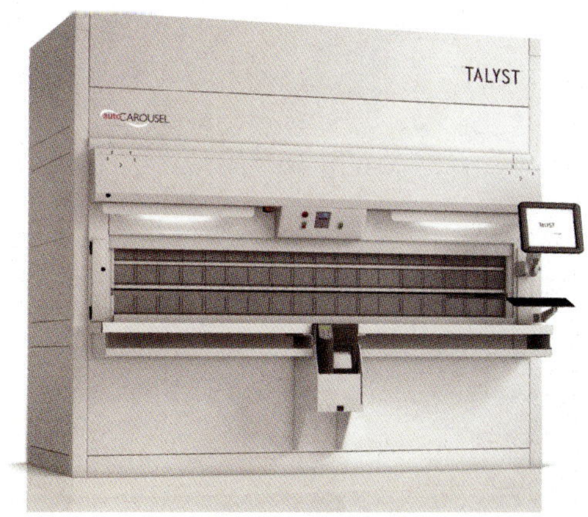

Talyst AutoCarousel
Photo courtesy of Talyst.

ORDERING

Ordering systems involve automated and manual activities.

Much of the work is done by computer systems. However, manual checking, editing, and confirmation are still essential.

AUTOMATED ORDERING

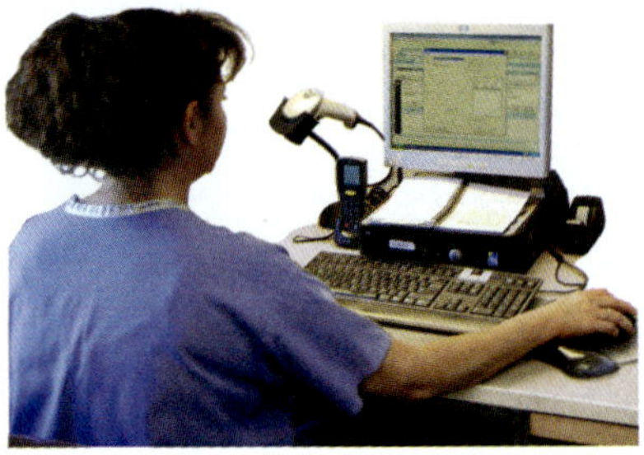

Orders can be generated using an order entry device or automatically generated by the system based on stock levels and reorder points. These reports must be checked and confirmed. If changes are needed, they can be made manually. The system then produces a revised order, which should again be checked and edited until it is ready for sending to the supplier.

When an order is ready, the ordering system and the supplier's system are usually connected via the Internet so the order can be downloaded from one system to the other.

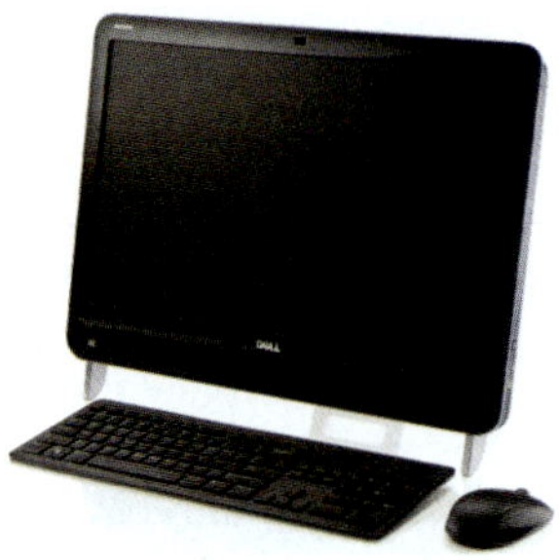

Photo courtesy Dell, Inc.

The supplier's computer system analyzes the order line by line to determine if there is enough inventory to fill the order as requested. If there is more than one warehouse in the system, it may check multiple locations.

- If the order can be filled as ordered, a message will automatically be sent to the purchaser, confirming the order. This confirmation can be read on screen but should also be printed.
- If the order cannot be filled exactly as ordered, a message will be sent listing the exceptions. This report should be printed and appropriate action taken to fill the order. It may be necessary to create a second purchase order, talk with the supplier personally, or find an alternative supplier. Some common reasons for omissions are: temporary out-of-stocks, back-ordered drugs, or the item may no longer be carried.

Rx safety you should know

Good ordering practices set up checks and balances so that the same person does not perform both ordering and receiving. This is especially important with controlled substances.

Material Safety Data Sheets (MSDS) OSHA required notices on hazardous substances that provide hazard, handling, clean-up, and first aid information.

ORDER DETAILS

Shipping

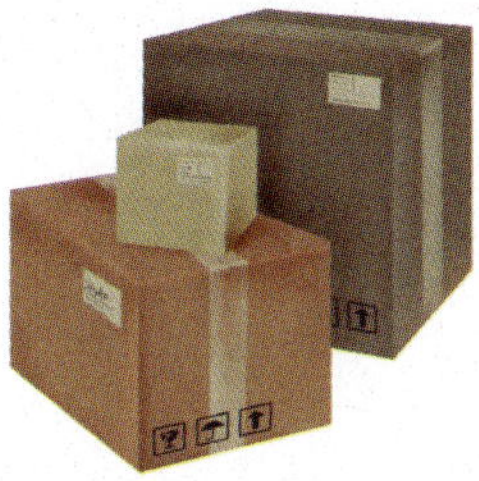

The type of shipping indicated by the purchaser determines the time and cost of shipping. Orders may be delivered in single or multiple shipments. For example, if a supplier does not have all the items ordered, a partial shipment may later come from another distribution center.

Material Safety Data Sheets (MSDS) indicate when special shipping is required for hazardous substances such as chemotherapeutic agents. The U.S. Postal Service, Federal Express, UPS, and others each have their own policies for shipping hazardous substances. In addition, the Federal Aviation Administration (FAA) will not allow some substances to be shipped by plane; often these drugs are shipped via a courier.

Credits/Returns

Each supplier has policies and procedures that must be followed in order to receive the credit on returns. Documentation must be carefully checked item by item. A printed copy must be kept on file.

Companies known as reverse distributors specialize in returns to the manufacturer of expired and discontinued drugs. They complete each manufacturer's return form and then package, mail, and track the drugs. They also return and fill out the paper work for C-II drugs and other controlled substances. Their fee is usually a percentage of the return credit that is deducted automatically from the refund.

Receiving Chemotherapy Drugs

The National Institute for Occupational Safety and Health (NIOSH) publishes very detailed guidelines on how to safely and legally handle chemotherapy and other hazardous drugs.

NIOSH Publication No. 2004-165: *Preventing Occupational Exposure to Antineoplastic and Other Hazardous Drugs* can be downloaded from www.cdc.gov/niosh/docs/2004-165/.

Receiving

Accuracy is essential in checking in medications received from suppliers. Be alert for drugs that have been incorrectly picked or are damaged, outdated, or missing entirely from the supplier. In many settings, items are stickered with bar codes that can be scanned to do an automatic count.

- ✔ Shipments, invoices, and purchase orders must be reconciled item by item.
- ✔ The strength and amount of each item must be checked to make sure they are correct. A common mistake is an item sent in bulk instead of unit dose (or the reverse).
- ✔ Shipment prices on the supplier invoice should match the purchase order exactly. Individual price changes must be identified and may have to be entered into the pharmacy system manually to make sure the system has the correct information.
- ✔ Broken or damaged stock must be brought to the attention of the supplier. They should be removed, bagged, or otherwise separated to help prevent contamination or damage to other stock.
- ✔ If there are any discrepancies, the supplier should generally be notified immediately; most wholesalers require that a completed form describing the problem be faxed to them.

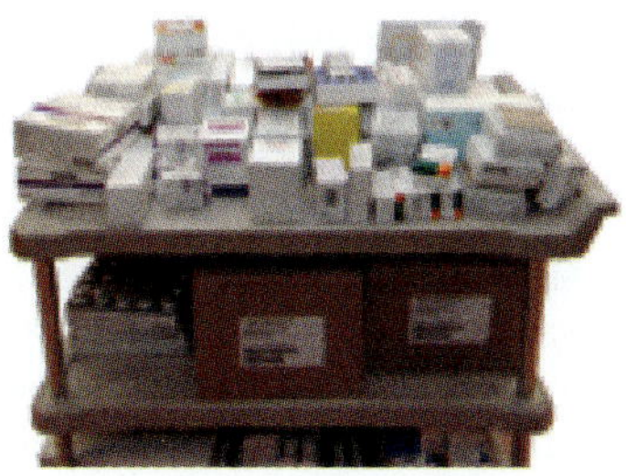

Ordering and Receiving Controlled Substances

Schedule I and II drugs require a special order form, DEA Form 222. An electronic system called CSOS (Controlled Substance Ordering System) is available through the DEA at www.deaecom.gov. This system allows secure electronic transmission of Schedule I-V controlled substance orders without having to send the supporting paper version of Form 222.

Controlled substances are shipped separately and should be checked in by a pharmacist.

FORMS

The Online Ordering Screen

Online ordering systems generally contain abbreviated descriptions of drug products in the formulary. The technician uses a "Select" (or similar) function to choose products and may then "Add" it to an order. Quantities may be manually entered or edited—if they have been automatically recorded by the system.

The system automatically assigns to each order a ***purchase order number*** for identification. Once the order is finished, checked, and ready, it is sent to the supplier's system.

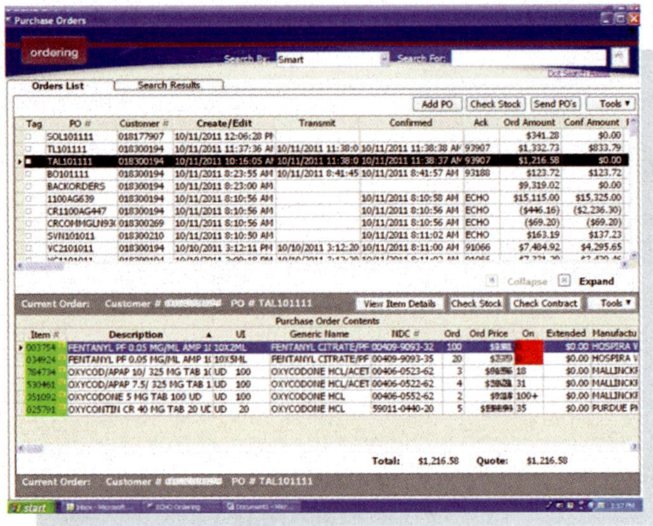

The Confirmation Printout

When an online purchase order is received by the supplier, the supplier's system checks the order to see what items are available. Next, a confirmation of the order is sent back to the purchaser's system. This confirmation indicates which items will be shipped, which are unavailable, the cost of the items, and any related costs. An order confirmation is saved on the system and a copy is printed out so that a hard copy is available for checking.

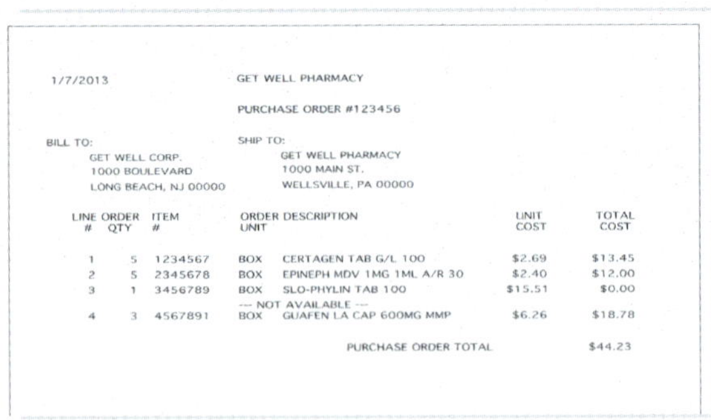

1/7/2013

GET WELL PHARMACY

PURCHASE ORDER #123456

BILL TO:
GET WELL CORP.
1000 BOULEVARD
LONG BEACH, NJ 00000

SHIP TO:
GET WELL PHARMACY
1000 MAIN ST.
WELLSVILLE, PA 00000

LINE #	ORDER QTY	ITEM #	ORDER UNIT	DESCRIPTION	UNIT COST	TOTAL COST
1	5	1234567	BOX	CERTAGEN TAB G/L 100	$2.69	$13.45
2	5	2345678	BOX	EPINEPH MDV 1MG 1ML A/R 30	$2.40	$12.00
3	1	3456789	BOX	SLO-PHYLIN TAB 100	$15.51	$0.00
			--- NOT AVAILABLE ---			
4	3	4567891	BOX	GUAFEN LA CAP 600MG MMP	$6.26	$18.78
				PURCHASE ORDER TOTAL		$44.23

purchase order number the number assigned to each order for identification.

The Shipping Invoice

When the items are shipped, the supplier includes an invoice listing the items in the shipment, items that may be shipped separately, items that are unavailable, and the cost of the shipment. The invoice must be checked item by item against the items in the shipment to make certain nothing is missing.

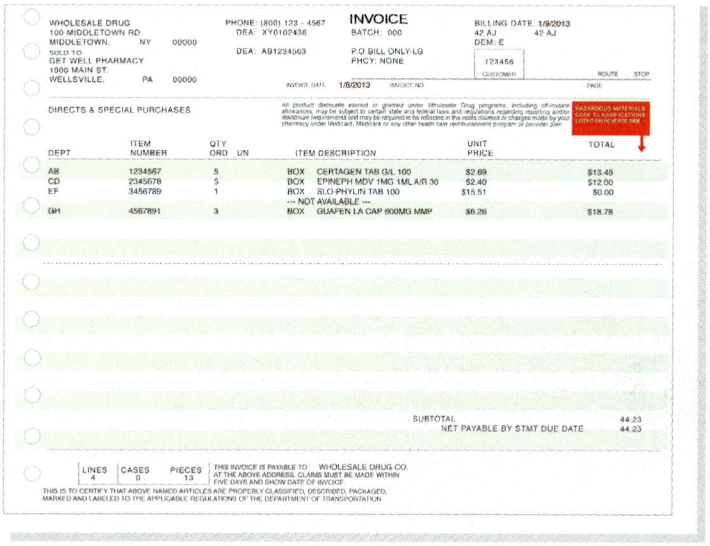

WHOLESALE DRUG
100 MIDDLETOWN RD.
MIDDLETOWN, NY 00000
SOLD TO
GET WELL PHARMACY
1000 MAIN ST.
WELLSVILLE, PA 00000

PHONE: (800) 123 - 4567
DEA: XY0102436
DEA: AB1234563

INVOICE
BATCH: 000
P.O.BILL ONLY-LG
PHCY: NONE

BILLING DATE: 1/9/2013
42 AJ 42 AJ
DEM: E
123456 CUSTOMER
ROUTE STOP
INVOICE DATE 1/8/2013 INVOICE NO PAGE

DIRECTS & SPECIAL PURCHASES

All product discounts earned or granted under Wholesale Drug programs, including off-invoice allowances, may be subject to certain state and federal laws and regulations regarding reporting and/or disclosure requirements and may be required to be reflected in the costs claimed or charges made by your pharmacy under Medicaid, Medicare or any other health care reimbursement program or provider plan.

HAZARDOUS MATERIALS CODE CLASSIFICATIONS LISTED ON REVERSE SIDE

DEPT	ITEM NUMBER	QTY ORD	UN	ITEM DESCRIPTION	UNIT PRICE	TOTAL
AB	1234567	5		BOX CERTAGEN TAB G/L 100	$2.69	$13.45
CD	2345678	5		BOX EPINEPH MDV 1MG 1ML A/R 30	$2.40	$12.00
EF	3456789	1		BOX SLO-PHYLIN TAB 100 --- NOT AVAILABLE ---	$15.51	$0.00
GH	4567891	3		BOX GUAFEN LA CAP 600MG MMP	$6.26	$18.78

SUBTOTAL 44.23
NET PAYABLE BY STMT DUE DATE 44.23

LINES	CASES	PIECES
4	0	13

THIS INVOICE IS PAYABLE TO WHOLESALE DRUG CO. AT THE ABOVE ADDRESS. CLAIMS MUST BE MADE WITHIN FIVE DAYS AND SHOW DATE OF INVOICE.

THIS IS TO CERTIFY THAT ABOVE NAMED ARTICLES ARE PROPERLY CLASSIFIED, DESCRIBED, PACKAGED, MARKED AND LABELED TO THE APPLICABLE REGULATIONS OF THE DEPARTMENT OF TRANSPORTATION.

The Returns Form

Preprinted, multipart forms are often used for returns, though some computer inventory systems generate their own. When returning items, the following information is usually required:

- original p.o. number
- item number
- quantity
- reason for return

Reasons for returning products can include over shipments, damaged or expired products, or changed needs.

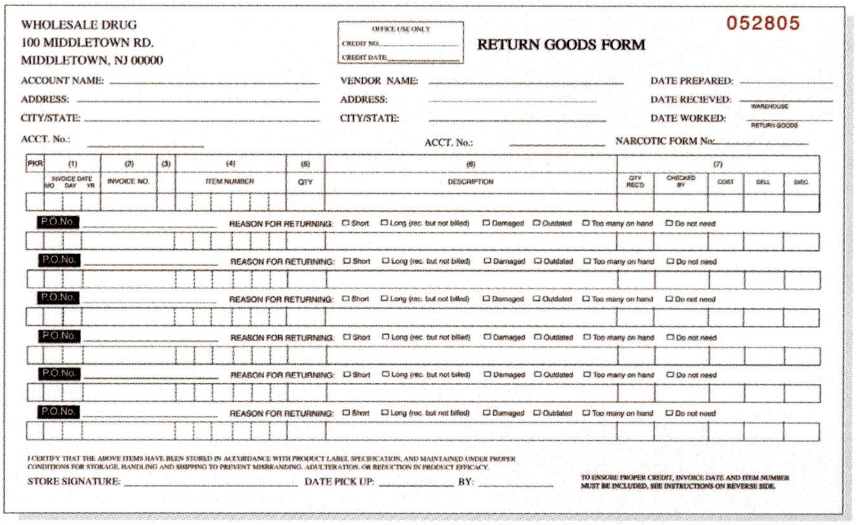

WHOLESALE DRUG
100 MIDDLETOWN RD.
MIDDLETOWN, NJ 00000

OFFICE USE ONLY
CREDIT NO.
CREDIT DATE

RETURN GOODS FORM

052805

ACCOUNT NAME: VENDOR NAME: DATE PREPARED:
ADDRESS: ADDRESS: DATE RECIEVED: WAREHOUSE
CITY/STATE: CITY/STATE: DATE WORKED: RETURN GOODS
ACCT. No.: ACCT. No.: NARCOTIC FORM No.:

PKR	(1) INVOICE DATE MO DAY YR	(2) INVOICE NO.	(3)	(4) ITEM NUMBER	(5) QTY	(6) DESCRIPTION	(7) QTY REC'D	CHECKED BY	COST	SELL	DISC.

P.O.No. REASON FOR RETURNING: ☐ Short ☐ Long (rec. but not billed) ☐ Damaged ☐ Outdated ☐ Too many on hand ☐ Do not need

P.O.No. REASON FOR RETURNING: ☐ Short ☐ Long (rec. but not billed) ☐ Damaged ☐ Outdated ☐ Too many on hand ☐ Do not need

P.O.No. REASON FOR RETURNING: ☐ Short ☐ Long (rec. but not billed) ☐ Damaged ☐ Outdated ☐ Too many on hand ☐ Do not need

P.O.No. REASON FOR RETURNING: ☐ Short ☐ Long (rec. but not billed) ☐ Damaged ☐ Outdated ☐ Too many on hand ☐ Do not need

P.O.No. REASON FOR RETURNING: ☐ Short ☐ Long (rec. but not billed) ☐ Damaged ☐ Outdated ☐ Too many on hand ☐ Do not need

P.O.No. REASON FOR RETURNING: ☐ Short ☐ Long (rec. but not billed) ☐ Damaged ☐ Outdated ☐ Too many on hand ☐ Do not need

I CERTIFY THAT THE ABOVE ITEMS HAVE BEEN STORED IN ACCORDANCE WITH PRODUCT LABEL SPECIFICATION, AND MAINTAINED UNDER PROPER CONDITIONS FOR STORAGE, HANDLING AND SHIPPING TO PREVENT MISBRANDING, ADULTERATION, OR REDUCTION IN PRODUCT EFFICACY.

STORE SIGNATURE: DATE PICK UP: BY:

TO ENSURE PROPER CREDIT, INVOICE DATE AND ITEM NUMBER MUST BE INCLUDED, SEE INSTRUCTIONS ON REVERSE SIDE.

STOCKING & STORING

Most medications are received from suppliers in bulk stock bottles whose labels have information required by the FDA.

This information includes the brand name, generic name, prescription legend, storage requirements, dosage form, quantity, controlled substance mark, manufacturer's name, lot number, expiration date, and NDC (National Drug Code) number.

In hospitals, medications are often packaged in individual doses called *unit-dose packaging*.

Because the dose information is on each dose, it is easily checked before leaving the pharmacy. In many settings, technicians prepare unit-dose packaging under the supervision of a pharmacist.

The USP and state laws provide regulations for repackaging medications.

Many states follow USP guidelines, which require using the manufacturer's original expiration date or an expiration date no more than 12 months from the date the medication is repackaged, whichever is shorter. A repackaging log must be maintained, depending on state law, to track all repackaged medications back to their original manufacture and lot number.

Drugs must be stored according to the manufacturer's specifications.

Most drugs are kept in a fairly constant room temperature of 59°–86°F (and not below, unless stated by the manufacturer to do so). The storage room and drug shelves must have adequate ventilation and air distribution to allow for proper air flow around the medications.

Bar codes are used to quickly identify a product.

For most medications, the bar code includes the product's NDC number, which in turn identifies the product and package size. Many computer systems use the bar codes as a double check for pharmacists and technicians when filling prescriptions. Bar codes are also used in hospitals for Bedside Medication Verification (BMV): When administering a medication, a nurse scans his or her own bar-coded name badge, the patient's bar-coded arm band, and the medication bar code; the computer thus verifies that the correct medication is given to the patient.

PACKAGING

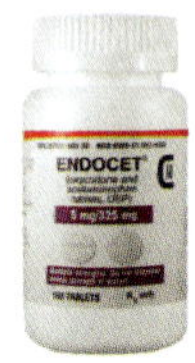

a bulk stock bottle

Unit-Dose Packaging

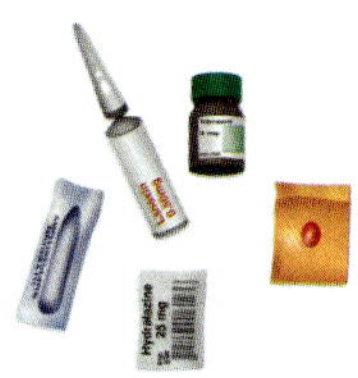

Unit-dose packaging can take many forms: plastic packs, vials, tubes, ampules, etc. Some are packaged in individual bubbles on cards containing 10 or more doses. Each unit-dose package contains the name of the drug, its strength, and the expiration date. All unit-dose containers must comply with USP requirements.

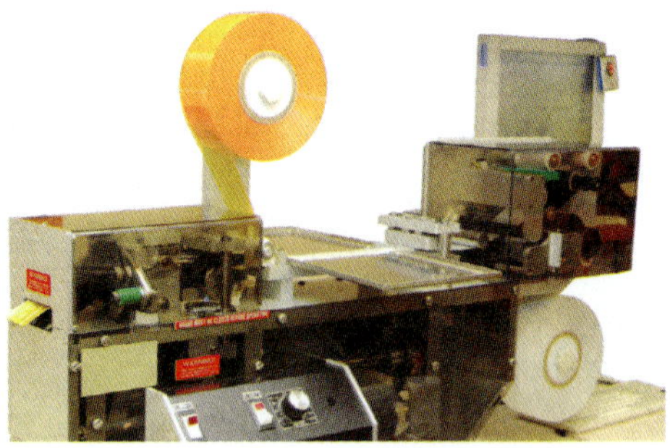

a unit-dose packaging machine

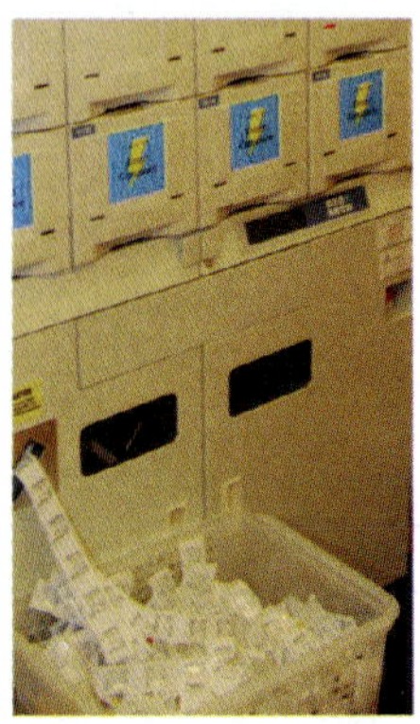

canister unit dose system

unit-dose packaging a package containing a single dose of a medication.

STORAGE

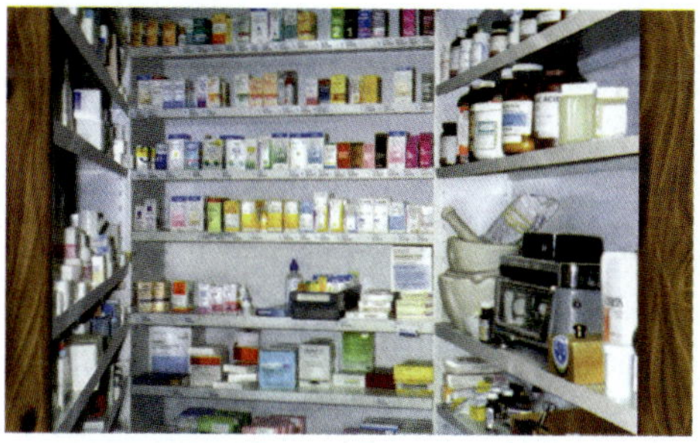

Physical Organization

Drugs can be organized by manufacturer and brand name or alphabetically by generic name. In alpha-generic organization, cimetidine and Tagamet®, for example, would be placed together.

Whatever the overall organization, the following basic guidelines should be met:

- ✔ Each medication should be organized such that the oldest items are dispensed first.
- ✔ Enough space should be provided to minimize breakage and to help prevent accidentally selecting the wrong medication.
- ✔ To help prevent errors, drugs with similar names should not be on the shelf next to each other. Example: Hydroxazine and Hydralazine.

Consignment Stock

Some high cost medications are on consignment, meaning the pharmacy does not pay for them until a patient purchases them. There is usually a higher price for these medications, but the consignment company carries the cost of the product until it is sold and is also financially responsible for any outdated drugs. These items need to be monitored closely to make sure the patient is charged correctly and also to prevent theft. Some facilities use RFI (Radio-Frequency Identification), a wireless technology that tracks movement from storage and automatically places reorders for these medications.

Controlled Substances

Schedule II–V substances can either be stocked separately in a locked cabinet or with noncontrolled drugs. Controlled substances stock must be continually monitored and documented. All records must be kept on hand for two years, unless state law requires a longer time frame.

Refrigeration

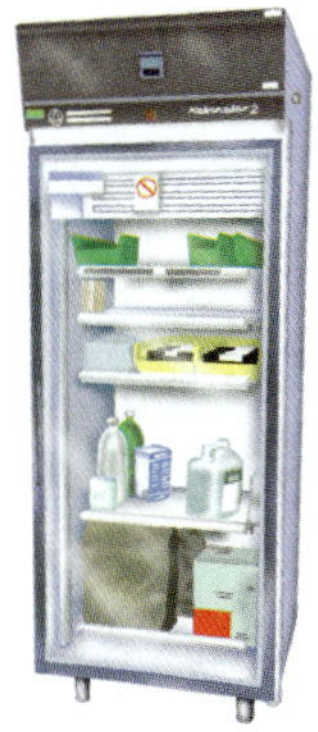

Some drugs must be stored at a constant temperature in a controlled commercial refrigerator or freezer designed for medications. These units have internal temperature gauges mounted on the outside for monitoring. Refrigeration temperatures should generally be 36°–46°F.

Refrigerators and freezers should be plugged into a wall receptacle that is marked for emergency use and will switch to emergency power generators if there is a power failure.

If refrigerated or frozen medications are left out for too long as per the corresponding literature, they may break down chemically and/or lose potency, and should be discarded.

Durable and Nondurable Equipment Supplies

Durable medical equipment (DME) includes items such as walkers, wheel chairs, crutches, and bedpans. Because these products are often bulky they are sometimes ordered on a next-day basis from wholesalers. In hospitals, these items are found in central supply or distribution departments.

Nondurable equipment includes items such as syringes, needles, and ostomy supplies.

Point-of-Use Stations

In hospitals and other settings, medications are stocked throughout the facility in dispensing units called supply stations or med-stations. Since they are at the point-of-use, they greatly simplify the dispensing of medications to patients.

Items stocked in these stations differ based upon the needs of the patients. For example, a station in an operating room would contain many anesthetics.

All withdrawals and restocks of stations are recorded just as they would be from a central dispensary. Some stations may be linked to the facility's computing system so that inventory information is automatically communicated.

REVIEW

KEY CONCEPTS

INVENTORY MANAGEMENT

- ✔ Good inventory management ensures that drugs that are likely to be needed are both on hand and usable—that is, not expired, damaged, contaminated, or otherwise unfit for use.
- ✔ An open formulary is one that allows purchase of any medication that is prescribed. A closed formulary is a limited list of approved medications.
- ✔ Formularies must be routinely reviewed to evaluate newer products as well as safety profiles for current medications.
- ✔ More than three-quarters of pharmaceutical manufacturers' sales are directly to drug wholesalers, which in turn resell their inventory to hospitals, pharmacies, and other pharmaceutical dispensers.

INVENTORY SYSTEMS

- ✔ A perpetual inventory system maintains a continuous record of every item in inventory so that it always shows the stock on hand.
- ✔ Turnover is the rate at which inventory is used.
- ✔ Pharmacy operations generally use a point-of-sale system in which the item is deducted from inventory as it is sold or dispensed.
- ✔ Drug reorder points are maximum and minimum inventory levels for each drug.
- ✔ Important reports (especially purchase orders) should be regularly printed out and filed as hard copy both for convenience and as a backup record-keeping system.

COMPUTERS AND INVENTORY

- ✔ Pharmacy computer files must be regularly backed up or copied to an appropriate storage media.
- ✔ In a computerized inventory system, orders can be generated using an order entry device or automatically generated by the system based on stock levels and reorder points.

ORDERING

- ✔ In an online ordering system, if an order can be filled as ordered, a message from the supplier will automatically confirm the order to the ordering system. The system automatically assigns to each order a purchase order number for identification.
- ✔ Schedule II substances require a special order form for reordering.
- ✔ Controlled substances are shipped separately and should be checked in by a pharmacist.
- ✔ Material Safety Data Sheets (MSDS) for hazardous substances such as chemotherapeutic agents indicate when special handling and shipping is required.
- ✔ Good ordering practices assign separate personnel for ordering and receiving steps or processes.

STOCKING AND STORING

- ✔ Most medications are received from the supplier in bulk stock bottles.
- ✔ Drugs must be stored according to manufacturer's specifications.
- ✔ Most drugs are kept in a fairly constant room temperature of 59°–86° F. The temperature of refrigeration should generally be 36°–46°F.

STOCKING AND STORING (cont'd)

✔ Schedule II substances may be stocked separately or with regular stock; their stock must be continually monitored and documented.

✔ Medications should be organized in a way that will dispense the oldest items first.

✔ In hospitals and other settings, medications are stocked in dispensing units throughout the facility that may be called supply stations or automated dispensing machines.

SELF-TEST

the answer key begins on page 569

MATCH THE TERMS

1. automated dispensing machine _____
2. closed formulary _____
3. database _____
4. formulary _____
5. inventory _____
6. Material Safety Data Sheets (MSDS) _____
7. open formulary _____
8. perpetual inventory _____
9. point-of-sale system (POS) _____
10. purchase order number ____
11. reorder points _____
12. therapeutic equivalent ____
13. turnover _____
14. unit-dose packaging _____

a. a system that allows purchase of any medication that is prescribed.
b. a limited list of approved medications.
c. the rate at which inventory is used, generally expressed in number of days.
d. an inventory system in which the item is deducted from inventory as it is sold or dispensed.
e. minimum and maximum stock levels that determine when a reorder is placed and for how much.
f. a collection of information structured so that specific information within it can easily be retrieved and used.
g. OSHA required notices that provide hazard, handling, clean-up, and first aid information.
h. identification number assigned to orders.
i. a package containing a single dose of a medication.
j. a system that maintains a continuous record of every item in inventory so that it always shows the stock on hand.
k. a list of goods or items a business uses in its normal operations.
l. pharmaceutical equivalents that produce the same effects in patients.
m. a system in which medications are dispensed at their point of use upon confirmation of an order communicated from a centralized computer system.
n. a list of medications approved for use.

REVIEW

CHOOSE THE BEST ANSWER

1. A goal of inventory management is
   a. to ensure that drugs are available when they are needed.
   b. to maintain MSDS sheets.
   c. to develop closed formularies.
   d. to increase use of wholesalers.

2. A list of the goods or items a business will use in its normal operation is called a(an)
   a. purchase order.
   b. inventory.
   c. open formulary.
   d. closed formulary.

3. In an open formulary, when a medication is ordered that is not on the formulary
   a. the medication may be ordered without obtaining additional permission.
   b. the patient must obtain the medication at another pharmacy.
   c. the physician must first receive permission to use the medication.
   d. the pharmacist is required to choose a therapeutic equivalent.

4. Formulary medications are routinely reviewed to
   a. add more of the same product.
   b. review safety of older products and evaluate newer products.
   c. make room on the shelves.
   d. add a product upon request of the manufacturer.

5. A therapeutically equivalent drug is
   a. chemically the same.
   b. chemically different but with similar actions and effects.
   c. the generic version of a trade drug.
   d. a drug that a physician must get approval to use.

6. Wholesalers that provide medications to hospitals, pharmacies, and other medication dispensers account for about __________ of pharmaceutical manufacturers' sales.
   a. half
   b. one-quarter
   c. three-quarters
   d. one-third

7. As an expiration date approaches, the pharmacy technician should be aware that it must be ____________ before the expiration date passes.
   a. returned to the manufacturer for credit
   b. dispensed
   c. used
   d. returned to the wholesaler for credit

8. Proper disposal or destruction of nonreturnable medications includes
   a. placement in regular trash.
   b. flushing down sink or water system.
   c. using a company that meets EPA regulations.
   d. selling the medications at a discount.

9. If a supplier's terms are 30 days net,
   a. it would be best to have a turnover less than 30 days.
   b. it would be best to have a turnover equal to 30 days.
   c. it would be best to have a turnover greater than 30 days.
   d. none of the above.

10. "Fast Movers" account for approximately what percent of a pharmacy's orders and prescriptions?
    a. 5%
    b. 30%
    c. 40%
    d. 80%

11. The 340B Drug Pricing program is
    a. a purchasing program open to any store.
    b. a purchasing program for qualified clinics and hospitals.
    c. a subsection of the DEA concerning diversion.
    d. NDC numbers associated with retail pharmacy.

12. ______________________ is an inventory system in which the item is deducted from inventory as it is sold or dispensed.
    a. Point-of-sale system
    b. Turnover
    c. Automated reports
    d. Reorder point system

13. Minimum and maximum stock levels used to determine when a reorder is placed and for how much are
    a. reorder points.
    b. automatic ordering.
    c. POS.
    d. turnovers.

14. A generic term used for computerized medication dispensing machines used in hospitals is a/an
    a. ADM.
    b. CART.
    c. Pyxis®.
    d. PAR.

15. Checking of order reports to ensure the order contains no gross errors is done
    a. by computer.
    b. manually.
    c. by the corporate office.
    d. by the wholesaler.

16. All of the following are used to store medications except
    a. automated dispensing machines.
    b. carousels.
    c. glove boxes.
    d. Pyxis® machines.

17. Best practices for ordering medications include
    a. having the same person place the order and check it in.
    b. having different people place the order and check it in.
    c. having the pharmacy manager check in all products.
    d. having anyone available place and receive orders.

18. Material Safety Data Sheets (MSDS) provide
    a. protocols for fire hazards in the pharmacy setting.
    b. safety codes by OSHA in the storage of inventory.
    c. information concerning hazardous substances.
    d. none of the above.

19. Safe handling of chemotherapy medications can be found in a publication by
    a. the DEA.
    b. TJC.
    c. SAFRX.
    d. NIOSH.

20. In receiving an order, it is important to be alert for drugs that have been incorrectly picked, received damaged, are outdated, or missing, so orders are reconciled
    a. once per month.
    b. item by item.
    c. every two years.
    d. once per year.

REVIEW

21. When reconciling an order, if a technician detects discrepancies, the supplier should be notified
    a. immediately.
    b. before the end of the current reporting period.
    c. before the end of the month.
    d. before the end of the week.

22. A purchase order number is
    a. a number that is used to identify the pharmacy.
    b. is the same on all orders from a given pharmacy.
    c. is assigned by the FDA.
    d. a number used to identify an order.

23. Hard copies of order reports
    a. are only needed if there is a computer failure.
    b. are not needed since everything is on the computer.
    c. are kept for an established amount of time for business and legal reasons.
    d. are only needed if there is a power failure.

24. Most drugs are kept at room temperature between
    a. 36°–46°F.
    b. 33°–45°C.
    c. 59°–86°F.
    d. 33°–45°F.

25. A bar code on a manufacturer's product
    a. indicates the medication's price.
    b. ensures the patient receives the correct medication.
    c. keeps count of the medications stocked.
    d. includes the product's NDC number.

26. A package that contains a single dose of a medication is called a(an)
    a. MSDS package.
    b. single-use package.
    c. POS package.
    d. unit-dose package.

27. In an alpha-generic organization, drugs are stored alphabetically by
    a. generic name with corresponding trade versions placed next to the generic drug.
    b. trade name with the corresponding generic version placed next to it.
    c. manufacturer.
    d. drug classification.

28. Consignment stock is:
    a. stock purchased by the pharmacy at a discount.
    b. medications ordered through the GPO.
    c. durable medical equipment.
    d. items stocked in the pharmacy not paid for until used or dispensed to a patient.

29. How would a pharmacy technician store controlled substances?
    a. Only in locked areas.
    b. Stored in locked areas or within the regular stock.
    c. Stored in one location within the pharmacy on an open shelf.
    d. Only in computerized inventory machines.

30. The temperature of a refrigerator in a pharmacy should generally be
    a. 36°–46°F.
    b. 28°–32°C.
    c. 36°–46°C.
    d. 28°–32°F.

31. An example of durable medical equipment (DME) could be
    a. ostomy supplies.
    b. crutches.
    c. syringes.
    d. antiseptics.

CRITICAL THINKING QUESTIONS

1. You find a medication on the shelf and realize it should be refrigerated. What do you do with the drug?
2. You notice no special procedures are followed while a coworker is checking in a C-II medication. What should you do?
3. You are told to place the drug order for the day. Should you just order whatever the pharmacist has used for the day?

THINKING IT THROUGH WRAP-UP

1. Checking in the order is done electronically using a device that scans the bar code on each product to verify it was ordered by the pharmacy. You need to notify the wholesaler of any errors. Depending on the wholesaler's policies, you may need to call in the problem or fax a copy of the invoice documenting the problem. The wholesaler will then check their system to see if perhaps the item was manually pulled and missed by their system.
2. As you stock each item, verify that the correct product is in the correct place on the shelf, that it is in-date, and that it is undamaged. Remove any outdated or soon-to-be outdated medication. Put the newer stock in back of the older stock so that the oldest stock is pulled first.
3. The minimum and maximum values for each item in the pharmacy should be reviewed while putting the order together. Any seasonal changes should also be considered to adjust the order amount, such as with Tamiflu® during flu season.
4. Follow these steps: 1) Scan the shelf sticker for the drugs at or below the minimum. 2) Transmit the order to the wholesaler or warehouse. 3) Note any shortages and try to find an alternative.

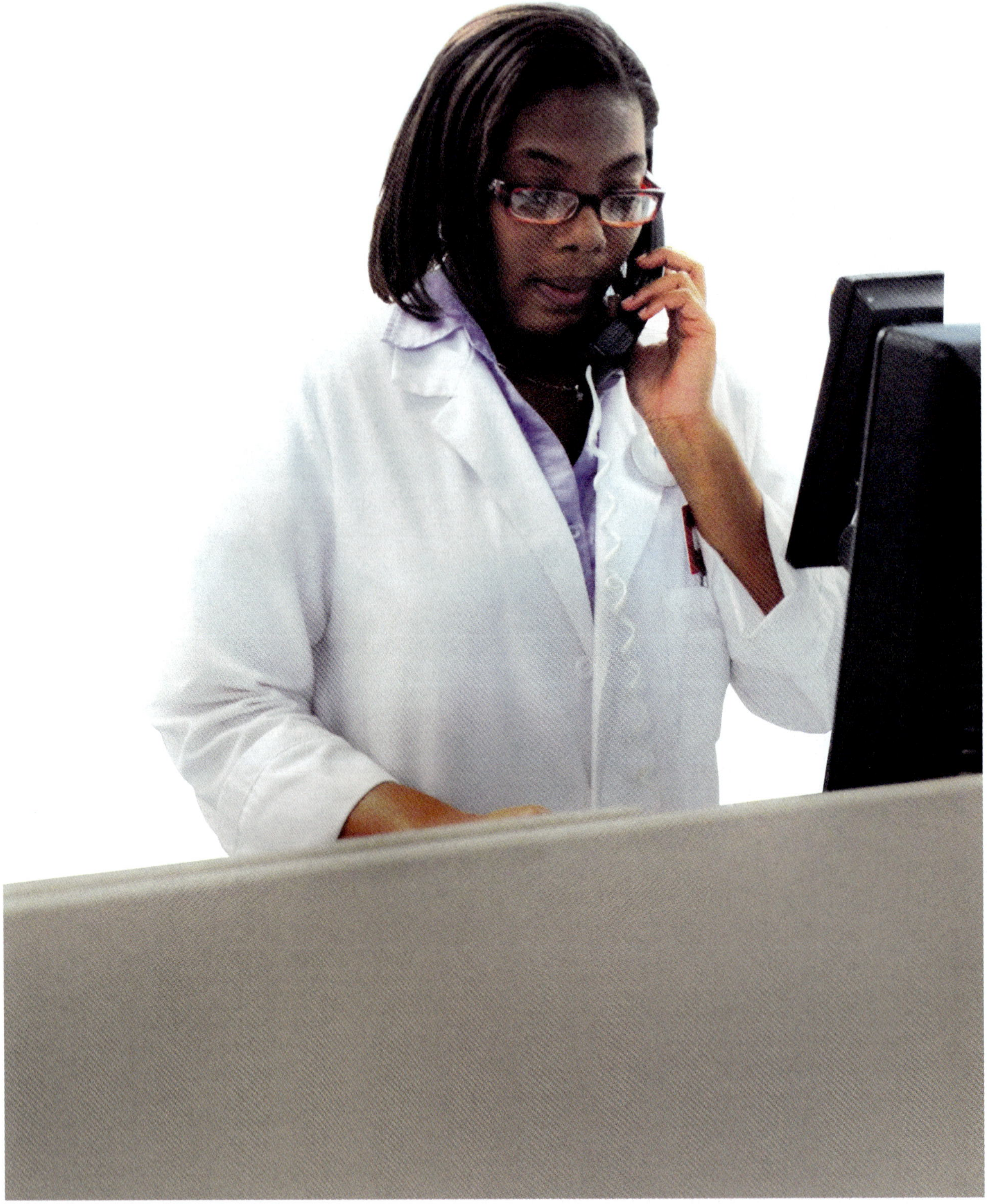

14

FINANCIAL ISSUES

LEARNING OBJECTIVES

At the completion of study, the student will:

- ✔ describe how medication prices have changed over time.
- ✔ describe the role of third-party programs and pharmacy benefit managers in pharmacy.
- ✔ compare different types of managed care programs: HMOs, POSs, and PPOs.
- ✔ define Medicare and Medicaid.
- ✔ describe online adjudication.
- ✔ explain how a pharmacy technician can resolve rejected third-party claims.
- ✔ describe billing procedures for Medication Therapy Management services.

THINKING IT THROUGH

In her job as a pharmacy technician at a community pharmacy, Jennifer has worked with patients who have a variety of types of third-party insurance coverage for their prescriptions: Some patients are covered through an HMO; some are covered through their employers as well as workers' compensation; some are covered through Medicaid; and others have coverage through Medicare.

As you read this chapter, consider the following questions:

1. How does an HMO differ from other types of managed care programs?
2. What are the differences between Medicaid and Medicare?
3. What types of medications can be billed through workers' compensation?

FINANCIAL ISSUES

Financial issues have a substantial influence on health care and pharmacy practice.

In 1985, the average prescription price was approximately \$10. By 2011 the average prescription price was \$84, the average brand-name retail price was \$268, and the average generic price was \$33. The increase is due to a number of reasons, including inflation and the aging of the population. It is also due to the use of new medications that enhance the quality of health care, but which are often costly.

The use of third-party programs to pay for prescriptions has also increased dramatically.

Third-party programs are simply another party besides the patient or the pharmacy that pays for some or all of the cost of medication: essentially, an insurer. Most people have some form of public or private health insurance. These include both public programs such as Medicaid and Medicare and private programs such as HMOs and basic health insurance. Many but not all such programs include prescription drug coverage. While the growth of these programs is largely a response to the rising costs of health care, in many cases third-party programs allow patients to benefit from new and often more expensive drug therapies than they would otherwise be able to afford.

Because of the pharmacy technician's role in the prescription filling process, he or she must understand the different types of health insurance and how drug benefits differ among the programs.

A patient's prescription drug program determines important considerations for filling their prescription. Generic substitution may be required. There may be limits on the quantity dispensed (tablets, capsules, etc.) per fill, or on the frequency and number of refills, and so on.

PHARMACY BENEFIT MANAGERS

Regardless of how the claims are submitted and processed, participating pharmacies must sign contracts with insurers or pharmacy benefit managers before patients can get their prescriptions filled at that pharmacy and billed to their insurer or pharmacy benefit manager. A ***pharmacy benefit manager (PBM)*** is a company that administers drug benefit programs. Many insurance companies, HMOs, and self-insured employers use the services of more than 50 PBMs to manage drug benefit coverage for employees and health-plan members. The following are the names of some pharmacy benefit managers (PBMs).

- Argus
- Catamaran
- Cigna Healthcare
- CVS/Caremark
- Express Scripts
- Humana Pharmacy Solutions
- MedImpact
- SXC

co-insurance an agreement for cost-sharing between the insurer and the insured.

co-pay the portion of the price of medication that the patient is required to pay.

dual co-pay co-pays that have two prices: one for generic and one for brand medications.

maximum allowable cost (MAC) the maximum price per tablet (or other dispensing unit) an insurer or PBM will pay for a given product.

online adjudication the resolution of prescription coverage through the communication of the pharmacy computer with the third-party computer.

pharmacy benefit managers companies that administer drug benefit programs.

U&C or UCR the maximum amount of payment for a given prescription, determined by the insurer to be a usual and customary (and reasonable) price.

COMPUTERS AND THIRD-PARTY BILLING

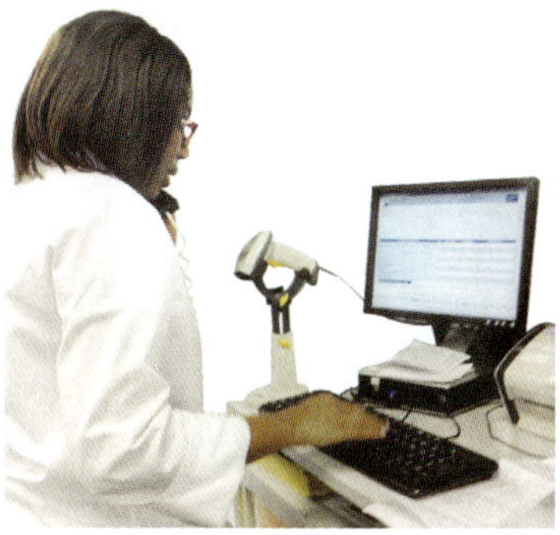

Procedures used by pharmacies to submit third-party claims vary. Most insurers or pharmacy benefit managers mail checks to pharmacies (or their accounts receivable departments) at regular intervals along with listings of the prescriptions covered and those not covered (i.e., rejected).

Before the computer age, prescriptions were billed to third parties using paper claims. Although paper claims are still used, most claims are now filed electronically by online claim submission and ***online adjudication*** of claims. This electronic submission and adjudication process benefits both third-party programs as well as pharmacies. The online communication between the prescription-filling computer in the pharmacy and the claim-processing computer of the insurer or pharmacy benefit manager results in improved accuracy and control. It is also much faster and more direct than processing paper claims. The benefits of computerizing the claims process have also been a factor in the rise of third-party programs.

CO-PAYS

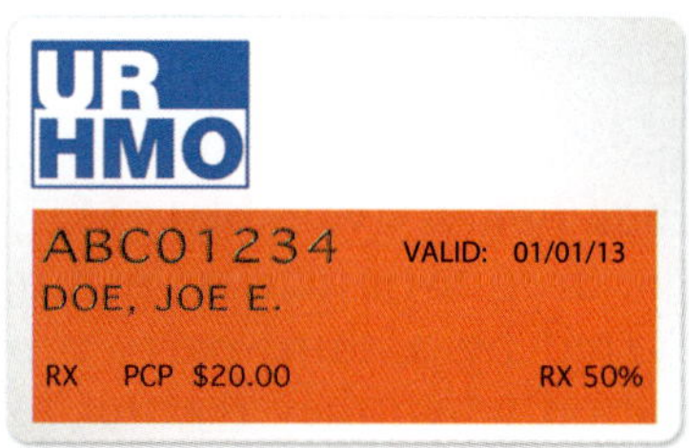

One of the common aspects of many third-party programs is ***co-insurance***, which is essentially an agreement between the insurer and the insured to share costs. One aspect of this is the requirement for the patient to ***co-pay*** for the filled prescription. That is, the patient must pay a portion of the price of the medication and the insurance company is billed for the remainder.

The amount paid by the insurer is not equal to the retail price normally charged, but is determined by a formula described in a contract between the insurer and the pharmacy. There is a ***maximum allowable cost (MAC)*** per tablet or other dispensing unit that an insurer or PBM will pay for a given product. This is often determined by survey of the ***usual and customary (U&C)*** prices for a prescription within a given geographic area. This is also referred to as the ***UCR (usual, customary, and reasonable)*** price for the prescription.

Many third-party plans have ***dual co-pays***, which means that a lower co-pay applies to prescriptions filled with generic drugs and a higher co-pay applies to prescriptions filled with brand name drugs that have no generic equivalent. Some plans have three different co-pays: The lowest co-pay applies to prescriptions filled with tier one drugs that are usually generics; a higher co-pay applies to prescriptions usually filled with brand name drugs from a listing of tier two drugs; and a third higher co-pay applies to brand name drugs from a listing of tier three drugs.

THIRD-PARTY PROGRAMS

PRIVATE HEALTH INSURANCE

Basic private health insurance policies may pay for prescribed expenses (such as prescriptions) when the patient is covered by a supplementary comprehensive major medical policy or when the patient's coverage includes an additional prescription drug benefit. Patients covered by comprehensive major medical policies pay out-of-pocket for their prescriptions. Once a *deductible* is met, the insurer may pay a portion of the cost of prescriptions filled the rest of the year. In other words, once a patient has paid a certain dollar amount for prescribed medical expenses (usually including prescriptions), the insurance company will reimburse a portion of the cost of filled prescriptions for the rest of the year. Whether or not a patient is required to get generic drugs when they are available is determined by individual plans and may not be obvious before filling the prescription. Major medical claims frequently involve paper claims. However, the use of electronic claim processing for major medical claims is growing.

Prescription Drug Coverage

Some traditional health insurance policies have the added benefit of prescription drug coverage. Patients with prescription drug coverage through a private insurance company are issued *prescription drug benefit cards* to carry in their wallets. These cards contain necessary billing information for pharmacies, including the patient's identification number, group number, and co-pay amount.

As with other prescription plans, there may be various types of co-pays and patients may be required to get generic drugs (when available). Many third-party programs for prescription drugs have drug formularies. A drug *formulary* is a list of medications that are covered by a third-party program; patients are given their formulary information when they register for benefits. Additionally, some third-party programs have different *tiers,* or categories, of drugs with corresponding differences in co-pays, depending on which tier a specific drug is in.

Most prescription claims are processed through online adjudication: the pharmacy computer communicates with the insurer's or PBM's computer to determine the prescription drug benefit. When the claim is adjudicated or processed by the insurer or pharmacy benefit manager it becomes obvious if generic substitution is mandatory.

deductible a set amount that must be paid by the patient for each benefit period before the insurer will cover additional expenses.

formulary a list of medications covered by third-party plans.

prescription drug benefit cards cards that contain third-party billing information for prescription drug purchases.

tier categories of medications that are covered by third-party plans.

MANAGED CARE PROGRAMS

Managed care programs include health maintenance organizations (HMOs), point-of-service programs (POS), and preferred provider organizations (PPOs). Managed care programs provide all necessary medical services (usually including prescription coverage) in return for a monthly premium and co-pays. Most managed care prescription drug plans require generic substitution when a generic is available. Some managed care plans have single co-pays, some have dual co-pays, and some have three types of co-pays.

HMOs are made of a network of providers who are either employed by the HMO or have signed contracts to abide by the policies of the HMO. HMOs usually will not cover expenses incurred outside their participating network. HMOs often require generic substitution.

POS programs are made of a network of providers contracted by the insurer. Patients enrolled in a POS choose a primary care physician (PCP) who is a provider in the insurer's network. Patients may receive care outside of the POS network, but the primary care physician is required to make referrals for such care. POSs often partially reimburse expenses incurred outside of their network. POSs usually require generic substitution.

PPOs are also a network of providers contracted by the insurer. Of the managed care options, PPOs offer the most flexibility for their members. PPOs often partially reimburse expenses incurred outside of their participating network and do not require a primary care physician within their network to make referrals. PPOs usually require generic substitution.

Patients with prescription drug coverage through managed care organizations are issued prescription drug benefit cards with billing and co-pay information. Most claims for these programs are processed through online adjudication. Many HMOs, POSs, and PPOs use pharmacy benefit managers (PBMs) to manage drug benefit coverage.

HMO a network of providers for which costs are covered inside but not outside of the network.

POS a network of providers where the patient's primary care physician must be a member and costs outside the network may be partially reimbursed.

PPO a network of providers where costs outside the network may be partially reimbursed and the patient's primary care physician need not be a member.

THIRD-PARTY PROGRAMS (cont'd)

PUBLIC HEALTH INSURANCE

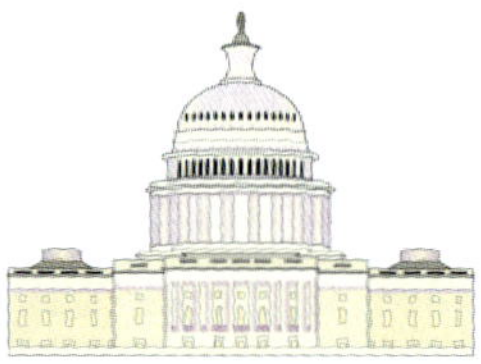

The largest public health insurance plans in the United States are Medicare and Medicaid.

Medicare is a federal program covering people aged 65 and over, as well as disabled people under age 65 and people with kidney failure. Medicare Part A basically covers inpatient hospital expenses for patients who meet certain conditions, and it may also cover some hospice expenses. Medicare Part B basically covers doctors' services as well as some other medical services that are not covered by Part A. Medicare beneficiaries who pay a monthly premium for this medical coverage are covered by Medicare Part B.

Medicare beneficiaries may enroll in the Medicare Prescription Drug Plan, also known as Medicare Part D. This plan requires participants to pay a monthly premium and also meet certain deductibles and co-payments. Medicare beneficiaries that do not participate in the Medicare Prescription Drug Plan may have prescription drug coverage through a current or former employer. Some Medicare beneficiaries may not have any prescription drug coverage if they do not participate in either the Medicare Drug Plan or a prescription drug plan from a current or previous employer. Furthermore, some Medicare beneficiaries may qualify for Medication Therapy Management (MTM) services provided by pharmacists.

Medicaid is a federal–state program for eligible individuals and families with low incomes. State welfare departments usually operate Medicaid. Each state decides who is eligible for Medicaid benefits and what services will be covered. A prescription drug formulary is a listing of the drugs that are covered by Medicaid. Prescription drug formularies for Medicaid recipients are determined by each state. Medicaid programs do not automatically cover drugs that are not on the state formulary. Completion of a prior authorization form is sometimes required to justify the need for a medication that is not on the state Medicaid formulary; however, completion of the form does not imply the drug will be covered. Medicaid recipients can also qualify for HMO programs.

Medicaid a federal–state program, administered by the states, providing health care for the needy.

Medicare a federal program providing health care to people with certain disabilities or who are over age 65; it includes basic hospital insurance, voluntary medical insurance, and voluntary prescription drug insurance.

patient assistance programs manufacturer sponsored prescription drug programs for the needy.

workers' compensation an employer compensation program for employees accidentally injured on the job.

OTHER PROGRAMS

Workers' Compensation

In the United States, the federal government and every state have enacted *workers' compensation* laws. Under workers' compensation legislation, procedures for compensation for employees accidentally injured on-the-job are established. Administrative guidelines require that accidents be reported to a public board that grants compensation awards to injured workers.

In recent years, state workers' compensation programs have been broadened to provide for coverage of occupational diseases. Prescriptions related to the occupational injury or disease can be billed to the state's bureau of workers' compensation or to the employer (if the employer is self-insured). Many workers' compensation claims can be processed through online adjudication. However, some claims require paper claims. It is important to realize the billing procedure can be slightly different for self-insured claims. Pharmacy benefit managers (PBMs) may administer workers' compensation prescription drug benefits.

Patient Assistance Programs

Patient assistance programs are programs offered by some pharmaceutical manufacturers to help needy patients who require medication they cannot afford and do not have insurance coverage. Patient assistance programs require patients and their physicians to complete applications and submit them to the pharmaceutical manufacturer offering the program. Patients who qualify for patient assistance programs are often given cards issued by pharmacy benefit managers.

COORDINATION OF BENEFITS

Many households with two adults who are spouses or domestic partners have two different health insurance plans. A growing number of employers are requiring both adults to subscribe to the health insurance plans that are available, which could result in the adults as well as any dependent children having coverage on two different plans. When this happens, there is need for coordination of benefits.

Coordination of benefits allows for patients to have maximum coverage for health-care expenses through both health insurance plans. The rules for coordination of benefits ensure that the benefit coverage for a claim does not exceed 100% of the total cost. An example of coordination of benefits in pharmacy is if one pharmacy benefit plan is billed for a prescription and a second pharmacy benefit plan is billed for the co-pay or coinsurance.

ONLINE ADJUDICATION

In online adjudication, the technician uses the computer to determine the appropriate third-party's exact coverage for each prescription. The pharmacy computer communicates with the insurer's or pharmacy benefit manager's computer to determine this. Most community pharmacy computer programs are designed so the prescription label does not print until confirmation of payment is received from the insurer or PBM.

THE ONLINE PROCESS

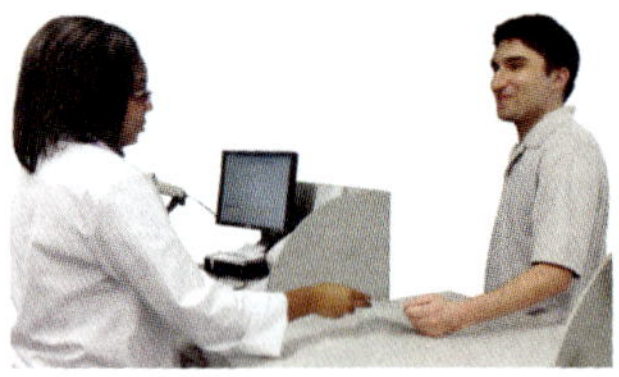

While non-patient information (NPI number, prices, co-pay, etc.) is provided by the computer system, it is generally the pharmacy technician's responsibility to obtain the patient, prescription, and billing information. In a typical community pharmacy, a patient presents a prescription (and often a prescription drug card) to a technician who must then obtain all of the patient and billing information required to enter the prescription and claim. If the patient has had prescriptions filled previously at the pharmacy, much of this information will be in the system already (though it is important for the technician to verify that this information is still correct).

Photos courtesy Dell, Inc.

Once the necessary information is obtained, the pharmacy technician enters it into the pharmacy computer. Billing information for the prescription is then transmitted to a processing computer for the insurer or PBM. If all information has been entered correctly and is in agreement with data on file with the insurer, the prescription claim is processed using online adjudication and an online response is received in less than one minute in the pharmacy. The claim-processing computer instantly determines the dollar amount of the drug benefit and the appropriate co-pay.

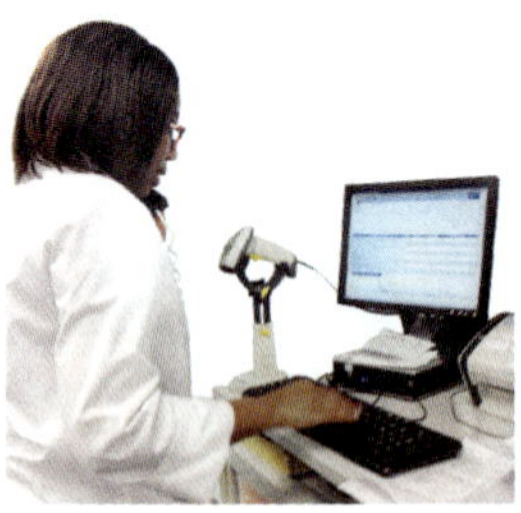

The pharmacy technician usually has an opportunity to review the data provided by the claim-processing computer before giving the OK for the prescription label and receipt to print in the pharmacy. The receipt indicates how much of the price of the prescription the patient must pay as determined by the insurer. The prescription can then be filled. The pharmacy technician should carefully review this adjudication information before proceeding to make sure the claim was processed properly. The pharmacy may be underpaid if the drug dispensed has a generic equivalent. The pharmacy technician should also look for claim processing messages such as drug or disease interaction alerts.

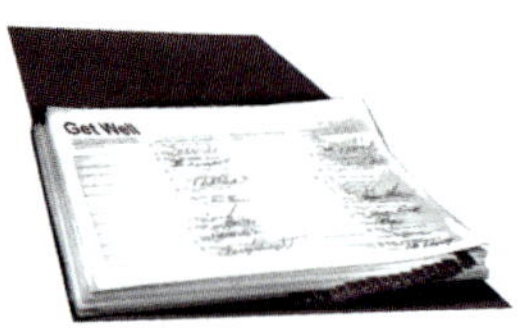

When prescriptions are billed online, pharmacies must keep records to verify that prescriptions were actually dispensed. Insurers or PBMs require pharmacies to maintain hard copies of each prescription that must be readily retrievable upon request. Insurers or PBMs also require pharmacies to maintain signature logs for all claims submitted electronically that must be readily retrievable upon request.

ONLINE CLAIM INFORMATION

Although there are many different types of health-care insurance, the information required for online processing of claims is remarkably similar. The following information is usually required for online claim processing:

- cardholder identification number
- group number (a number assigned by the insurer to the employer of the cardholder)
- name of patient
- birth date
- sex (M or F)
- relationship to cardholder, i.e., cardholder (C), spouse (S), dependent (D), other (O)
- date Rx written
- date Rx dispensed
- is this a new or refill prescription
- national drug code (NDC) of drug
- DAW indicator
- amount or quantity dispensed
- days supply
- identification number of prescribing physician
- identification of the pharmacy/National Provider Identifier (NPI)
- ingredient cost
- dispensing fee
- total price
- deductible or co-pay amount
- balance due

Dispense As Written (DAW)

When entering patient and prescription information, it is important to verify whether the patient's plan covers the brand name of a particular drug or if the patient is required to get generic drugs. When brand name drugs are dispensed, numbers corresponding to the reason for submitting the claim with brand name drugs are entered in a DAW (Dispense as Written) indicator field. Most health plan members have a choice between brand and generic drugs.

The following lists DAW indicators.

0 No DAW (No Dispense As Written)
1 DAW handwritten on the prescription by the prescriber
2 Patient requested brand
3 Pharmacist selected brand
4 Generic not in stock
5 Brand name dispensed but priced as generic
6 N/A
7 Substitution not allowed; brand mandated by law
8 Generic not available
9 Other

In some programs, if a patient receives a brand name drug when a generic is available, the patient must pay the difference between the cost of the brand and the cost of the generic.

Rx tip

Billing special medications such as compounded prescriptions requires somewhat different procedures. These procedures are different for each insurer or PBM. When billing compounded medications or special medications the pharmacy technician should refer to informational booklets provided to the pharmacy by the insurer or PBM or call the pharmacy help desk as listed on the prescription drug card.

REJECTED CLAIMS

In the online adjudication process, the insurer sometimes rejects the claim as submitted.

This occurs before the prescription is dispensed and provides an opportunity to resolve the problem before it becomes larger. There are various reasons for rejections, and most problems can be resolved by telephoning a representative of the insurer or discussing the rejection with the patient. Rejections are best resolved during normal business hours.

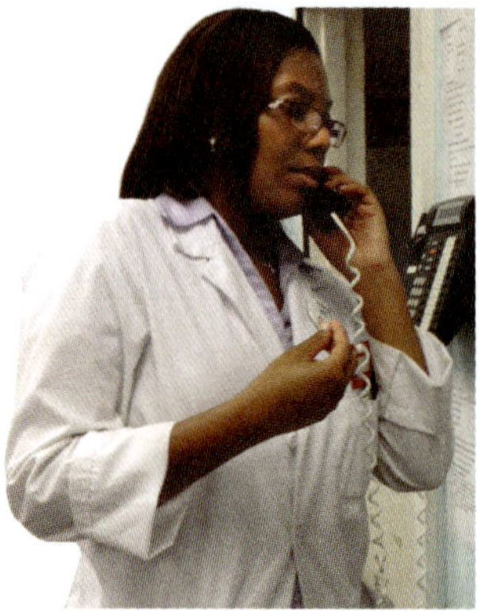

Resolving Rejections

When there is a question on coverage, the pharmacy technician can telephone the insurance plan's pharmacy help desk to determine if the patient is eligible for coverage. Pharmacy help desk personnel are often very helpful in resolving problems. If an employer has changed insurers, sometimes pharmacy help desk personnel can advise the pharmacy technician who the new insurer is. Many pharmacies maintain a list of phone numbers for insurers and their processors. If the prescription drug card is not available, the pharmacy technician can obtain the phone number of the insurer from this list.

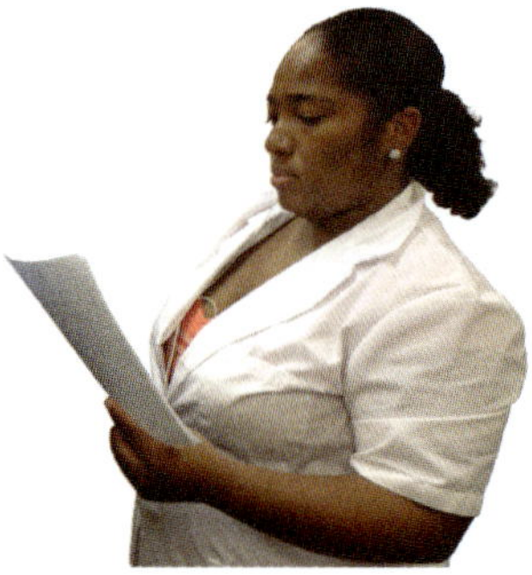

Handling Paper Claim Rejects

When paper claims are rejected by third parties, rejections often do not appear for several weeks after the claim was submitted. Rejections of paper claims are almost always accompanied by an explanation of the rejection and give details on what the technician can do to obtain successful payment of the claim. In many cases, the paper claim form was not completed correctly, information is missing, and the technician needs to only complete the missing information and resubmit the claim. Sometimes a telephone call must be made to the patient and/or the insurer to resolve the problem.

COMMON REASONS FOR THIRD-PARTY CLAIM REJECTIONS

Dependent exceeds plan's age limit

Many prescription drug plans have age limitations for children or dependents of the cardholder. Often, full-time college students are eligible for coverage as long as appropriate paperwork is on file with the insurer.

Invalid birth date

The birth date submitted by the pharmacy sometimes does not match the birth date in the insurer's computer. To solve this problem, first double-check that you have the correct birth date for the patient.

Invalid person code

The person code (e.g., 00,01,02,03) does not match the person code for the patient with the same sex and birth date information in the insurer's computer.

Invalid sex

The sex (M or F) submitted by the pharmacy does not match the sex in the insurer's computer for the patient. To solve this problem, change the sex code (if M change to F) and resubmit the claim.

Prescriber is not a network provider

This type of reject is common to Medicaid programs and is sometimes seen with HMO programs. Simply stated, only prescriptions issued by network prescribers are covered by the insurer.

Unable to connect with insurer's computer

Sometimes, due to computer problems, an insurer's computer may be unavailable for claim processing. If this happens, the technician must follow their employer's guidelines.

Patient not covered (coverage terminated)

This can occur when a patient has a new insurance card, whether the new card is issued by the same insurer or a new one. If the insurer has not changed, perhaps billing numbers have changed (new cardholder identification number, group number, etc.).

Refill too soon

Most third-party plans require that most of the medication has been taken before the plan will cover another dispensing of the same medication. Early refills should always be brought to the attention of the pharmacist. If the pharmacist thinks it is appropriate to dispense a refill early (for example, if a patient is going on vacation), the next step is to contact the insurer to determine if it will pay for an early refill.

Refills not covered

Many managed care health programs require mail order pharmacies to fill prescriptions for maintenance medications. Patients often are not aware of mail order requirements of their prescription drug coverage. Ideally, the employer is responsible to explain mail order requirements if their employees are required to use mail order for maintenance medications. Sometimes, patients do not realize this restriction until prescription claims are rejected at their community pharmacy. In such cases, the pharmacy technician will have to contact the insurer to determine if emergency refills are covered at the community pharmacy.

NDC not covered

This type of rejection is common with state Medicaid programs and managed care programs with closed formularies. Ideally, the patient is aware that the insurer has a limited formulary for prescription drug coverage. However, often patients are not aware of how this works. The pharmacy technician can call the pharmacy help desk for specific information about drug coverage. Sometimes, the insurer will consider prior authorization to cover medications that are not on the formulary. Sometimes, the insurer will not cover the prescribed medication and a pharmacist may determine what should be done next.

OTHER BILLING PROCEDURES

PAPER CLAIMS FOR BILLING PRESCRIPTIONS

Processing paper claims usually involves the pharmacy and the patient completing a form that has been issued by the insurer. Most insurers require completion of a form that they provide. A ***universal claim form (UCF)*** is a standardized form accepted by many insurers. Before online claim submission, most pharmacy third-party claims were submitted on universal claim forms. Instructions for completing paper claims (insurer provided forms as well as universal claim forms) are printed on the claim forms so that anyone can complete the forms as long as they have access to the required information. Usually there is a requirement for signature by the patient and the pharmacist or health-care provider. Incomplete forms or forms that have not been completed following directions printed on the forms are returned to the pharmacy for correction before the insurer will consider paying the claim. Generally, the same type of information required for online claims is also required for paper claim processing.

IN-HOUSE BILLING PROCEDURES

Pharmacy billing is not limited to billing insurers. Some pharmacies have in-house billing procedures. For example, the finances of an elderly or disabled patient may be handled by a family member or legal representative who does not live with the patient. In these cases, a monthly bill is mailed to the family member or legal representative, who then pays the pharmacy. Most pharmacies do not have in-house billing. When a pharmacy does do in-house billing, the pharmacy technician must carefully follow the policies and procedures of the employer.

DISEASE STATE MANAGEMENT SERVICES

Disease state management services are evolving as a component of pharmaceutical care. PBMs are selling disease management services to employers and health plans. Conditions most often targeted for disease state management include diabetes, hypertension, asthma, smoking cessation, and cholesterol management.

Both electronic and paper billing systems can be used for billing disease state management services; however, a growing number of claims are submitted electronically. Pharmacy technicians must properly document services as well as submit and follow up on paper claims. Note that the paper claims for these services are submitted to a department within an insurance company or PBM that is different from the department that processes claims for prescription drugs. The claims should include a cover letter, a copy of the order for the service from the physician (also known as the statement of medical necessity), an appropriate billing form (usually the standard *CMS-1500 form*, formerly named the HCFA 1500 form, shown at right), and accurate documentation of the services provided by the pharmacy.

CMS-1500 form the standard form used by health-care providers to bill for services, including disease state management services.

universal claim form (UCF) a standard claim form accepted by many insurers.

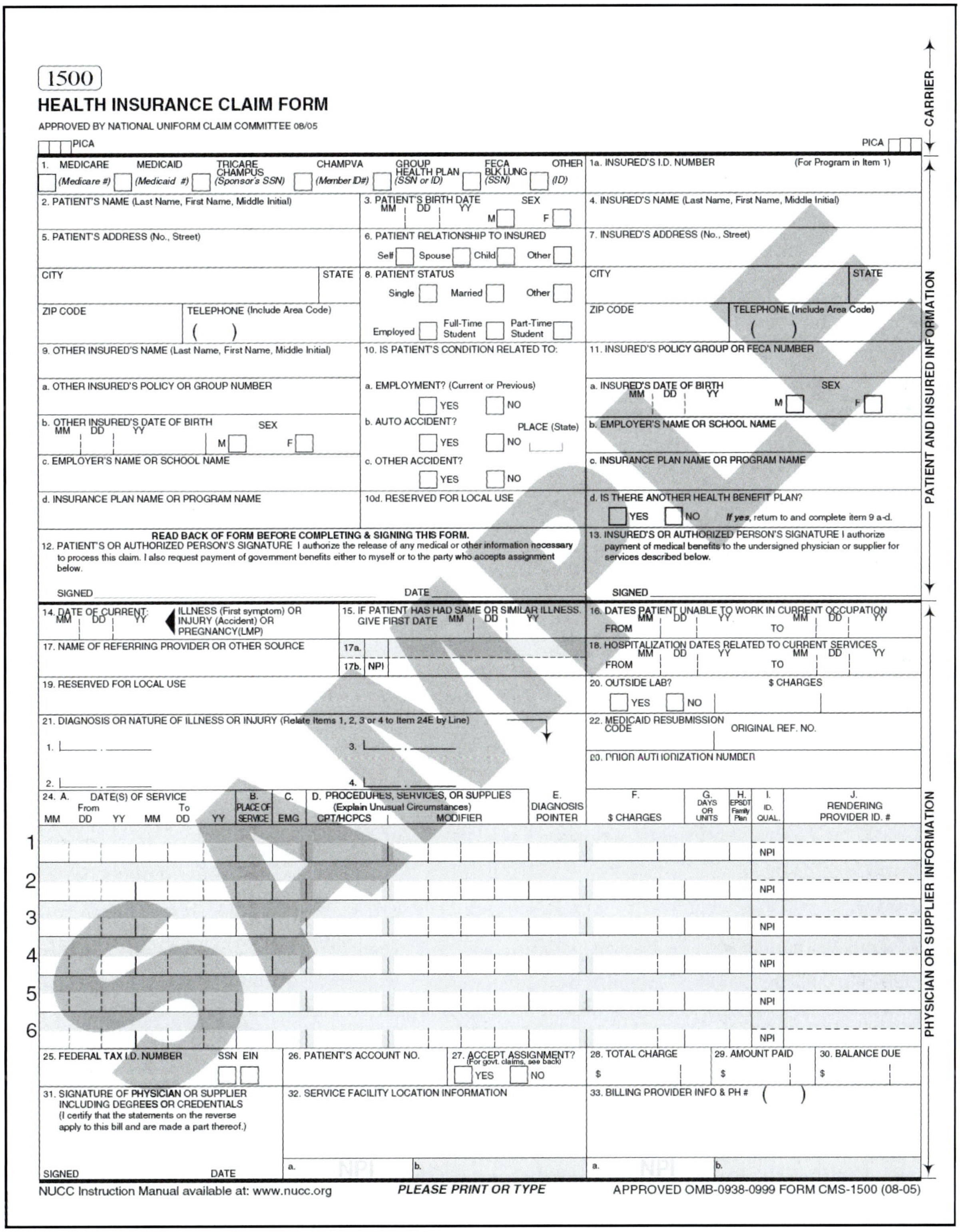
1500

HEALTH INSURANCE CLAIM FORM

APPROVED BY NATIONAL UNIFORM CLAIM COMMITTEE 08/05

PICA ☐☐☐ PICA ☐☐☐ — CARRIER

1. MEDICARE ☐ (Medicare #) MEDICAID ☐ (Medicaid #) TRICARE CHAMPUS ☐ (Sponsor's SSN) CHAMPVA ☐ (Member ID#) GROUP HEALTH PLAN ☐ (SSN or ID) FECA BLK LUNG ☐ (SSN) OTHER ☐ (ID)

1a. INSURED'S I.D. NUMBER (For Program in Item 1)

2. PATIENT'S NAME (Last Name, First Name, Middle Initial)

3. PATIENT'S BIRTH DATE MM DD YY SEX M ☐ F ☐

4. INSURED'S NAME (Last Name, First Name, Middle Initial)

5. PATIENT'S ADDRESS (No., Street)

6. PATIENT RELATIONSHIP TO INSURED Self ☐ Spouse ☐ Child ☐ Other ☐

7. INSURED'S ADDRESS (No., Street)

CITY STATE

8. PATIENT STATUS Single ☐ Married ☐ Other ☐

CITY STATE

ZIP CODE TELEPHONE (Include Area Code) ( )

Employed ☐ Full-Time Student ☐ Part-Time Student ☐

ZIP CODE TELEPHONE (Include Area Code) ( )

9. OTHER INSURED'S NAME (Last Name, First Name, Middle Initial)

10. IS PATIENT'S CONDITION RELATED TO:

11. INSURED'S POLICY GROUP OR FECA NUMBER

a. OTHER INSURED'S POLICY OR GROUP NUMBER

a. EMPLOYMENT? (Current or Previous) ☐ YES ☐ NO

a. INSURED'S DATE OF BIRTH MM DD YY SEX M ☐ F ☐

b. OTHER INSURED'S DATE OF BIRTH MM DD YY SEX M ☐ F ☐

b. AUTO ACCIDENT? ☐ YES ☐ NO PLACE (State)

b. EMPLOYER'S NAME OR SCHOOL NAME

c. EMPLOYER'S NAME OR SCHOOL NAME

c. OTHER ACCIDENT? ☐ YES ☐ NO

c. INSURANCE PLAN NAME OR PROGRAM NAME

d. INSURANCE PLAN NAME OR PROGRAM NAME

10d. RESERVED FOR LOCAL USE

d. IS THERE ANOTHER HEALTH BENEFIT PLAN? ☐ YES ☐ NO *If yes,* return to and complete item 9 a-d.

READ BACK OF FORM BEFORE COMPLETING & SIGNING THIS FORM.

12. PATIENT'S OR AUTHORIZED PERSON'S SIGNATURE I authorize the release of any medical or other information necessary to process this claim. I also request payment of government benefits either to myself or to the party who accepts assignment below.

SIGNED DATE

13. INSURED'S OR AUTHORIZED PERSON'S SIGNATURE I authorize payment of medical benefits to the undersigned physician or supplier for services described below.

SIGNED

— PATIENT AND INSURED INFORMATION —

14. DATE OF CURRENT: MM DD YY ◀ ILLNESS (First symptom) OR INJURY (Accident) OR PREGNANCY(LMP)

15. IF PATIENT HAS HAD SAME OR SIMILAR ILLNESS. GIVE FIRST DATE MM DD YY

16. DATES PATIENT UNABLE TO WORK IN CURRENT OCCUPATION MM DD YY FROM TO

17. NAME OF REFERRING PROVIDER OR OTHER SOURCE

17a.

17b. NPI

18. HOSPITALIZATION DATES RELATED TO CURRENT SERVICES MM DD YY FROM TO

19. RESERVED FOR LOCAL USE

20. OUTSIDE LAB? ☐ YES ☐ NO $ CHARGES

21. DIAGNOSIS OR NATURE OF ILLNESS OR INJURY (Relate Items 1, 2, 3 or 4 to Item 24E by Line)

1. ___ . ___ 3. ___ . ___

2. ___ . ___ 4. ___ . ___

22. MEDICAID RESUBMISSION CODE ORIGINAL REF. NO.

23. PRIOR AUTHORIZATION NUMBER

	24. A. DATE(S) OF SERVICE From MM DD YY	To MM DD YY	B. PLACE OF SERVICE	C. EMG	D. PROCEDURES, SERVICES, OR SUPPLIES (Explain Unusual Circumstances) CPT/HCPCS MODIFIER	E. DIAGNOSIS POINTER	F. $ CHARGES	G. DAYS OR UNITS	H. EPSDT Family Plan	I. ID. QUAL.	J. RENDERING PROVIDER ID. #
1										NPI	
2										NPI	
3										NPI	
4										NPI	
5										NPI	
6										NPI	

25. FEDERAL TAX I.D. NUMBER SSN EIN ☐☐

26. PATIENT'S ACCOUNT NO.

27. ACCEPT ASSIGNMENT? (For govt. claims, see back) ☐ YES ☐ NO

28. TOTAL CHARGE $

29. AMOUNT PAID $

30. BALANCE DUE $

31. SIGNATURE OF PHYSICIAN OR SUPPLIER INCLUDING DEGREES OR CREDENTIALS (I certify that the statements on the reverse apply to this bill and are made a part thereof.)

SIGNED DATE

32. SERVICE FACILITY LOCATION INFORMATION

a. NPI b.

33. BILLING PROVIDER INFO & PH # ( )

a. NPI b.

— PHYSICIAN OR SUPPLIER INFORMATION —

NUCC Instruction Manual available at: www.nucc.org *PLEASE PRINT OR TYPE* APPROVED OMB-0938-0999 FORM CMS-1500 (08-05)

SAMPLE

Source: www.cms.hhs.gov/cmsforms/downloads/cms1500805.pdf.

OTHER BILLING PROCEDURES (cont'd)

MEDICATION THERAPY MANAGEMENT SERVICES

Medicare Part D provides opportunities for pharmacists to provide *Medication Therapy Management (MTM) services* to some Medicare beneficiaries that are taking multiple medications or have certain diseases. Pharmacy technicians have an important responsibility for billing these services, maintaining necessary documentation, and ensuring that payment is received. The CMS-1500 form is especially important for billing MTM services through *Prescription Drug Plans (PDPs)*.

In order to bill prescription drug plans for MTM services using the CMS-1500 form, the pharmacist or pharmacy offering the services must be enrolled as a provider for the patient's PDP and also have a *National Provider Identifier (NPI)*. Applying for a NPI can be done online using the web-based NPI process (https://nppes.cms.hhs.gov) or by mailing the completed *CMS-10114 form* to NPI Enumerator.

When completing the CMS-1500 form, the diagnosis code is needed and can be obtained from the physician. When billing MTM services, *Current Procedural Terminology codes (CPT codes)* provide a systematic way to bill for the services provided. Three different CPT codes can be used to bill prescription drug plans for MTM services provided by pharmacists: 99605, 99606, and 99607. Also, it is essential that documentation for services provided is carefully maintained.

CPT Codes for Pharmacist-Provided Services	
➡ 99605	Used for a first encounter with a patient and may be billed in 1–15 minute increments.
➡ 99606	Used for follow-up encounters and may be billed in 1–15 minute increments.
➡ 99607	An add-on CPT code to be used with 99605 or 99606 when additional 15 minute increments of time are spent face-to-face with a patient.

Rx tip

OutcomesMTM (http://www.outcomesmtm.com/), RxTherapy Management (http://rxtm.org/Pharmacists.aspx), and Mirixa (http://www.mirixa.com/) are three online platforms for MTMs. Some MTM-billable services are Comprehensive Medication Reviews (CMR), prescriber consultations for cost efficacy management and/or drug therapy problems, as well as patient consultations for compliance, education and/or monitoring.

CMS-10114 form the standard six-page form used by health care providers to apply for a national provider identifier (NPI).

Current Procedural Terminology codes (CPT codes) identifiers used for billing pharmacist-provided MTM services.

Medication Therapy Management (MTM) services services provided to some Medicare beneficiaries who are enrolled in Medicare Part D and who are taking multiple medications or have certain diseases.

National Provider Identifier (NPI) the code assigned to recognized health-care providers; needed to bill MTM services.

Prescription Drug Plans (PDPs) third-party programs for Medicare Part D.

DEPARTMENT OF HEALTH AND HUMAN SERVICES
CENTERS FOR MEDICARE & MEDICAID SERVICES

Form Approved
OMB No. 0938-0931

NATIONAL PROVIDER IDENTIFIER (NPI) APPLICATION/UPDATE FORM

Please PRINT or TYPE all information so it is legible. Do not use pencil. Failure to provide complete and accurate information may cause your application to be returned and delay processing of your application. In addition, you may experience problems being recognized by insurers if the records in their systems do not match the information you have furnished on this form.

SECTION 1 – BASIC INFORMATION

A. Reason For Submittal Of This Form (Check the appropriate box)

1. ❑ Initial Application
2. ❑ Change of Information (See instructions)
   NPI No.________________
3. Deactivation NPI No.________________
   REASON (Check one of the following)
   ❑ Death ❑ Business Dissolved
   ❑ Other ________________

B. Entity Type (Check the appropriate box)

1. ❑ An individual who renders health care. (Complete Sections 2A, 3, 4A and 5)
2. ❑ An organization that renders health care. (Complete Sections 2B, 3, 4B and 5)

SECTION 2 – IDENTIFYING INFORMATION

A. Individuals

1. Prefix (e.g.,Major, Mrs.)	2. First	3. Middle	4. Last
5. Suffix (e.g., Jr., Sr.)		6. Credential (e.g., M.D., D.O.)	

Other Name Information (If applicable. Use additional sheets of paper if necessary)

7. Prefix (e.g.,Major, Mrs.)	8. First	9. Middle	10. Last
11. Suffix (e.g., Jr., Sr.)		12. Credential (e.g., M.D., D.O.)	

13. Type of other Name
❑ Former Name ❑ Professional Name ❑ Other (Describe) ________________

14. Date of Birth (mm/dd/yyyy)	15. State of Birth (U.S. only)	16. Country of Birth (If other than U.S.)

17. Gender
❑ Male ❑ Female

18. Social Security Number (SSN)	19. IRS Individual Taxpayer Identification Number

B. Organizations and Groups

1. Name (Legal Business Name)	2. Employer Identification Number (EIN) or SSN

3. Other Name (Use additional sheets of paper if necessary)

4. Type of Other Name
❑ Former Legal Business Name ❑ D/B/A Name ❑ Other (Describe) ________________

Form CMS-10114 (02/05) EF (05/2005) 1

Page one of the CMS-10114 Form. Available by calling EPI Enumerator at 1-800-465-3203.

REVIEW

KEY CONCEPTS

FINANCIAL ISSUES

- ✔ Third-party programs are simply another party besides the patient or the pharmacy that pays for some or all of the cost of medication: essentially, an insurer.
- ✔ A pharmacy benefit manager (PBM) is a company that administers drug benefit programs for insurance companies, HMOs, and self-insured employers.
- ✔ Co-insurance is essentially an agreement between the insurer and the insured to share costs. One aspect of it is the requirement for patients to co-pay a portion of the cost of prescriptions.
- ✔ The amount paid by insurers for prescriptions is not equal to the retail price normally charged, but is determined by a formula described in a contract between the insurer and the pharmacy.

THIRD-PARTY PROGRAMS

- ✔ Prescription drug benefit cards contain necessary billing information for pharmacies, including the patient's identification number, group number, and co-pay amount.
- ✔ HMOs usually will not cover expenses incurred outside their participating network and often require generic substitution.
- ✔ POSs often partially reimburse expenses incurred outside of their network and usually require generic substitution.
- ✔ PPOs usually require generic substitution.
- ✔ Workers' compensation is compensation for employees accidentally injured on the job.
- ✔ Medicare covers people age 65 and over, disabled people under age 65, and people with kidney failure.
- ✔ Medicaid is a federal–state program for the needy.

ONLINE ADJUDICATION

- ✔ In online adjudication, the technician uses the computer to determine the exact coverage for each prescription with the appropriate third party.
- ✔ When brand name drugs are dispensed, numbers corresponding to the reason for submitting the claim with brand name drugs are entered in a DAW (Dispense as Written) indicator field in the prescription system.

REJECTED CLAIMS

- ✔ Many prescription drug plans have age limitations for children or dependents of the cardholder.
- ✔ Most third-party plans require that most of the medication has been taken before the plan will cover a refill of the same medication.
- ✔ Many managed care health programs require mail order pharmacies to fill prescriptions for maintenance medications.

OTHER BILLING PROCEDURES

- ✔ When a claim is rejected, the pharmacy technician can telephone the insurance plan's pharmacy help desk to determine if the patient is eligible for coverage.
- ✔ Claims for disease state management services can be submitted using a paper system and often require follow up.

SELF TEST

the answer key begins on page 569

MATCH THE TERMS: I

1. CMS-1500 form ____
2. CMS-10114 form ____
3. co-insurance ____
4. co-pay ____
5. Current Procedural Terminology codes (CPT codes) ____
6. deductible ____
7. dual co-pay ____
8. formulary ____
9. HMOs ____
10. maximum allowable cost (MAC) ____
11. Medicaid ____
12. Medicare ____
13. Medication Therapy Management (MTM) services ____
14. National Provider Identifier (NPI) ____
15. online adjudication ____

a. the resolution of prescription coverage through the communication of the pharmacy computer with the third-party computer.

b. the portion of the price of medication that the patient is required to pay.

c. the maximum price per tablet (or other dispensing unit) an insurer or PBM will pay for a given product.

d. a federal–state program, administered by the states, providing health care for the needy.

e. a cost-sharing agreement between the insurer and the insured.

f. co-pays that have two prices: one for generic and one for brand medications.

g. a set amount that must be paid by the patient for each benefit period before the insurer will cover additional expenses.

h. a network of providers for which costs are covered inside but not outside of the network.

i. the standard form used by health-care providers, such as physicians, to bill for services. It can be used to bill for disease state management services.

j. a federal program providing health care to people with certain disabilities over age 65.

k. services provided to some Medicare beneficiaries who are enrolled in Medicare Part D and who are taking multiple medications or have certain diseases.

l. the code assigned to recognized health care providers; needed to bill MTM services.

m. identifiers used for billing pharmacist-provided MTM services.

n. the standard form used by health-care providers to apply for a National Provider Identifier (NPI).

o. a list of medications covered by a third-party plan.

REVIEW

MATCH THE TERMS: II

1. patient assistance programs ____
2. pharmacy benefit managers ____
3. POSs ____
4. PPOs ____
5. prescription drug benefit cards ____
6. Prescription Drug Plans (PDPs) ____
7. tier ____
8. U&C or UCR ____
9. universal claim form _____
10. worker's compensation _____

a. companies that administer drug benefit programs.
b. a standard paper claim form accepted by many insurers.
c. the maximum amount of payment for a given prescription, determined by the insurer to be a usual and customary (and reasonable) price.
d. manufacturer sponsored prescription drug programs for the needy.
e. cards that contain third-party billing information for prescription drug purchases.
f. a network of providers where the patient's primary care physician must be a member and costs outside the network may be partially reimbursed.
g. a network of providers where costs outside the network may be partially reimbursed and the patient's primary care physician need not be a member.
h. an employer compensation program for employees accidentally injured on the job.
i. third-party programs for Medicare Part D.
j. categories of medications that are covered by a third-party plan.

CHOOSE THE BEST ANSWER

1. Companies that administer drug benefit programs are called
   a. pharmacy benefit managers.
   b. MACs.
   c. HMOs.
   d. employers.

2. Another party, besides the patient or the pharmacy, that pays some or all of the cost of the medication is a(an)
   a. third-party.
   b. co-insurance.
   c. MAC.
   d. UCR.

3. An agreement for cost sharing between the insurer and the insured is called
   a. MAC.
   b. dual co-pay.
   c. co-insurance.
   d. co-pay.

4. The prescription drug co-pay is paid by
   a. the insurance company.
   b. the patient.
   c. the patient's employer.
   d. Medicaid.

5. Third-party plans reimburse pharmacies for the actual retail price of all prescriptions.
   a. True
   b. False

6. Plans in which the patient pays a different amount depending on whether a generic or brand name medication is dispensed have
   a. dual co-pays.
   b. MAC.
   c. duplicate pricing.
   d. UCR.

7. If a third-party plan has a dual co-pay, the patient usually pays __________ for generic drugs compared to brand name drugs.
   a. the same amount
   b. less
   c. more

8. Generic drugs are usually in tier
   a. one.
   b. two.
   c. three.
   d. four.

9. A(an) ______________ is a network of providers for which costs are covered inside, but not outside of the network.
   a. POS
   b. HMO
   c. MAC
   d. PPO

10. A(an) ____________ is a network of providers where costs outside the network may be partially reimbursed and the patient's primary care physician need not be a member.
   a. PPO
   b. HMO
   c. POS
   d. MAC

11. Which type of managed care program is least likely to require generic substitution?
   a. Medicare
   b. PPO
   c. Medicaid
   d. HMO

12. A drug formulary is
   a. a list of medications that are covered by a third-party program.
   b. an official compendium of the FDA.
   c. a list of ingredients in a prescription.
   d. the price of a prescription under a third-party program.

13. Medicare Part D covers
   a. prescription drugs.
   b. inpatient hospital expenses.
   c. doctors' services.
   d. hospice expenses.

14. Closed formulary programs, such as Medicaid, may cover drugs not on the formulary through a process called
   a. dual co-pay.
   b. co-insurance.
   c. POS.
   d. prior authorization.

REVIEW

15. The rules for coordination of benefits ensure that the benefit coverage for a claim does not exceed _______ of the total cost.
    a. 25%
    b. 33%
    c. 50%
    d. 100%

16. Which of the following information is generally not required in online claim processing?
    a. birth date
    b. weight
    c. sex
    d. group number

17. The DAW indicator that is appropriate for online adjudication if a physician has handwritten DAW on the prescription is
    a. 4.
    b. 2.
    c. 1.
    d. 3.

18. When there is a question on insurance coverage for an online claim, the pharmacy technician can
    a. telephone the insurance plan's pharmacy help desk.
    b. immediately refer the problem to the pharmacist.
    c. contact the prescriber.
    d. contact the county health department.

19. When a technician receives a rejected claim "NDC Not Covered," this probably means
    a. the insurance plan has a closed formulary.
    b. the insurance plan has an open formulary.
    c. the birth date submitted does not match the birth date in the insurer's computer.
    d. the patient has mail order.

20. When a technician receives a rejected claim "Invalid Person Code," this probably means
    a. the patient is on Medicare.
    b. the patient has a mail order program.
    c. the person code entered does not match the birth date and/or sex in the insurer's computer.
    d. the patient is on Medicaid.

21. When a technician receives a rejected claim "Unable to Connect," this probably means
    a. the insurer has an incorrect birth date for the patient.
    b. the patient's coverage has expired.
    c. the connection with the insurer's computer is temporarily unavailable due to computer problems.
    d. the insurer has a closed formulary.

22. A standard form used by health-care providers to bill for services is
    a. a universal claim form (UCF).
    b. a pdf.
    c. an NDC.
    d. CMS-1500.

23. The CPT codes for billing Medication Therapy Management services provided by pharmacists are
    a. ICD-9.
    b. MAC.
    c. PPO.
    d. 99605, 99606, and 99607.

CRITICAL THINKING QUESTIONS

1. Discuss reasons why pharmacy technicians are well-suited to be the experts in the pharmacy for pharmacy billing and reimbursement.
2. Why is it important that pharmacy technicians are able to resolve rejected claims?
3. What are the advantages for patients having coverage through Medicare Part D?

THINKING IT THROUGH WRAP-UP

1. HMOs have more restrictions on eligible providers and levels of coverage. They generally provide coverage within the HMO network but providers out of network are typically not covered.
2. Medicaid is a federal–state program to provide medical assistance for individuals and families with low incomes. Medicare is a federal program for people age 65 and over as well as some disabled people under 65 who have kidney disease. Some people with Medicare also qualify for Medicaid.
3. Only medications used to treat covered work-related injuries can be billed to workers' compensation. Medications that were not prescribed for the work-related injury cannot be billed to worker's compensation.

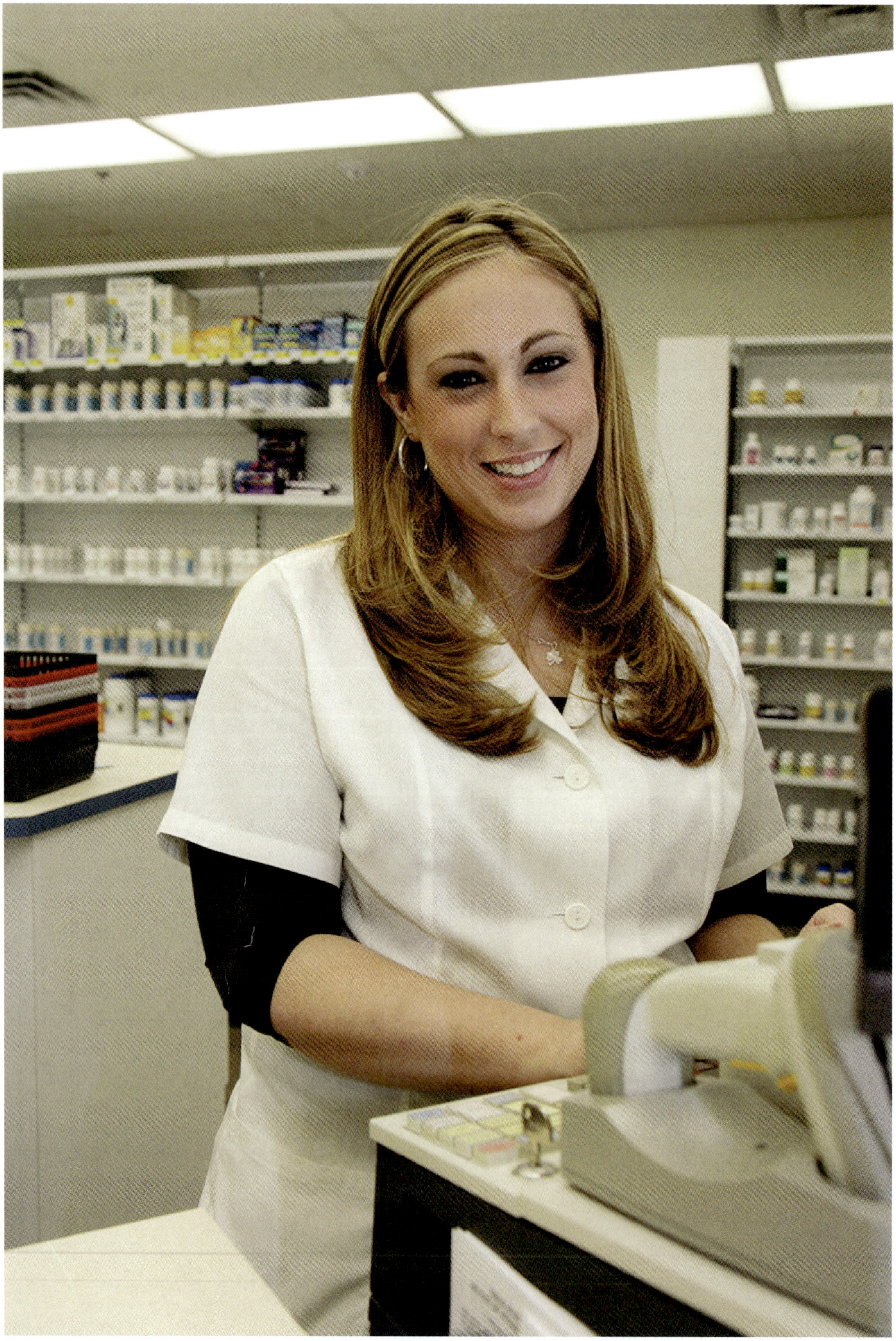

15

COMMUNITY PHARMACY

LEARNING OBJECTIVES

At the completion of study, the student will:

- ✔ have a basic understanding of pharmacy practice in the community setting.
- ✔ be familiar with the setup of a community pharmacy.
- ✔ understand basic customer service principles.
- ✔ understand the basics of prescription processing in a community pharmacy.
- ✔ understand the general duties of a pharmacy technician in the community pharmacy practice setting.

THINKING IT THROUGH

As you read this chapter, consider what you would do in the following situations:

1. A customer is dissatisfied with having to wait for their prescription.
2. An elderly customer tells you that because of her arthritis she has a hard time opening her medication bottles. She also tells you in conversation that it was difficult for her to get to the pharmacy because she doesn't drive.
3. A customer is asking what she can purchase over-the-counter to treat her cough and cold symptoms.

COMMUNITY PHARMACY

Community or retail pharmacy practice is the practice of providing prescription services to the public.

Community pharmacies also sell over-the-counter medications and health and beauty products. A community pharmacy may be owned independently or by a chain. Chains may specialize in pharmacy or be part of a broader mass merchandise or food store business.

Almost two-thirds of all prescription drugs in the United States are dispensed by community pharmacies.

As a result, more pharmacists and technicians are employed in community pharmacy than any other area. The role of the community pharmacist in counseling and educating patients has also been steadily increasing, which in turn has expanded the role of the pharmacy technician in assisting with dispensing prescriptions. Community pharmacy practice provides great opportunity for employment as a pharmacy technician and also as a way to serve the community.

One of the key characteristics of community pharmacy is the close interaction with patients.

In contrast to institutional and other environments, technicians in the community pharmacy constantly interact with patients as customers. It is important to remember that the patient is a customer who has many alternatives for where they can bring their business. As a result, customer service is a major area of importance in the community pharmacy and technicians employed there must have strong *interpersonal skills*.

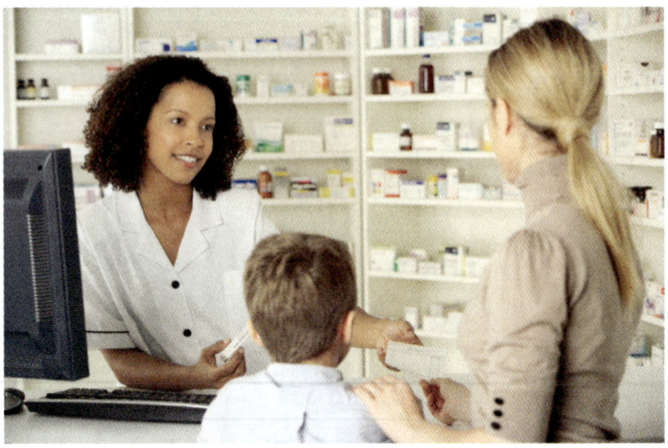

Strong interpersonal skills and good customer service are essential in the community pharmacy environment.

TYPES OF COMMUNITY PHARMACIES

There are about 60,000 community pharmacies in the United States that provide convenient access to medications and medication information. They are found in a variety of settings:

- **Independent Pharmacies**
  Individually owned local pharmacies.
- **Chain Pharmacies**
  Regional or national pharmacy chains such as CVS, Rite-Aid, Walgreens, and others.
- **Mass Merchandiser Pharmacies**
  Regional or national chains such as Walmart, KMart, Costco, Target, and others that sell mass merchandise and have in-store pharmacies.
- **Food Store Pharmacies**
  Regional or national food store chains such as A&P, Giant Eagle, Kroger's, Pathmark, and others that have in-store pharmacies.

interpersonal skills skills involving relationships between people.

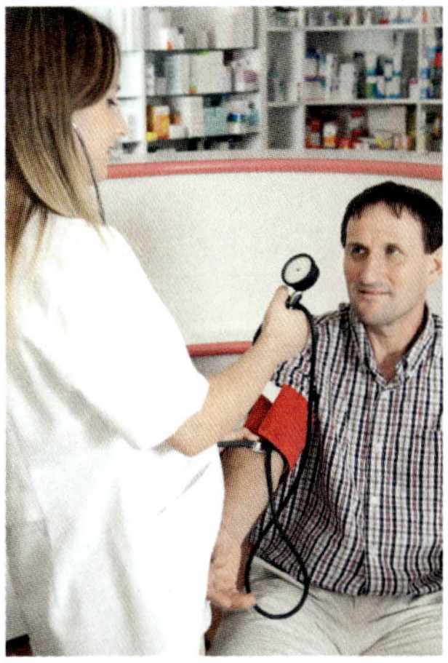

a pharmacist taking a patient's blood pressure

Rapidly growing aspects of community pharmacies are disease state management (DSM) programs, Medication Therapy Management (MTM) services, and other clinical services and programs.

DSM programs provide one-on-one pharmacist-patient consultation sessions to help manage chronic diseases or conditions such as diabetes. For example, the pharmacist may teach diabetes patients how to properly use blood glucose monitoring devices or the pharmacist may analyze a patient's blood-glucose readings on an on-going basis and recommend medication changes to the patient's physician as needed. These programs are also offered for asthma/chronic obstructive pulmonary disease (COPD), anticoagulation, weight loss, smoking cessation, and cholesterol reduction.

Some Medicare patients are eligible for Medication Therapy Management (MTM) services provided by pharmacists.

MTM services are similar to DSM, but tailored to the provisions of Medicare Part D. MTM includes five core elements: medication therapy review (MTR), personal medication record (PMR), medication-related action plan (MAP), intervention and/or referral, and documentation and follow-up.

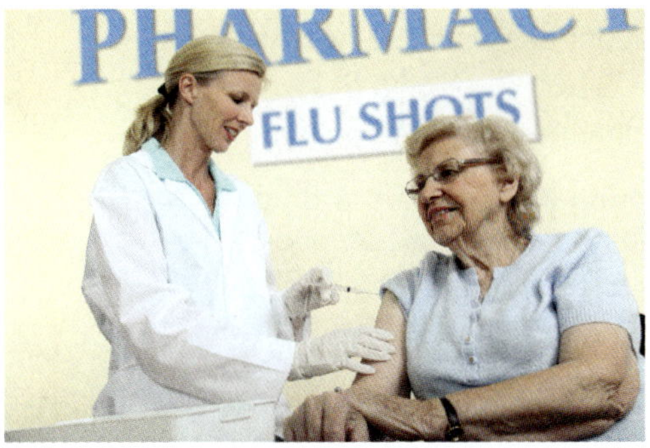

a pharmacist giving a flu shot

Pharmacies may also have walk-in clinics such as *Minute Clinics* at some CVS locations and *Take Care* clinics at some Walgreens locations.

These clinics are staffed by a nurse practitioner who can provide treatment for a limited number of common conditions such as colds and minor injuries. Depending on state laws, they may possibly also write prescriptions for some medications and administer routine vaccinations. Some of the growing number of vaccines that pharmacists are administering include influenza, herpes zoster, and pneumococcal vaccines.

Pharmacy technicians help with these services by coordinating billing with the patient's insurance company, scheduling appointments, and taking patient information.

As with all patient-related medical information, HIPAA regulations mandate complete confidentiality regarding these services.

REGULATIONS

There are many regulations that affect the community pharmacy practice.

Pharmacy technicians must be knowledgeable regarding these regulations.

Federal Regulations

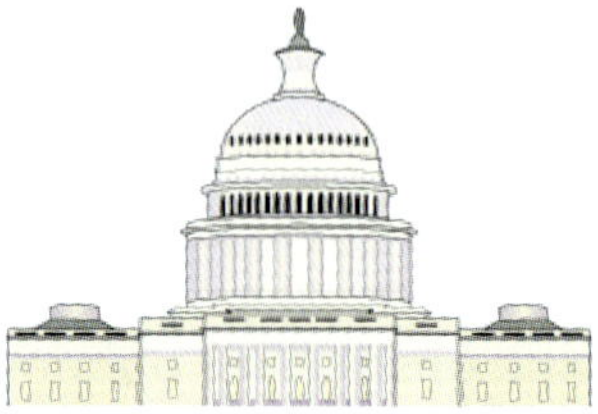

The 1990 ***Omnibus Budget and Reconciliation Act (OBRA)*** requires community pharmacists to offer Medicaid patients counseling and instruction regarding prescription drug dosage, route of administration, and duration of administration; special directions; common severe side effects or interactions and therapeutic contraindications; proper storage; what to do if a dose is missed; and refill information.

The 1996 ***Health Insurance Portability and Accountability Act (HIPAA)*** requires all health-care professionals to protect patients' privacy. Any information related to a patient or their medical condition is considered protected health information and must be kept confidential. This information includes, but is not limited to, the patient's name and address, date of birth, diagnosis, medical history, and medications.

Some practical ways of protecting patients' privacy include:

- Never discussing patients outside of the pharmacy setting;
- shredding documents, papers, or labels with patient information (instead of discarding in regular trash);
- speaking to patients, or about patients to other authorized health-care professionals, in the most private area possible;
- and never discussing patients with any individual unless the patient has provided written authorization to do so.

When working in any pharmacy, be sure to read and understand the pharmacy's HIPAA policy.

The 2003 ***Medicare Prescription Drug Improvement and Modernization Act*** provides a drug benefit program to senior citizens. Known as Medicare Part D, it relies on private prescription drug plan (PDP) companies to provide coverage to Medicare eligible individuals. The PDP's must operate within very detailed government guidelines but can design their own programs and compete with each other. PDP's use their own formularies or lists of covered drugs, non-covered drugs, and sometimes preferred drugs that may carry a lower copayment. Pharmacists and pharmacy technicians must know how to assist patients when a drug is not covered, be involved with prescribers when making drug changes to the formulary, and be familiar with online billing procedures for these plans.

Pharmacist-provided Medication Therapy Management (MTM) is also part of the Medicare Modernization Act. OutcomesMTM, RxTherapy Management, and Mirixa are three of the online platforms for MTM. Technicians can learn more about MTM at their websites http://www.outcomesmtm.com/, http://rxtm.org/Pharmacists.aspx, and http://www.mirixa.com/.

The 2005 ***Combat Methamphetamine Epidemic Act*** limits the sales of all over-the-counter products in any form that contains the methamphetamine precursor chemicals pseudoephedrine (PSE), ephedrine, or phenylpropanolamine. Specific requirements under this law are:

- Retail sales may not exceed 3.6 grams PSE per day per purchaser, regardless of the number of transactions.
- Individuals are prohibited from purchasing more than 9 grams PSE per 30-day period.

Combat Methamphetamine Act (CMEA) federal legislation enacted to regulate over-the-counter sales of ephedrine and pseudoephedrine.

Health Insurance Portability and Accountability Act (HIPAA) federal legislation designed to protect patients' personal and medical information and also to encourage use of electronic data interchange in the U.S.

- All nonliquid forms (including gel caps) of PSE products must be sold in blister packs with no more than two dosages or in unit-dose packets or pouches.
- Mail-order companies may not sell more than 7.5 grams to any single customer within a 30-day period.
- All PSE products must be placed in a locked display case or behind a counter (any counter, not necessarily the pharmacy counter) that is not accessible to consumers. Retailers must give the product directly to the purchaser.
- Retailers must maintain a written or electronic logbook of all transactions involving products with more than 60 mg of PSE. The logbook must contain the purchaser's signature, name and address; date and time of sale; name of product sold; and quantity sold.
- The retailer must check the information entered by the purchaser against their photo ID. Logbooks must provide notice to purchasers that entering false statements or misrepresentations may subject them to criminal penalties. Each entry must be maintained for two years following the date of entry.
- Retailers must train applicable sales personnel to ensure that they understand the requirements of PSE product sales and submit self-certifications of training to the attorney general. The Drug Enforcement Administration is responsible for issuing regulations on the training criteria.

In 2007, the Federal Trade Commission (FTC) enacted provisions known jointly as the ***Red Flag Rule*** to help prevent identity theft from financial and medical institutions, including pharmacies, that maintain patient accounts for billing. Institutions that meet the definition of a "creditor" may be required to develop policies, procedures, and employee training to prevent customer identity theft.

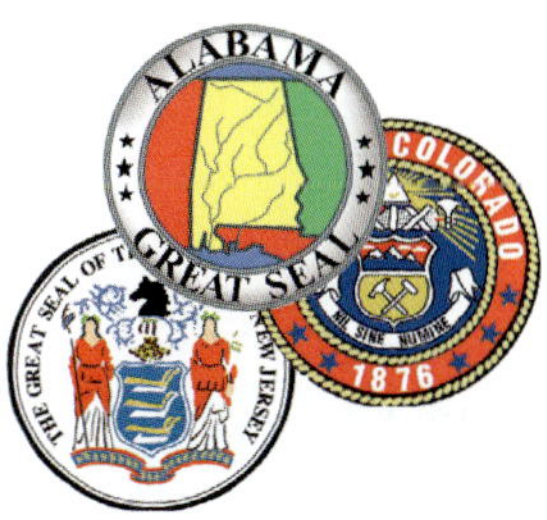

State Regulations

Community pharmacies are most closely regulated at the state level. Each state has a board of pharmacy that establishes and enforces regulations for their state. For example, many states have mandated OBRA '90 counseling requirements for all patients, not just those on Medicaid. Also, states are increasingly requiring that technicians attain national pharmacy technician certification or they may have their own certifying process, which may include registration with the state's board of pharmacy. States also regulate such things as the ratio of pharmacists to technicians, scope of technician practice, record keeping, required equipment, work area requirements, and the scope of medication compounding. A pharmacy can be inspected at any time by a state inspector for compliance with regulations.

Medicare Prescription Drug Improvement and Modernization Act federal legislation that created Medicare Part D and made allowance for Medicare recipients to receive Medicare medical coverage through private health insurance plans.

Omnibus Budget Reconciliation Act (OBRA) federal legislation requiring pharmacists to provide counseling to Medicaid patients receiving new prescriptions.

Red Flag Rule a set of provisions created by the Federal Trade Commission (FTC) to help prevent identity theft from patient billing accounts maintained by medical and financial institutions.

ORGANIZATION

Prescription processing areas may be organized differently from one community pharmacy to another, but they generally contain the same elements.

Note also that a number of space and equipment decisions are dictated by state regulations.

Transaction Windows

Every pharmacy will have an area designated for dropping off and picking up prescriptions. Sometimes pharmacies will have separate counters for intake and dispensing. Additionally, most pharmacies will have some type of private or semiprivate area for pharmacist-patient consultation. In accordance with HIPAA, ***transaction windows*** should be positioned so as to provide privacy for the patient.

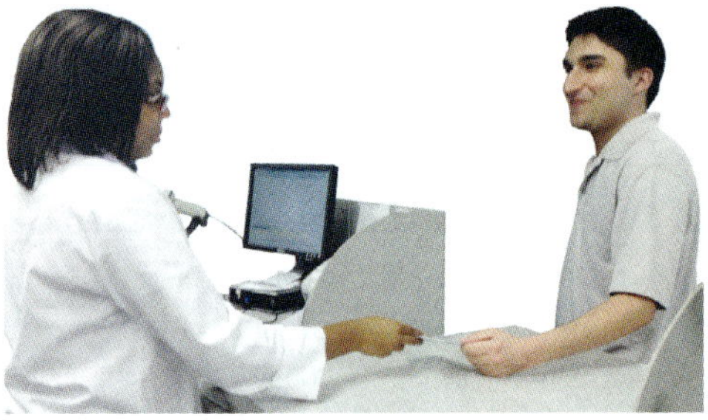

pharmacy technician receiving a prescription from a patient

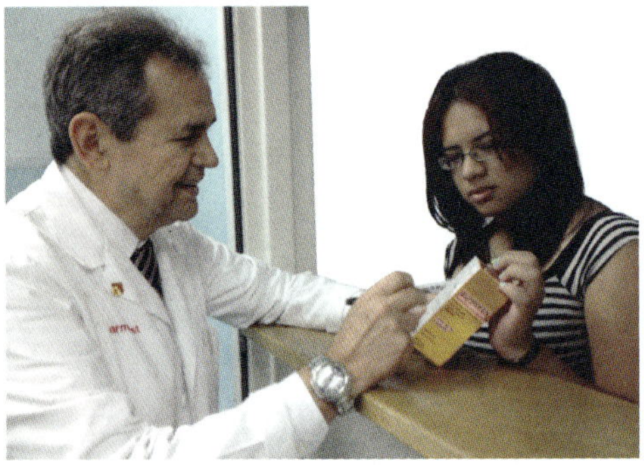

pharmacist-patient consultation area

Storage

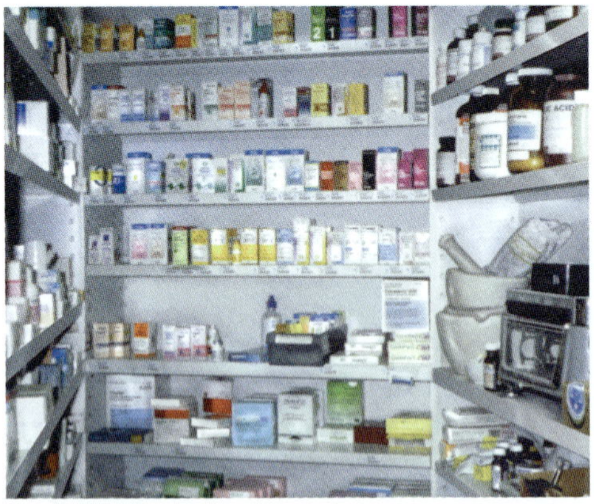

There must be adequate shelving, cabinets, or drawers for storage of medications. The medications may be arranged on the shelves alphabetically according to generic name or they may be arranged according to brand, or trade name.

Within whichever overall organizational system is used there will be specific areas for each type of dosage form. Such dosage form categories include stock bottles of tablets and capsules; syrups and suspensions; creams, ointments, and other topical products; eye drops and ear drops; rectal and vaginal suppositories; injectable drugs; and inhalers and nebulized medications. Schedule II controlled substances must be kept in a separate locked storage area while Schedule III, IV, and V controlled substances may mixed with other products on the regular storage shelves.

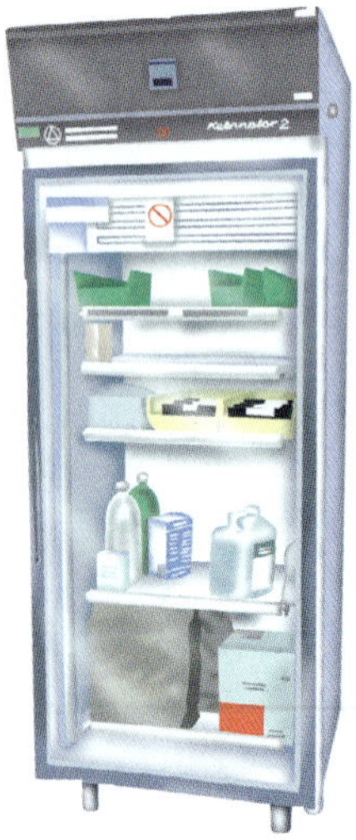

A refrigerator is required to store medications that must remain between 2° and 8° Celsius. The refrigerator must be designated for drugs only. No food products are allowed to be stored in the same refrigerator.

transaction windows counter areas designated for taking prescriptions and for dispensing them to patients.

Prescription Counter

There will be at least one counter designated for preparing noncompounded prescriptions. Equipment used in this area includes counting trays, vials, labels, and auxiliary or precautionary labels. This counter should be kept clean and orderly at all times.

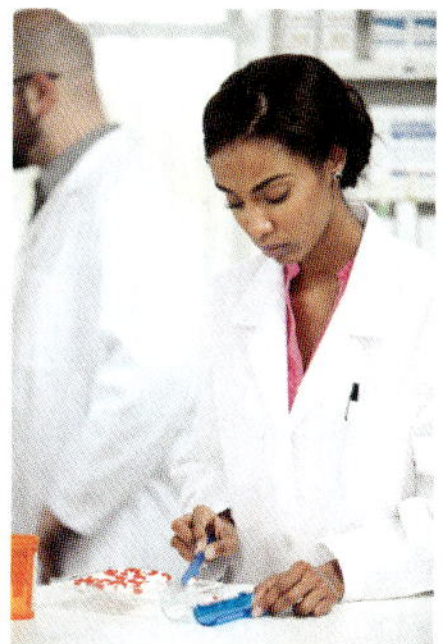

Compounding Area

The pharmacy will also include a compounding area. This is for prescriptions requiring mixing or other preparation. There must be an easily accessible sink in this area, kept clean at all times.

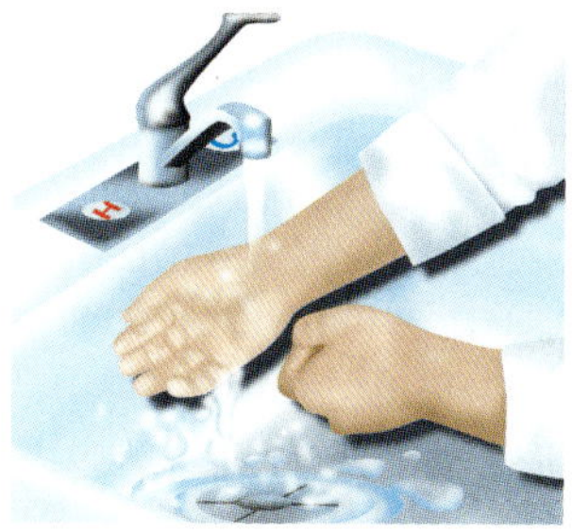

Compounding equipment includes a prescription balance, a set of metric weights, a glass mortar and pestle, glass funnels, stirring rods, graduates for measuring liquids, spatulas, an ointment board or parchment paper, etc. Some community pharmacies also have a clean room for making sterile compounds.

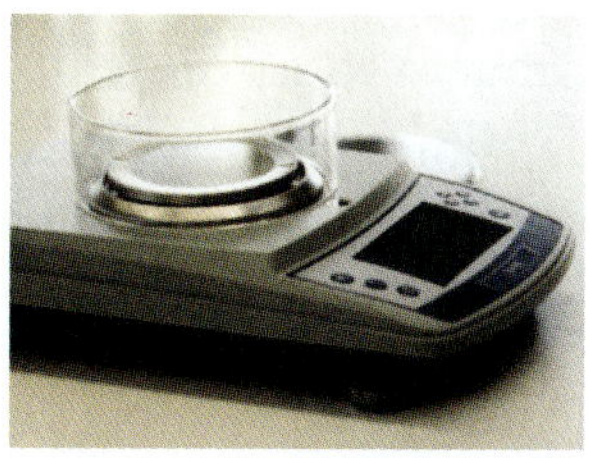

Prescription Bins or Shelves

Completed prescriptions are generally placed in bins or shelves alphabetized by the customer's last name.

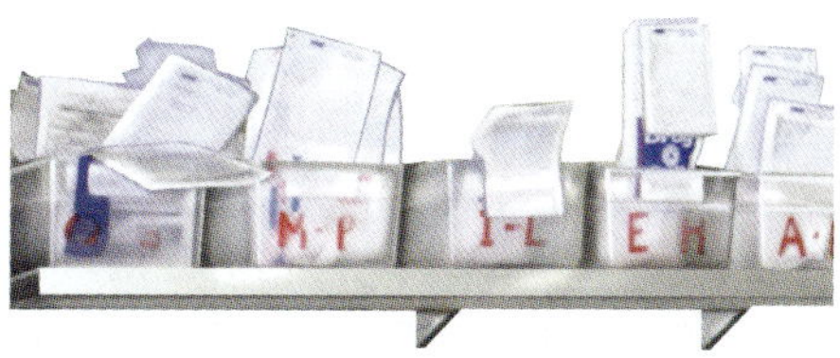

CUSTOMER SERVICE

Customer satisfaction is the goal of customer service.

Good customer service requires presenting yourself to customers in a calm, courteous, and professional manner. It requires listening to and understanding customer requests for service and fulfilling those requests accurately or explaining to the customer's satisfaction why the request cannot be serviced.

The health of customers is a significant factor in their experience of community pharmacy service.

Customers may often feel sick or irritable and need their medication quickly. Having to wait in a line may be physically difficult or emotionally upsetting. The cost of the medication may be an additional worry. Consequently, though customer service is important in any type of retail store, it is particularly important in the community pharmacy setting.

It is important to respond to customers in a positive way at all times.

In any situation where a customer is angry, frustrated, or otherwise dissatisfied, it is especially important to give a positive response. This can be done in part by listening intently and making eye contact with the customer. Restating what the customer has said is also important, since it demonstrates that you have listened to their complaint. Use positive, not negative, terms to tell the customer what you can do, not what you can't do to solve their problem.

Involve the pharmacist in all difficult situations.

If after spending some time with the customer, you have been unable to resolve the problem, you should inform the pharmacist. This should be done immediately for serious complaints regarding problems with prescriptions. Remember that employees who possess well-developed interpersonal skills are good for business and will be appreciated by employers.

℞ safety you should know

A pharmacy technician must know when to refer a customer to the pharmacist. It is a good idea to discuss such situations with the pharmacist regularly. Any time you are uncertain of whether a question requires the pharmacist's judgment, refer the question to the pharmacist.

CUSTOMER SATISFACTION, PRODUCTIVITY, AND EFFICIENCY

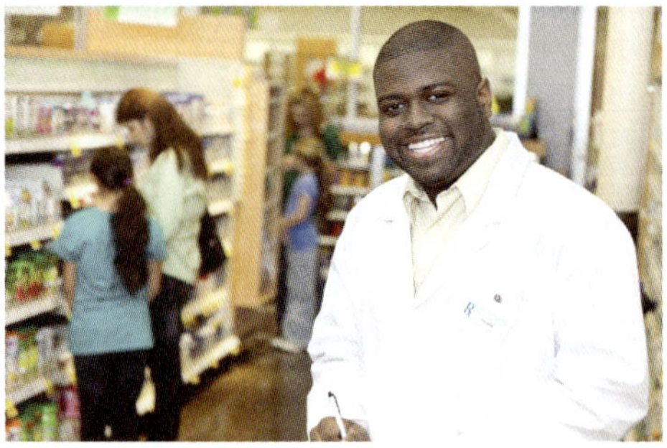

Since pharmacy technicians are generally responsible for handling the pharmacy counter, they have direct contact with customers and play a key role in assisting customers with their needs.

This involves taking in new and refill prescriptions, but also includes directing customers to requested over-the-counter products or answering other questions that do not require the pharmacist's judgment. The technician should be familiar with the layout of the store and know where various types of over-the-counter products are located so they can help customers find products quickly.

Technicians should be aware of any programs that their pharmacy may have to measure customer satisfaction, such as surveys or compliment and complaint programs, as well as any practices, such a recording phone calls, to ensure quality.

Some pharmacies will also have programs in place for recording productivity and efficiency that may have to do with, for example, the number of prescriptions processed within a given time, overall sales, or amounts of inventory ordered.

ON THE TELEPHONE

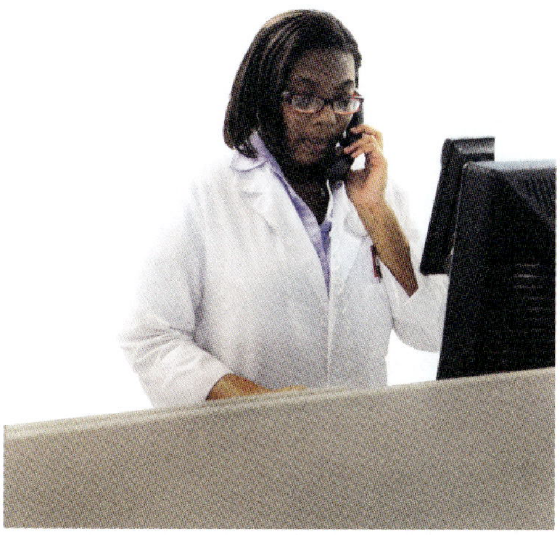

A significant part of the pharmacy technician's responsibilities includes answering the telephone. Calls must be answered in a pleasant and courteous manner, following a standard format that should be indicated by the store manager or pharmacist. Generally, this begins with stating the name of the pharmacy and your name. An example:

"Main Street Pharmacy, Joan speaking, may I help you?"

Many calls will concern the price or stock availability of prescription and over-the-counter products. Some will be to place refill requests. In that case, the same process is followed as when taking refill requests at the counter, except that the technician should also ask the patient when they plan to pick up the prescription.

Some calls will require the pharmacist's judgment. These should be directed immediately to the pharmacist. This applies to questions regarding medication or general health-related questions. When patients raise such questions, politely ask them to hold on the line while you get the pharmacist.

INTERPERSONAL TECHNIQUES

At the Counter

Techniques for interacting with customers at the counter include:

- listening carefully
- making eye contact
- repeating what the customer said
- using positive rather than negative language to describe what you can do
- calling the patient by name

On the Phone

Techniques for interacting with customers on the telephone include:

- using a pleasant voice and courteous manner
- stating the name of the pharmacy and your name
- following the standard procedure indicated for your pharmacy
- referring all calls that require a pharmacist's judgment to the pharmacist

PROCESSING PRESCRIPTIONS

A major pharmacy technician responsibility is to process new and refill prescriptions.

This is done using the pharmacy's computerized prescription system. Different pharmacies will use different systems. The pharmacist or another pharmacy technician will usually provide training on the system that is used. Learning to process prescriptions efficiently and accurately on the system is essential and will take some time and commitment.

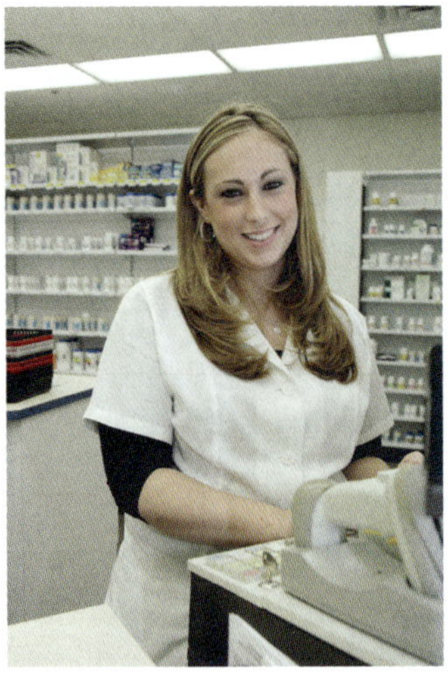

Prescription In-Take

The drop off area, which may also be a drive through window, is where customers will come to drop off new prescriptions or order refills. Greeting customers in a friendly and professional manner is a crucial function that makes customers want to remain loyal patrons.

Prescriptions may also be faxed, sent electronically as an e-script to the pharmacy's computer system, or called in to the pharmacist. For phone orders, the pharmacist will transcribe the prescription to a telephone prescription pad and give it to the technician to enter into the system.

Insurance information

The patient's insurance card has the following information:

- ✔ name of plan
- ✔ patient's ID number
- ✔ group number—identifies the patient's employer or association
- ✔ pharmacy BIN number—a six-digit bank identification number that is necessary to correctly route online claims for payment.
- ✔ person code—(indicates if the patient is the primary cardholder (01), the spouse (02), or a dependent child (03 and following)
- ✔ provider services phone number—the insurance company's (or other provider's) phone number

ENTERING PATIENT PROFILE INFORMATION

The initial part of the prescription filling process is entering new patient information into the computer system and, for existing patients, verifying and updating information. This information, known as the patient profile, includes the patient's:

- ➥ name (check for correct spelling)
- ➥ date of birth
- ➥ current address
- ➥ telephone number(s)
- ➥ allergies to medications
- ➥ insurance information (see left)
- ➥ service preferences such as childproof caps or easy-open tops
- ➥ whether the patient will wait for the prescription or when they will return to pick it up

Other service options that might be offered, and entered into the computer system, depending on individual pharmacy programs and policies are:

- ➥ automatic refills as they are due
- ➥ messaging when a prescription order is ready
- ➥ delivery

℞ tip

Accuracy in filling prescriptions is of utmost importance. When using the computer system always be sure you are working in the correct patient profile. Because different patients may have similar or even identical names, always verify the patient's date of birth and address.

safety you should know

Most computer systems will flag drug interactions and allergy conflicts. Always alert the pharmacist to any flag so that he or she can evaluate its significance. The pharmacist may say it is okay to proceed or they may stop the process to consult the patient or prescriber.

ENTERING PRESCRIPTION INFORMATION

The pharmacy technician will key the following prescription information into the appropriate fields on the computer screen:

Physician's name

Physician's DEA number
Enter if required by third-party payor or if dispensing a controlled substance.

Directions for use (the sig)
Here the directions are to take one tablet daily.

Number of authorized refills
Here the prescriber gives three refills.

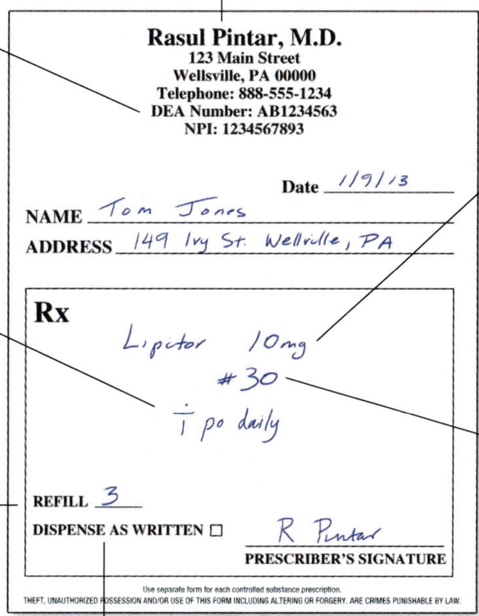
Rasul Pintar, M.D.
123 Main Street
Wellsville, PA 00000
Telephone: 888-555-1234
DEA Number: AB1234563
NPI: 1234567893

Date 1/9/13
NAME Tom Jones
ADDRESS 149 Ivy St. Wellville, PA

Rx
Lipitor 10mg
#30
i po daily

REFILL 3
DISPENSE AS WRITTEN ☐
R Pintar
PRESCRIBER'S SIGNATURE

Use separate form for each controlled substance prescription.
THEFT, UNAUTHORIZED POSSESSION AND/OR USE OF THIS FORM INCLUDING ALTERING OR FORGERY, ARE CRIMES PUNISHABLE BY LAW.

Correct drug and strength
Most pharmacy computer systems will automatically suggest a generic drug when one is available. For instance, if the technician enters Lipitor® 10 mg, the computer will suggest 10 mg atorvastatin, the generic equivalent.

Quantity
In this prescription the prescriber indicates a customary one month's supply of 30 tablets.

Dispense as Written (DAW)/Dispensing Code
The prescriber checks the DAW box if a substitution is not allowed. Based on this and other information, such as whether a brand drug is mandated by law or a generic substitution is not available, the technician enters one of the dispensing codes listed below.

Dispensing Codes

0. No product selection indicated.
1. Substitution not allowed by prescriber—prescriber checked "Dispense as Written" (DAW) box on prescription.
2. Substitution allowed—patient requested product dispensed.
3. Substitution allowed—pharmacist selected product dispensed.
4. Substitution allowed—generic drug not in stock.
5. Substitution allowed—brand drug dispensed as generic.
6. Override.
7. Substitution not allowed—brand drug mandated by law.
8. Substitution allowed—generic drug not available in marketplace.
9. Other.

PROCESSING PRESCRIPTIONS (cont'd)

REFILLS

Every prescription will have been assigned a prescription number by the pharmacy computer system when it is first filled. Refills of the prescription will carry the same prescription number.

Most refills are looked up either by the prescription number or by looking in the patient's profile for the requested medication.

The technician must first check to make sure that there are refills available. Most computer systems will indicate when no refills are available, in which case the pharmacy technician can offer to fax a refill request to the prescriber or ask the pharmacist to call the doctor for authorization.

The technician should also check to see if it is too early to refill the medication. If it is more than a week early, many third-party plans will reject the claim. Refills for controlled substance medications should not be refilled early since they have the potential for abuse; if a patient requests an early refill of a controlled substance, check with the pharmacist immediately.

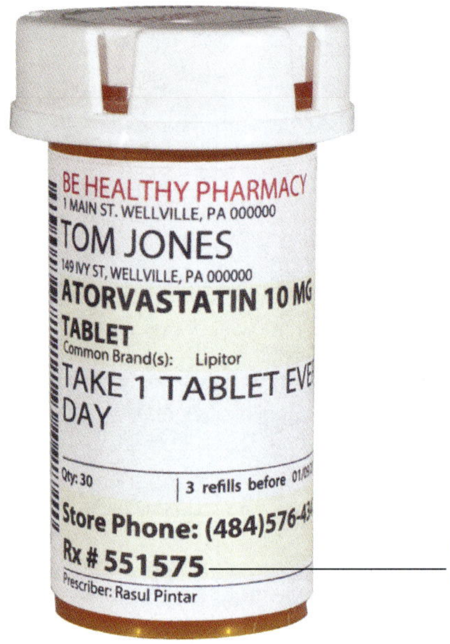

ONLINE BILLING

Today's pharmacy dispensing systems will generally "fill and bill" at the same time: As a prescription is entered into the system, the system sends a claim to the patient's insurance company or other third-party payor. The third party then responds online within a few moments either stating that the claim has been paid or has been rejected. The system will also indicate the co-pay amount if one is required. If the claim is rejected, there will be a general message regarding why the claim has not been paid. Sometimes resolving insurance rejections requires calling the third party to see what can be done to have the medication covered, such as switching from a brand to a generic drug.

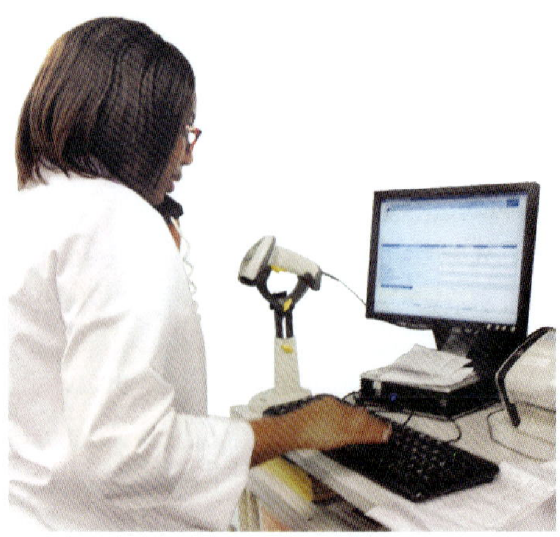

FILING

When a patient brings in a new prescription on paper, it is known as an original hard copy prescription. Original hard copies must be filed, usually by prescription number, for a specified length of time in accordance with state and federal laws.

Faxed, phoned, and electronic prescriptions must also be printed or transcribed onto a paper hard copy and filed.

State laws vary, but most require that prescriptions for Class II controlled substances are filed separately. Again depending on state law, Class III, IV, and V prescriptions may be filed with or separately from prescriptions for noncontrolled substances; if they are filed with noncontrolled substance prescriptions, they may need to be stamped or marked with a red "C".

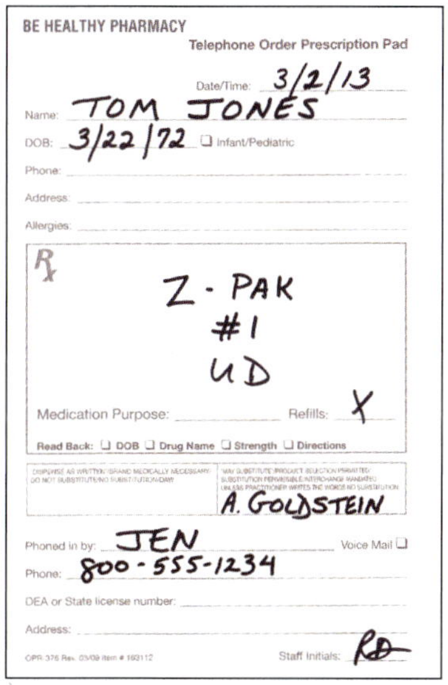

BE HEALTHY PHARMACY
Telephone Order Prescription Pad

Date/Time: 3/2/13
Name: TOM JONES
DOB: 3/22/72 ☐ Infant/Pediatric
Phone:
Address:
Allergies:

℞
Z - PAK
#1
UD

Medication Purpose: Refills: X
Read Back: ☐ DOB ☐ Drug Name ☐ Strength ☐ Directions

A. GOLDSTEIN

Phoned in by: JEN Voice Mail ☐
Phone: 800-555-1234
DEA or State license number:
Address:
Staff Initials: RD

a transcribed telephone prescription

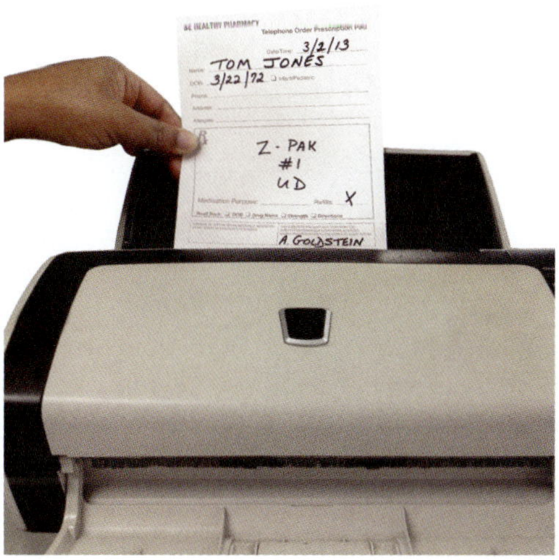

Scanning a hard copy prescription

For accuracy and improved record keeping, many pharmacies also scan the prescription into the pharmacy dispensing system.

PREPARING THE PRESCRIPTION

Once the patient and prescription information has been correctly entered into the computer system, there are several steps in preparing the prescription.

These include generating the label; retrieving the correct medication from stock; counting, measuring, and otherwise preparing the medication; placing the prescription label on the container; and organizing the prescription and medication for final check by the pharmacist.

GENERATING THE LABEL AND RETRIEVING THE PRODUCT

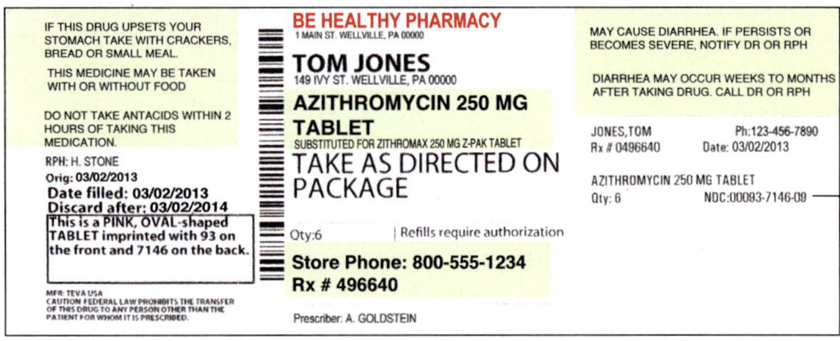

After all the prescription information has been entered into the system, use the computer's print function to generate a label. The label will include the product's National Drug Code (NDC) number, an eleven-digit number unique not only to the drug but also to the particular strength and form of the drug product. Scanning the NDC number on the drug product selected from the stock shelves, or checking it manually, will confirm that it is the same as the prescribed product.

CONTAINERS

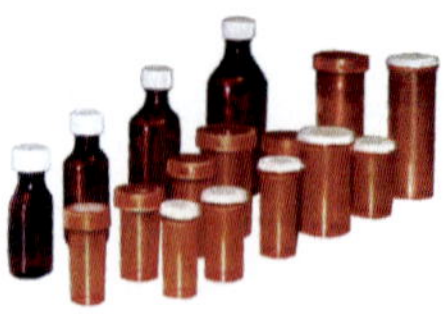

Pills and tablets are usually placed in plastic amber containers while liquids are poured into glass amber bottles. The dark amber color is designed to protect the drug from light, which can adversely affect the quality and effectiveness of some drugs.

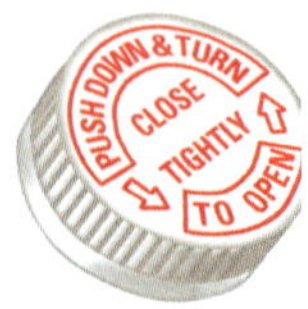

All prescription vials and bottles must have a ***safety cap*** or child resistant cap, unless the patient requests an easy-open cap. As discussed earlier, most computer systems have a field for recording the patient's preference. It is important to pay attention to which cap is indicated as some elderly or arthritic patients have extreme difficulty opening child-resistant caps.

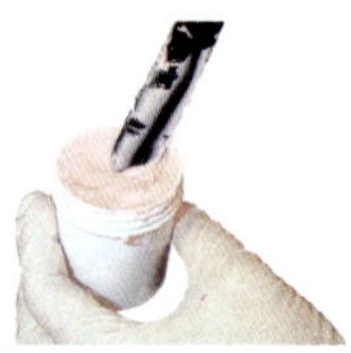

Creams and ointments that are not prepackaged are transferred with a spatula to an ointment jar of the correct size.

automated filling and dispensing machines automated machines that fill and label pill bottles with correct quantities of ordered drugs.

counting tray a tray designed for counting pills from a stock bottle into a prescription vial.

safety cap a child-resistant cap.

COUNTING PILLS AND TABLETS

One way to count capsules and tablets is using a ***counting tray***.

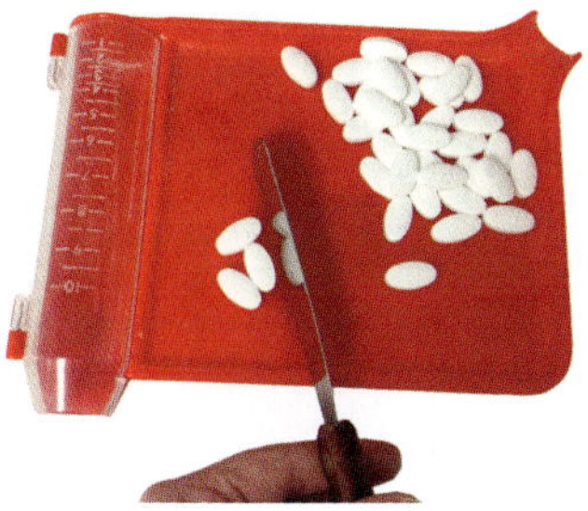

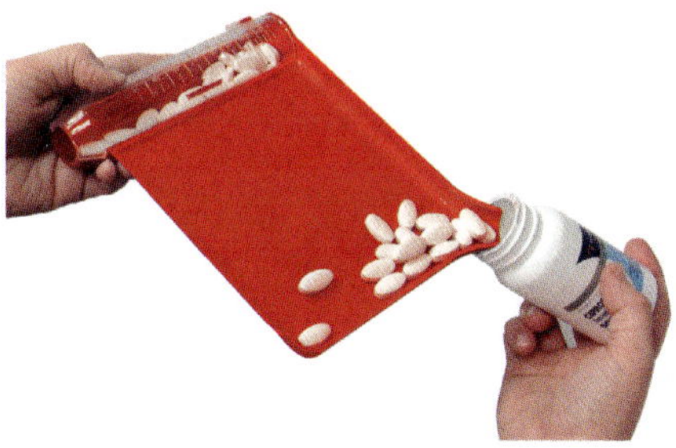

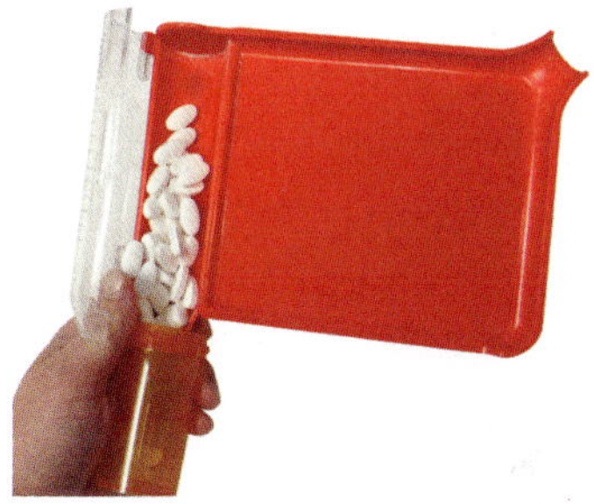

Place several pills or tablets on a counting tray and use a spatula to move pills two, three, or five at a time into the cylinder on the left until reaching the correct number. Return the extra pills to the stock bottle via the guide at the top right of the tray. Finally, slide the pills from the cylinder into the appropriately sized amber prescription vial.

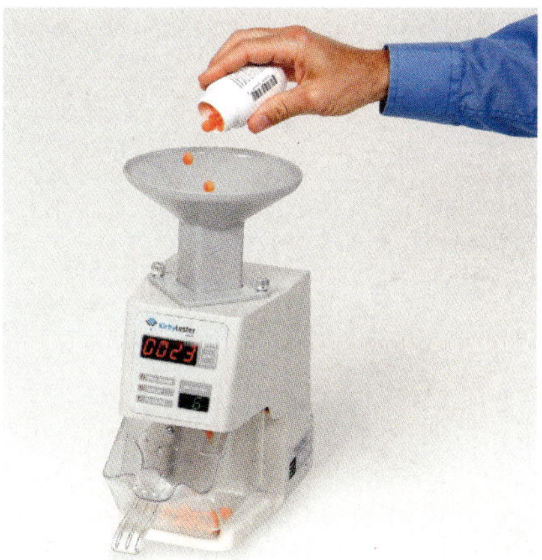

Automatic pill counting devices are frequently used to help a technician count medications. Pill counters like the Kirby Lester® KL1 (shown at left) are more accurate and usually much faster that using a counting tray. Pour the tablets or capsules through the top funnel of the pill counter, which records the number of pieces falling through. Stop when you reach the desired quantity, and transfer the counted medications into the appropriately sized vial.

(Image courtesy Kirby-Lester, LLC)

AUTOMATED FILLING MACHINES

Mid- to high-volume pharmacies may use ***automated filling and dispensing machines*** such as the Parata Max® (shown at right) for their fastest-moving drugs in capsule or tablet form. These machines automatically fill prescription bottles with correct quantities and label them. The pharmacy technician needs to maintain these machines on a daily basis by adding inventory to each cell, making sure the machine has a supply of labels, and keeping the machine clean. Note that a pharmacist must still check the final product even when dispensed by an automated filling machine.

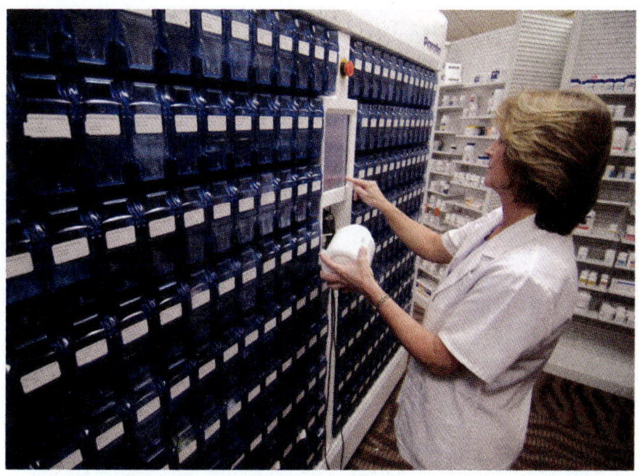

A pharmacy technician prepares to load a drug into Parata Max®.

(Photo courtesy of Parata Systems, LLC)

PREPARING THE PRESCRIPTION (cont'd)

MEASURING LIQUIDS

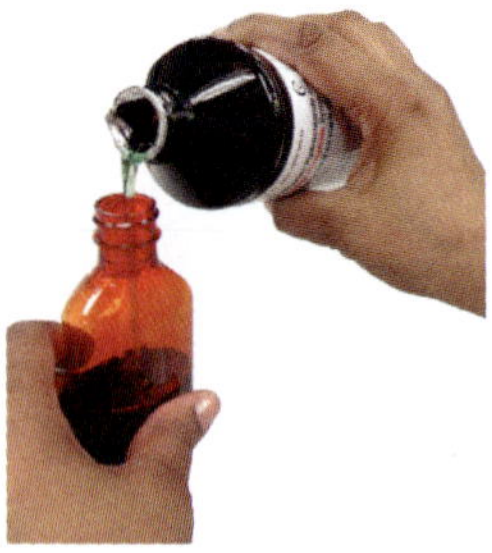

If the product is liquid, pour the correct metric quantity from the stock bottle into an appropriately sized amber bottle. Amber bottles come in the following sizes: 2 ounce (60 ml), 4 ounce (120 ml), 6 ounce (180 ml), 8 ounce (240 ml), 12 ounce (360 ml), and 16 ounce (480 ml). Each fluid ounce is equivalent to 30 milliliters.

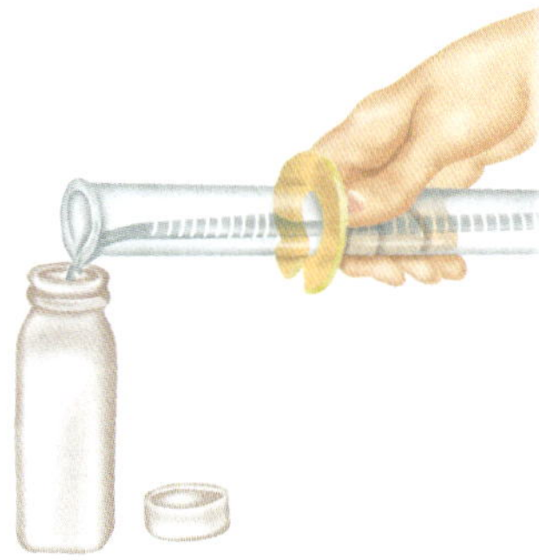

Some powder products will need to be reconstituted or mixed with distilled water prior to dispensing. The stock bottle will indicate the number of milliliters of water needed, which should be measured using a graduate. Once measured, the technician should pour the water into the bottle and shake well.

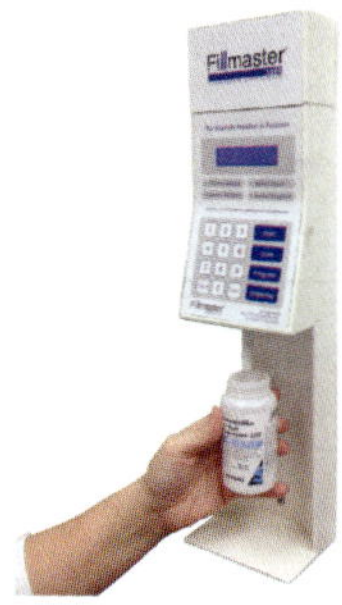

Some pharmacies may have an automated device such as a Fillmaster® that dispenses the exact amount of distilled water into the bottle.

PREPACKAGED MEDICATIONS

Some products are prepackaged and ready to dispense. These include eye and ear drops; creams, ointments, and gels; inhalers; oral contraceptives; and insulin vials. With these products, the prescription label is affixed directly on the package or container.

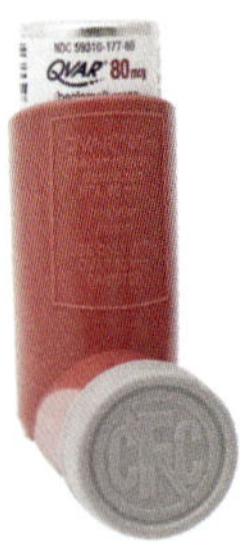

prepackaged inhaler

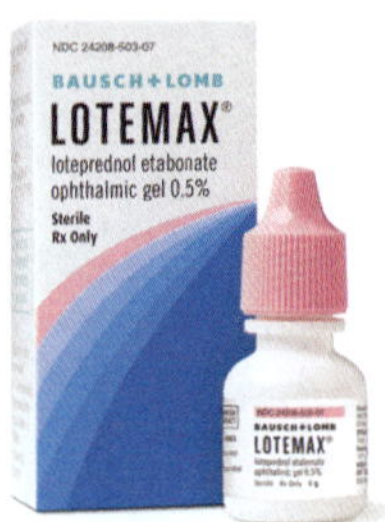

prepackaged eye drops

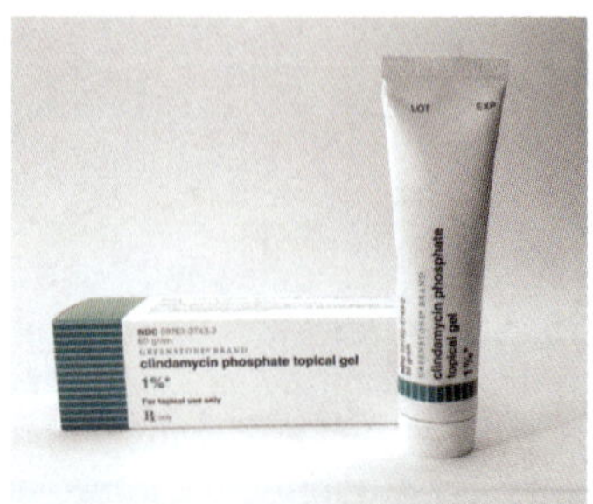

prepackaged cream

auxiliary labels labels regarding specific warnings, foods or medications to avoid, potential side effects, and other cautionary interactions.

LABELS

Once the desired pills or other product is put in an appropriate container, the finished prescription label is placed on the product along with any ***auxiliary labels*** that may be necessary. These labels identify important usage information, including specific warnings or alerts on:

- administration
- proper storage
- possible side effects
- potential food and drug interactions

Examples include "take with food," "may cause drowsiness," and others shown at right. Some computer systems automatically identify which auxiliary labels are needed. If this is not the case, ask the pharmacist which labels should be applied.

Some medications such as oral contraceptives require Patient Package Inserts (PPI). Medication Guides (MedGuides) may also be provided voluntarily by some manufacturers. Both PPIs and MedGuides provide information on how to safely use medications and are part of FDA-approved labeling.

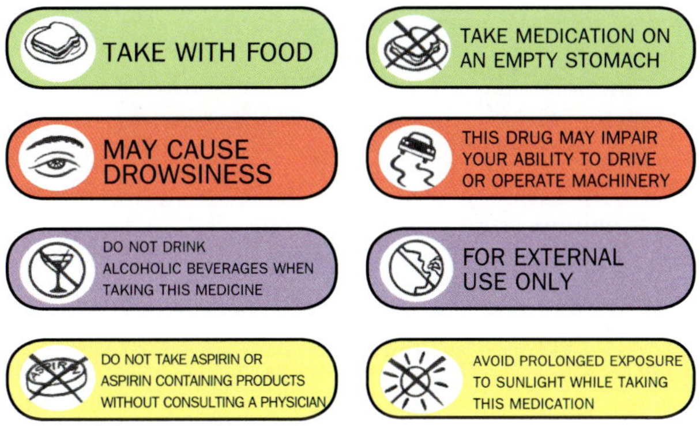

sample auxiliary labels

FINAL CHECK BY THE PHARMACIST

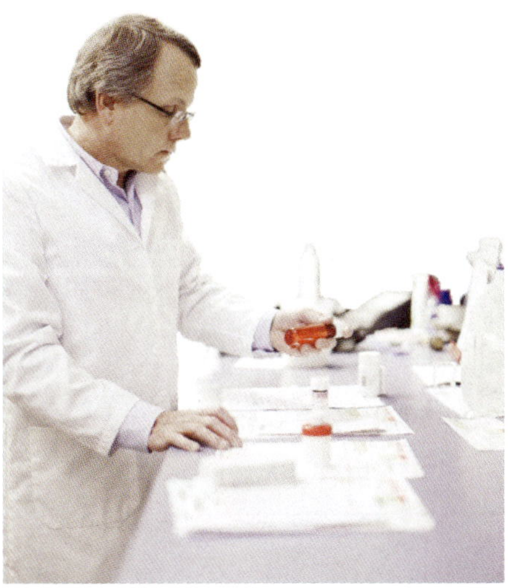

As the final step of the preparation process, organize the completed product for the pharmacist's final check. Leave stock bottles or other packaging next to the final product so the pharmacist can see that the correct product was chosen from stock.

After the pharmacist has checked the prescription, the pharmacy technician returns any products used to their proper place on the shelf, cabinet, or drawer. Finally, the technician places the prescription in a prescription bag with the receipt attached.

safety you should know

Schedule II controlled substances must be checked and signed for by the pharmacist.

CUSTOMER PICK-UP

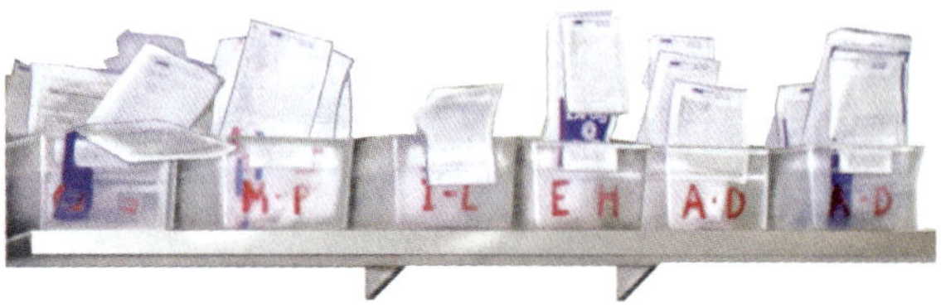

alphabetized prescription bins

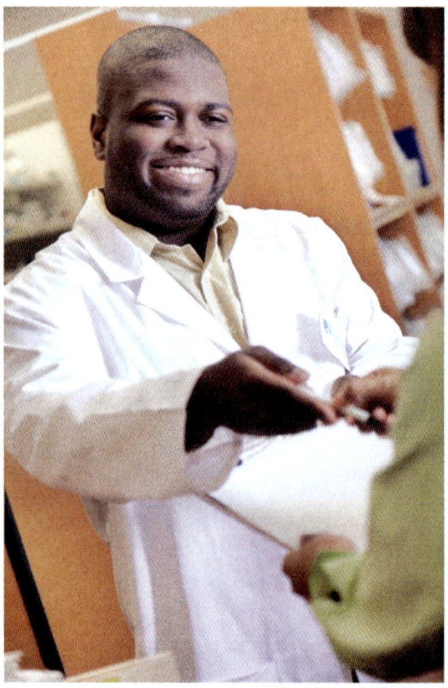

A technician asks a customer to sign the prescription pickup log.

Picking Up the Prescription

Completed prescriptions are usually filed alphabetically by the patient's last name either in bins or another storage area. Always be sensitive to the confidential nature of prescription information and be sure to follow HIPAA privacy regulations. Always speak in a quiet voice in the area specifically designated for prescription pick ups and be careful not to inadvertently give out protected information. For instance, do not ask, "Would you also like to pick up your daughter's prescription while you're here?" Though this may seem helpful, it is a breach of HIPAA privacy regulations. Provide only the prescription that was requested.

Signature Logs

Most community pharmacies have customers sign a log to record that the prescription was picked up. This serves as proof to a third-party payer such as Medicaid or a private insurer that the prescription was dispensed to the patient. Third-party payers commonly review the ***signature log*** when conducting pharmacy audits.

The log may also record that patient medication counselling was offered. The usual process is to ask the patient if they would like the pharmacist to speak with them regarding their prescription. The patient is then asked to sign that they have either accepted or declined.

In addition, pharmacies may require a person picking up a Schedule II, and sometimes also a Schedule III, IV, or V prescription, to show a driver's license. The driver's license number will be recorded either in the log or on the back of the prescription. This information will help in the event that the drug is used unlawfully.

Note that some companies may be using hard copy paper log books while others may be utilizing electronic signature capture technology.

signature log a book which patients sign for the prescriptions they receive, for legal and insurance purposes; may be electronic.

USING A CASH REGISTER

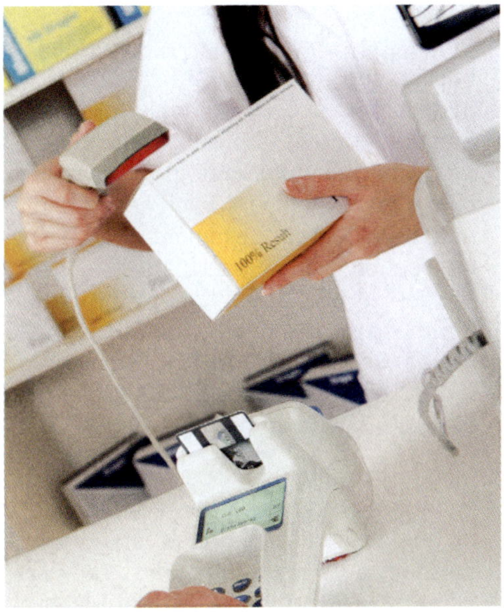

scanning a price

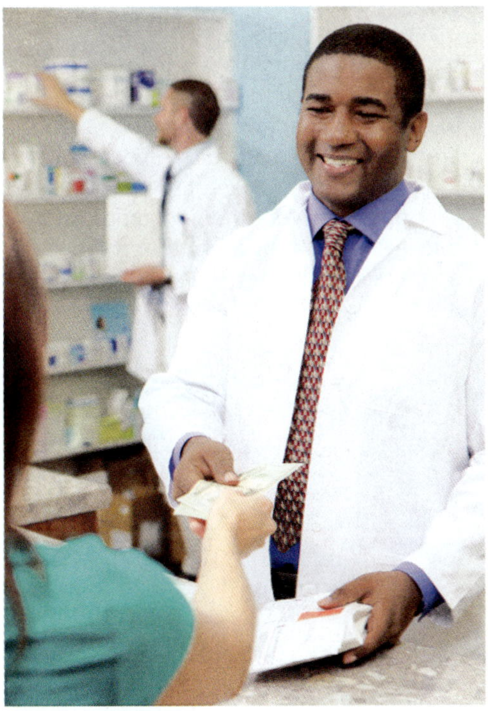

handling a cash payment

Pharmacy technicians often ring up purchases into the cash register and accept payment for prescriptions and over-the-counter products. Cash registers are integrated into the pharmacy's computerized system so prices for products can be automatically entered by using bar-code scanners. Scanners can be hand-held or built into the counter. The scanner beam is targeted at the bar code and identifies the product for the register. The product's price (or discounted price if there is a prescription plan discount) is automatically entered into the register. If a mistake is made between the pricing on the product or shelf and the amount in the system, changes can be made manually, though each system is different, and technicians need to know and follow the procedures used at their pharmacy.

Operating a cash register also requires handling payments properly. When cash payment is made, it is important to count the payment within the customer's line of sight and to confirm the amount orally to the customer. This will avoid misunderstandings over what the customer thought they gave you. If change is necessary, the amount should be counted out loud and placed into the customer's hand. An example of such a transaction would be:

- A twenty dollar bill is given as payment for a bill of $14.50.
- The bill should be held or placed within the customer's line of sight and the amount confirmed as, "That's twenty dollars."
- The amount is then entered into the register and a receipt is produced.
- The change is counted out as it is placed into the customer's hand, e.g., "Fifty cents makes fifteen dollars, and five dollars makes twenty dollars."
- After the customer has received their change and is given the receipt, the twenty dollar bill is placed into the register drawer.

Following this general procedure will avoid disputes, either out of confusion or intent to deceive, over whether a larger bill was tendered or the correct change given.

The pharmacy technician must also be able to handle checks, credit cards, and debit cards appropriately. Be sure to check the identification of the customer as instructed by the store manager or pharmacist for these forms of payments.

Finally, the technician must also know procedures for accepting coupons and gift cards

OTHER DUTIES

The pharmacy technician should know the names and locations of the various over-the-counter products carried in the pharmacy.

The technician should be able to direct customers to any OTC product. Examples include cough and cold preparations, laxatives, antidiarrheals, medications for the treatment of indigestion, analgesics, vitamins, herbal and dietary supplements, first aid supplies, dental and denture care products, and infant care products. Additionally, many pharmacies sell durable medical equipment such as canes, walkers, and wheelchairs.

However, the technician should not recommend OTC products to pharmacy customers.

With the exception of behind-the-counter medications, OTC products may be bought freely by customers. (See the discussion of PSE drugs earlier in this chapter, pages 396-397, as well as in Chapter 3, pages 46-47.) However, they are not without risks. Incorrect dosages and drug-drug interactions with OTC products can produce significant adverse effects. For example, many cough and cold preparations contain ingredients that may increase blood pressure and worsen a diabetic condition. Therefore, the technician should refer to the pharmacist patients' questions about OTC products.

Pharmacy technicians are responsible for reordering stock as needed.

The technician must know which products are used more frequently than others and reorder in appropriate quantities. For instance, a popular antihypertensive medication should be kept well stocked, while medications that are not as popular do not need to be available in large quantities.

The pharmacy technician is also generally responsible for keeping the pharmacy clean, neat, and in proper working order.

Periodically, the counting trays and the pharmacy counter should be wiped with alcohol. Pharmacy supplies, such as prescription bags, prescription vials and bottles, prescription labels, printer paper, and cash register receipts must be stocked regularly. The stock bottles should periodically be rearranged so that all labels face front. At least monthly, the pharmacy technician should check all bottles for outdated expiration dates because it is unlawful to dispense outdated medications. Expired drugs must be sent back to the wholesaler or be destroyed.

RETAIL CONCEPTS

Community pharmacies are also retail businesses that sell over-the-counter medications and various other products. To make a profit, the retailer sells the products at a ***markup*** from the purchase price they paid wholesalers and manufacturers. For example, if an OTC medication is purchased from a manufacturer at $5.00 and has a 50% markup, the retailer's price to the consumer will be: $5.00 plus the $2.50 markup ($5.00 times 50%), or $7.50. This is the price stickered on the product.

Markups are generally calculated by the pharmacy computer system and based on business costs (building, equipment, salaries, etc.) and profit goals. They will differ by pharmacy and can also differ by product.

Shelf Stickers

OTC products have ***shelf-stickers*** that can be scanned for inventory identification. They also indicate ***unit price*** information for consumers. A unit price is the price of a unit of medication (such as an ounce of a liquid cold remedy), rather than the price of the entire package. Unit prices protect the consumer from packaging that suggests that more is contained in the item than actually is.

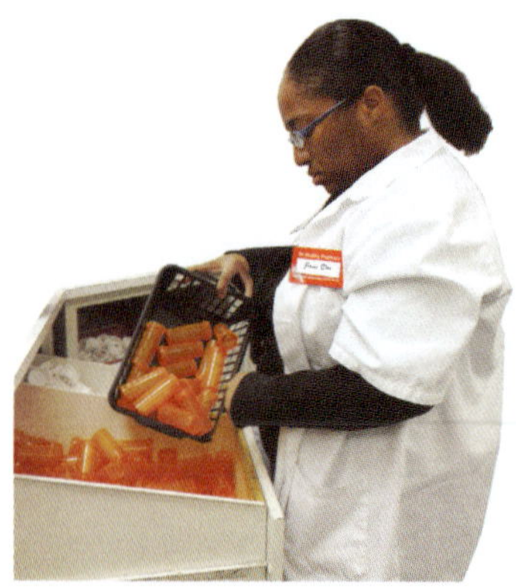

stocking prescription vials

markup the difference between the retailer's purchase price and their sale price.

shelf stickers stickers with bar codes that can be scanned for inventory identification.

unit price the price of a unit of medication, such as one ounce of a liquid cold remedy.

PRODUCT STOCK DUTIES

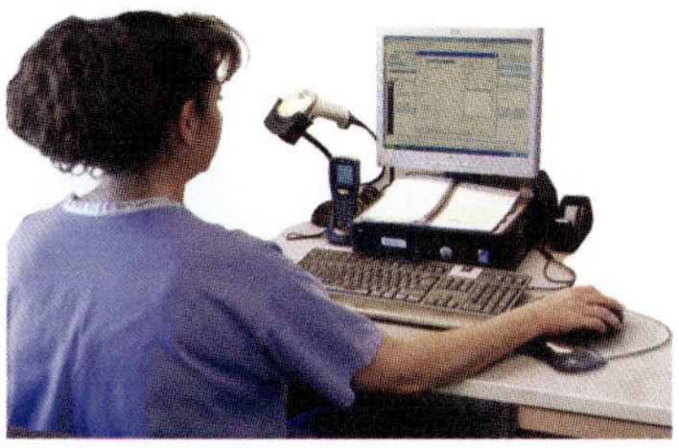

Ordering

Stock orders in most pharmacies are transmitted electronically to a drug wholesaler by either scanning or manually entering the product's stock number into a computer.

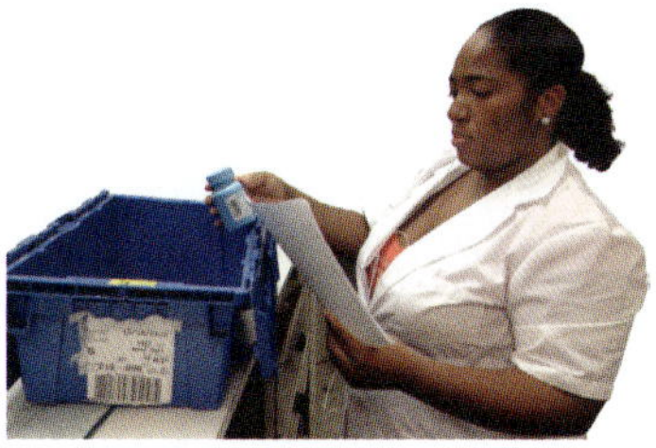

Receiving

The pharmacy technician is usually responsible for unpacking the order and checking that all items on the invoice have been received. Each item must be checked to make sure the following are as ordered:

- ✔ drug product
- ✔ strength
- ✔ packaging
- ✔ quantity

In addition items must be inspected for:

- ✔ damage
- ✔ expiration dates

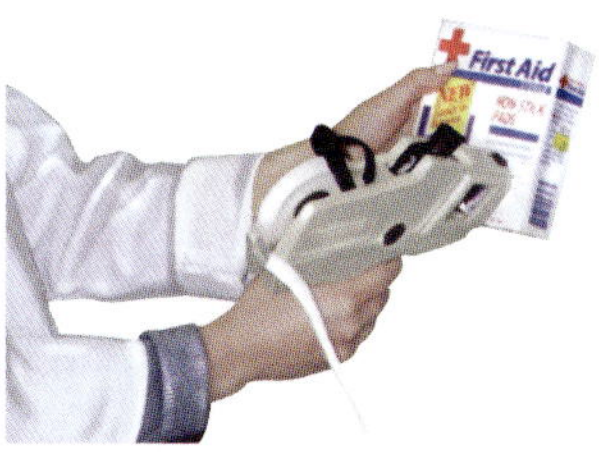

Stickering, Shelving, and Filing Invoices

Products are often stickered with pricing information and reorder numbers. These stickers may be applied with a stickering gun or by hand. Then the items need to be put on the shelves in their proper places. The invoices will also need to be filed for reference.

Resolving Problems

Finally, a pharmacy technician should know whom to go to within their pharmacy organization to resolve problems and issues such as product recalls or shortages. In some pharmacies, this may be the pharmacist in charge, while in others it may be a district manager or the head a specific department.

SEPARATION AND REMOVAL OF TRASH

- In accordance with HIPAA laws, pharmacies must separate from the regular trash any documents, reports, unused prescription labels, printouts or hand-written notes containing protected health information. Protected health information includes any patient specifics such as names, addresses, phone numbers, medications, medical history, etc. All documents with protected health information must be shredded or separated in a receptacle to be picked up by an outside vendor contracted to shred trash.
- Many pharmacies separate empty drug stock bottles from regular trash to be picked up by an outside vendor for recycling.
- Regular trash must be removed in accordance with the pharmacy's established procedure.

REVIEW

KEY CONCEPTS

COMMUNITY PHARMACY

- ✔ In addition to prescription drugs, community pharmacies sell over-the-counter medications as well as other health and beauty products.
- ✔ The community pharmacist's role in counseling and educating patients has been steadily increasing.

REGULATIONS

- ✔ Pharmacists and pharmacy technicians must be knowledgeable regarding the many federal and state regulations that affect the practice of pharmacy.

ORGANIZATION

- ✔ Pharmacies have basic space and equipment requirements that may vary slightly from state to state but generally include a prescription counter to work on, proper storage areas for drugs, designated refrigerators for drugs, equipment for compounding, a sink, computer system, and areas for dispensing prescriptions.

CUSTOMER SERVICE

- ✔ Technicians should always respond to customers in a positive and courteous way.

PROCESSING PRESCRIPTIONS

- ✔ In the case of a patient requesting an early refill of a controlled substance, involve the pharmacist right away.
- ✔ Processing new prescriptions involves entering patient information and prescription drug information, as well as billing information.

PREPARING THE PRESCRIPTION

- ✔ Whenever the prescription system flags drug interactions and allergy conflicts, alert the pharmacist so that he or she can evaluate the significance of the flag.
- ✔ Every drug product has a unique, 11-digit national drug code (NDC) number that can be used when filling a prescription to verify the correct product has been retrieved from stock.
- ✔ All dispensed prescription vials and bottles must have a safety cap or child-resistant cap, unless the patient requests an easy-open or non-child-resistant cap.
- ✔ Auxiliary labels identify important usage information, including specific warnings or alerts on: administration, proper storage, possible side effects, and potential food and drug interactions.
- ✔ As a final step of the preparation process, the final product and all paperwork, including the original prescription, is organized for the pharmacist's final check.

CUSTOMER PICK UP

- ✔ Customer signatures in a log are required for Medicaid and most third-party insurers or HMO prescriptions, along with Schedule V controlled substances, poisons, and certain other prescriptions (depending upon the state).

OTHER DUTIES

- ✔ With the exception of behind-the-counter OTC medications (see Chapter 3), OTC products may be bought freely by customers, but they are not without risks. The technician may direct customers to a product but should involve the pharmacist when making recommendations.
- ✔ Ordering stock is often a responsibility of the pharmacy technician.
- ✔ The pharmacy technician is generally responsible for keeping the pharmacy clean, neat, and in proper working order.

SELF TEST

the answer key begins on page 569

MATCH THE TERMS

1. automated filling and dispensing machines ____
2. auxiliary labels ____
3. Combat Methamphetamine Epidemic Act (CMEA) _____
4. counting tray _____
5. Health Insurance Portability and Accountability Act (HIPAA) _____
6. interpersonal skills ____
7. markup ____
8. Medicare Prescription Drug Improvement and Modernization Act _____
9. Omnibus Budget and Reconciliation Act (OBRA)
10. Red Flag Rule _____
11. safety caps ____
12. shelf stickers ____
13. signature log ____
14. transaction windows ____
15. unit price ____

a. skills involving relationships between people.

b. counter areas designated for taking prescriptions and for dispensing them to patients.

c. a child-resistant cap.

d. the price of a unit of medication (such as an ounce of a liquid cold remedy).

e. a tray designed for counting pills.

f. specific warnings that are placed on filled prescriptions.

g. book which patients sign for the prescriptions they receive, for legal and insurance purposes; may be electronic.

h. the amount of the retailer's sale price minus their purchase price.

i. stickers with bar codes that can be scanned for inventory identification.

j. automated machines that fill and label pill bottles with correct quantities of ordered drugs.

k. federal legislation enacted to regulate over-the-counter sales of ephedrine and pseudoephedrine.

l. federal legislation designed to protect patients' personal and medical information and also to encourage use of electronic data interchange in the United States.

m. federal legislation requiring pharmacists to provide counseling to Medicaid patients who are receiving new prescriptions.

n. a set of provisions created by the Federal Trade Commission (FTC) to help prevent identity theft from patient billing accounts maintained by medical and financial institutions.

o. federal legislation that created Medicare Part D and made allowance for Medicare recipients to receive Medicare medical coverage through private health insurance plans.

REVIEW

CHOOSE THE BEST ANSWER

1. ______________________________ are skills involving relationships between people.
   a. Computer skills
   b. Data management skills
   c. Transaction skills
   d. Interpersonal skills

2. More technicians and pharmacists are employed in ________________ than any other type of pharmacy.
   a. community pharmacy
   b. hospital pharmacy
   c. mail order pharmacy
   d. long-term care

3. Community pharmacies that are individually owned local pharmacies are
   a. food store pharmacies.
   b. mass merchandiser pharmacies.
   c. chain pharmacies.
   d. independent pharmacies.

4. Community pharmacies, such as CVS and Walgreens, that are part of regional or national pharmacy chains are
   a. independent pharmacies.
   b. food store pharmacies.
   c. chain pharmacies.
   d. mass merchandiser pharmacies.

5. Examples of pharmacist clinical services programs include
   a. teaching diabetic patients to use a blood glucose meter.
   b. recommending a medication change to a patient's physician.
   c. administering a vaccination to a patient.
   d. all of the above.

6. _____________________ require(s) community pharmacists to offer counseling to Medicaid patients regarding medications.
   a. Medicare Part D
   b. The 1990 Omnibus Budget and Reconciliation Act (OBRA)
   c. HIPAA
   d. The DEA

7. The HIPAA laws
   a. require pharmacists to provide counselling on all new medications.
   b. requires that health information be kept confidential.
   c. allows pharmacy staff to discuss a patient's health information outside the pharmacy.
   d. none of the above.

8. The Combat Methamphetamine Epidemic Act limits the over-the-counter sales of
   a. acetaminophen.
   b. aspirin.
   c. pseudoephedrine.
   d. laxatives.

9. Individual states
   a. do not regulate pharmacy practice.
   b. may require national pharmacy technician certification or may have their own certification process.
   c. regulate the scope of pharmacy technician practice, including the ratio of pharmacists to technicians.
   d. b & c

10. The refrigerator in a community pharmacy may be used to store
    a. drugs only.
    b. drugs as well as lunches of pharmacy personnel.
    c. drugs and sealed containers of soda pop.
    d. drugs and the pharmacist's lunch.

11. Completed prescriptions are generally placed in bins or on shelves
    a. alphabetically by the name of the drug being dispensed.
    b. alphabetically by the customer's last name.
    c. randomly.
    d. in the same order in which they were completed.

12. Pharmacy technicians
    a. must be calm and courteous when interacting with customers.
    b. must know when to refer a customer complaint or customer question to the pharmacist.
    c. must be familiar with the layout of the store.
    d. all of the above.

13. Good interpersonal skills include
    a. making eye contact.
    b. calling the customer by name.
    c. listening carefully.
    d. all of the above.

14. A patient's questions regarding medications or general health
    a. can be handled by the technician.
    b. should be referred to the pharmacist.
    c. can be answered by the pharmacy technician or by the pharmacist, depending on state regulations.
    d. can sometimes be answered by the pharmacy technician and sometimes by the pharmacist, depending on the technician's judgement.

15. The patient profile information
    a. includes the patient's name, date of birth, and current address.
    b. can be bypassed by the pharmacy technician if the customer is in a rush.
    c. may include the customer's preferences such as child-proof caps or easy-open caps.
    d. a and c

16. When entering a new prescription into the pharmacy computer, the technician must enter the following information:
    a. the prescription number
    b. the dispensing code
    c. the sig
    d. b and c

17. An NDC number
    a. is nine-digits long and is the same for some drugs.
    b. is the same as the prescription number
    c. is an 11-digit number unique to each product.
    d. None of the above.

REVIEW

18. All dispensed prescriptions must have a ________________ cap unless that patient specifies a _______________ cap.
    a. child-resistant, non-child-resistant
    b. child-resistant, child-resistant
    c. non-child-resistant, non-child-resistant
    d. non-child-resistant, child-resistant

19. A Kirby-Lester® is
    a. a medication specially mixed by a pharmacist.
    b. a machine to measure liquids such as syrups.
    c. an automatic pill counter.
    d. a counting tray.

20. The pharmacist _______ check the final product dispensed by an automated filling machine.
    a. must
    b. may
    c. does not need to

21. Products such as eye drops, insulin vials, and inhalers are all examples of
    a. prepackaged medications.
    b. unpackaged medications.
    c. unlabeled medications.
    d. none of the above.

22. Labels that are placed on the prescription container in addition to the prescription label and provide specific warnings are called
    a. poison labels.
    b. flags.
    c. prescription labels.
    d. auxiliary labels.

23. The pharmacist always checks the prescription
    a. after it is filled by the technician.
    b. when the patient signs the log.
    c. after it is rung on the cash register.
    d. as it is given to the patient.

24. A(n) ___________________ is a book that patients sign for prescriptions they receive.
    a. exempt narcotic book.
    b. patient register book.
    c. patient compliance book.
    d. signature log.

25. A few of the many tasks that pharmacy technicians are responsible for include
    a. keeping the pharmacy in clean, neat, and proper working order.
    b. entering new and refill prescriptions into the computer.
    c. both A and B.
    d. none of the above.

26. Ordering stock is a responsibility of the
    a. computer system.
    b. prescription counter.
    c. pharmacy technician.
    d. third party.

27. Operating a cash register generally requires
    a. handling cash payments.
    b. handling credit cards and checks.
    c. using a bar-code scanner.
    d. all of the above.

28. Unit price information is found on shelf stickers for
    a. Schedule III, IV, and V medications.
    b. Schedule II medications.
    c. OTC products.
    d. legend drugs.

29. All unused documents and labels containing protected health information
    a. can be used as scrap paper.
    b. must be shredded.
    c. can be removed from the pharmacy daily in the regular trash.
    d. must be disposed of in sharps containers.

CRITICAL THINKING QUESTIONS

1. When entering a new prescription into the pharmacy computer system, what are two parameters a technician should verify first to ensure that the prescription is being entered in the correct patient profile?
2. A new prescription calls for 150 ml of ibuprofen suspension for a child. How should the technician prepare the prescription for dispensing?
3. A prescription calls for cyclobenzaprine 10 mg tablets to be taken three times daily as needed for back spasm. The quantity ordered by the doctor is 90 tablets. How would a pharmacy technician use a counting tray to count out ninety tablets?

THINKING IT THROUGH WRAP-UP

1. In this situation the customer will appreciate an empathetic pharmacy technician who acknowledges that it can be difficult to wait for medications that are being prepared, especially when the customer is not feeling well. Positive responses, including intent listening, making eye contact, and restating what the customer has said will show him or her that you do care and are doing your best to understand and help.
2. This elderly arthritic person will be greatly relieved by being asked if she would like her prescriptions dispensed with easy-off, flip-open caps. Additionally, if the pharmacy offers delivery services, offering to deliver her prescriptions to her home will be of great convenience.
3. This customer should be courteously told, "I'll get the pharmacist to help you select the right product."

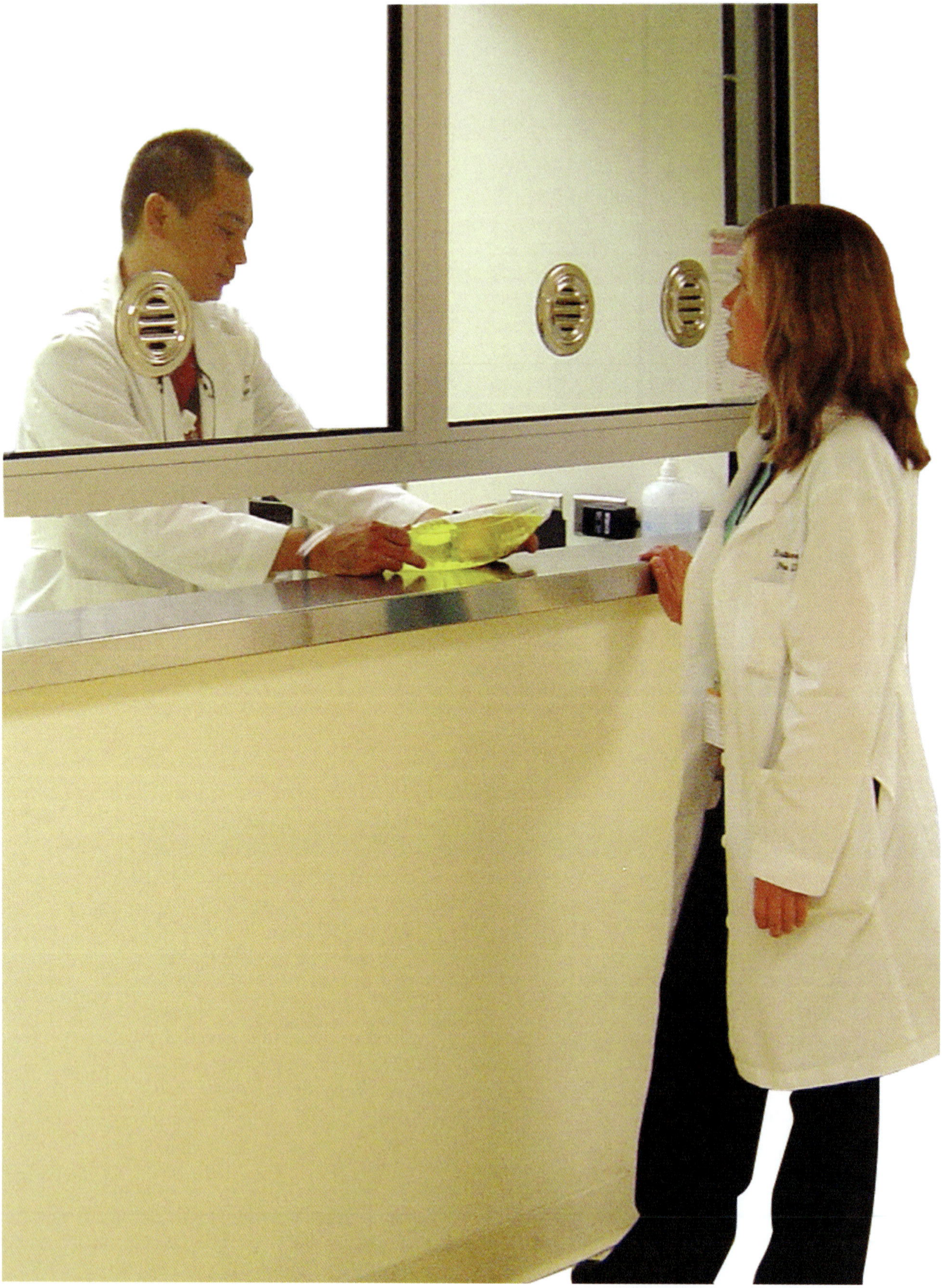

16

HOSPITAL PHARMACY

LEARNING OBJECTIVES

At the completion of study, the student will be able to:

- ✔ list various members of the health-care team.
- ✔ identify the variety of roles of a pharmacy technician.
- ✔ define hospital formulary and therapeutic exchange.
- ✔ summarize why unit dose medications are used in the hospital setting.
- ✔ discuss the components of a patient chart and/or electronic medical record.
- ✔ compare and contrast hospital medication orders with outpatient prescriptions.
- ✔ differentiate manual versus automated order processing.
- ✔ outline the process for hospital drug inventory ordering and receiving.
- ✔ compare the difference between single and multi-dose medication vials.
- ✔ explain the importance of Material Safety Data Sheets (MSDS).
- ✔ demonstrate an understanding of hospital pharmacy calculations.

THINKING IT THROUGH

Sam is a hospital pharmacy technician working in the oncology pharmacy satellite at Metropolitan Hospital. Dr. Stewart calls from the bone marrow transplant unit (BMTU) to give a telephone order for a STAT intravenous potassium chloride dose. Sam tells Dr. Stewart the pharmacist is on the other line. Dr. Stewart replies impatiently that he is in a hurry.

As you read this chapter, consider the following questions:

1. How should Sam respond to the doctor?
2. Can a pharmacy technician take a doctor's telephone order in this situation?
3. What information should Sam look up in the computer system to help?

HOSPITAL PHARMACY

Pharmacy technicians in the hospital work under the direct supervision of a pharmacist or supervising technician and play a vital role in the preparation, storage, and delivery of medications to patients.

Most hospitals require a high school diploma or equivalent and a current state pharmacy technician license; however, some hospitals will train a person while in the process of applying for licensure. Training requirements may vary by state and hospital, but hospitals are increasingly seeking technicians who already have received certification (CPhT).

To better understand the hospital pharmacy technician's roles and responsibilities, it is important to become familiar with the details of a hospital.

Though they may be organized differently, hospitals generally contain the same elements. Patient rooms are divided into groups called nursing units or patient care units. Patients with similar problems are usually located on the same unit. Often, names of specific units are referred to by their abbreviations. For example, a patient being treated for a heart attack would be treated in the cardiac care unit (CCU) and a woman about to give birth would be admitted to the obstetrics (OB) ward.

The work station for medical personnel on a nursing unit is called the *nurses' station*.

The nurses' station is a communication center for patient care in each hospital unit. This area stores various items required for care of the patients on the unit, including medications.

There are several other areas of the hospital, called ancillary areas, that also provide patient care.

Each hospital has different ancillary areas, but some common ones are radiology, the cardiac catheterization lab, and the emergency room. These areas use medications and are serviced by the pharmacy department.

nurses' station work station for medical personnel located on a nursing unit.

SOME HOSPITAL UNIT ABBREVIATIONS

- BMTU: Bone Marrow Transplant Unit
- CCU: Cardiac Care Unit or Coronary Care Unit
- ED: Emergency Department
- ER: Emergency Room
- ICU: Intensive Care Unit
- CT-ICU: Cardiothoracic ICU
- NICU: Neonatal ICU or Neurological ICU
- PICU: Pediatric ICU
- SICU: Surgical ICU
- OB: Obstetrics
- OR: Operating Room
- PAR: Post-Anesthesia Recovery
- PACU: Post-Anesthesia Care Unit
- PEDS: Pediatrics

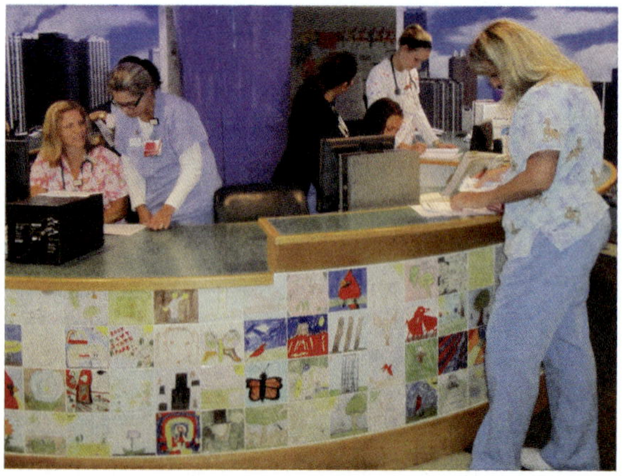

The nurses' station is a central storage and communication center for patient care in the hospital.

THE HEALTH-CARE TEAM

It takes a team of many different types of health-care professionals to meet patients' medication needs, and individual patients generally receive care from a variety of these professionals. Most health-care personnel are identified by abbreviations that indicate their discipline. Each individual profession plays a part on the multidisciplinary health-care team. Their common objective is to care for patients and assist in their recovery. Pharmacy technicians interact with many of the following professions.

Physician

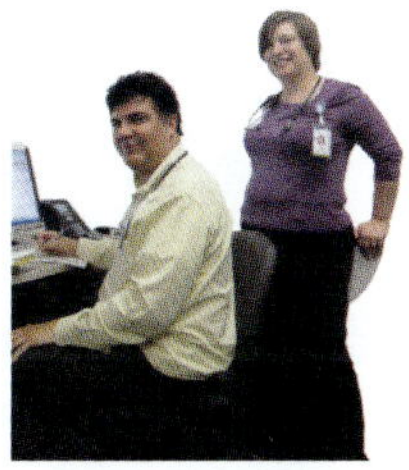

M.D., Medical Doctor

An M.D. examines patients, orders and interprets lab tests, diagnoses illnesses, and prescribes and administers treatments for people suffering from injury or disease. M.D.s write the majority of all medication orders.

D.O., Doctor of Osteopathy

A osteopathic physician has the same responsibilities as an M.D. but practices a "whole person" approach to medicine.

Other Staff

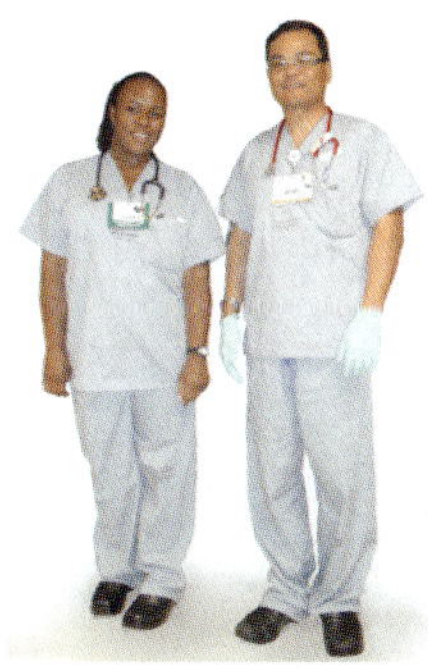

R.T., Respiratory Therapist

A respiratory therapist assists in the evaluation, treatment, and care of patients with breathing problems or illnesses. They may also administer respiratory drug treatments to patients.

P.A., Physician Assistant

A physician assistant coordinates care for patients under the close supervision of a M.D. or D.O. They are allowed to prescribe certain medications.

P.C.T., Patient Care Technician

A patient care technician works as a unit clerk or assists nurses in patient care activities. P.C.T.s are often sent to the pharmacy to pick up patient medications in between pharmacy deliveries.

M.S.W., Master's of Social Work

A social worker is concerned with patient social factors such as child protection, coping capacities of patients and their families, and patients' ability to pay for medications.

Nursing

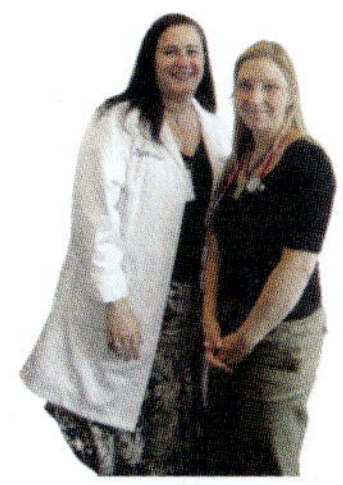

N.P., Nurse Practitioner or A.P.N., Advanced Practice Nurse

A nurse practitioner or advanced practice nurse provides basic primary health care or can do further training to specialize in a specific area. The N.P. works closely with doctors and can prescribe various medications in most states.

R.N., Registered Nurse

A registered nurse provides bedside care, assists physicians in various procedures, and administers medication regimens to patients.

L.P.N., Licensed Practical Nurse

A licensed practical nurse provides basic bedside care under the supervision of an R.N. An L.P.N. may administer medication to patients.

Pharmacy

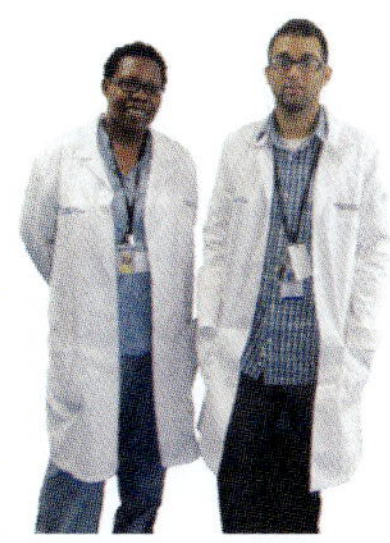

R.Ph., Registered Pharmacist

A registered pharmacist is licensed to work by the state. Duties include reviewing patient drug regimens, dispensing medications, and advising the medical staff on the selection of drugs. An R.Ph. may have a bachelor of science in pharmacy (B.S.Pharm.) or a Doctor of Pharmacy (Pharm.D.) degree.

Pharm.D., Doctor of Pharmacy

A Pharm.D. is a pharmacist with a doctorate in pharmacy. Pharm.D. degree requirements include more clinical science courses and more experiential training than do B.S.Pharm. degree requirements.

TECHNICIAN ROLES

The hospital pharmacy technician has many responsibilities. Most pharmacy technicians are cross-trained. This allows the technician to work in different areas of the pharmacy as needed. Some responsibilities may overlap between the different roles. Listed below are examples of various duties a pharmacy technician may have in the hospital setting.

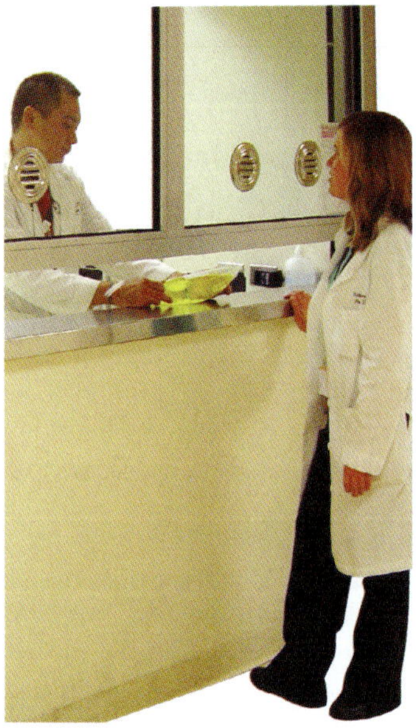

Front Counter

Hospital pharmacy technicians are often assigned to work the front counter in the main pharmacy. Here the technician is responsible for answering phone calls, helping other health-care professionals, filling first doses of oral medications, and other duties as needed. Many of the phone calls to the pharmacy include missing medications, automated dispensing cabinet issues, intravenous compatibility, and drug information questions. The pharmacy technician may answer questions about missing medications and troubleshoot automated dispensing cabinet problems; however, compatibility and drug information questions must be answered by a pharmacist.

Satellite Pharmacies

Some hospitals have a main pharmacy along with smaller satellite pharmacies located in different areas of the hospital. Hospital pharmacy technicians need to complete more specific training to work in pharmacy satellites and may rotate through the different areas (e.g., pediatrics, oncology, operating room, etc.).

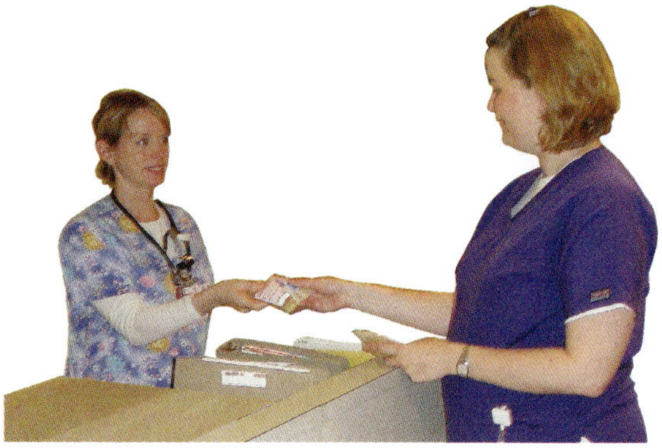

Delivery

A delivery technician is responsible for transporting medications and other pharmacy supplies from the pharmacy to nursing units, other ancillary areas of the hospital, and/or outpatient clinics. This role may include picking up new orders and bringing discontinued medications back to the pharmacy.

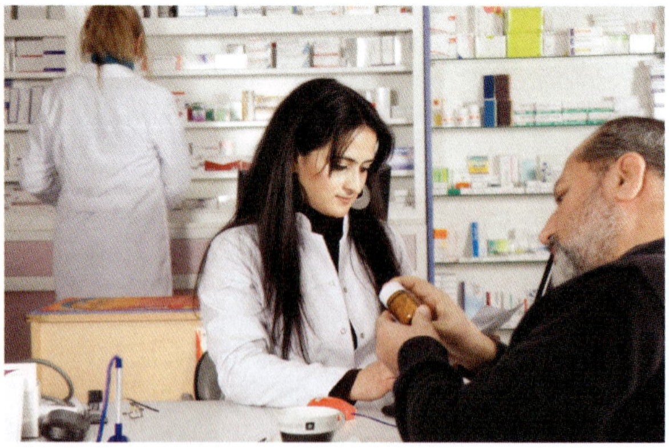

Outpatient Pharmacy

The outpatient pharmacy technician assists the pharmacist in processing prescriptions for patients leaving the hospital or visiting their doctor.

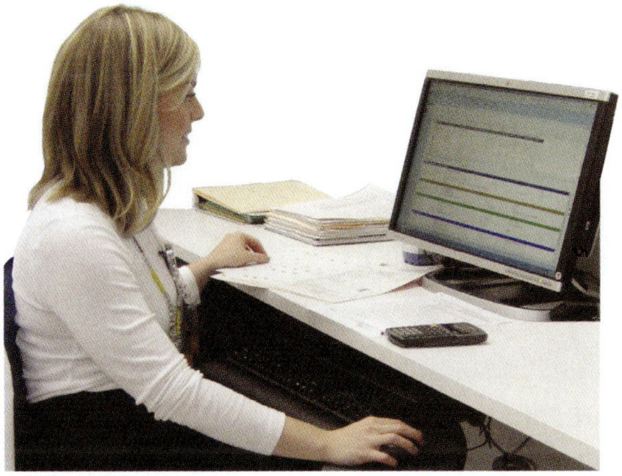

Order Processing

Order processing is another role often assigned to pharmacy technicians. In some hospitals, the technician is responsible for entering written medication orders in the computer system. While entering orders, the technician may assist the pharmacist by screening the patient profile for allergies, duplicate therapies, and pertinent labs. By bringing this information to the pharmacist's attention, the technician can help prevent medication errors.

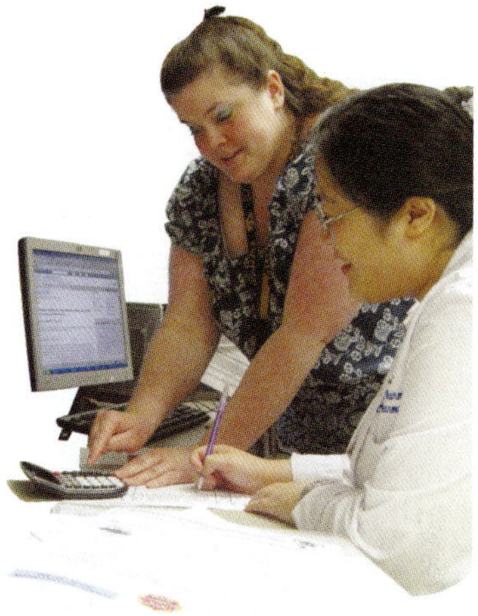

Monitoring Drug Therapy

A pharmacy technician is sometimes assigned to assist a pharmacist in monitoring patients' drug therapies. This entails retrieving drug levels, labs values, or other patient specific information (e.g., blood pressure, fever, etc.) from patient charts or from the hospital computer system. The technician may also be asked to run reports of patients who are on medications, such as vancomycin, that require drug monitoring.

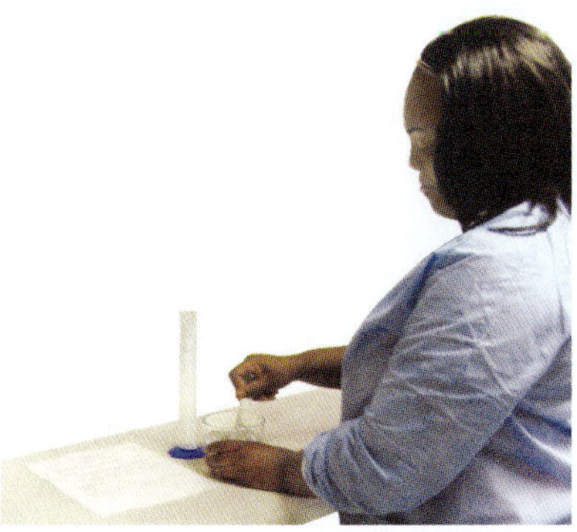

Compounding/ Unit Dosing

A pharmacy technician assigned to compounding is responsible for making medication formulations that are not available from a manufacturer. This is done by using specific recipes provided by the pharmacy. Duties also include reconstituting bottles of commercially available medications and drawing up unit doses from bulk medication bottles. This role can also include operating a prepacking machine to package unit doses of oral capsules and tablets from bulk bottles.

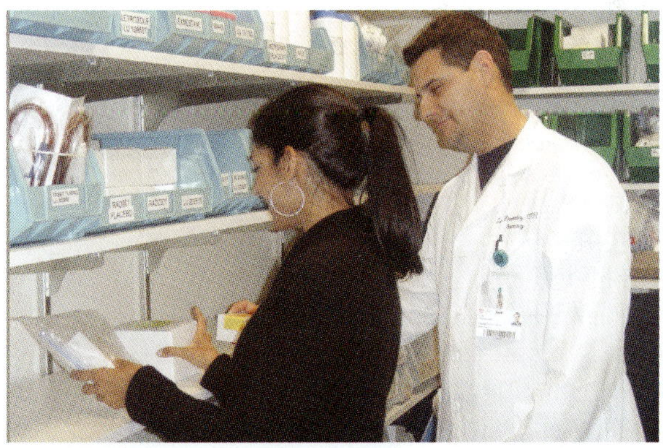

Investigational Drug Service

In hospitals that conduct drug studies, a pharmacy technician often assists the investigational drug pharmacist by preparing and delivering study medications for patients enrolled in drug studies. Investigational medications require a great deal of paperwork; technicians working in this area frequently help the pharmacist with the large amount of required documentation.

TECHNICIAN ROLES (cont'd)

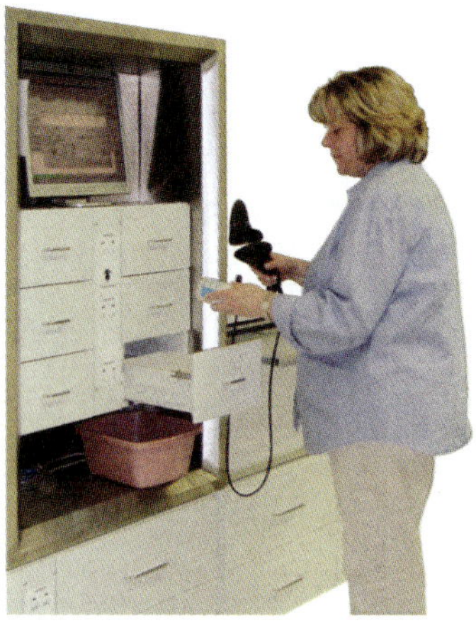

Inventory Control

An inventory technician is responsible for maintaining the pharmacy stock. Duties include ordering medications and checking pharmacy invoices. Inventory technicians also assist in handling drug recalls, shortages, and emergency drug procurement. In some hospitals, inventory technicians may also be responsible for filling automated dispensing cabinets in nursing and ancillary areas. Drug shortages have become a major issue in many hospitals. The inventory control technician plays a vital role in maintaining inventory for these drugs or ordering a substitution (alternative medication) while a drug is in short supply.

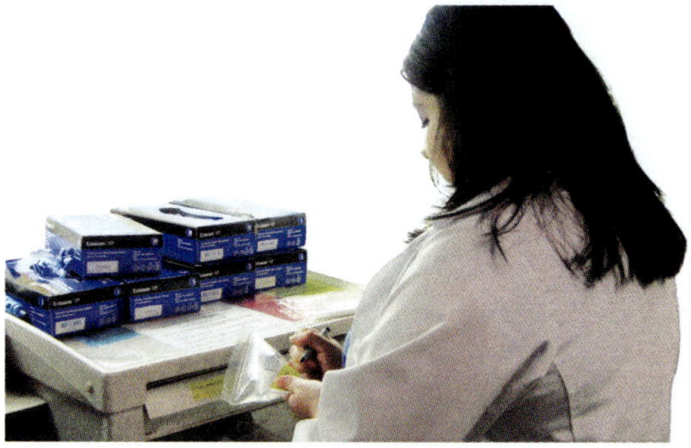

Cart Fill

In hospitals with manual cart fills, technicians fill the medication carts. These carts contain a 24-hour supply of patient medications in patient-specific cassettes or drawers. In hospitals with automated dispensing cabinets or a robot, the cart fill position may not exist or it may be limited to filling only the few medications not already stored in the automated dispensing cabinet or robot.

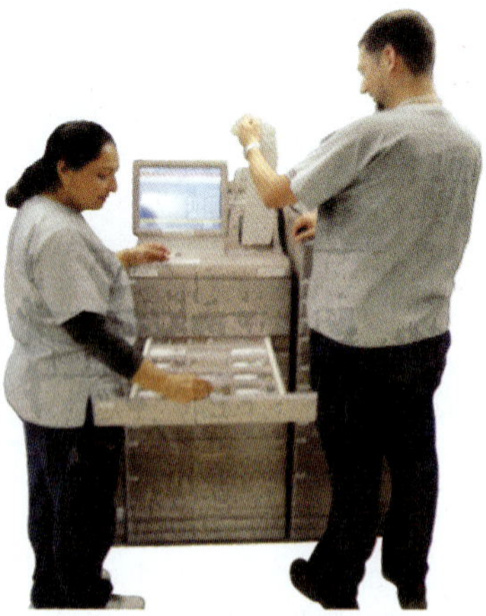

Narcotics/ Controlled Substances

Many hospitals have a pharmacy technician who helps coordinate narcotic drug distribution. This involves ensuring the security of narcotics when receiving, preparing, and delivering them to nursing units or automated dispensing cabinets. The technician also reviews inventory reports, completes audits, reviews discrepancy reports, and confirms the hospital's compliance with state and federal controlled substances laws.

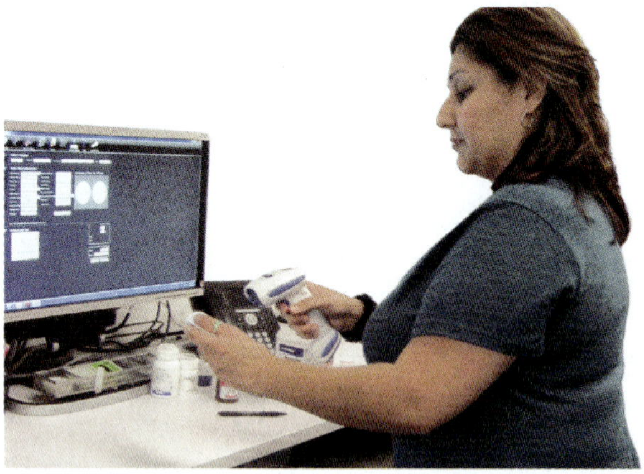

Automation

An automation technician is responsible for providing technical support for pharmacy systems. This role may entail operating a pharmacy robot, assisting health-care providers with use of automated dispensing cabinets, and assigning new user names and passwords. The automation technician often becomes an expert at using the automated systems and can be called on to troubleshoot problems with them.

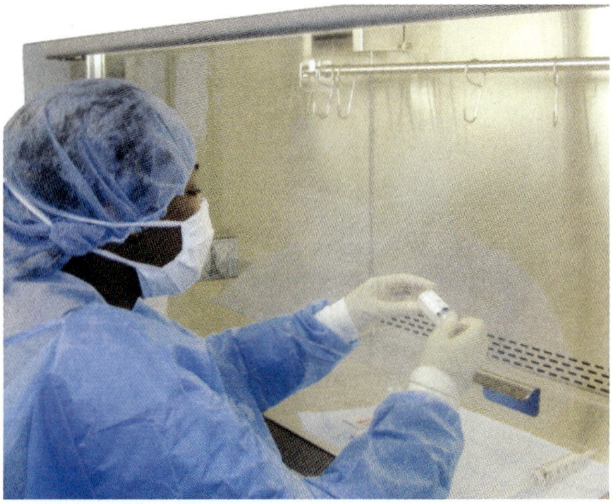

IV/Clean Room

The main responsibility of the IV/Clean room technician is to prepare sterile intravenous medications. Special training is often required prior to working in the clean room. This role may also include preparation of chemotherapy and parenteral nutrition.

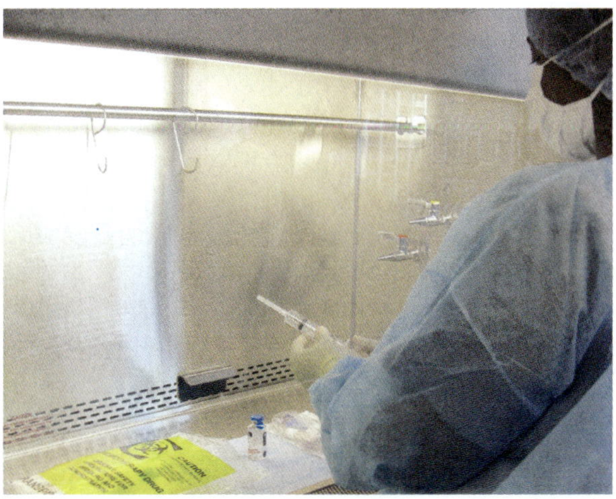

Chemotherapy

A chemotherapy technician receives additional training on handling and preparing chemotherapeutic agents and other hazardous drugs. Knowledge regarding decontamination and management of spills is essential. Often, a technician supervisor will administer a special skills test before the technician is allowed to prepare chemotherapy.

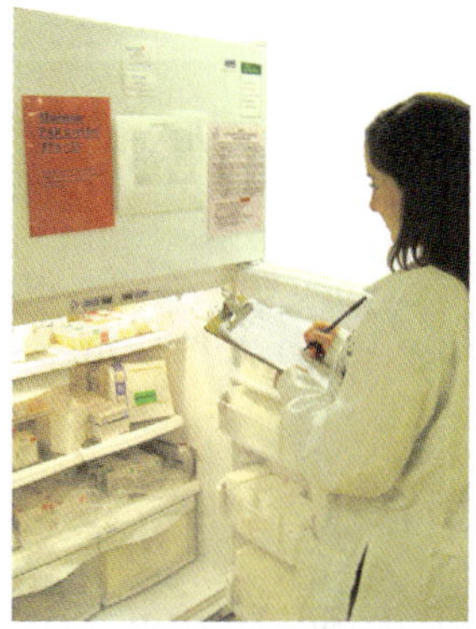

Quality Assurance (QA)

The quality assurance technician conducts inspections of nursing units and other areas of the hospital that store medications. During inspections, the technician makes sure that medications are stored and handled in compliance with hospital policy. This position may also include serving on various hospital committees (e.g., Medication Safety, Quality Committee). This role may also include investigating why a pharmacy medication error occurred, and developing a procedure to prevent the same type of error from happening again.

Pharmacy Technician Supervisor

This leadership role includes managing a team of hospital pharmacy technicians. The supervisor is often responsible for training technicians, creating work schedules, and completing annual evaluations for all technicians.

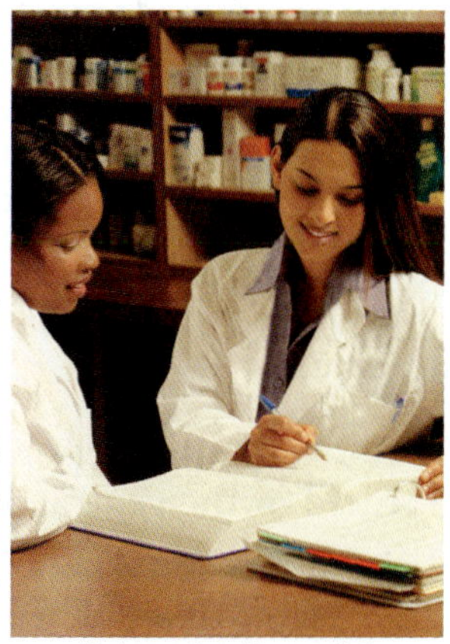

Photo courtesy Hanson Ng/ Design Pics/Getty Images

Staff Development

The goal of staff development is to improve the knowledge and skills of pharmacy technicians by providing staff training materials, reading assignments, demonstrations, and written or practical tests. Other staff development opportunities may include discussion groups and seminars on topics pertaining to hospital pharmacy.

HOSPITAL PHARMACY AREAS

The *inpatient pharmacy* is the area of the hospital responsible for medication preparation and distribution.

Some hospitals may also have *pharmacy satellites* located in different areas of the hospital. A pharmacy satellite is a branch of the inpatient pharmacy dedicated to serving a particular group of hospitalized patients. Satellites are often located in the same area as the patient care units they are servicing (e.g., pediatrics, operating room). Satellites are responsible for providing first doses of new medications ordered, all emergency medications, and replacing any missing or lost doses. They have a limited supply of medications that are specific to the patient care areas they service. Satellite pharmacies may be open 24 hours a day or have limited hours (e.g., 7 a.m.–10 p.m.).

In hospitals that have satellite pharmacies, the main inpatient pharmacy is called the *central pharmacy*.

The central pharmacy houses the bulk of the hospital's inventory of medications. The central pharmacy is generally responsible for preparation and delivery of unit-dose patient medication carts, *batching* of medications, and covering service areas not covered by pharmacy satellites. The central pharmacy also conducts a variety of packaging functions in order to keep other areas in the hospital supplied with the drugs they need.

In most hospitals, the central pharmacy is open 24 hours a day.

When a pharmacy satellite is closed, the central pharmacy will take over responsibility for servicing these areas as well.

The sterile product area, or *clean room*, is usually located in the central pharmacy.

Laminar flow hoods are located in the central pharmacy since this is where the majority of intravenous medications are prepared.

USP <797>

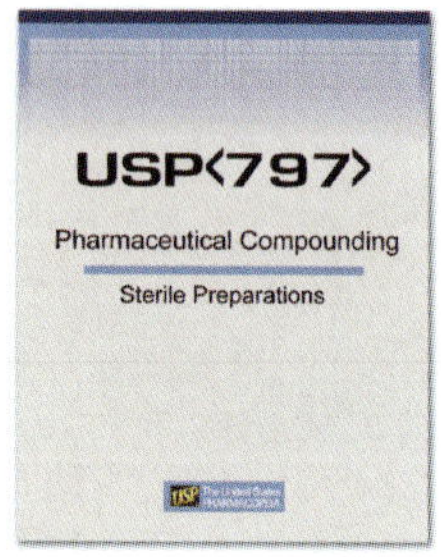

USP <797> is a set of regulations issued by the U.S. Pharmacopoeia. These regulations include a strict set of policies and practices that must be followed by any pharmacy that prepares compounded sterile products. The policies are intended to decrease infections transmitted to patients through drug preparation and better protect staff in their exposure to pharmaceuticals. All hospitals accredited by The Joint Commission (TJC) must be compliant with USP <797> standards.

batching preparation of large quantities of unit-dose oral solutions/ suspensions or small volume parenterals for future use.

central pharmacy the main inpatient pharmacy in a hospital that has pharmacy satellites. It is the place where most of the hospital's medications are prepared and stored.

clean room area designed for the preparation of sterile products.

inpatient pharmacy a pharmacy located in a hospital that services only those patients in the hospital and its ancillary areas.

outpatient pharmacy a pharmacy attached to a hospital that services patients who have left the hospital or who are visiting doctors in a hospital outpatient clinic.

pharmacy satellite a branch of the inpatient pharmacy responsible for preparing, dispensing, and monitoring medication for specific patient areas.

unit inspection a review of a nursing unit to ensure compliance with hospital medication policies.

See Chapter 9 for more on compounding sterile products.

SOME PHARMACY SATELLITES

Pediatric satellite: Special considerations must be taken into account when dosing and preparing medications for pediatric patients. Pediatric doses are often individually calculated based on a patient's weight and frequently require special dilutions since they are much smaller doses than for adults. Pharmacists and pharmacy technicians in the pediatric satellite carefully review and monitor pediatric patient medications and prepare individualized doses of IV and oral medications.

Operating room (OR) satellite: The OR is a dynamic environment where it is difficult for physicians and nurses to track medications prepared and given to patients. Pharmacists and pharmacy technicians in an OR satellite help oversee and control drug distribution for all operating rooms, decrease controlled substance loss and waste, reduce inventory expenses, and improve documentation of patient medication charges.

Oncology satellite: Chemotherapy medications require special preparation and precautions since they can be toxic to the person preparing them if not managed appropriately. The oncology satellite reviews, prepares, and delivers antineoplastic agents (chemotherapy) for hospital patients. Pharmacy technicians in the oncology satellite require special training and chemotherapy certification from the pharmacy department.

tip

Many large academic hospitals often have a separate drug information center with resources for answering drug-related questions. Other hospitals may set up a designated area in the pharmacy for drug references. See Chapter 12 for more on information sources.

A centralized area for storage of drug product or inventory may also be a part of the pharmacy department.

In larger hospitals this area requires an entire staff of its own that deals only with the order and delivery of drug products for the other pharmacy areas. Technicians often make up a large portion of this staff and may be in charge of running the area.

A number of hospitals have an investigational drug service, which is a specialized pharmacy subsection that deals solely with clinical drug trials.

These drug studies require a great deal of paperwork and special documentation of all doses of study medication. The investigational drug service may provide study drugs to patients located in the hospital and those treated in outpatient clinics, but only those patients enrolled in an investigational drug study or trial.

Quality assurance is another area in which pharmacy technicians are involved.

A pharmacy technician may be assigned to a specific area of the pharmacy to remove any outdated or expired medications. Another responsibility may be making sure refrigerators and freezers are maintained at correct temperatures and completing a daily log of temperatures. Pharmacy technicians may also be assigned to do unit inspections. A ***unit inspection*** is a review of a nursing unit to ensure compliance with hospital medication policies. This may include replacing expired medications, eliminating medications that should not be on the unit, and citing the unit for not adhering to policies.

Doctor's offices or clinics along with an *outpatient pharmacy* are often located near hospitals.

These pharmacies provide prescription medications to patients visiting their doctor. They are run very similarly to a retail pharmacy, but hospital technicians may be required to staff in these areas in addition to their inpatient responsibilities. Although an outpatient pharmacy may be located within a hospital, it does not supply inpatient medications. It only provides medications for patients who have obtained prescriptions from their doctors at the clinic or upon leaving the hospital.

HOSPITAL FORMULARY

Because hospitals cannot afford to stock every medication that is available, many maintain a hospital *formulary*.

A formulary is a list of drugs that have been selected by health-care professionals at the hospital based on therapeutic factors as well as cost. It is the responsibility of the Pharmacy and Therapeutics Committee (or P&T Committee) to set up, add, remove, and periodically evaluate medications listed on the hospital formulary. It is important for anyone who orders, prepares, or dispenses medications to know the medications currently on the formulary.

A *closed formulary* means that the hospital carries only formulary medications and physicians must order from this list.

Of course, some exceptions apply and the pharmacy will have a section of "non-formulary" drugs. *Non-formulary* drugs may require a special form stating why the physician requires that specific medication. Since a non-formulary drug is not stocked by the pharmacy, there may be a delay in the patient receiving the drug. Once the non-formulary drug is approved by the pharmacist, the inventory technician must order the medication. Since it may take several days to arrive, it is important for the technician to let the pharmacist know when the drug is scheduled to be delivered so the physician and patient can be made aware.

The Pharmacy and Therapeutics Committee consists of doctors, pharmacists, nurses, and other health-care professionals.

They work as a team to review medications for the hospital formulary; evaluate medication use, adverse drug reactions, and drug-related errors in the hospital; and provide guidelines and protocols for medication use throughout the institution.

---

closed formulary a type of formulary that requires physicians to order only those medications on the formulary list. (Some exceptions may apply.)

formulary a list of drugs stocked at the hospital that have been selected based on therapeutic factors as well as cost.

non-formulary drugs not on the formulary list and not regularly stocked in the pharmacy.

COMMON HOSPITAL IV MEDICATIONS

Emergency Medications

- Adenosine (Adenocard®)
- Atropine (AtroPen®)
- Epinephrine (Adrenalin®, Epi-pen®)

Critical Care Medications

- Dopamine (generic)
- Dobutamine (Dobutrex®)
- Fentanyl (Sublimaze®)
- Fosphenytoin (Cerebyx®)
- Heparin (generic)
- Midazolam (Versed®)
- Milrinone (Primacor®)
- Nitroprusside (Nipride®, Nitropress®)
- Norepinephrine (Levophed®)
- Phenylephrine (Neo-synephrine®)
- Phenytoin (Dilantin®)
- Propofol (Diprivan®)
- Vecuronium (Nocuron®)

Intravenous Electrolytes

- Calcium gluconate
- Magnesium sulfate
- Potassium chloride
- Sodium phosphate

Intravenous Anti-infectives

- Acyclovir (Zovirax®)
- Ampicillin-sulbactam (Unasyn®)
- Cefazolin (Ancef®, Kefzol®)
- Ceftriaxone (Rocephin®)
- Clindamycin (Cleocin®)
- Fluconazole (Diflucan®)
- Ganciclovir (Cytovene®)
- Gentamicin (Geramycin®)
- Imipenem-cilastatin (Primaxin®)
- Metronidazole (Flagyl®)
- Piperacillin-sulbactam (Zosyn®)
- Vancomycin (Vancocin®)

therapeutic interchange a policy approved by the hospital P&T Committee that allows the pharmacist to change a medication order to a therapeutically equivalent formulary medication.

THERAPEUTIC INTERCHANGE

sample therapeutic interchange protocol

Therapeutic Interchange Protocol
H-2 Receptor Antagonists

Background:
The purpose of this protocol is to optimize patient care while considering cost containment and cost-effectiveness. This protocol defines the equivalent doses of the H-2 Receptor Antagonists. This protocol has been approved by the Pharmacy and Therapeutics Committee (P&TC) and the Medical Executive Committee (MEC).

Statement:
The P&TC will establish which H-2 receptor antagonists will be on formulary.
Pharmacists are permitted to convert orders according to the following protocol.

Protocol:

1) **Ranitidine (Zantac) is the only formulary agent.**
2) **Orders for nonformulary agents will be converted to the equivalent dose of ranitidine. The dosage regimens across each row are equivalent.**

Oral Conversion Table

Ranitidine (Zantac®)	Cimetidine (Tagamet®)	Famotidine (Pepcid®)	Nizatidine (Axid®)
150 mg PO BID	300 mg PO QID	20 mg PO BID	150 mg PO BID
150 mg PO BID	400 mg PO BID	20 mg PO BID	150 mg PO BID
150 mg PO BID	400 mg PO TID	20 mg PO BID	150 mg PO BID
300 mg PO HS	800 mg PO HS	40 mg PO HS	300 mg PO HS
150 mg PO QD	300 mg PO BID	20 mg PO QD	150 mg PO QD

Intravenous Conversion Table

Ranitidine (Zantac®)	Cimetidine (Tagamet®)	Famotidine (Pepcid®)
50 mg IV x 1	300 mg IV x 1	20 mg IV x 1
50 mg IV Q8H	300 mg IV Q6H	20 mg IV Q12H
50 mg IV Q12H	300 mg IV Q8H	20 mg IV Q24H
50 mg IV Q24H	300 mg IV Q12H	20 mg IV Q24H

*Nizatidine (Axid®) is not available IV.

Most hospital formularies include only a few medications in each specific class. This means that a patient who is admitted to the hospital may be taking a medication at home that is not included on the hospital formulary. In many of these cases there is another drug on the formulary that is in the same therapeutic class and works the same way but is a different drug entity (and usually of a different dose). The pharmacist is knowledgeable about therapeutic equivalence of drugs in the same class and can recommend the appropriate interchange for the doctor to order. Some hospitals have a formal ***therapeutic interchange*** program that allows the pharmacist to automatically change an order for a certain number of drugs without notifying the physician. In these cases a preset list of conditions must be fulfilled and the pharmacist must follow a strict protocol that includes entering into the computer an order for the formulary drug that was exchanged for the non-formulary drug.

COMMUNICATION

In order to coordinate patient care, there must be communication between the various departments within the hospital.

Written and computer-generated medication orders are the routine method for letting the pharmacy know a medication is needed, but they are not the only ways pharmacy personnel interact with staff from other departments.

The pharmacy technician is often responsible for answering and directing phone calls.

When answering the phone, the technician should identify him/herself and use good etiquette. Any drug information questions that require the pharmacist's knowledge should be given to the pharmacist, but technicians should handle other phone calls related to their own job function.

Some information must be written or printed.

Fax machines and computer-generated printouts are often used to quickly transmit written information such as drug orders from one area to another.

Some hospitals have advanced systems that allow for electronically transmitted communication.

Some systems can scan written medication orders into the computer system on the nursing unit and then transmit them as an electronic image to the pharmacy or other location. Computerized order entry systems allow medication orders to be put directly into the computer and transmitted to the pharmacy. They may also allow health-care workers to send electronic messages to other areas of the hospital. For example, a nurse may send an electronic message to notify the pharmacy staff of a missing medication, or new medication order that is needed right away, or that medication supplies are low. The pharmacy technician is often responsible for checking these messages. In addition, e-mail has become an effective way of communicating information about new policies, medication recalls and shortages, changes in the formulary, or other administrative business.

pneumatic tube a system that shuttles objects through a tube using compressed air as the force; commonly used in hospitals for delivery of medication.

PNEUMATIC TUBE SYSTEMS

A system that allows for the mechanical transfer of written communications and drugs is the ***pneumatic tube***.

In the pneumatic tube system, medication orders and drugs are transferred via plastic capsules to and from stations in the pharmacy and other areas of the hospital. A destination is programmed into the tube station and in minutes the shuttle arrives at the desired location. Some limitations of the system are that it may not be used with unstable medications (e.g., albumin, insulin, IVIG), those that are too large for the tubes, and those restricted by hospital policy (e.g., narcotics).

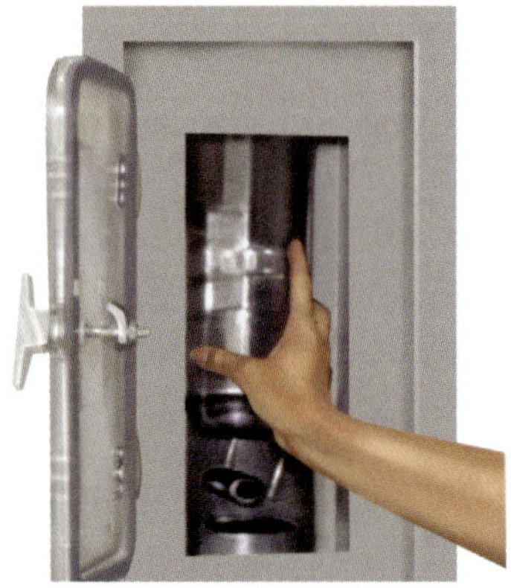

pneumatic tube and capsule

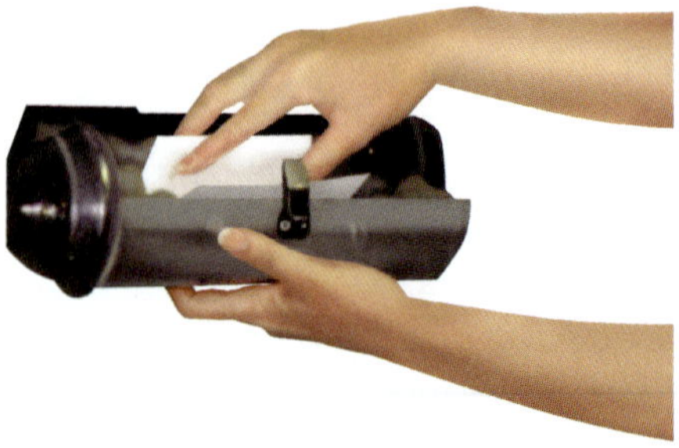

pneumatic capsule with document and medications

COMPUTER SYSTEMS

16

Most hospital information and documentation are computerized.

Information systems can integrate patient information, history of medications, laboratory data, general care of the patient, billing, and many other types of information. However, each hospital system is customized to its own needs and therefore different. Individual systems may or may not integrate various areas of the hospital.

Hospital pharmacies rely heavily on computerized systems.

Knowledge of the hospital's pharmacy information system will be a large part of the initial training for a hospital pharmacy technician, since they must rely on it to perform many of their daily tasks including ordering pharmaceuticals, inventory control, and medication order processes.

An important responsibility for the pharmacist is to provide information on medications and their use to patients and other health-care professionals.

Previously, much of this information was found in written form such as *Facts and Comparisons*. Newer hospital information systems link drug information directly with the pharmacy computer system allowing information on patients' specific medications to be viewed online. In addition, many drug references are available using wireless Internet and smartphones.

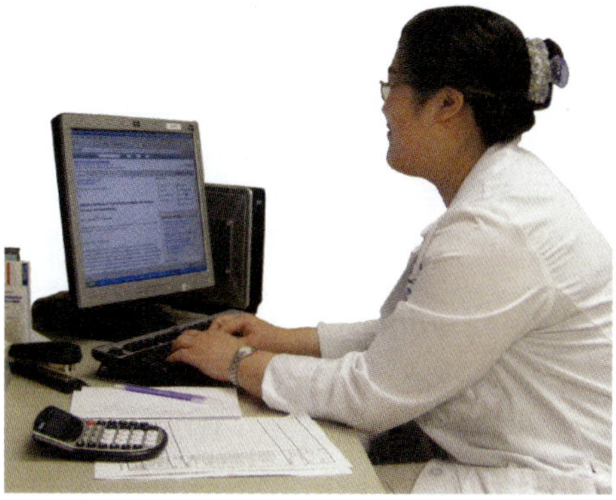

Among their many functions, hospital information systems provide the pharmacist with quick access to medication information.

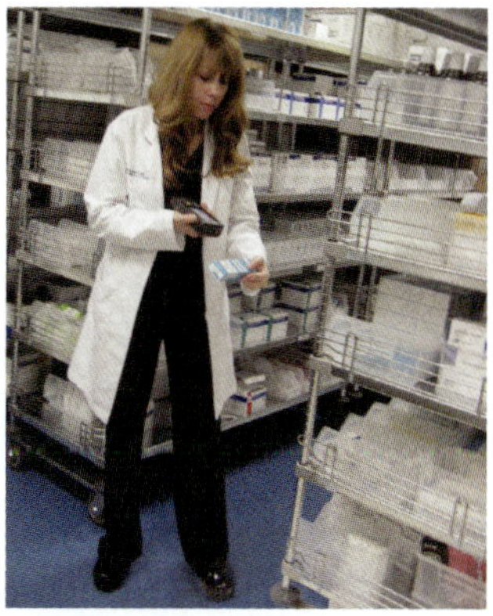

a technician using a hand held entry device for a computerized inventory system

Confidentiality and Security

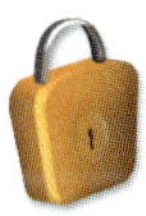

The information contained on a hospital information system is highly confidential. In many cases (especially with patient information), it is illegal to give the information to anyone except those who are authorized to have it. As a result, access to the computer system is limited by password or other security measures. Passwords should never be shared and technicians should always sign off the system each time they leave the work station so no one else will have access to their sign on.

The Health Insurance Portability and Accountability Act (HIPAA) is a federal privacy law enacted to safeguard a patient's protected information when it is spoken, written, or transferred electronically. It includes regulations regarding privacy, confidentiality, assessing and releasing patient information, and complying with patients' rights. Technicians should never look at a patient's chart or computer profile unless specifically required to fulfill an assigned task. Likewise, technicians should not provide information to anyone unless specifically directed by the pharmacist.

MEDICAL RECORDS

Medical records or health records are detailed, chronological accounts of a patient's medical history and care.

They provide information on the continuity of care, which helps health care providers make the most appropriate, individualized decisions on the current care of a patient.

The medical record typically includes notes from doctors and other health-care providers.

It includes a detailed account of a patient's medical complaints and history, physical exams, current and past medications, laboratory results, diagnostic tests and procedures, and treatment plans. In a hospital setting, the medical record will also include daily progress notes and flow sheets that track the care of the patient while admitted to the hospital.

Medical records are traditionally compiled using paper charts and folders, but can also be created using paperless *electronic medical records (EMR)* or *electronic health records (EHR)*.

Electronic medical records integrate patient medical records with billing as well as patient appointments and allow authorized health-care providers to access a patient's medical information from any secure location. Most hospitals use a combination of both paper and electronic charts with some information located in a physical chart and other information stored in the computer record.

It is important for the pharmacy technician to know the components of a medical record since they may be asked to find information for the pharmacist.

It is just as important that a pharmacy technician views only the areas of the chart that are absolutely necessary; viewing other information would be breaking confidentiality rules set forth by HIPAA, and may lead to termination of their job.

electronic medical record (EMR) or electronic health record (EHR) a computerized patient medical record.

MILITARY TIME

Most hospitals use a 24–hour clock, or military time, to indicate when medications are due, as well as when they expire. The day is divided into 24 hours: Midnight begins the clock at 00:00 and it goes until 23:59 before starting over.

12–hour clock	24–hour clock
Midnight	**00:00**
1 a.m.	01:00
2 a.m.	02:00
3 a.m.	03:00
4 a.m.	04:00
5 a.m.	05:00
6 a.m.	06:00
7 a.m.	07:00
8 a.m.	08:00
9 a.m.	09:00
10 a.m.	10:00
11 a.m.	11:00
Noon	**12:00**
1 p.m.	13:00
2 p.m.	14:00
3 p.m.	15:00
4 p.m.	16:00
5 p.m.	17:00
6 p.m.	18:00
7 p.m.	19:00
8 p.m.	20:00
9 p.m.	21:00
10 p.m.	22:00
11 p.m.	23:00

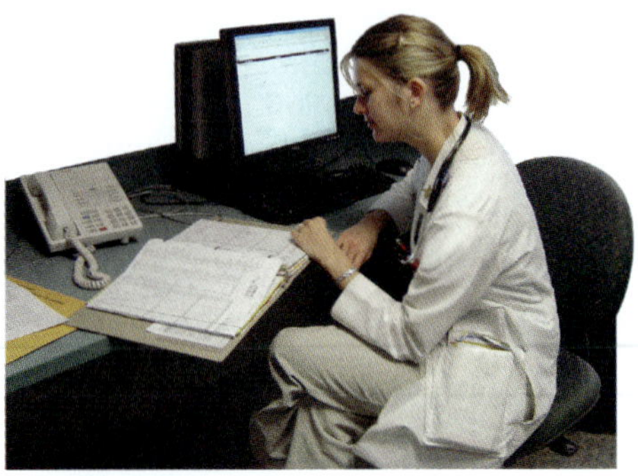

A physician reads a medical chart.

Encounters | Labs | Microbiology | Imaging | Procedures | ECG | Other Orders | Medications | Episodes | Letters | Notes | Misc Reports

Clear All

Back

CHEMISTRY PANEL

Status: **Final result** MyChart: **Not Shared** Next appt with me: **None** Dx: **Essential hypertension, benign**

	Range	2/3/2013	1/14/2013	10/30/2012	09/05/2012	09/09/2011
Sodium	135 - 145 mEq/L	140	140	145	139	144
Potassium	3.6 - 4.8 mEq/L	3.9	4.0	4.6	4.5	4.4
Calcium	8.9 - 10.1 mg/dL	8.9	9.0	9.4	8.9	9.9
Phosphorus	2.5 - 4.5 mg/dL	3.5	3.9	4.0	4.0	3.8
Creatinine	0.8 - 1.2 mg/dL	1.0	1.0	1.0	1.2	1.4 (A)
AST/SGOT	12 - 31 U/L	31	35 (A)	35 (A)	35 (A)	45 (A)
Alk phos	98 - 251 U/L	125	125	175	185	146
Total bilirubin	0.1 - 1.1 mg/dL	0.9	1.0	1.0	0.9	.89
Glucose	70 - 100 mg/dL	105 (A)	110 (A)	115 (A)	125 (A)	130 (A)
Cholesterol	250 mg/dL	220	230	240	245	250
Protein (plasma)	6.3 - 7.9 g/dL	6.9	6.9	7.0	6.9	6.9
Albumin	3.5 - 5.0 g/dL	3.5	3.9	4.1	3.9	3.9

Lab Flowsheet
Order Details View Encounter Lab and Collection Details Routing Result History
Specimen Collected: 02/03/13 Last Resulted: 02/03/13

Reviewed by List
Marty E Seeger, M.D. on 02/05/13 2:17 PM

An example of an **electronic medical record.**

A patient's medical chart and/or electronic medical record include many different sections:

- **Demographics:** personal identification information about the patient that is not medical. This includes the patient's phone numbers, addresses, and emergency contact information but may also contain the patient's religion, race, occupation, and insurance information.
- **Allergies:** list of drug and/or food allergies and the allergic response experienced (e.g., rash, anaphylaxis). NKA or NKDA are common abbreviations for "no known allergy" and "no known drug allergy."
- **Medical history:** list of present medical conditions or disease states as well as previous illnesses, surgeries, pregnancies, vaccinations, significant family and social history. A summary of prescription, over-the-counter, and herbal medications taken at home may also be located here or in a separate section.
- **Medication orders:** orders written by a physician or agent of a physician for medication to be given to a patient. The order specifies the name of the drug, the dose, the route of administration, how often it is to be administered, and may include how long that order is to last.
- **Medication administration record:** a computerized or handwritten form that tracks the medications given to a patient, what time they were given, and who administered them.
- **Lab/test results:** results for blood tests (e.g., blood sugar, drug levels), radiology exams (e.g., X-rays), microbiology (e.g., blood culture), and other specialized testing (e.g., biopsy).
- **Documentation flow sheet:** form filled out by nursing that tracks a patient's vitals on an hourly or scheduled basis, hourly rates of large volume IVs and medication drips, ventilator settings or other respiratory support, patient intake, urine output, pain scores, and other nursing notes.
- **Progress notes:** notes that detail the current progress of a patient and include any patient complaints, laboratory data, physical exam findings, overall assessment and plan for the patient. Usually written by physicians on a daily basis while the patient is in the hospital. Other health-care professionals may also write notes (nurse, social worker, pharmacist, etc.)

MEDICATION ORDERS

Several different types of professionals have authority to write medication orders in the hospital setting.

The most obvious of these is the doctor. However, both nurses and pharmacists may write orders if they are directly instructed to do so by a doctor in person or over the telephone. These are referred to as verbal orders or telephone orders and must be cosigned by the physician who approved them. In some hospitals, specialized health-care providers with advanced training can write orders without the signature of a physician. These people include physician assistants and nurse practitioners.

In the hospital, all written orders for a patient are done on a medication order form and not a prescription blank as seen in a community pharmacy.

Medication order forms are an all-purpose communication tool used by the various members of the health care team. Orders for various procedures, laboratory tests, and X-rays may be written on the form in addition to medication orders. Several medication orders may be written on one medication order form. These forms are traditionally prepared in duplicate or triplicate so that the original remains in the medical chart and only copies are sent to other areas of the hospital for processing.

An alternative to the traditional written order is computerized physician order entry (*CPOE*).

CPOE is a system in which the doctor or agent of the doctor enters orders directly into the hospital computer system. This helps eliminate errors due to illegible handwriting and also expedites orders to the pharmacy, lab, radiology, etc. When a physician enters a medication order, a copy is sent electronically to the pharmacy or a printout is generated for review by a pharmacist before the medication is dispensed.

There are several types of medication orders.

Standard medication orders for patients to receive a certain drug at scheduled intervals throughout the day are called *standing orders* (or scheduled orders). Orders for medications that are administered only on an as needed basis are called *PRN orders*. A third type of order for a medication needed right away is a *STAT order*.

MEDICATION ORDER FORMS

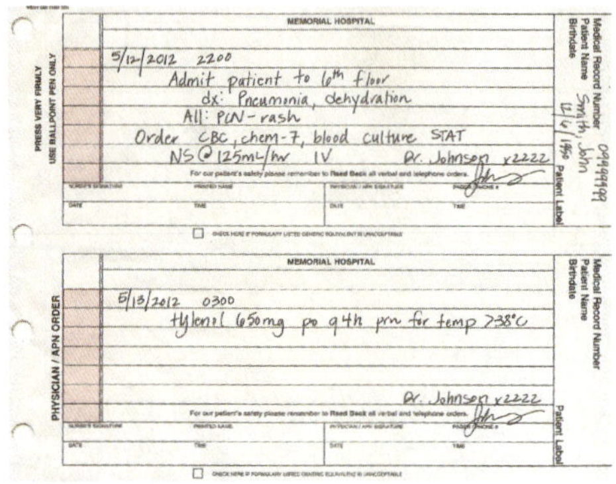
MEMORIAL HOSPITAL

5/12/2012 2200
Admit patient to 6th floor
dx: Pneumonia, dehydration
All: PCN - rash
Order CBC, chem-7, blood culture STAT
NS @ 125mL/hr IV Dr. Johnson x2222

MEMORIAL HOSPITAL

5/13/2012 0300
Tylenol 650mg po q4h prn for temp >38°C
Dr. Johnson x2222

sample medication order form

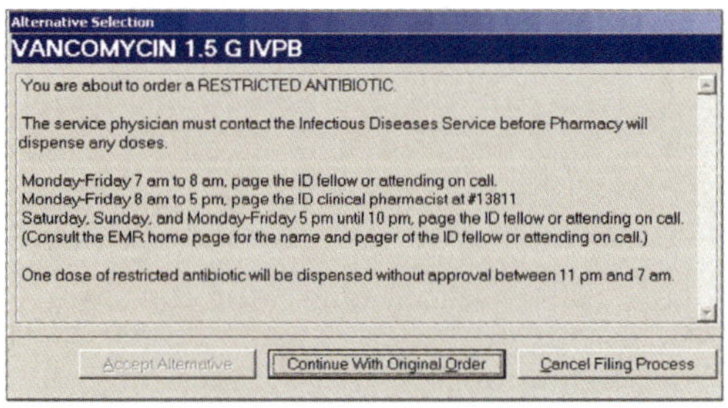

Some medications are restricted and require approval from a specific hospital service before they can be dispensed from the pharmacy. © 2013 Epic Systems Corporation. Used with permission.

CPOE a system in which the physician or agent of the physician enters orders directly into the hospital computer system.

medication administration record (MAR) a form that tracks the medications administered to a patient.

PRN order an order for medication to be administered only on an as needed basis (e.g., 1 tablet every 4 to 6 hours as needed for pain).

Common abbreviations for medication orders can be found on page 89 and pages 100-101.

MEDICATION ADMINISTRATION RECORDS

Nurses record and track medication orders using the ***medication administration record (MAR)***. The MAR may be a written or computer generated form or may be electronic.

The MAR records every medication ordered for a patient over a 24-hour period, as well as the time the medications were administered and the person who gave each dose. Whether handwritten by the nursing staff or generated by the pharmacy computer system, the accuracy of this document is crucial.

In some hospitals, nurses may chart medications directly into the computer. Alternatively, the nurse may scan the medication bar code at the patients' bedside; this information will then be processed onto a computerized MAR.

COMMUNITY HOSPITAL
Medication Administration Record

Room/Bed: 675-01
Patient: SMITH, JOHN
Account #: 099999999
Sex: M
Age: 48Y
Doctor: JOHNSON, P.

From 0730 **on** 02/01/13 **to** 0700 **on** 02/02/13
Diagnosis: PNEUMONIA; DEHYDRATION
Height: 5'11" **weight:** 75KG
Verified By: Susie Smith, RN

Allergies: PENICILLIN-->RASH

	0730–1530	1600–2300	2330–0700
5% DEXTROSE/0.9% SODIUM CHLORIDE 1 LITER BAG DOSE 125 ML/HR IV Q 8 HRS ORDER #2	800 JD	1600 SS	2400
MULTIVITAMIN TABLET DOSE: 1 TABLET P.O. DAILY ORDER #4	1000 Given @ 9AM JD		
CLARITHROMYCIN 500 MG TABLET DOSE: 500MG P.O. Q 12 HRS ORDER #5	1000 JD	2200 SS	

a sample medication administration record

standing order a standard medication order for patients to receive medication at scheduled intervals (e.g., 1 tablet every 8 hours).

STAT order an order for medication to be administered immediately.

Order entry into a computer system may be performed by a unit clerk, pharmacy technician, pharmacist, nurse, or prescriber.

Before entering orders, technicians will require specialized training in the interpretation of medical orders as well as on how to use the pharmacy's computerized order-entry system. Each medication order must contain the medication name, dose, route, and frequency. The order may also include the duration of therapy.

The technician must also be aware of any specialized protocols the hospital has in place such as restricted medications or automatic stop orders.

In order to ensure safety and appropriateness as well as contain costs, some medications may be restricted by certain services in the hospital (e.g., infectious diseases, hematology). Such restricted medications cannot be dispensed until the appropriate service approves the order. Other medications can only be ordered by a physician with a specialty in the area that the medication is used. For example, many hospitals will only allow an oncologist to order chemotherapy. Automatic stop orders are used for certain classes of medications, such as antibiotics or narcotics. These orders are active for only a limited period of time, after which a new medication order is required to continue. Automatic stop orders help ensure that the patient's therapy is continually reassessed and monitored.

The hospital pharmacy technician plays an important role in assisting the pharmacist in making sure a medication and its dose are appropriate for each individual patient.

The pharmacist may ask the technician to get such information as weight, allergies, or home medications from a patient's nurse or chart. The technician may also need to obtain laboratory or microbiology data from the hospital computer system.

The pharmacy technician may also screen medication orders for any that seem inappropriate.

For example, if a drug that is usually given once a day is ordered to be given four times a day, the technician should alert the pharmacist of the potential error. Although the pharmacist is required to review all orders before they are fully processed, the technician can serve as a valuable team member by flagging orders with potential problems.

ORDER PROCESSING

Once the medication order is approved by the pharmacist, the order needs to be filled.

There are several steps involved in this process.

Since many medications look similar and the same drugs may come in several different doses, the technician must be vigilant in making sure the right medication and dose are being filled.

The technician should pay close attention to the following when preparing a medication for the final check by a pharmacist: drug, dosage form, concentration or strength, quantity, expiration date, base solution, and volume.

After the medication has been prepared, the technician must prepare and initial the medication label.

Some medications require special auxiliary labels (e.g., "Refrigeration," "High Risk Medication"), and should be affixed to the product by the pharmacy technician. Also, some intravenous medications (e.g., mannitol, phenytoin) require a ***final filter*** for the nursing staff to use upon administration. The pharmacy is usually responsible for providing the nursing staff with the filter.

In most states, medications must be checked by a pharmacist before being sent to the nursing units.

However, at least nine states currently allow a process called tech-check-tech in hospital settings. Using this process, a specially trained technician can check another technician's work. Each state has specific training and auditing requirements for tech-check-tech.

Medications may be delivered to patient care areas by pharmacy technicians, hospital delivery staff, or a pneumatic tube system.

Often these deliveries, or rounds, are done on an hourly basis. While on rounds, the technician is often required to pick up medication returns and credit them to the patient.

safety you should know

Receipt of controlled substances must be witnessed by someone on the nursing unit. This can be done with a paper or electronic signature log.

MANUAL ORDER PROCESSING

✔ The medication order is written in the patient chart.

↓

✔ A copy of the medication order is removed from the chart.

↓

✔ The order is picked up at the nursing station by a pharmacy technician or is faxed or tubed to the pharmacy.

↓

✔ The medication order is entered into the pharmacy computer system.

↓

✔ The pharmacist reviews and verifies the medication order.

↓

✔ The medication order is filled by a pharmacy technician and then checked by a pharmacist.

↓

✔ Patient-specific medication is manually delivered or tubed to the nursing unit.

AUTOMATED ORDER PROCESSING

✔ The physician or physician's agent enters the medication order directly into the hospital computer system, which then automatically communicates the order to the pharmacy.

↓

✔ The pharmacist reviews and verifies the medication order.

↓

✔ The R.N. retrieves the medication from a point-of-use automated station.

↓

✔ The pharmacy technician refills inventory as supplies fall below par.

Automated order processing may include only part of the above process. For instance, even though order processing may start with physician order entry directly into a computer, a hospital may not have point-of-use automated machines. In this case, the medication would still be manually delivered or tubed to the nursing station.

Missing doses of medications for patients can be a challenge at hospitals.

Missing doses are medications that should have already been delivered to the nursing unit but cannot be located. If a missing medication is requested, the technician should ask the following questions in order to ensure the patient receives the medication in a timely manner while minimizing duplication of work by the pharmacy staff:

- Is there a current order for the medication?
- Did the nurse check the correct area for the medication, such as the refrigerator or automated dispensing cabinet?
- When was the medication last dispensed by the pharmacy? (If a label for that medication was printed recently, the medication may still be in the pharmacy.)
- Was the patient transferred from a different unit in the hospital?

If the medication cannot be located, the technician should print another label and make sure the missing dose is sent to the nursing unit.

Hospital technicians often perform *drip rounds*.

This means the pharmacy technician will go to specific nursing units (mainly intensive care units) and track what intravenous drips will be needed later that day. The technician may need to communicate with the nursing staff to find out if an IV infusion (e.g., dopamine, fentanyl) will be discontinued, expire soon, or run out in a few hours. The purpose of drip rounds is to reduce the number of STAT medications and decrease the workload on other pharmacy shifts.

drip rounds a process in which the pharmacy technician goes to specific nursing units to find out what IV drips will be needed later that day.

final filter a device used to remove particulate matter. The filter should be placed at the end point of an IV line just before it enters a patient's vein.

INVENTORY CONTROL

Pharmacy technicians may also be responsible for inventory control.

Ensuring that adequate supplies of medications are available for all areas of the hospital is the primary responsibility for staff in this area. This is especially important in the hospital setting, where having a medication may be a matter of life and death. Inventory duties may include ordering medication, storing medication in proper areas, checking the pharmacy order invoice, and dealing with *drug recalls* and shortages.

The pharmacy inventory is usually ordered through a special computer program that communicates with the distributor/wholesaler.

To make ordering inventory more accurate and cost-effective, many hospitals use bar-coding technology for maintenance of the pharmacy inventory.

One way the pharmacy technician knows what to order is by using *par* levels for each drug product.

Par is the quantity of drug that should be kept on the shelf. Each drug product has its own par. Par levels may also be assigned to drug products in automated dispensing cabinets.

When a pharmacy shipment arrives, the pharmacy technician checks the order against the invoice.

If something is on the invoice but not in the shipment, the technician should notify his/her supervisor. When all items are accounted for, the technician places the medications in the appropriate location (e.g., refrigerator, overstock area, etc.).

A primary area of concern for inventory control is narcotics, or controlled substances.

Controlled substances require an exact record of the amount and location of every item, and must be ordered in a particular way according to state and federal laws. There are several systems for controlling narcotic inventory. Some are manual and others involve electronic equipment. Many hospitals require two people to count narcotic inventory before it is stored. Also, if a narcotic medication is damaged for any reason, two people must sign a form to witness the disposal.

INVENTORY

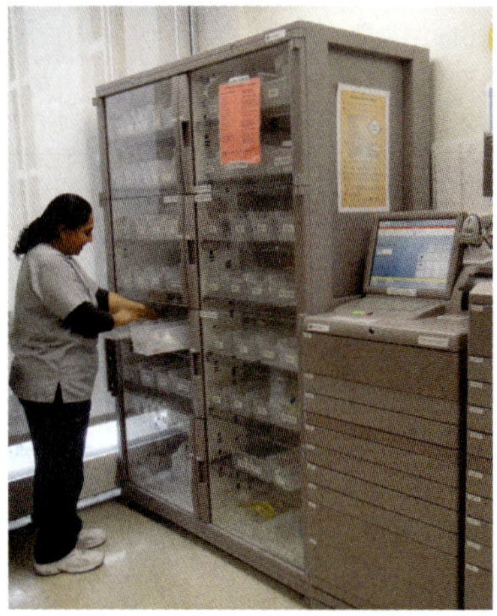

an automated dispensing system

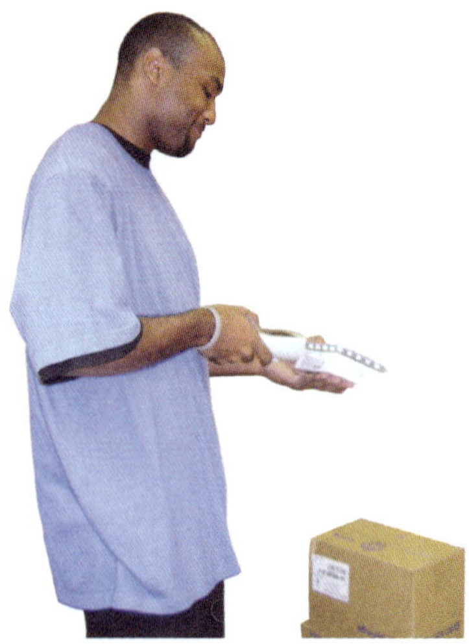

bar coding assists in inventory management

See Chapter 13 for more information on inventory systems.

RISK EVALUATION AND MITIGATION STRATEGY (REMS)

Under the Food and Drug Administration Amendments Act of 2007, the FDA requires manufacturers of drugs with serious safety concerns to complete a Risk Evaluation and Mitigation Strategy (REMS).

As part of REMS, manufacturers of such drugs must develop one or more of the following: (1) a Medication Guide or Patient Package Insert, (2) a Communication Plan for health-care providers, (3) an Element to Assure Safe Use (ETASU), and/or (4) an Implementation Plan.

An ETASU may require a drug's prescribers to complete specific training and certification, only allow the drug to be dispensed in certain health-care settings, require patients to receive specific monitoring (e.g., blood tests, pregnancy tests), and/or require patients to register for use.

Implementation plans may require pharmacies and hospitals to show documentation of certification and safe use conditions, and require manufacturers to monitor, evaluate, and assess the implementation process.

Some drugs that require REMS are:

- Tracleer® (bosentan)
- Aranesp® (darbopoetin alfa)
- Tikosyn® (dofetilide)
- Epogen®/Procrit® (epoetin alfa)
- Botox/Botox Cosmetic® (onabotulinumtoxin A)
- Thalomid® (thalidomide)

Although there is usually a sufficient supply of drug products in the United States, shortages may occur due to manufacturing shortages or a discontinuation of one brand, which then creates a shortage of another brand.

If not enough medication can be stocked, the inventory technician may have to go outside of their usual distributor. This may include using a secondary distributor, directly contacting the company that makes the drug product, or buying from a group purchasing organization. If it still is not possible to obtain enough drug product, the inventory technician notifies a pharmacist of the shortage and pharmacists work together in recommending alternatives to those medications. Sometimes, this alternative may not be on formulary. In these cases, the non-formulary drug will be stocked unrestricted until the formulary product is available again.

The pharmacy inventory staff is often responsible for removal of drug recalls from the inventory.

A drug may be recalled by the manufacturer for unknown reasons, or may be mandated by the FDA due to safety concerns.

Sometimes a medication that is not stocked by the pharmacy may be needed in an emergency.

In these cases the inventory technician may call other local hospitals to borrow a short-term supply or be asked to order an emergency shipment from a wholesaler or drug manufacturer. This is called *emergency drug procurement*.

drug recall the voluntary or involuntary removal of a drug product by the manufacturer. It usually only pertains to a particular shipment or lot number.

emergency drug procurement to quickly obtain a medication not currently in stock in the pharmacy in situations where the drug is urgently needed.

par the amount of drug product that should be kept on the pharmacy shelf. Each drug product may have a different par value. Par levels may also be assigned to drug products in automated dispensing cabinets.

ORGANIZATION OF MEDICATIONS

In most hospital pharmacies, medications are organized according to a precise system.

First, medications are usually categorized and placed in defined areas of the pharmacy based on the specific route of administration such as intravenous, oral, ophthalmic, topical, etc. Intravenous medications may be further separated by vials, small volume parenterals, and large volume parenterals. Oral drugs may be further divided into solid dosage forms (capsules, tablets) and liquids (suspensions, solutions) and placed in separate areas.

The second way medications are generally organized is in alphabetical order using the generic name of each drug.

This is different than most retail pharmacies, which place drugs in order of brand name. Since both the generic and brand name may be on a medication label, it is important for the hospital pharmacy technician to have a good knowledge of brand vs. generic names. (See Chapter 18 for examples of common hospital drugs.)

Some medications require refrigeration or freezing.

It is imperative that the technician identify these items and promptly put them in the correct place so that the medications retain their stability. For example, most vaccines require refrigeration. If left at room temperature for too long, they may lose some of their effectiveness.

Narcotics and other controlled substances are often stored in a secure area of the pharmacy.

They may be stored in a locked cabinet or automated dispensing cabinet that requires a personal code and password. Some pharmacies will also have video surveillance of this area to decrease risk of diversion or mishandling of these medications. It is mandatory for hospital pharmacies to lock CII medications in a secure area. CIII–CV medications are stored according to each institution's policy. Other pharmacies choose to keep them all in a secure area.

EXTEMPORANEOUS COMPOUNDING

When required to prepare an ***extemporaneous compound***, the pharmacy technician will follow a recipe for the compound. All of the ingredients and supplies needed to make the drug solution should be collected and brought to the oral compounding area. Prior to preparing the medication, pharmacy technicians must first wash their hands and clean the surface to be used.

Once the medication is compounded, a record of the preparation and ingredients must be put in a ***bulk compounding log***. Information must include a list of all the ingredients, amounts used, manufacturer, lot numbers, and expiration dates of each specific ingredient. Also, the bulk bottle needs to be labeled with the compounded drug name, its concentration, a lot number specific to the hospital, the expiration date, and the initials of the pharmacist after he/she checks the preparation.

Examples of Refrigerated and Frozen Medications

Refrigerator: 2° to 8°C (36°–46°F)

- Caspofungin (Cancidas®)
- Epoetin alfa (Epogen®, Procrit®)
- Filgrastim (Neupogen®)
- Fosphenytoin (Cerebyx®)
- Tobramycin for oral inhalation (Tobi®)
- Most vaccinations

Freezer: -10° to -20°C (Av -15°C, 5°F)

- Measles, Mumps, Rubella, and Varicella combination vaccine (Proquad®)
- Varicella (chickenpox) vaccine (Varivax®)
- Zoster (shingles) vaccine (Zostavax®)

See Chapter 8 for more information on compounding.

Most hospital pharmacies have a special area for compounding oral solutions and suspensions.

In this area, bulk amounts of nonspecific patient supplies are often compounded in advance for future needs of the hospitalized patients.

Some oral solutions and suspensions are available commercially but must be *reconstituted* before use.

These medications usually have a short stability (i.e., they expire in 10–14 days after they have been made). It is essential that the pharmacy technician labels the date of reconstitution and/or the date the reconstituted medication will expire. The technician should also place any other necessary labels on the bottle (e.g., "Refrigerate," "Shake Well Before Using," etc.). The pharmacist will check the technician's work and initial the bottle. The technician can then draw specific doses of the medication in oral syringes or put the medication in the proper storage area (i.e., a refrigerator).

If an oral medication is needed in liquid form but is not available commercially, it may be extemporaneously compounded.

Recipes or instructions on how to prepare extemporaneous compounds are usually stored in a binder or on a computer. The directions must be followed exactly since stability data is based on the precise preparation instructions that are listed. In the oral compounding area, the pharmacy technician should find the materials and ingredients commonly used in the preparation of extemporaneous compounds, including mortar and pestles, calibrated measuring devices, and common ingredients (e.g., sterile water, simple syrup, glycerin).

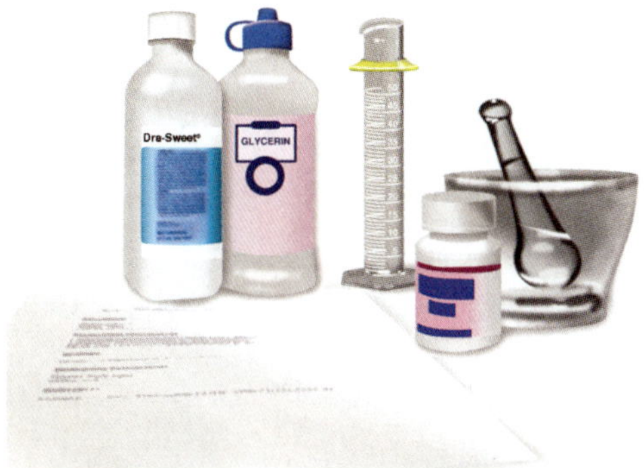

supplies gathered for preparation of an extemporaneous compound

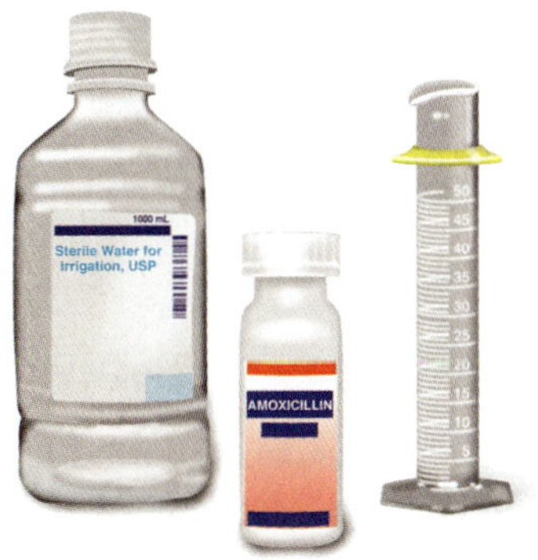

amoxicillin suspension for reconstitution

bulk compounding log a record of medications that are compounded in the pharmacy for nonspecific patients. Information must include a list of all the ingredients, amounts used, manufacturer, lot numbers and expiration dates of each specific ingredient.

extemporaneous compounds medications that must be prepared following a specific recipe or formula, usually because they are not available commercially.

reconstitute addition of water or other diluent to commercially made drug bottles or vials in order to make a solution or suspension from a premade powder form of the drug. This may include oral or parenteral products.

UNIT DOSE SYSTEM

Oral medications are commonly provided to the nursing unit in medication carts containing 24-hour dosages for each patient.

These carts have an individual drawer or tray for each patient on the nursing unit. Medications in the cart are packaged in individual containers holding the amount of drug required for one dose. This system is referred to as *unit dose* medication packaging. By preparing medication this way, nurses are not required to select medication from large bulk bottles, decreasing the chance of making an error.

Technicians play a large role in filling the medication carts.

Computer generated drug profiles are printed daily for each patient. Based on this, the technician places the appropriate amount of medications for the 24-hour period into each patient's tray, which is labeled with the patient's name and room number.

Some medications such as eye drops, creams, and metered-dose inhalers cannot be divided into unit dose increments.

In these cases, the bulk item is filled only once and then used for the patient throughout his/her stay.

Some nursing stations have *automated dispensing systems* that contain the most common unit-dose medications used in that patient care area.

This allows the nurse to obtain medications much more quickly. However, the nurse can access most of the medications only after a pharmacist reviews and verifies the order. A few emergency medications may be obtained without pharmacist verification, and this is governed by each hospital's policy.

Some hospitals do not have 24-hour cart fills because the automated dispensing systems are used for all the doses during the length of the patient's stay in a hospital.

However, it is often the responsibility of the pharmacy technician to make sure the automated dispensing systems remain stocked.

CART FILLING

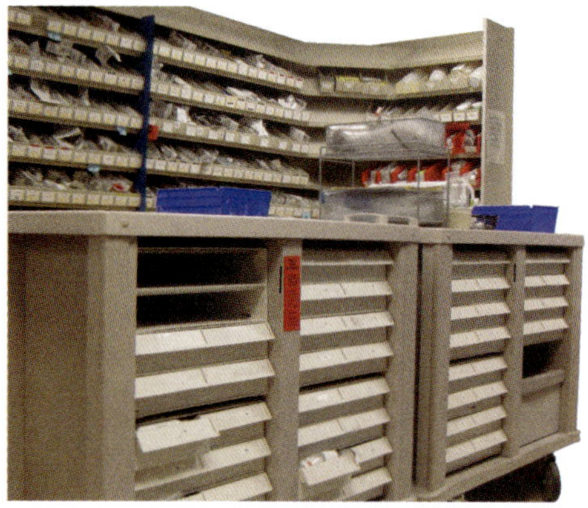

the cart filling area of a hospital pharmacy

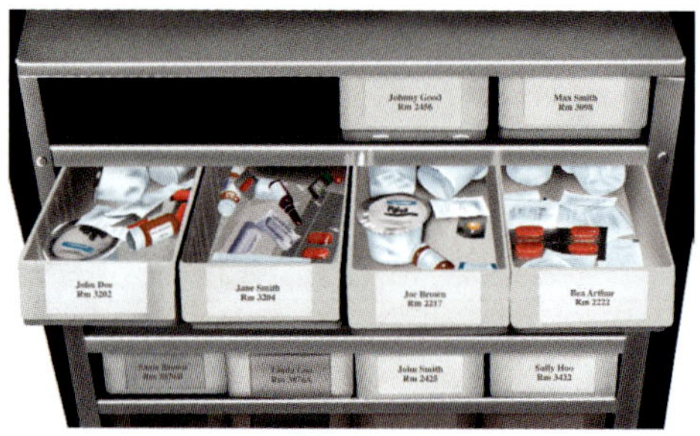

patient-specific trays

automated dispensing system a system in which medications are dispensed from an automated unit at the point of use.

unit dose a package containing the amount of a drug required for one dose.

Cart Filling Robots

Several machines referred to as robots have been developed to assist in the cart filling process. While this reduces the manual filling responsibilities of technicians, some medications, such as those stored in the refrigerator, must still be hand filled. Additionally, robots require a large amount of special packaging that technicians, who would traditionally be hand filling trays, are often required to stock. Because cart filling robots are very expensive and require a large amount of space within the pharmacy area, they are usually seen only in larger hospitals.

UNIT DOSE PACKAGING

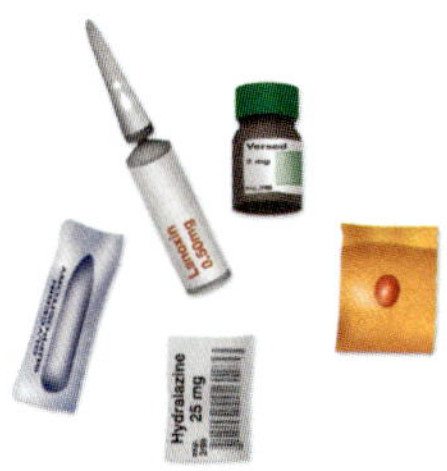

Unit Dose Package Types	
Type	Used for
plastic blister	tablets/capsules
foil blister	tablets/capsules
packet	powder
tube	ointment/cream
foil/plastic cup	oral liquid
cartridge	injection
vial	injection
ampule	injection
foil/plastic	suppository
IV syringe	injections
oral syringe	oral liquids

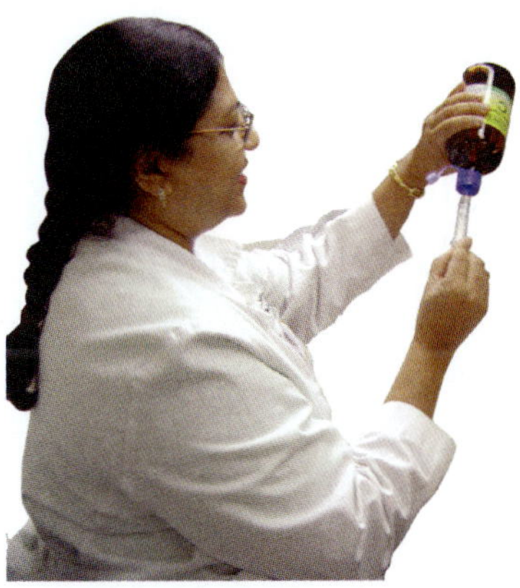

A technician prepares unit doses of an oral solution.

Many hospital pharmacies use machines to automate unit dose packaging.

These systems are generally used for prepacking oral solid medications (i.e., tablets and capsules). They label each unit dose package with information required by the institution. The pharmacy technician is often responsible for keeping these machines stocked and for documenting all bulk bottles that are put into the system.

Separate technologies exist that can draw up oral unit dose syringes.

Otherwise, oral liquids need to be manually drawn into unit dose syringes and labeled by the technician. It is important for the pharmacy technician to always use oral syringes when drawing up oral liquids. Oral syringes differ from IV syringes because they are not able to accept a needle. This protects a patient from accidentally receiving an oral dosage form intravenously.

After a medication has been prepacked, it is checked by a pharmacist.

Pharmacies keep documentation logs of prepacked medications. The documentation logs have the medication name, manufacturer, dose, expiration date, lot number, and pharmacist's initials.

Unit dose labels may also contain bar codes for identification and control.

Bar-coded medications help to improve patient safety and can help with inventory management. Some computer systems require the nursing staff to scan a patient's arm band and then the medication before giving the medication to the patient. If the medication is not on the patient's profile, the computer will alarm.

prepack label with bar code

STERILE PRODUCTS

A large portion of the medication used in the hospital is administered intravenously.

The hospital pharmacy technician plays a large role in preparing these products. IV admixtures may include small and large volume parenterals (SVPs and LVPs), parenteral nutrition therapy, or chemotherapy. Preparation of these products requires special training and use of laminar flow hoods or ventilated glove boxes. Most parenterals can be prepared in a horizontal hood. Chemotherapy and cytotoxic drugs, however, must be prepared in a biological safety cabinet or vertical flow hood, which offers more protection.

There are several steps involved in preparing a parenteral medication correctly.

- The technician calculates the amount of drug needed for the *IVPB (intravenous piggyback)*.
- The required equipment is gathered: medication vial, base solution bag, syringes, needles, and alcohol swabs.
- Prior to preparation, hands should be washed, gloves and gown worn (if required), and laminar flow hood cleaned.
- The IVPB is prepared using proper aseptic technique to ensure sterility.
- A double check should always be completed: check for correct drug, concentration, volume, base solution, and all calculations.
- The technician should write his initials on the label and add an expiration date and time prior to placing the label on the IVPB.
- Then the vial and syringes used in preparation are placed next to the IVPB for the pharmacist to check.
- All supplies used for product preparation should be disposed of in the proper bins as required by the hospital pharmacy.

epidural a sterile, preservative-free medication administered into a patient's epidural space (located near the spinal cord and backbone).

IVPB (intravenous piggyback) a small volume parenteral that will be added into or "piggybacked" into a large volume parenteral (LVP).

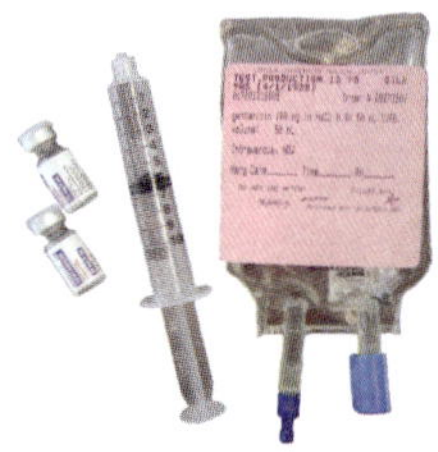

a small volume IVPB to be checked by a pharmacist

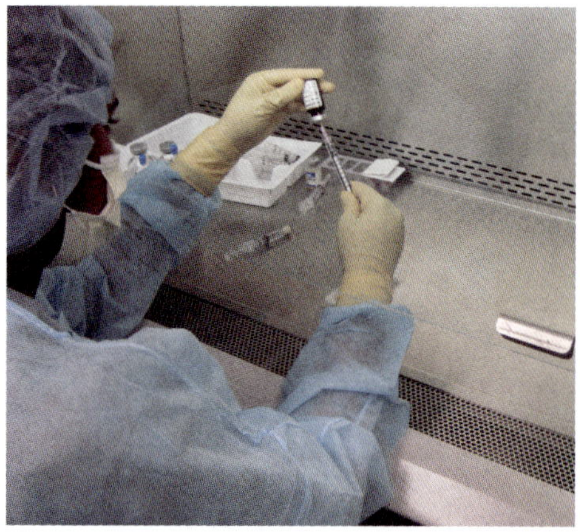

A pharmacy technician prepares IV products in a horizontal flow hood.

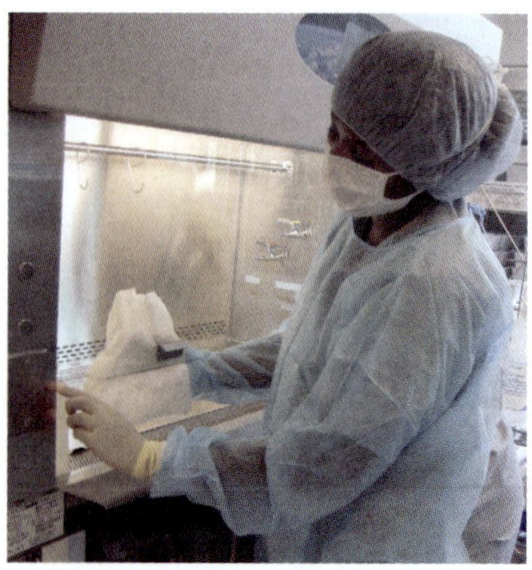

cleaning a vertical laminar flow hood (biological safety cabinet)

See Chapter 9 for more information on sterile techniques and preparing parenterals.

TPN PREPARATION

If a patient cannot eat or receive enteral feeds he or she may need to receive nutrition intravenously. ***Total parenteral nutrition (TPN)*** contains protein, carbohydrates, and essential nutrients to be given to the patient through an IV line. It may also contain fat emulsion (3 in 1) or fat emulsion may be given separately (2 in 1). TPNs can be prepared by the inpatient pharmacy or can be outsourced.

TPNs are often prepared on a TPN compounder. The TPN compounder is a machine that pumps all the components of the TPN into a sterile empty bag. Pharmacy technicians are often responsible for running the compounder.

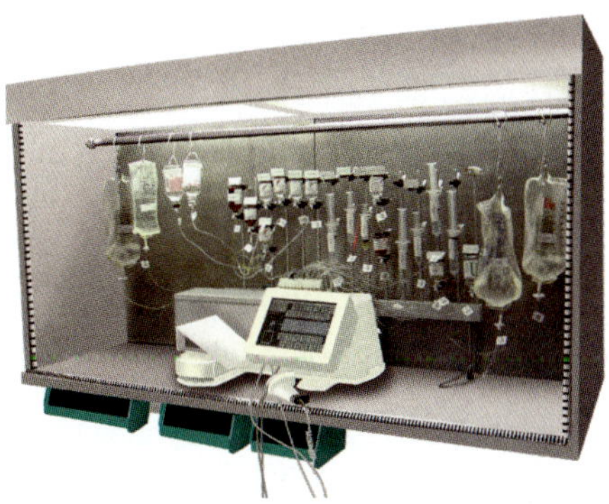

The pharmacy technician is often responsible for setting up the TPN compounder.

short stability medication that will expire soon after preparation (i.e., within 1–6 hours after preparation).

total parenteral nutrition (TPN) protein, carbohydrates and essential nutrients to be given to the patient through an IV line.

When selecting medication vials for preparing IV products, it is important to pay attention to the type of vial.

Medication vials can be single dose (one time use only) or multiple dose (multiple doses in one vial). Single dose vials are preservative-free while multi-dose vials contain preservatives. Technicians must visually inspect multi-dose vials for particulate matter prior to each use.

Final preparations should also be inspected for physical and chemical incompatibilities.

Many medications are not compatible in certain solutions. For example, amphotericin B is an antifungal drug that is not compatible in sodium chloride solutions and will precipitate if mixed with them. Other solutions may develop particulate matter for no known reason.

Some medications require special preparation.

Epidurals and intrathecal medications are to be administered into the epidural or intrathecal space of a patient's back (located near the spinal cord and backbone). Epidural and intrathecal medication cannot contain preservatives and must be sterile.

Certain IV medications have *short stability* or expire soon after preparation (e.g., sulfamethoxazole/trimethoprim, phenytoin).

Short stability medications are prepared shortly before the medication is due for the patient. Hospital IV rooms often have a box where they keep patient labels for medications with short stability. Often, it is the IV technician's responsibility to periodically check the short stability box and prepare the medications shortly before they are due.

Hospital pharmacies have policies in place for end product testing and validation.

The department will periodically take a sample of a prepared IVPB or LVP. The sample is sent to the laboratory and tested for contamination.

Advanced IV Preparation Technology

Robotics are used in some IV product preparation. IntelliFill™, for example, prepares patient-specific small volume parenterals. Other robotics can fill patient-specific IV syringes.

GENERAL HOSPITAL ISSUES

Hospital employees are required to meet some conditions of employment that may not be required in other pharmacy settings.

First, in addition to interviewing with the pharmacy department, prospective employees are usually required to interview with the Human Resources department. This department oversees the hiring process for the entire hospital.

All hospital employees are required to undergo a physical exam and often drug testing.

In addition, employees who may be exposed to blood products, which may or may not be the case for a pharmacy technician, are encouraged to receive the hepatitis B vaccine series. Many hospitals provide this vaccine, as well as flu shots, free of charge to employees.

New employees are required to attend a hospital-wide orientation.

In this session, information is given about employee benefits, rules and regulations, and safety training for various situations such as fires, bomb threats, exposure to blood-borne pathogens, and chemical spills. This is in addition to the training that the pharmacy department provides.

Even if a technician has previous experience working in a hospital pharmacy, he or she will go through training and a probationary period.

The probationary period gives the hospital time to assess whether the employee is actually suitable and qualified for the job. An employee may be terminated at any time during the probationary period. At the end of the probation, the employee's status may be changed to permanent, they may be terminated, or they may be placed on an additional three month probation.

All permanent employees receive an annual or semiannual performance review.

Technicians are rated on technical skills and interpersonal skills, as well as issues such as tardiness, dress code, and ability to complete tasks on time.

---

code cart a locked cart of medications and other medical equipment designed for emergency use only.

REGULATORY AGENCIES

Several different regulatory bodies oversee all aspects of hospital operations, including the pharmacy department.

- **The Joint Commission (TJC)**

  TJC surveys and accredits healthcare organizations at a minimum every 24-39 months, laying out specific guidelines for each hospital department. Although this survey is not required, CMS and several insurance providers require TJC accreditation for reimbursement.

- **Centers for Medicare and Medicaid Services (CMS)**

  CMS surveys and approves hospitals to provide care for Medicare and Medicaid patients. CMS approval is required to receive reimbursement for these patients.

- **The Department of Public Health (DPH)**

  The DPH is a state organization overseeing hospitals, including the pharmacy department, to assure compliance with hospital practice standards.

- **The State Board of Pharmacy (BOP)**

  The BOP registers pharmacists and technicians. While they do not have the authority to govern hospital pharmacy departments, they do regulate the registration of the pharmacists and technicians that work there.

- **United States Pharmacopoeia (USP)**

  The USP creates standards to assure the quality of medicines, dietary supplements, and related products that are available to the public.

- **Drug Enforcement Administration (DEA)**

  A federal regulatory agency for controlled substances (CI–CV). The DEA ensures that hospitals follow controlled substances laws.

SAFETY

All patient care areas are required to have ***code carts*** in case of a medical emergency on the floor.

These carts contain different medications and equipment commonly used in emergency situations. Each code cart has a special lock that can be broken when the cart needs to be used. Once a lock is broken, it cannot be reused and the medication drawer must be replaced. The pharmacy is responsible for maintaining these medication drawers. The technician refills the medication trays and charges the missing medications to the appropriate patient.

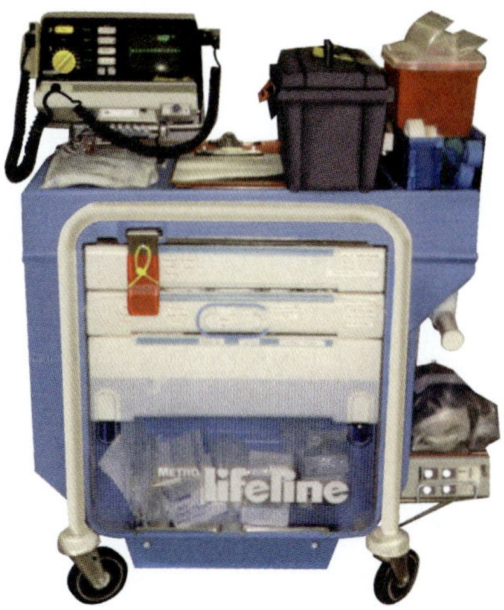

A code cart—note that the plastic yellow tie-lock must be broken to use the cart.

The Policy and Procedure Manual

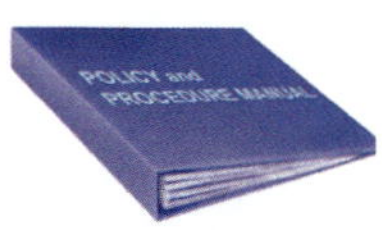

All departments within the hospital are required to maintain a policy and procedures manual from regulating agencies. This document contains information about every aspect of the job from dress codes to disciplinary actions as well as step-by-step directions on how to perform various tasks. It is absolutely essential that technicians know what they must and must not do in their job, as outlined in their institution's policy and procedure manual.

During safety training, employees learn universal precautions and how to handle hazardous substance spills.

Universal precautions are practices and guidelines that reduce the probability of exposure to blood-borne pathogens and explain what to do if an exposure occurs. These precautions include the use of protective barriers (gloves, gowns, masks, and protective eye wear) and how to prevent injuries from needle sticks. Even employees who may not have direct contact with blood products must be trained in universal precautions.

Some medications can be hazardous to personnel.

In cases of hazardous substance spills (e.g., cytotoxic drugs, harmful chemicals or drugs), special procedures are required that involve identifying the hazardous substance, containing the spill, and disposing of the waste. The Material Safety Data Sheets (MSDS) contain information regarding safe handling procedures, signs and symptoms of exposure, and exposure limits. The technician should know where the MSDS are located since these will explain how to proceed if a spill occurs.

Proper waste disposal is extremely important.

Red bags are usually used for items containing blood or infectious wastes. Soiled linen, scrubs, and items such as cleaning rags are cleaned rather than disposed of in red bags. Needles or other items that may cut or puncture the skin should always be thrown away in designated sharps containers.

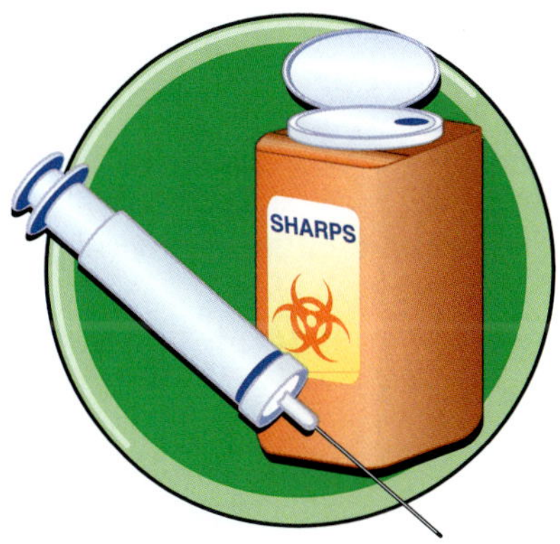

sharps container

CALCULATIONS

1

$\frac{1}{4}$

0.1

1%

Many different types of calculations are performed by hospital pharmacy technicians on a daily basis.

Some hospitals require technicians to pass a calculations test prior to completing their training.

Example—Drawing Up a Unit Dose Oral Syringe

When pharmacy technicians have to manually draw up unit dose oral syringes, there are important calculations involved. For example, a medication order reads: Gabapentin 300 mg ng t.i.d.

Question 1: If Gabapentin is available in a 50 mg/ml concentration, how many ml(s) of drug should be drawn up per dose?

Solution:

$$300 \text{ mg} \div 50 \text{ mg/ml} = 6 \text{ ml}$$

Or, solving for X: $\frac{300 \text{ mg}}{X} = \frac{50 \text{ mg}}{1 \text{ ml}}$ $\quad X = 6 \text{ ml}$

Question 2: How many syringes are needed for a 24-hour supply?

Answer: Since t.i.d. stands for three times daily, you would need 3 syringes.

Example—Flow Rate Calculation

Calculating flow rates can help prevent errors, decrease pharmacy waste, and help keep IV drips from running out before a new one arrives.

A medication order reads: Milrinone 0.75 mcg/kg/min; patient wt = 154 lbs. Milrinone is available as a premade IVPB with a concentration of 200 mcg/ml. Remember: 1 kg = 2.2 lbs. (wt = 154 lbs = 70 kg).

Question: How long will a 100 ml vs. a 200 ml ready-to-use (RTU) IVPB last?

Step 1: Calculate rate in ml/hr:

$$\frac{0.75 \text{ mcg}}{\text{kg x min}} \text{ x } 70 \text{ kg x } \frac{60 \text{ min}}{1 \text{ hr}} \text{ x } \frac{1 \text{ ml}}{200 \text{ mcg}} = 15.75 \text{ ml/hr}$$

Step 2: Calculate how long the 100 ml vs. 200 ml bag will last:

100 ml IVPB

$$\frac{100 \text{ ml}}{15.75 \text{ ml/hr}} = 6.3 \text{ hrs}$$

200 ml IVPB

$$\frac{200 \text{ ml}}{15.75 \text{ ml/hr}} = 12.6 \text{ hrs}$$

Answer: In this case it may be more advantageous to use a 200 ml bag since it will need to be replaced only every 12 hours instead of every 6 hours.

See Chapter 6 for more information on calculations.

Example—Timing of Medications

A nurse calls at 4 p.m. (military time 16:00) regarding a missing dose of Gentamicin for a patient. The patient has an active medication order for Gentamicin 100 mg IV q 8H. The last dose was given at noon. IV batch deliveries are made daily at 06:00 and 18:00.

Question: How should the pharmacy technician handle this phone call?

Step 1: Check to see when the last dose was given: 12:00 (noon).

Step 2: Verify the dose interval: every 8 hours.

Step 3: Calculate when the next dose is due:

12:00 + 8 hrs = 20:00 (8 p.m.).

Answer: The medication is not missing since it is not due until 20:00 (8 p.m.). The technician should let the nurse know the medication will arrive with IV batch delivery at 18:00 (6 p.m.).

Example—Percent Calculation

The IV technician receives an order for 500 ml of dextrose 12.5%. The pharmacy has a stock solution of dextrose 70% and sterile water to prepare the fluid.

Question: How many ml of dextrose 70% and how many ml of sterile water should the technician use to prepare the solution properly?

Step 1: Calculate the number of grams of dextrose needed to prepare 500 ml of D12.5W (dextrose 12.5% in water). Remember: weight-to-volume % = grams/100 ml (g/100 ml):

$$\frac{12.5 \text{ g dextrose}}{100 \text{ ml}} = \frac{X}{500 \text{ ml}} \qquad X = 62.5 \text{ g dextrose}$$

Step 2: Calculate how many ml of dextrose 70% is needed to give 62.5 g dextrose:

$$\frac{62.5 \text{ g dextrose}}{X} = \frac{70 \text{ g dextrose}}{100 \text{ ml}} \qquad X = 89.3 \text{ ml of D70W}$$

Step 3: Calculate the volume of sterile water needed. Remember: the total volume of solution will be 500 ml.

500 ml − 89.3 ml = 410.7 ml of sterile water

Step 4: Double check your calculations:

$$\frac{62.5 \text{ g dextrose}}{89.3 \text{ ml (D70W)} + 410.7 \text{ ml (Sterile Water)}} = \frac{62.5 \text{ g}}{500 \text{ ml}} = \frac{12.5 \text{ g}}{100 \text{ ml}} = 12.5\%$$

CALCULATIONS (cont'd)

Example—Drip Rate Calculation

While on drip rounds in the Pediatric ICU, a technician notices that a drip containing insulin 100 units in 100 ml and is running at 13.5 ml/hr. The technician thinks that this rate seems high. The patient is 12 years old and weighs 198 pounds. The technician knows that the usual dose of an insulin drip is between 0.05–0.2 units/kg/hr.

Question: What dose of insulin (in units/kg/hr) is the patient receiving?

Step 1: Convert the patient's weight from pounds to kg. (Remember: 1 kg = 2.2 pounds):

$$198 \text{ pounds} \times \frac{1 \text{ kg}}{2.2 \text{ pounds}} = 90 \text{ kg}$$

Step 2: Calculate how much the insulin drip is delivering in units/kg/hr:

$$\frac{13.5 \text{ ml}}{\text{hr}} \times \frac{100 \text{ units}}{100 \text{ ml}} = 13.5 \text{ units/hr} \div 90 \text{ kg} = 0.15 \text{ units/kg/hr}$$

After calculating the rate of infusion, the technician realizes the dose is within normal limits.

Example—Intravenous Order and Calculation

The pharmacy receives a written order for "Magnesium 2 gram IV rider over 3 hours" for a patient in the Cardiac Care Unit (CCU). It is part of the technician's job to type the order into the pharmacy computer system.

Question 1: How should the technician proceed?

Step 1: The technician should check the patient's magnesium (Mg^{++}) level so the pharmacist can evaluate if the order is appropriate.

Step 2: The technician must enter the order in the computer system with the dose of the drug and the volume of the IV solution. The technician knows the final concentration should be 40 mg/ml. From this information, he can calculate how much fluid should be ordered:

First, set up the ratio:

$$\frac{2{,}000 \text{ mg}}{X} = \frac{40 \text{ mg}}{\text{ml}}$$

Second, solve for X:

$$X = 50 \text{ ml}$$

OR

Calculate the volume needed as follows:

$$2{,}000 \text{ mg} \div 40 \text{ mg/ml} = 50 \text{ ml}$$

Question 2: At what rate should the magnesium rider be infused (in ml/hr)?

Answer: 50 ml ÷ 3 hours = 16.7 ml/hr

Example—Preparing a Small Volume Parenteral

Several calculations are required when preparing small volume parenterals. If the calculations are not performed correctly, this could lead to an overdose (if too much is given) or underdose (if too little is given).

A medication order reads: Cefazolin (Ancef®) 750 mg in NaCl 0.9% 50 ml

Problem: Cefazolin is available as a 1 gram powder vial. The directions on the vial state to add 4.5 ml sterile water to give a final product of 1 gram/5 ml. Reconstitute vial as directed. Remember: 1 g = 1,000 mg.

Question: What is the amount needed (in ml) to make 750 mg:

Step 1: First, set up the ratio:

$$\frac{750 \text{ mg}}{X} = \frac{1000 \text{ mg}}{5 \text{ ml}}$$

Second, solve for X:

$$X = 3.75 \text{ ml}$$

OR

First, figure out the concentration of drug per ml:

$$\frac{1000 \text{ mg}}{5 \text{ ml}} = 200 \text{ mg/ml}$$

Second, calculate ml needed:

$$750 \text{ mg} \div 200 \text{ mg/ml} = 3.75 \text{ ml drug}$$

Step 2: Add 3.75 ml of the reconstituted drug to a 50 ml bag of NaCl 0.9%.

Step 3: Initial the medication label and write the expiration date/time.

Example—Dilution Calculation

The pharmacy needs to prepare a furosemide IV dilution of 1 mg/ml. Furosemide is commercially available as 10 mg/ml.

Question: How many ml of drug is needed to prepare 20 ml of injection dilution at a concentration of 1 mg/ml? How many ml of diluent is needed?

Step 1: Calculate the amount of drug (in mg) needed for 20 ml of 1 mg/ml concentration:

$$\frac{X}{20 \text{ ml}} = \frac{1 \text{ mg}}{\text{ml}} \quad X = 20 \text{ mg} \quad \textbf{OR} \quad 20 \text{ ml} \div 1 \text{ mg/ml} = 20 \text{ mg}$$

Step 2: Calculate the volume (in ml) of the commercially available drug needed for 20 mg:

$$\frac{10 \text{ mg}}{1 \text{ ml}} = \frac{20 \text{ mg}}{X} \quad X = 2 \text{ ml} \quad \textbf{OR} \quad 20 \text{ mg} \div 10 \text{ mg/ml} = 2 \text{ ml}$$

Step 3: Subtract the volume of drug from the total volume to calculate diluent volume:

20 ml (total volume) − 2 ml (drug volume) = 18 ml diluent

Answer: The technician would draw up 2 ml of commercially available furosemide and add it to 18 ml of diluent to make 20 mg/20 ml (which = 1 mg/ml).

REVIEW

KEY CONCEPTS

HOSPITAL PHARMACY

✔ Patient rooms are divided into groups called nursing units or patient care units; patients with similar problems are often located on the same unit.

HOSPITAL TECHNICIAN ROLES

✔ Hospital pharmacy technicians have many roles and responsibilities and are often cross-trained to work in different areas of the pharmacy.

HOSPITAL PHARMACY AREAS

✔ The inpatient pharmacy is responsible for medication preparation and distribution.

HOSPITAL FORMULARY

✔ Since hospitals cannot stock every medication available, most have a hospital formulary, which is a list of medications the pharmacy keeps on its shelves and from which doctors can order.

COMMUNICATION AND COMPUTER SYSTEMS

✔ There are several ways the pharmacy communicates with other areas of the hospital, including telephones, fax machines, computerized printouts, pneumatic tubes, and in person.

MEDICAL RECORDS

✔ Medical records are detailed chronological accounts of a patient's medical history and care received. The medical record may be in the form of a paper chart or electronic system.

MEDICATION ORDERS

✔ In the hospital, all drugs ordered for a patient are written on a medication order form or are electronically entered through a computerized physician order entry (CPOE) system.

ORDER PROCESSING

✔ When preparing a medication, the technician must pay close attention to the drug name, dosage form, concentration or strength, quantity, and expiration date; and for IV's, solution and volume.

INVENTORY CONTROL

✔ To assist in the process of ordering inventory, par levels are assigned to each drug. Par is the quantity of drug that should be kept on the pharmacy shelf or in automated dispensing systems.

ORGANIZATION OF MEDICATIONS

✔ In hospital pharmacies, medications are organized in alphabetical order using generic names.

UNIT DOSE SYSTEM

✔ In the hospital, medications are often packed in individual packets that contain the amount of medication needed for each individual dose, called a unit dose.

STERILE PRODUCTS

✔ Technicians may be responsible for preparing small and large volume parenterals, parenteral nutrition therapy, and chemotherapy.

GENERAL HOSPITAL ISSUES

✔ Needles or other items that may cut or puncture the skin should always be thrown away in designated sharps containers.

HOSPITAL PHARMACY CALCULATIONS

✔ Hospital pharmacy technicians perform many calculations on a daily basis, all of which are critically important to a patient's health and safety. Some examples include calculations for preparing small volume parenterals, calculations for timing medications, and flow rate calculations.

SELF TEST

the answer key begins on page 569

MATCH THE TERMS: I

1. automated dispensing system ____
2. batching ____
3. bulk compounding log ____
4. central pharmacy ____
5. clean room ____
6. closed formulary ____
7. code cart ____
8. CPOE _____
9. drip rounds ____
10. drug recall ____
11. electronic medical record (EMR) ____
12. emergency drug procurement ____
13. epidural ____
14. extemporaneous compounds _____
15. final filter _____

a. the process of quickly obtaining an out-of-stock medication in an urgent situation.
b. area designed for the preparation of sterile products.
c. a system in which medications are dispensed from an automated unit at the point of use.
d. the main inpatient pharmacy in a hospital that has pharmacy satellites.
e. advance preparation of large quantities of unit-dose oral solutions/suspensions or small volume parenterals for future use.
f. a record of medications compounded in the pharmacy.
g. medications that must be prepared by following a specific recipe or formula, usually because they are not available commercially.
h. a type of formulary that requires physicians to order only the medications on the formulary list.
i. a computerized patient medical record; also known as an electronic health record (EHR).
j. a device placed at the end of an IV line that is used to remove particulate matter.
k. a process in which the pharmacy technician goes to specific nursing units to find out what IV drips will be needed later that day.
l. a system in which the physician or the physician's agent enters orders directly into the hospital computer system.
m. a sterile, preservative-free medication administered into a patient's epidural space.
n. voluntary or involuntary removal of a drug product by the manufacturer, usually pertaining to a particular shipment or lot number.
o. a locked cart of medications and other medical equipment for emergency use only.

REVIEW

MATCH THE TERMS: II

1. formulary ____
2. inpatient pharmacy ____
3. intravenous piggyback (IVPB) ____
4. medication administration record ____
5. non-formulary drugs ____
6. nurses' station ______
7. outpatient pharmacy ____
8. par ____
9. pharmacy satellite ____
10. pneumatic tube ____
11. PRN order ____
12. reconstitute ____
13. short stability _____
14. standing order _____
15. STAT order _____
16. therapeutic interchange _____
17. total parenteral nutrition (TPN) ____
18. unit dose ____
19. unit inspection _____

a. a form that tracks medications that have been administered to a patient.

b. the amount of a drug product that should be kept on the pharmacy shelf.

c. protein, carbohydrates, and essential nutrients given to the patient through an IV line.

d. a branch of the inpatient pharmacy responsible for preparing, dispensing, and monitoring medications for specific patient areas.

e. a system that shuttles objects through a tube using compressed air as the force.

f. an order for medication to be administered only on an as-needed basis.

g. a hospital pharmacy that services patients who have left the hospital or who are visiting doctors in a hospital outpatient clinic.

h. making a solution or suspension by adding water or other diluent to a premade powder form of a drug in a drug bottle or vial.

i. medication that will expire soon after preparation (i.e., within 1–6 hours after preparation).

j. an order to give medication at scheduled intervals.

k. an order to administer medication immediately.

l. a package containing the amount of a drug required for one dose.

m. drugs not on the formulary list and not regularly stocked in the pharmacy.

n. work station for medical personal on a nursing unit.

o. a review of a nursing unit to ensure compliance with hospital medication policies.

p. a policy approved by the hospital P&T Committee allowing the pharmacist to change a medication order to a therapeutically equivalent formulary medication.

q. a small volume parenteral added into or piggybacked onto a large volume parenteral (LVP).

r. a pharmacy located in a hospital that services only those patients in the hospital and its ancillary areas.

s. a list of drugs stocked at the hospital that have been selected based on therapeutic factors as well as cost.

CHOOSE THE BEST ANSWER

1. In a hospital, patients are admitted to different nursing units based on similar
   a. medical insurance.
   b. medical problems.
   c. demographics.
   d. income.

2. The main responsibilities of a pharmacy technician may include all of the following EXCEPT:
   a. preparing medications orders.
   b. conducting unit inspections.
   c. administering medications to patients.
   d. monitoring patients drug therapy.

3. A pharmacy technician who is working in the clean room may be responsible for preparing
   a. parenteral nutrition.
   b. oral medications.
   c. extemporaneous oral compounds.
   d. enteral nutrition.

4. Non-formulary medications
   a. must always be stocked in the pharmacy.
   b. may not be in supply and could take several days before they can be stocked in the pharmacy.
   c. are commonly used when a hospital has a closed formulary.
   d. are always inexpensive.

5. HIPAA is a federal law that protects a patient's private information when it is
   a. spoken.
   b. written.
   c. electronically transferred.
   d. all of the above

6. An IVPB is due at 2 p.m. What time would that be using military time?
   a. 02:00
   b. 12:00
   c. 14:00
   d. 20:00

7. In order to determine what rate a patient's dopamine drip is running, the pharmacy technician must look in the ________________ section of a patient's medical chart.
   a. lab/test results
   b. demographics
   c. progress notes
   d. documentation flow sheet

8. A(n) __________ order is an order for a medication to be administered as needed.
   a. PRN
   b. STAT
   c. Routine
   d. NPO

9. Nurses track medication administration on a(an)
   a. PCU.
   b. PRN.
   c. STAT.
   d. MAR.

10. Automatic stop orders
    a. can only be ordered by certain physicians in a hospital.
    b. limit the period of time the order will remain active.
    c. require approval from the appropriate service before the medication can be dispensed.
    d. allow medications to be ordered for long periods of time.

REVIEW

11. A medication order reads, "Ciprofloxacin 400 mg q 12 hours X 7 days." What essential information is missing from this order?
    a. dose
    b. route
    c. drug interactions
    d. timing

12. If a medication has been dispensed by the pharmacy and the nurse calls stating the medication is missing, where might the medication be found?
    a. In the automated dispensing cabinet.
    b. On another unit from which the patient was recently transferred.
    c. In the pharmacy ready to be delivered.
    d. All of the above.

13. Hepatitis B vaccine requires refrigeration. This means it must be kept between
    a. 2°–8°C.
    b. 8°–15°C.
    c. 15°–25°C.
    d. 25°–30°C.

14. Bulk bottles used for extemporaneous oral compounding MUST be labeled with the name of drug, expiration date, and
    a. concentration, lot number specific to the hospital, and pharmacist initials.
    b. concentration, lot numbers for all ingredients used in the preparation of the product, and pharmacist initials.
    c. manufacturer for all ingredients used in the preparation of the product, and pharmacist initials.
    d. manufacturer for all ingredients used in the preparation of the product, and technician initials.

15. When the pharmacy technician prepacks oral liquids the syringes MUST be
    a. amber colored.
    b. at least 5 ml in volume.
    c. able to accept a needle.
    d. unable to accept a needle.

16. A single dose vial
    a. can be used for 30 days after opening.
    b. should never be used in a hospital.
    c. contains no preservative.
    d. must always be reconstituted.

17. A code cart
    a. should never be locked.
    b. is where Material Safety Data Sheets (MSDS) should be stored.
    c. contains different medications and equipment commonly used in emergency situations.
    d. is a cart used for pharmacy technicians to delivery medications throughout the hospital.

18. If a patient's current rate of NaCl 0.9% is 125 ml/hr, how many one liter intravenous bags will be necessary to fill a 24-hour supply?
    a. 2
    b. 3
    c. 5
    d. 4

19. How many doses of amoxicillin 500 mg can be drawn up from a 250 ml bottle of amoxicillin 250 mg/5ml oral suspension?
    a. 10
    b. 50
    c. 25
    d. 20

20. A medication order reads: gentamicin 120 mg iv 8 hours. The last dose was given to the patient at 16:00. When is the next dose due?
    a. 14:00
    b. 18:00
    c. 12:00
    d. 00:00

21. Ampicillin/sulbactam (Unasyn®) 3 grams is reconstituted with 6.4 ml to give a final concentration of 375 mg/ml. How many ml are required to give a dose of 2 grams?
    a. 4.3 ml
    b. 5.3 ml
    c. 6.4 ml
    d. 7.5 ml

22. An IV infusion order calls for dopamine 800 mg in 250 ml of D5W to be infused at 10 mcg/kg/min. The patient weighs 55 kg. What will the flow rate be in ml/hr?
    a. 0.2 ml/hr
    b. 10.3 ml/hr
    c. 22.7 ml/hr
    d. 105.6 ml/hr

23. An order arrives in the IV room for 1,000 ml of dextrose 15%. How many ml of dextrose 70% will be needed to be added to sterile water make this solution?
    a. 184 ml
    b. 214 ml
    c. 150 ml
    d. 70 ml

CRITICAL THINKING QUESTIONS

1. Meropenem is a broad spectrum antibiotic on an infectious disease restriction list at Community Hospital. Explain what must occur in order to dispense this medication from the hospital pharmacy.
2. A nurse calls the pharmacy stating she is missing a 14:00 dose of tobramycin. Describe steps the pharmacy technician should take to determine if the pharmacy should dispense the dose again.
3. Kelly is a pharmacy technician at Mercy Hospital. While on duty in the main pharmacy, she receives a phone call from a coworker who says her brother was just admitted to the hospital for kidney failure. The coworker asks Kelly to look into the computer system to get her brother's most recent lab values. How should Kelly respond to her coworker?

THINKING IT THROUGH WRAP-UP

1. Sam should ask Dr. Stewart if he can hold until the pharmacist is available. If he cannot, Sam should ask Dr. Stewart for his pager or phone number so the pharmacist call him immediately after he/she is off the phone.
2. No, Sam cannot take a verbal order for a medication from the doctor. A pharmacist must take verbal orders for medication. Depending on hospital policy, registered nurses may also take verbal orders for medications.
3. Sam can ask Dr. Stewart for the patient's medical record number to bring up the patient in the computer system. Since Sam knows the order is for potassium chloride, he can look up the patient's last potassium level, which will help the pharmacist process the order quickly.

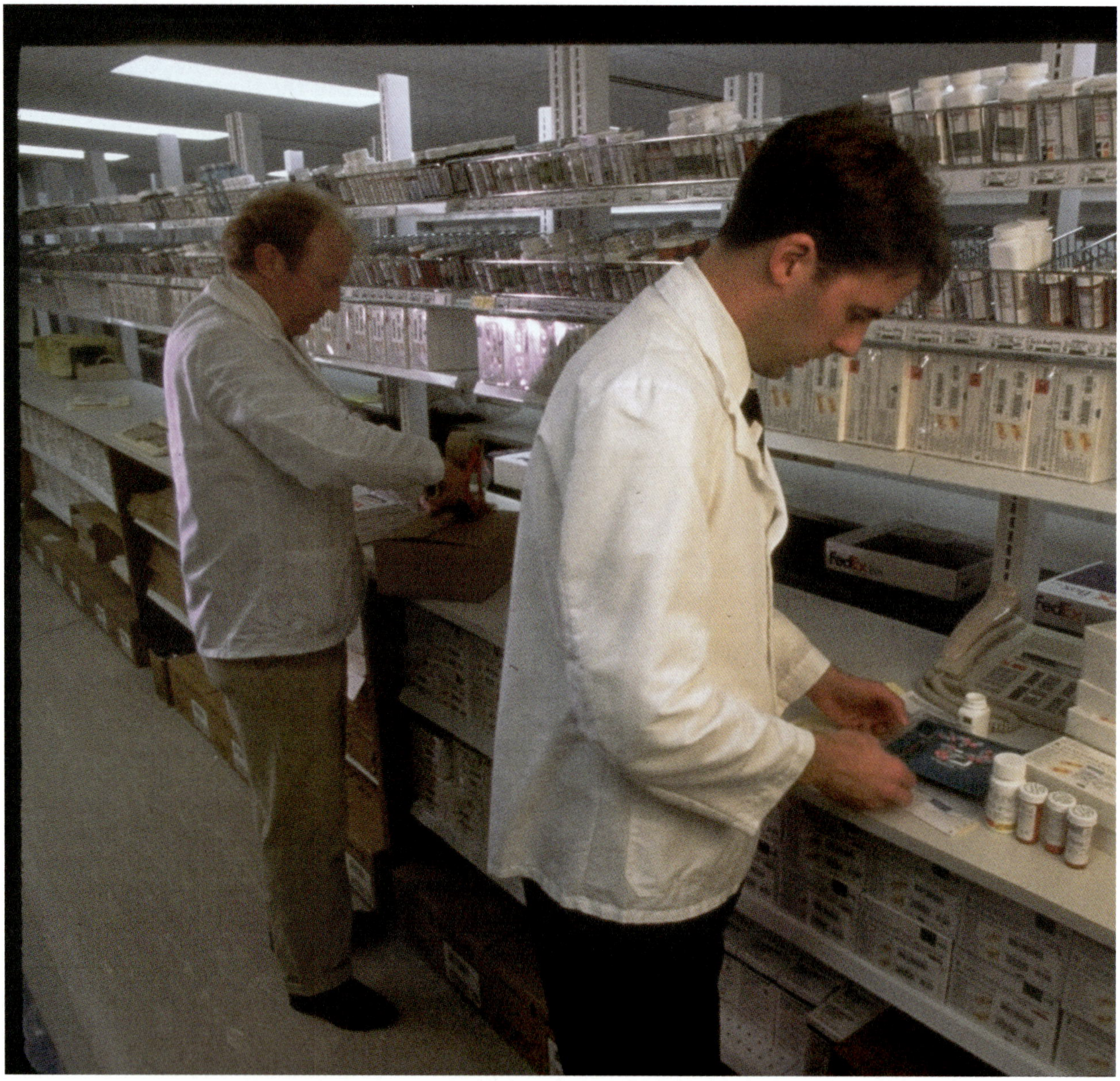

17

OTHER ENVIRONMENTS

LEARNING OBJECTIVES

At the completion of study, the student will:

- ✔ know for which kind of prescription mail-order pharmacy is most often used.
- ✔ understand the importance of automated systems in mail-order pharmacy.
- ✔ be aware of how state and federal laws apply to mail-order pharmacy.
- ✔ understand how long-term care organizations handle pharmacy services.
- ✔ be aware of the different types of home infusion therapies and what rules govern preparing home infusion admixtures.
- ✔ be aware of the role of nuclear pharmacies in health care.

THINKING IT THROUGH

Sarah has been looking through the classified ads in the newspaper for a job opening as a pharmacy technician. She noticed several different jobs in today's paper: one is for pharmacy technician at North American Mail Order Pharmacy, another is at Happy Valley Long Term Care, and a third is at MetroWest Health Systems Parenteral Solutions.

As you read through the chapter keep in mind the following questions:

1. Which of these opportunities would Sarah be qualified for if Sarah has no experience working in an IV room or with unit-dose medications?
2. Which of these environments is likely to have the most automation?

MAIL ORDER PHARMACY

Chain community pharmacies are the largest segment of the retail pharmacy market, but mail order pharmacy is the fastest growing.

A mail order pharmacy sends medications to patients through mail or other delivery services. They have staffs of pharmacists, registered nurses, and technicians and can offer all the services of a community pharmacy, including compounding.

Because mail order medications involve a delivery time of at least 24–48 hours, they are used in situations where the need for the medication is known in advance.

This is true of *chronic conditions* like diabetes, high blood pressure, or depression, where the need for medication can be predicted and the supply can be easily maintained by mail delivery. This type of medication is called a *maintenance medication*, because it is used to maintain the patient with a chronic condition. By comparison, if a patient has an *acute condition*, such as a sudden infection, they would go to their community pharmacy to obtain the prescribed medication immediately after receiving their diagnosis.

Because they use the mail, mail order pharmacies can serve broad geographic areas.

In the United States, for example, they can provide services to all states. This means that they can operate at a high volume. In addition to high volume discounts, this provides mail order pharmacies with economies of scale. These and other factors allow them to sell their medications at lower costs than community pharmacies. For this reason, mail order pharmacies are increasingly popular with third-party insurers, a major source of their growth.

acute condition a sudden condition requiring immediate treatment.

chronic condition a continuing condition that requires ongoing treatment for a prolonged period.

maintenance medication a medication that is required on a continuing basis for the treatment of a chronic condition.

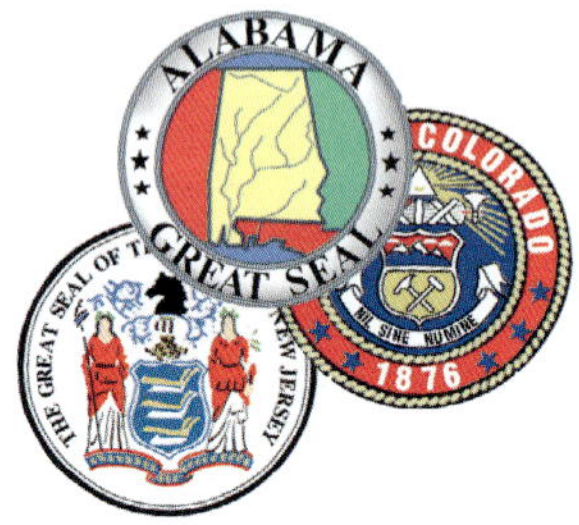

Regulation and Licensing

Though mail order pharmacies must follow federal and state requirements in processing prescriptions, they are not necessarily licensed in each state to which they send medications. As a condition for doing business there, some states now require that mail order pharmacies employ pharmacists licensed to practice in that state. However, not all do.

Online Drugstores

Online drugstores are a type of mail order pharmacy that use the Internet to advertise and take orders for drugs, which are then mailed to the customer. Some online drugstores also use traditional mail order marketing methods and, like mail order pharmacies, they have a full staff of pharmacists, technicians, and doctors employed to ensure proper filling of prescriptions as well as provide patient counseling regarding medications.

Drugs cost less in Canada and U.S. cross-border regulations allow Canadian pharmacies to fill individual prescriptions from U.S. consumers for small amounts of drugs. Because of this, the Canadian online drugstore industry has grown rapidly, and has been the subject of much consumer and political debate.

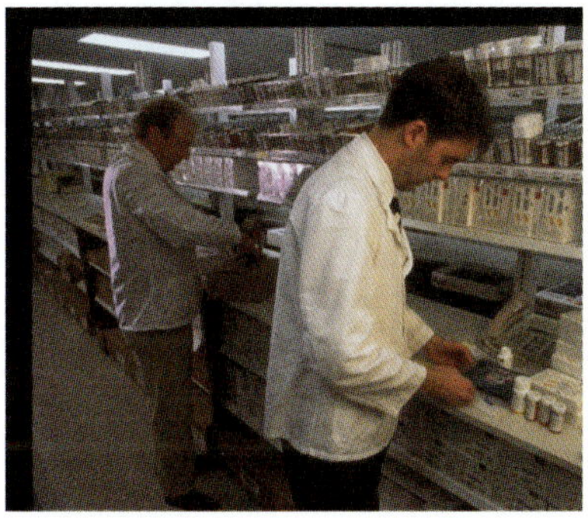

Automation and Quality Control

Mail order pharmacies are generally large-scale operations that are highly automated. They use assembly line processing in which each step in the prescription fill process is completed or managed by a person who specializes in that step. For example, one technician may be responsible for entering prescriptions into the system, another for running an automated dispensing machine to fill prescriptions, and another for preparing the prescription for shipping. There are also steps for pharmacists to review the prescription before and after filling. Bar coding of each prescription is used so that the prescription may be checked continually throughout the process against the information in the system. This ensures a high level of quality control. In fact, the increasing ability of automated systems to deliver a high-quality product is one of the key contributing factors in the growth of mail order pharmacy.

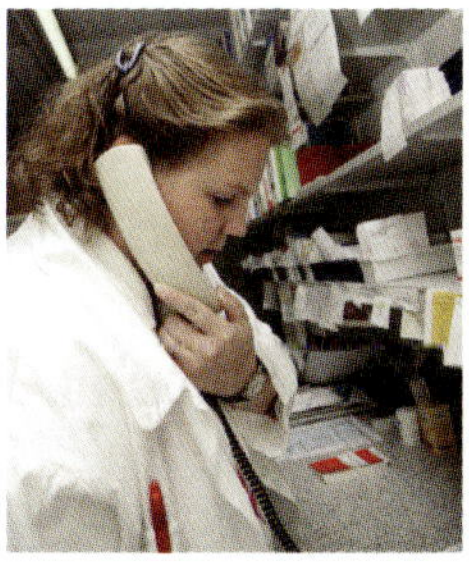

Counseling and Information

Mail order pharmacies have help desk or customer service numbers that patients can call when in need of counseling. Since calls may be related to medications, billing, or other issues, these areas can be staffed with a mix of pharmacists, nurses, and technicians. As in the community pharmacy, technicians may not answer any questions related to medications, but of course can answer questions regarding forms, claims, and other non-medication issues.

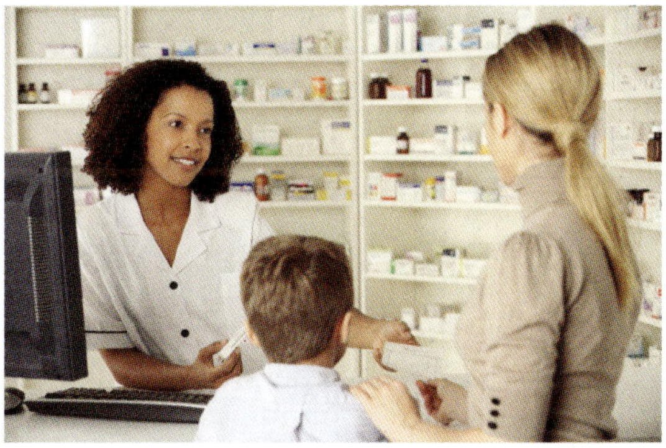

Mail Order and Community Pharmacy

Much of the growth of mail order pharmacy has come at the expense of community pharmacy, which has historically served all patients, including those with chronic conditions. The large scale and sophistication of mail order pharmacies gives them many advantages (price being an extremely important one), which will undoubtedly help them continue growing. At the same time, the personal availability of the pharmacist and the face-to-face interaction between pharmacist and patient in the community pharmacy are advantages likely to ensure their vital role in the health of their communities. Both areas offer excellent career opportunities to pharmacy technicians.

LONG-TERM CARE

Long-term care facilities provide care for people unable to care for themselves because of mental or physical impairment.

Patients may be of any age and include chronically ill elderly, impaired children, and permanently disabled adults whose families can no longer care for their needs. Nursing homes make up the majority of long-term care facilities, but others include psychiatric institutions, chronic disease, and rehabilitation facilities. The amount of time a patient may need long-term care can extend from months to years or even a lifetime.

Because of limited resources, most long-term care facilities contract out dispensing and clinical pharmacy services.

This means that they will pay for another company to take care of the majority of patient medicines. The licensed professional pharmacy or practice that provides medications and/or clinical services to long-term care facilities and their residents is called a long-term care pharmacy organization. Although a pharmacist or pharmacy technician does not have to physically be present at the facility during all hours, pharmacy services must be made available 24 hours a day (e.g., by phone pager).

Pharmacists perform two types of functions for long-term care: distributive and consultant.

The *distributive pharmacist* is responsible for making sure the patients are receiving the correct medicines that were ordered. This job is mainly done outside of the long-term care facility itself.

The *consultant pharmacist* is responsible for developing and maintaining an individualized pharmaceutical plan for every long-term care resident.

This is done by reviewing patient charts, assessing how a patient may receive optimal benefits from their medicines, and monitoring for drug-related problems. They interact with doctors, nurses, and other health professionals. An individual consultant pharmacist is usually responsible for several different nursing homes or other facilities and so may only visit each on certain weekly or monthly intervals. It is important to make the distinction between these types of responsibilities because the pharmacy technician working for a long-term care pharmacy organization may be assisting in these different tasks.

REGULATION

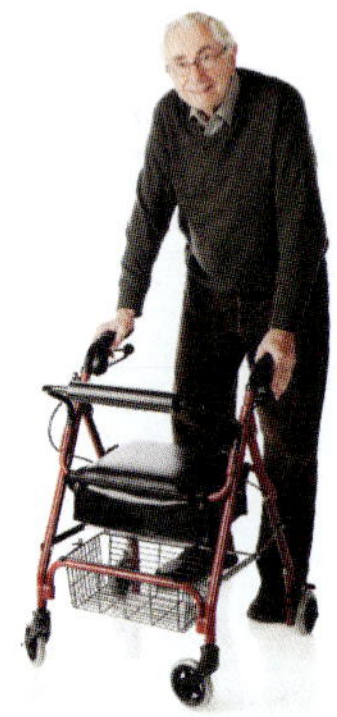

Nursing Homes

Most long-term care facilities are nursing homes that provide daily nursing care. Patients in this setting are generally referred to as residents.

Requirements for Pharmacy Services in Long-Term Care Facilities

The Code of Federal Regulations section 483.60 states the requirements for pharmacy services operating in long-term care facilities.

Long-term care facilities must provide pharmaceutical services to meet the needs of each resident. The pharmacy services must include service consultation by a licensed pharmacist. The pharmacy is also required to establish a system of records of receipt and disposition of all controlled drugs. Additionally, a licensed pharmacist must perform a drug regimen review for each resident at least once a month.

automated dispensing system a system in which medications are dispensed from an automated unit at the point of use upon confirmation of an order communicated by computer from a central system.

Many of the duties of pharmacy technicians in the long-term care pharmacy organization are similar to those in the hospital. These include filling medication carts, packaging prescriptions, mixing intravenous solutions, ordering medication stock, maintaining *automated dispensing systems* and emergency medication carts, and crediting returned medications. As in the hospital environment, the technician works under supervision of the pharmacist and must understand the limitations set forth by law.

In some facilities, the medication cart may be filled with enough medications to last for a week.

This is different from the hospital setting because there is much less medication and patients' drug therapies are not changed as frequently. However, if a patient receives a new medication order, there must be a system in place to make sure the appropriate drugs are received. To handle this, the pharmacy organization in charge of the facility may make arrangements with an alternative pharmacy or use an automated dispensing system. Copies of new medication orders may be faxed to an alternative pharmacy that will deliver the appropriate drugs. Some facilities may have a limited drug inventory stored in a secured location where only authorized personnel may obtain access, and pharmacy technicians may be required to keep track of inventory in these locations.

Emergency kits, or code carts, similar to those in hospitals are also located in long-term care facilities for emergency situations.

As in hospitals, if these emergency kits are opened, the appropriate patient must be charged for the medications used and the cart must be refilled. The technician is responsible for these duties and the pharmacist makes a final check before the cart is resealed. A pharmacy technician working with the pharmacist may also be responsible for the inventory of controlled substances stored in the long-term care facility.

consultant pharmacist develops and maintains an individual pharmaceutical plan for each long-term care patient.

distributive pharmacist makes sure long-term care patients receive the correct medications ordered.

Training

The orientation process at a long-term care pharmacy organization is comparable to the hospital setting. There is an initial orientation and training regarding performance of assigned functions and special requirements in the long-term care setting. Also, there is a written job description of the functions the pharmacy technicians may perform in accordance with specific regulations in the state. It is important to be aware of what the pharmacy technician is able to do or not do according to the law.

Changing Responsibilities

In addition to typical duties such as preparing, packaging, stocking, and delivering medications, new opportunities are emerging for pharmacy technicians in the long-term care environment. These include working closer with the consultant pharmacist to assist in the collection of data for patient assessment, compiling quality improvement data, maintaining computerized information between distributive and consultant pharmacists, performing reviews of drug use in individual long-term care facilities, and preparing pharmacy reports.

Automated Dispensing Systems

When a medication is needed suddenly, the time it takes for delivery from an outside supplier can present problems. Because of this, many nursing homes are turning to point-of-use automated dispensing systems. The medication order is communicated by computer to a central pharmacy system which then sends a confirmation of the order to the unit at the point-of-use. As soon as the unit receives this confirmation, a nurse can get the medication from the unit.

HOME INFUSION

Home care provides care in a patient's home that might otherwise be provided in an institutional setting or physician's office.

The primary providers of such care are ***home care agencies***. Care is supervised by a registered nurse who works with a physician, pharmacist, and others to administer a care plan that involves the patient or another caregiver. The primary advantage of home care over institutional care is a better quality of life, though in many cases it may also be less expensive.

The fastest growing area of home health care is home infusion.

Advances in infusion pump technology have made the infusion process more accurate and easier to administer and have been a major factor in the growth of home infusion. Pumps are available for specific therapies or multiple therapies. There are ambulatory pumps that can be worn by patients and allow freedom of movement compared to being restricted to an infusion pump attached to an administration pole.

The type of pump used depends on several factors.

These include the type of therapy or therapies, the ambulatory status of the patient, the involvement of caregivers, and so on. The supervising nurse and the pharmacist consult on the patient's care plan and choose the appropriate pump.

One of the fundamental activities of home care is patient education.

That is, the patient is educated about their therapy: how to self-administer, monitor, report problems, and so on. The supervising nurse is the primary person responsible for personally educating the patient or their caregiver about therapy. However, the pharmacist is responsible for providing medication information to the supervising nurse and the patient or caregiver. Patients or caregivers are generally required by law to sign a form indicating that they have received the appropriate information.

home care agencies home nursing care businesses that provide a range of health-care services, including infusion.

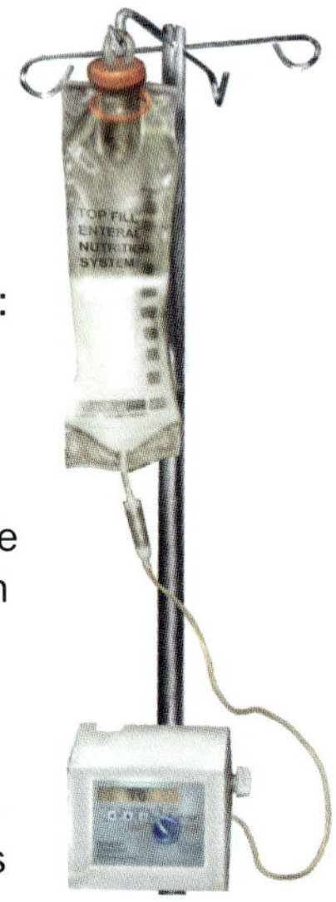

Primary Providers

The primary providers of home infusion services are:

- **Home Care Agencies:** These are essentially home nursing care businesses that provide a range of home health care services, which can include infusion.
- **Home Infusion Pharmacies:** These are specialized pharmacies that prepare admixtures, provide infusion pumps, and are involved in various aspects of the patient's care plan.
- **Hospitals:** Many hospitals offer home infusion therapies as a way to ensure continued therapy after patients are released.

Primary Home Infusion Therapies

The primary therapies provided by home infusion services are:

- **Antibiotic Therapy:** Antibiotic therapy is a common home infusion service used in treating AIDS-related and other infections.
- **Parenteral Nutrition:** Parenteral nutrition is often required for patients with various intestinal disorders or AIDS.
- **Pain Management:** This generally applies to the infusion of narcotics for patients with painful terminal illnesses or other types of severe chronic pain.
- **Chemotherapy:** In certain situations, chemotherapy is provided in the home, generally in conjunction with an oncology program at a hospital or clinic.

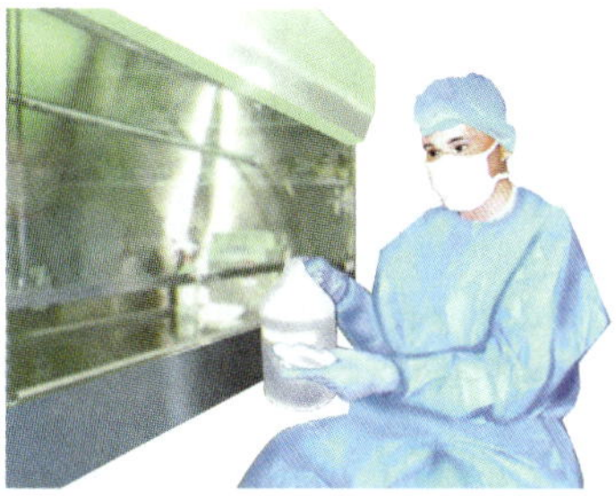

Compounding

The same rules apply to preparing parenteral admixtures in the home infusion setting as in the hospital. Compounding such admixtures requires the use of clean rooms, special equipment such as laminar flow hoods, and the use of aseptic practices. As with other parenteral admixtures, stability of the admixture for its intended use is a primary issue and storage a major concern. A complicating factor is that storage cannot be monitored as closely in a patient's home as in an institutional setting. This results in short stability time limits that along with storage conditions require special attention. It also sometimes results in the on-site preparation of certain therapies by the patient or caregiver. In addition, automated devices that mix parenteral nutrition formulations at the time of administration are sometimes used.

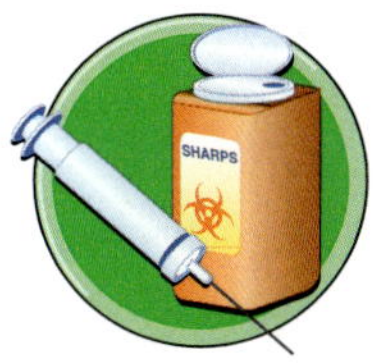

Hazardous Waste

Chemotherapy, the treatment of AIDS patients, and other infusion therapies involve the transportation, storage, and disposal of hazardous materials and is a primary area of concern. Home infusion personnel, patients and care givers must comply with all regulations governing such material. Compliance is a fundamental responsibility of home infusion personnel and is monitored by various regulatory agencies.

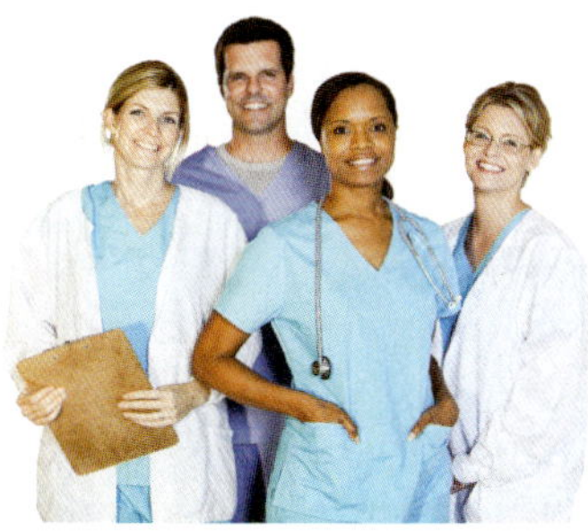

Home Care Team

The team that provides home health care includes the following:

Physician: The patient's physician orders the infusion therapy.

Registered Nurse: The nurse is responsible for coordinating and monitoring the care plan and the home care team, and for educating the patient.

Pharmacist: The pharmacist works with the supervising nurse to develop a pharmaceutical care plan, which includes selection of the infusion device, identification of potential adverse reactions and interventions, and monitoring practices.

Pharmacy Technician: The technician works under the pharmacist's supervision and may be involved with compounding, labeling, delivery, and other non-consulting activities.

Home Care Aide: Aides are nonprofessional staff employed by the home care agency who work under the supervision of the registered nurse. They assist in various aspects of a patient's care, but generally not in medication therapy.

NUCLEAR PHARMACY

Nuclear pharmacies are specially licensed and regulated pharmacies that prepare radioactive materials called radiopharmaceuticals that are used for diagnosis as well as treatment of diseases.

There are major nuclear pharmacy chains, such as Cardinal Health, GE Healthcare, PETNET Solutions, and Triad Isotopes, as well as independently-owned nuclear pharmacies. Pharmacists and pharmacy technicians who work in nuclear pharmacies obtain special training in order to safely work with radioactive materials.

Nuclear pharmacies are usually located for easy access to hospitals and clinics where most of the diagnostic testing takes place.

Nuclear pharmacies typically operate 24 hours a day, 7 days a week, 365 days a year. Nuclear pharmacies prepare and dispense most agents in the evenings so the agents can be delivered to hospitals and clinics before 6 a.m. daily. Some additional orders are received as STAT orders and prepared and delivered during the day.

Nuclear pharmacies have restricted and unrestricted areas.

The restricted areas are those areas where orders are entered, materials are compounded (including sterile products), and where the dispensing process occurs. The restricted areas are where radioactive materials are stored (including radioactive waste). The unrestricted areas are those areas with limited or no contact with radioactive materials.

USES FOR RADIO-PHARMACEUTICALS

There are more than 100 diagnostic tests that use radiopharmaceuticals, including brain scans, bone scans, cardiac tests, and thyroid studies. Patients are administered the radiopharmaceutical orally, intravenously, or by inhalation. Two of the most commonly used types of nuclear imaging are positron emission tomography (PET) scans and single photon emission computerized tomography (SPECT) scans.

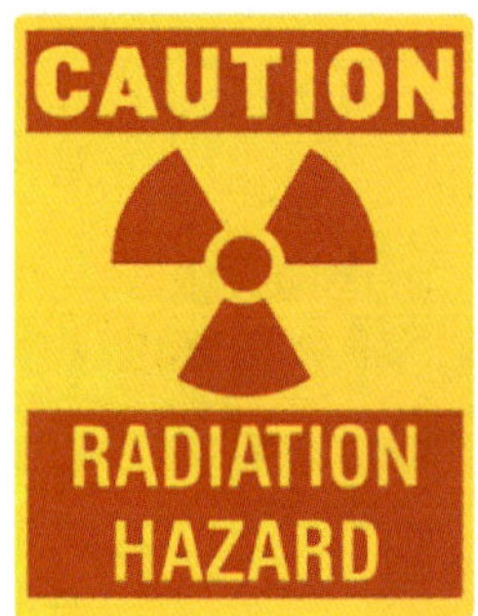

Some Examples of Radiopharmaceuticals Used in Diagnostic Tests

Disease or Condition	Radiopharmaceutical Used
Bone diseases	Sodium Fluoride F 18, Technetium Tc 99m Medronate, Technetium Tc 99m Oxidronate, Technetium Tc 99m Pyrophosphate, Technetium Tc 99m (Pyro- and trimeta-) Phosphates
Bone marrow diseases	Sodium Chromate Cr 51, Technetium Tc 99m Albumin Colloid, Technetium Tc 99m Sulfur Colloid
Brain diseases and tumors	Fludeoxyglucose F 18, Indium In 111 Pentetreotide, Iofetamine I 123, Sodium Pertechnetate Tc 99m, Technetium Tc 99m Exametazime, Technetium Tc 99m Gluceptate, Technetium Tc 99m Pentetate
Cancer; tumors	Fludeoxyglucose F 18, Gallium Citrate Ga 67, Indium In 111 Pentetreotide, Methionine C 11, Radioiodinated Iobenguane, Sodium Fluoride F 18, Technetium Tc 99m Arcitumomab, Technetium Tc 99m Nofetumomab Merpentan
Colorectal disease	Technetium Tc 99m Arcitumomab
Heart disease	Ammonia N 13, Fludeoxyglucose F 18, Rubidium Rb 82, Sodium Pertechnetate Tc 99m, Technetium Tc 99m Albumin, Technetium Tc 99m Sestamibi, Technetium Tc 99m Teboroxime, Technetium Tc 99m Tetrofosmin, Thallous Chloride Tl 201

RADIATION SAFETY

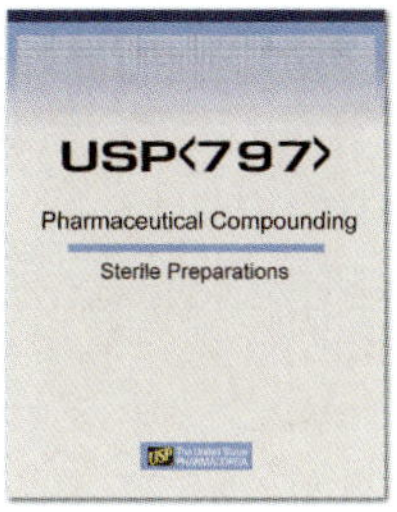

USP <795> and <797> provide guidelines for compounded products (see Chapters 8 and 9). Procedures to prepare radiopharmaceuticals also follow USP <795> and <797> standards.

Prescription orders for radiopharmaceuticals consist of four elements:

1. agent to be administered
2. amount of radioactivity
3. time of administration
4. patient name

Radiopharmaceuticals are typically dispensed as unit doses in 3–5 ml syringes and in a protective container that is often made of lead.

Radiopharmaceuticals are considered hazardous materials.

Their safe handling is regulated on the federal level by the Nuclear Regulatory Commission (NRC) in Part 10 of the Code of Federal Regulations (10 CFR) (see http://www.nrc.gov/reading-rm/doc-collections/cfr/). Additionally the Department of Transportation (DOT) has federal regulations for shipping and receiving radioactive materials. State boards of pharmacy also have rules for radiopharmaceuticals.

The federal government has annual limits for exposure to radioactive materials.

Employers sometimes have more strict limits than the federal government. Pregnant women have stricter limits.

Pharmacists and pharmacy technicians who work with radiopharmaceuticals are required to wear badges to monitor radiation exposure.

Ring badges are used to monitor extreme exposure and are monitored weekly. Body badges are worn on the shirt collar to monitor whole body exposure and are monitored monthly. Pregnant women wear an additional fetal badge near the belly.

Some Examples of Radiopharmaceuticals Used in Diagnostic Tests, cont'd

Disease or Condition	Radiopharmaceutical Used
Heart muscle damage (infarct)	Ammonia N 13, Fludeoxyglucose F 18, Rubidium Rb 82, Technetium Tc 99m Pyrophosphate, Technetium Tc 99m (Pyro- and trimeta-) Phosphates, Technetium Tc 99m Sestamibi, Technetium Tc 99m Teboroxime, Technetium Tc 99m Tetrofosmin, Thallous Chloride Tl 201
Kidney diseases	Iodohippurate Sodium I 123, Iodohippurate Sodium I 131, Iothalamate Sodium I 125, Technetium Tc 99m Gluceptate, Technetium Tc 99m Mertiatide, Technetium Tc 99m Pentetate, Technetium Tc 99m Succimer
Liver diseases	Ammonia N 13, Fludeoxyglucose F 18, Technetium Tc 99m Albumin Colloid, Technetium Tc 99m Disofenin, Technetium Tc 99m Lidofenin, Technetium Tc 99m Mebrofenin, Technetium Tc 99m Sulfur Colloid
Lung diseases	Krypton Kr 81m, Technetium Tc 99m Albumin Aggregated, Technetium Tc 99m Pentetate, Xenon Xe 127, Xenon Xe 133
Thyroid diseases; thyroid cancer	Fludeoxyglucose F 18, Indium In 111 Pentetreotide, Radioiodinated Iobenguane, Sodium Iodide I 123, Sodium Iodide I 131, Sodium Pertechnetate Tc 99m, Technetium Tc 99m Sestamibi

REVIEW

KEY CONCEPTS

MAIL ORDER PHARMACY

- ✔ Mail order pharmacy is used for maintenance therapy for such chronic conditions as depression, gastrointestinal disorders, heart disease, hypertension, and diabetes.
- ✔ Mail order pharmacies must follow federal and state requirements in processing prescriptions, but are not necessarily licensed in each state to which they send medications.
- ✔ Mail order pharmacies are generally large scale operations that are highly automated.
- ✔ Pharmacists review mail order prescriptions before and after filling.

LONG-TERM CARE

- ✔ Because of limited resources, most long-term care facilities contract out dispensing and clinical pharmacy services.

HOME INFUSION

- ✔ Home care is supervised by a registered nurse who works with a physician, pharmacist, and others to administer a care plan that involves the patient or another caregiver.
- ✔ The fastest growing area of home health care is home infusion.
- ✔ Infusion pumps are available for specific therapies or multiple therapies, and include ambulatory pumps that can be worn by patients.
- ✔ In home infusion, the patient or caregiver is educated about the therapy: how to self administer, monitor, report problems, and so on.
- ✔ The primary therapies provided by home infusion services are: antibiotic therapy, parenteral nutrition, pain management, and chemotherapy.
- ✔ The same rules apply to preparing parenteral admixtures in the home setting as in the hospital.

NUCLEAR PHARMACY

- ✔ Nuclear pharmacies prepare radiopharmaceuticals that are used for diagnosis and treatment of diseases.
- ✔ Nuclear pharmacies are typically located for easy access to hospitals and clinics where diagnostic testing is performed.
- ✔ Radiation safety is regulated on the federal level by the Nuclear Regulatory Commission (NRC) and the Department of Transportation (DOT).

SELF TEST

the answer key begins on page 569

MATCH THE TERMS: I

1. acute condition ____
2. antibiotic therapy ____
3. automated dispensing system ____
4. chronic condition ____

a. continuing condition that requires ongoing treatment for a prolonged period.

b. a sudden condition requiring immediate treatment.

c. a common home infusion service used in treating AIDS related and other infections.

d. a system in which medication orders are communicated electronically and dispensed from an automated unit at the point-of-use.

MATCH THE TERMS: II

1. consultant pharmacist ____
2. distributive pharmacist ____
3. home care agencies ____
4. maintenance medication ____

a. develops and maintains an individual pharmaceutical plan for each long-term care patient.
b. a medication that is required on a continuing basis for the treatment of a chronic condition.
c. businesses that provide a range of home nursing care services, including infusion.
d. makes sure long-term care patients receive the correct medications ordered.

CHOOSE THE BEST ANSWER

1. Mail order pharmacies are used for maintenance medications, for chronic conditions. Which of the following conditions would NOT be likely to require maintenance medication?
   a. root canal
   b. HIV/AIDS
   c. depression
   d. hypertension

2. The delivery time for mail order medications is at least
   a. 24 to 48 hours.
   b. 2 weeks.
   c. 4 weeks.
   d. 6 weeks.

3. A sudden condition requiring immediate treatment is a(an)
   a. chronic condition.
   b. PRN condition.
   c. acute condition.
   d. maintenance condition.

4. A continuing condition that requires ongoing treatment for a prolonged period is called a(an)
   a. chronic condition.
   b. acute condition.
   c. infectious condition.
   d. maintenance condition.

5. Mail order pharmacies must follow ____________ requirements.
   a. only state
   b. federal and state
   c. international
   d. only federal

6. The type of order processing used by mail order pharmacies in which each step in the prescription fill process is completed or managed by a person who specializes in that step is called
   a. extemporaneous processing.
   b. assembly line processing.
   c. bin fill processing.
   d. automated processing.

REVIEW

7. The majority of long-term care services are
   a. psychiatric institutions.
   b. rehabilitation facilities.
   c. nursing homes.
   d. urgent care centers.

8. Long-term care facilities must have pharmacy services available
   a. 9 am–5 pm.
   b. 7 am–7 pm.
   c. 7 am–11 pm.
   d. 24 hours a day.

9. The distributive pharmacist for a long-term care facility mainly works outside the facility.
   a. True
   b. False

10. A licensed pharmacist must perform a drug regimen review for each nursing home patient
    a. at least once a month.
    b. at least twice a month.
    c. at least three times a month.
    d. every week.

11. The requirement for pharmacy services in nursing homes to meet the needs of each patient is in the Code of Federal Regulations.
    a. True
    b. False

12. The type of infusion therapy associated with patients with digestive disorders or AIDS is called
    a. admixture therapy.
    b. PO.
    c. NPO.
    d. parenteral nutrition therapy.

13. The type of infusion therapy generally associated with an oncology program at a hospital or clinic is called
    a. chemotherapy.
    b. antibiotic therapy.
    c. PO.
    d. NPO.

14. Compounding parenteral admixtures for home infusion requires all of the following EXCEPT:
    a. aseptic practices.
    b. laminar flow hoods.
    c. ointment tiles.
    d. use of clean rooms.

15. Which member of the home care team orders the infusion therapy?
    a. R.Ph.
    b. physician
    c. Pharm.D.
    d. pharmacy technician

16. Which member of the home care team coordinates and monitors the care plan?
    a. home care aide
    b. registered nurse
    c. R.Ph.
    d. Pharm.D.

17. Which member of the home care team works with the supervising nurse to select the appropriate infusion device?
    a. home care aide
    b. physician
    c. pharmacy technician
    d. pharmacist

18. Which member of the home care team may be involved with compounding, labeling, delivery, and other non-consulting activities?
    a. R.Ph.
    b. home care aide
    c. pharmacy technician
    d. Pharm.D.

19. Which member of the home care team works under the supervision of the registered nurse?
    a. home care aide
    b. pharmacy technician
    c. R.Ph.
    d. Pharm.D.

20. Which member of the home care team is not involved in medication therapy?
    a. pharmacy technician
    b. nurse
    c. home care aide
    d. physician

21. Procedures to prepare radiopharmaceuticals follow ____________ standards.
    a. USP <102> and <104>
    b. USP <355> and <356>
    c. USP <795> and <797>
    d. none of the above

22. Prescription orders for radiopharmaceuticals consist of the agent to be administered, the amount of radioactivity, the time of administration , and __________.
    a. lot number
    b. expiration date
    c. patient name
    d. DEA number

23. Patients are administered radiopharmaceuticals by the intravenous route only.
    a. True
    b. False

CRITICAL THINKING QUESTIONS

1. What are some practical reasons why a medication for an acute condition should not be obtained through a mail order pharmacy?
2. What are the typical duties of a pharmacy technician in long-term care pharmacy? What are some of the emerging opportunities in the long-term care environment?
3. Why is home infusion pharmacy considered an area within home health care?

THINKING IT THROUGH WRAP-UP

1. Of the three different types of pharmacies, the mail order pharmacy is the only option that aligns with Sarah's set of experiences. Mail order pharmacies typically provide maintenance medications to patients in supplies that last a few months. There may be some opportunities for Sarah at the Long Term Care pharmacy performing data entry.
2. Mail order pharmacies process the largest volume of prescriptions and are likely to have the most automation.

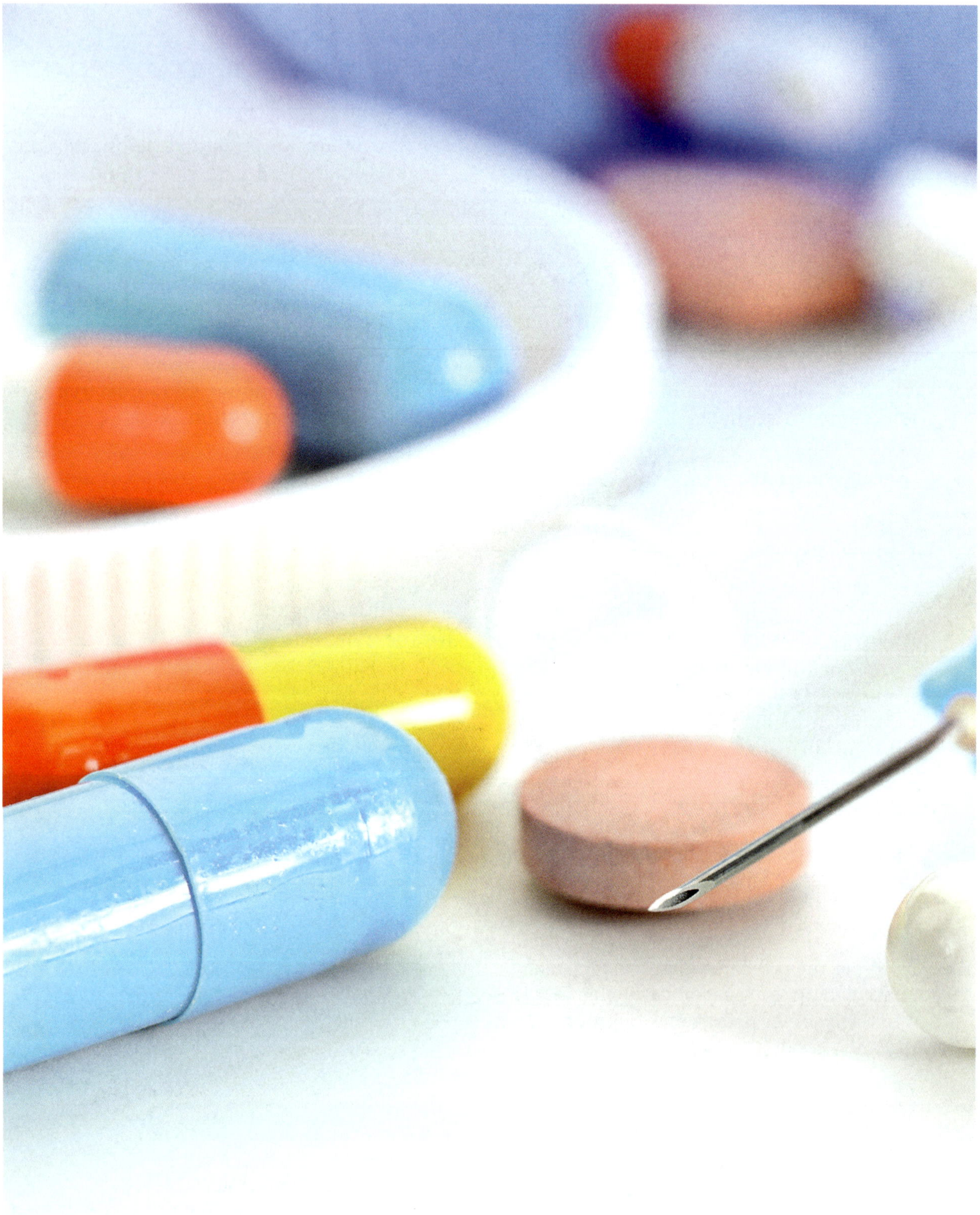

18

COMMON DRUGS & THEIR USES

LEARNING OBJECTIVES

At the completion of study, the student will:

- ✔ describe how drugs are named.
- ✔ describe how drugs are classified.
- ✔ list brand and generic names for commonly prescribed drugs.
- ✔ identify at least one medical use for drugs that are commonly prescribed.
- ✔ identify medication safety issues for commonly prescribed drugs.

THINKING IT THROUGH

Steven is a pharmacy technician who has just had a root canal. His dentist prescribed amoxicillin and ibuprofen. As you read this chapter, consider what you would do in the following situations:

1. Why would these two drugs be prescribed after a dental procedure?
2. What is another type of drug therapy that may have been used during his root canal procedure?
3. Why would it be important to start taking the amoxicillin right away?

DRUG NAMES & CLASSES

When a drug compound is first synthesized or isolated, it is known by its atomic composition: the types and numbers of atoms contained in it.

For example, the compound $C_{14}H_{19}Cl_2NO_2$ has 14 carbon atoms, 19 hydrogen atoms, 2 chlorine atoms, 1 nitrogen atom, and 2 oxygen atoms. Besides being awkward to pronounce, this kind of identification does not really describe the structure of the molecule.

A drug's name begins with a chemical name that describes its structure and its components.

These names identify a specific compound, but they are long and complicated and not useful for general communication. As a result, highly specific chemical names are shortened to less descriptive but more easily pronounceable ones.

While a potential drug is under development, the developer gives it a code number or a suggested nonproprietary name.

Once a suggested nonproprietary name is officially approved, it becomes the generic name of the drug compound. Many pharmaceutical companies will assign code numbers to their compounds in the earliest development stages, and then a suggested nonproprietary name if the compound shows promise of being effective as a drug. At that point, the sponsor will apply for a proprietary or trademark name from both the U.S. Patent Office and foreign agencies. If approved, the proprietary name will have the ® symbol next to it when used in interstate commerce.

While under patent protection, a drug has one nonproprietary name and one proprietary, or brand, name which belongs to the sponsor.

When a drug goes off-patent, other companies may market the same compound under their own brand names. For example, erythromycin is a generic drug that has been off patent for many years. It is available as EryTab® and PCE®, which are brand names used by different companies. But Viagra® (which has the generic name sildenafil) is available only under one brand name because the compound is still under patent protection. The point to remember is that there is only one nonproprietary (generic) name for a drug, but it may be sold under many different brand names once its patent protection has expired.

WHAT'S IN A NAME

USAN

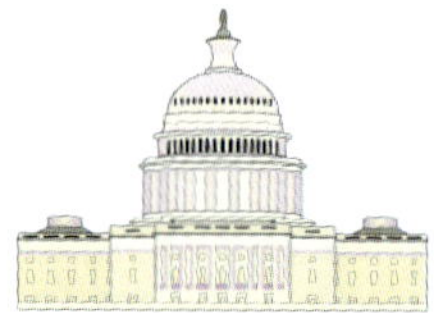

The United States Adopted Names Council (USAN) designates nonproprietary names for drugs. This council was organized in the early 1960s at the joint recommendation of the American Medical Association and the U. S. Pharmacopeial (USP) Convention. Other organizations, the American Pharmaceutical Association (now the American Pharmacists Association) and the FDA, were included in the Council during the latter part of the 1960s. There are publications that list official nonproprietary and proprietary names, as well as drug code designations, empirical names, chemical names, and show the molecular structures. The *USP Dictionary of USAN and International Drug Names* is such a reference.

Applying for a Name

To apply for a name, the sponsoring company initiates a request for a name. The USAN and the sponsor will arrive at a Proposed USAN that is suitable to both. This proposed name is then submitted for consideration to U.S. and foreign drug regulatory agencies. When approved by these different agencies, the name becomes the official name of the drug. The USAN guidelines for the recommendation of names include that the name should:

- be short and distinctive in sound and spelling and not be easily confused with existing names;
- indicate the general pharmacological or therapeutic class into which the substance falls, or the general chemical nature of the substance if the latter is associated with the specific pharmacological activity;
- embody the syllable(s) characteristic of a related group of compounds.

Drug classes are group names for drugs that have similar activities or are used for the same type of diseases and disorders.

The assignment of a drug to a drug class is proposed when the sponsor makes an application to the USAN Council for an adopted name. The USAN Council and the sponsor then agree to a pharmacological or therapeutic classification. Unlike the generic and brand names, this classification is not an "official" one, however, and the drug may be listed in different classifications by different sources. For example, drugs classified one way in this chapter may appear in other classifications in other reference works.

There are common stems or syllables that are used to identify the different drug classes.

The USAN Council approves the stems and syllables and recommends using them in making new nonproprietary names. There are always new stems and syllables being approved by the Council, so the list is ever changing. On this page is a list of some common stems and syllables and the drug class associated with them.

STEMS & CLASSES

Following are the USAN approved stems and the drug classes associated with them.

Stem	Drug Class
-alol	Combined alpha and beta blockers
-andr-	Androgens
-anserin	Serotonin 5-HT_2 receptor antagonists
-arabine	Antineoplastics (arabinofuranosyl derivatives)
-ase	Enzymes
-azepam	Antianxiety agents (diazepam type)
-azosin	Antihypertensives (prazosin type)
-bactam	Beta-lactamase inhibitors
-bamate	Tranquilizers/antiepileptics
-barb	Barbituric acid derivatives
-butazone	Anti-inflammatory analgesics (phenylbutazone type)
-caine	Local anesthetics
-cef	Cephalosporins
-cillin	Penicillins
-conazole	Antifungals (miconazole type)
-cort-	Cortisone derivatives
-curium	Neuromuscular blocking agents
-cycline	Antibiotics (tetracycline type)
-dralazine	Antihypertensives (hydrazine-phthalazines)
-erg-	Ergot alkaloid derivatives
estr-	Estrogens
-fibrate	Antihyperlipidemics
-flurane	Inhalation anesthetics
-gest-	Progestins
-irudin	Anticoagulants (hirudin type)
-leukin	Interleukin-2 derivatives
-lukast	Leukotriene antagonists
-mab	Monoclonal antibodies
-mantadine	Antivirals
-monam	Monobactam antibiotics
-mustine	Antineoplastics
-mycin	Antibiotics
-olol	Beta-blockers (propranolol type)
-olone	Steroids
-oxacin	Antibiotics (quinolone derivatives)
-pamide	Diuretics (sulfamoylbenzoic acid derivatives)

Stem	Drug Class
-pamil	Coronary vasodilators
-parin	Heparin derivatives
-peridol	Antipsychotics (haloperidol type)
-poetin	Erythropoietins
-pramine	Antidepressants (imipramine type)
-pred	Prednisone derivatives
-pril	Antihypertensives (ACE inhibitors)
-profen	Anti-inflammatory/analgesic agents (ibuprofen type)
-rubicin	Antineoplastic antibiotics (daunorubicin type)
-sartan	Angiotensin II receptor antagonists
-sertron	Serotonin 5-HT_3 receptor antagonists
-sulfa	Antibiotics (sulfonamide derivatives)
-terol	Bronchodilators (phenethylamine derivatives)
-thiazide	Diuretics (thiazide derivatives)
-tiazem	Calcium channel blockers (diltiazem derivatives)
-tocin	Oxytocin derivatives
-trexate	Antimetabolites (folic acid derivatives)
-triptyline	Antidepressants
-vastatin	Antihyperlipidemics (HMG-CoA inhibitors)

CLASSIFICATION SCHEMES

There are many systems for classifying drugs: by disorder, body system affected, type of receptor acted on, type of action, etc.

This text uses common classifications, but it is important to recognize that there is no standard classification system used in medicine.

A number of classifications are based on whether they influence the parasympathetic or sympathetic nervous system.

Most organs in the body are influenced by both the parasympathetic and sympathetic nervous systems. These systems generally stimulate opposing responses, which balances their effects and results in a normal state of ***homeostasis***. Drugs that act on the parasympathetic system are called cholinergic because acetylcholine is the ***neurotransmitter*** of this system. Drugs that act on the sympathetic nervous system are called adrenergic, because the neurotransmitters for this system (norepinephrine and epinephrine) are secreted from the adrenal glands.

Many classifications are also named for the type of interaction with the receptor.

Agonist or antagonist interaction is the primary basis for classification (e.g., cholinergic antagonist, etc.), but drugs may be classified based on specific receptor characteristics. For example, adrenergic receptor responses may be categorized as alpha (α) and beta (β).

Classification schemes have grown significantly as different types of receptors have been discovered.

Each type of receptor is responsible for a specific pharmacological effect. As drugs designed to interact with these receptors are developed, the complexity of classifications also increases.

There are also other factors that complicate classification schemes.

One factor for drugs that affect the autonomic nervous system is the use of prefixes or suffixes such as ***blocker***, -lytic, or anti- to mean antagonist, and ***mimetic*** to mean agonist. Another factor is the presence of neurotransmitters other than acetylcholine, norepinephrine, and epinephrine. These include serotonin, dopamine, histamine, gamma-amino butyric acid (GABA), etc. Each has subtypes, and each has agonists and antagonists that act by a variety of mechanisms.

CLASSIFICATIONS

Classification schemes for drugs can be highly complex. They can also vary greatly and any combination of terms or nomenclature schemes might be used. The classifications used in this text should provide insight into how and why the drugs in them are used, but are not the only way to classify these drugs.

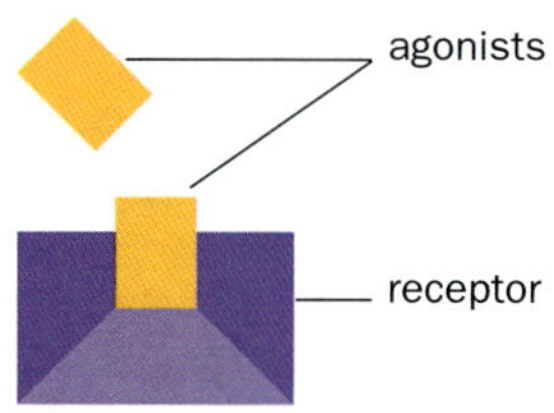

agonists activate receptors

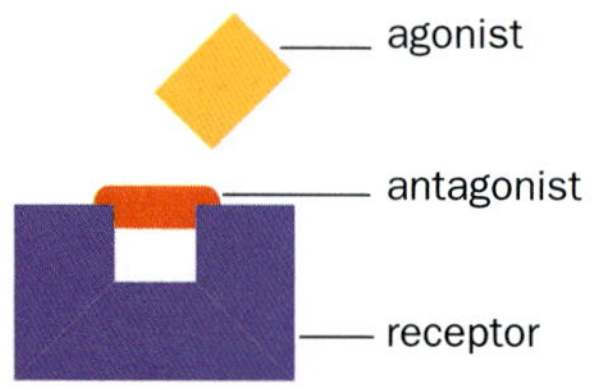

antagonists block receptors

blocker another term for an antagonist drug, because antagonists block the action of neurotransmitters.

homeostasis the state of equilibrium of the body.

mimetic another term for an agonist, because agonists imitate, or "mimic," the action of the neurotransmitter.

neurotransmitter chemicals released by nerves that interact with receptors to cause an effect.

Note: Throughout this chapter, drugs highlighted in green are parenteral drugs that are commonly found in hospitals and other institutional settings.

The Primary Classifications Used in this Text

- Analgesics
  - Salicylates
  - NSAIDs
  - Nonaspirin, non-NSAID
  - Opiates
- Anesthetic Agents
  - Local
  - General
- Anti-infectives
  - Antibiotics (antimicrobials)
  - Antivirals
  - Antifungals
  - Antimycobacterials
  - Antiprotozoals
  - Anthelmintics
- Antineoplastics
  - Antimetabolites
  - Alkylating agents
  - Plant alkaloids
  - Hormones
  - Antitumor antibiotics
  - Radioactive isotopes
- Cardiovascular Agents
  - Beta-blockers
  - Calcium channel blockers
  - Diuretics
  - ACE inhibitors
  - Vasodilators
  - Antianginals
  - Antiarrhythmics
  - Antihyperlipidemics
  - Antihypertensives
  - Thrombolytics/Anticoagulants
  - Vasopressors
- Dermatologicals
- Electrolytic Agents
- Gastrointestinal & Urinary Tract Agents
  - Enzymes
  - Antidiarrheals
  - Antiemetics
  - Antacid/antiulcer agents
  - Laxatives and stool softeners
  - Urinary tract agents
- Hematological Agents
  - Hematopoietic agents
  - Hemostatic agents
- Hormones & Modifiers
  - Thyroid & Parathyroid agents
  - Pituitary agents
  - Adrenal agents
  - Insulins
  - Oral antidiabetics
  - Androgens
  - Phosphodiesterase inhibitors
  - Progestins
  - Estrogens
  - Contraceptives
- Immunobiologic Agents
  - Immune globulins
  - Vaccines
- Musculoskeletal Agents
  - Anti-gout agents
  - Osteoporitics
  - Muscle relaxants
  - Antispasmodics
- Neurological Agents
  - Antiparkinsonian agents
  - Anti-Alzheimer's agents
  - Antiepileptics
  - Anti-migraine agents
- Ophthalmic and Otic Agents
  - Antiglaucoma agents
  - Other ophthalmics
  - Otics
- Psychotropic Agents
  - Antipsychotics
  - Sedatives & hypnotics
  - Antianxiety agents
  - Antidepressants
  - Drug dependency
- Respiratory Agents
  - Antihistamines
  - Decongestants
  - Antitussives
  - Expectorants & mucolytics
  - Bronchodilators

ANALGESICS

Analgesic drugs create a state called *analgesia* in which the pain from a painful medical condition is reduced or not felt.

Once pain has signaled the presence of a medical condition, its usefulness is generally complete and in most cases it can be safely blocked with the use of an analgesic.

There are several types of analgesics.

Two groups are used for mild to moderate pain, the nonsteroidal anti-inflammatory drugs (NSAIDs) and the salicylates. Acetaminophen is also a popular agent for treating mild to moderate pain that some consider an NSAID but others do not.

Opiate-type narcotic analgesics are used to treat severe pain.

The naturally occurring opiates (morphine and codeine) and the synthetic opioids such as meperidine are called narcotic analgesics and have a high abuse potential. In this section, we'll explore the types of analgesics and identify and describe common drug examples of each group.

The Transmission of Pain

Nerve fibers carry pain impulses from the body's receptor sites through the spinal cord and up to the thalamus and cerebral cortex. The cerebral cortex is the ridge-like neural tissue that covers the brain's hemispheres. Analgesics are thought to depress the thalamus and interfere with the transmission of pain impulses. In addition, the brain's interpretation of pain may be altered with the use of these drugs.

Opiate-type Drugs & the Brain

Three specific receptors in the brain have been identified to react to opiate and opioid drugs:

- Mu (μ): produces euphoria, respiratory depression, and physical dependence
- Kappa (κ): produces analgesia
- Sigma (σ): produces dysphoria and hallucinations

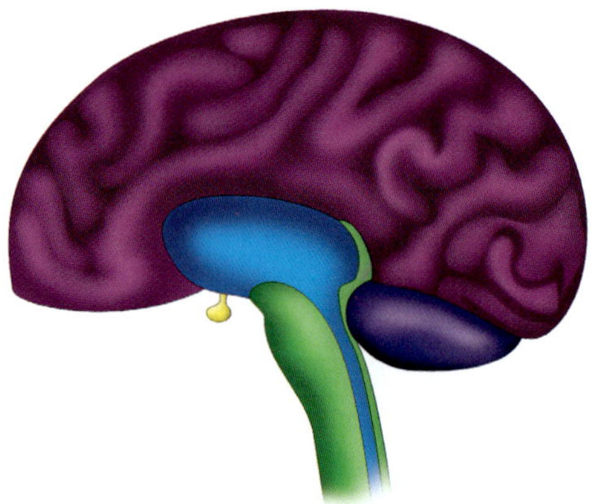

Some Common Analgesic Drugs

Type	Brand Name	Generic Name
Salicylates	Bayer	acetylsalicylic acid (aspirin)
Nonaspirin, non-NSAID	Tylenol, Ofirmev	acetaminophen
NSAID	Motrin, Advil	ibuprofen
NSAID	Naprosyn	naproxen
Opiates	MS Contin	morphine
Opiates	Demerol	meperidine

See Additional Common Drugs by Classification on pp 533-537 for more drugs in this class.

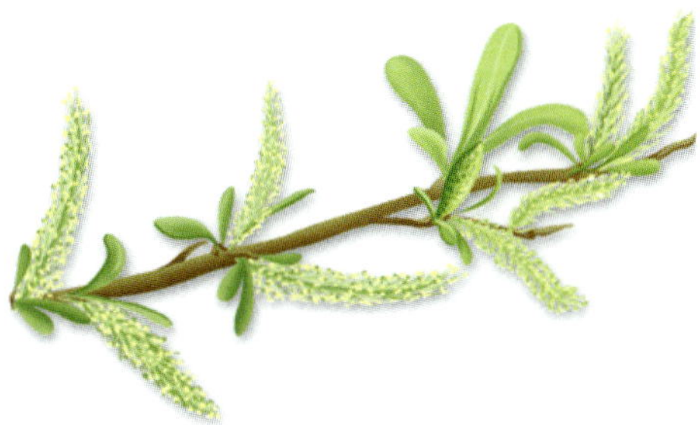

the white willow, a source of salicylic acid

Salicylates

- Relieves mild to moderate pain
- Anti-inflammatory
- Antipyretic

Acetaminophen

- Relieves mild to moderate pain
- Antipyretic

NSAIDs

- More potent than salicylates
- Relieve mild to moderate pain
- Anti-inflammatory
- Antipyretic

Opiate-type

- For severe pain
- Addicting

analgesia a state in which pain is not felt even though a painful condition exists.

antipyretic reduces fever.

An extract of willow bark, salicylic acid has been used as a pain reliever for thousands of years.

Hippocrates and other ancient physicians used plants such as gaultheria and the poplar tree to obtain natural salicylates. Today, nonaddicting analgesic products such as aspirin (acetylsalicylic acid) and methyl salicylate are widely used. Salicylates, acting both centrally and peripherally, are found effective as mild to moderate pain relievers, anti-inflammatory medications, and fever reducers (*antipyretics*).

Nonsteroidal anti-inflammatory drugs (NSAIDs) are both analgesic and anti-inflammatory.

They are generally more potent than the salicylates and serve to relieve mild to moderate pain, reduce fever, and treat rheumatic symptoms. At higher doses, NSAIDs inhibit the synthesis of prostaglandins, a chief contributor to the inflammation process. As a result, inflammation is slowed or reduced. The effect of lower doses is analgesic. The selection and dosing of these drugs is very patient specific as one NSAID may be more effective than another for any given patient. NSAIDs may also have an antipyretic quality by which they reduce fever. The temperature-regulating brain center is the hypothalamus and it is believed that some NSAIDs affect select areas of the hypothalamus to increase vasodilation, sweating, and encourage excess heat loss. Common drugs in this category include ibuprofen (Motrin®) and naproxen (Naprosyn®).

Taken from the poppy plant, Papaver Somniferum, opium was used in ancient times to relieve pain.

Opiate-type and opioid narcotics of today have been found to affect the CNS by reducing the awareness and perception of pain. They mimic the actions of the body's natural, narcotic-like substances called endorphins. The narcotic analgesics do not eradicate the pain, but rather alter the patient's perception of it. Therefore, these drugs are thought to be most helpful if given before the severe pain is present. Common, naturally occurring, opiate-type drugs include morphine and codeine, while common opioid drugs include meperidine (Demerol®).

ANESTHETIC AGENTS

Anesthetics cause an absence of sensation or pain.

They are classified into two groups: local and general.

Local anesthetics block pain conduction from peripheral nerves to the central nervous system without causing a loss of consciousness.

They do this by allowing the nerve's membrane to stabilize in a resting position and not respond to painful stimuli. Cocaine is credited by some sources as the first recognized local anesthetic, but it has a limited use today (e.g., topical application in eye and nasal surgery) and is a Schedule II substance.

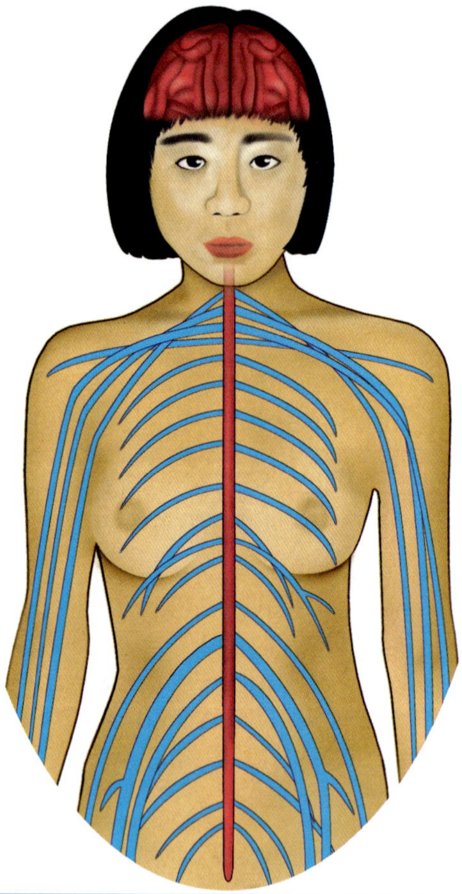

Note: Drugs highlighted in green in the text and tables are parenteral drugs commonly found in hospitals and other institutional settings.

LOCAL ANESTHETICS

Indications

Common indications for local anesthetics include:

- dental work or discomfort (topical or injection);
- birth pain (spinal, epidural, or caudal IV);
- sunburn, hemorrhoids, and skin irritations (topical).

Groups

Local anesthetics can be grouped by chemical structure as follows:

- **Esters**—metabolized by enzymes found in the blood or skin, short to moderate duration of effectiveness.
- **Amides**—metabolized in the liver and therefore longer acting.
- **Others**—agents suitable for patients with allergies to esthers or amides.

Blocking Pain

Pain is conducted from its local site through the Peripheral Nervous System (blue) to the Central Nervous System (red). Local anesthetics block pain conduction to the CNS, but do not affect the CNS, so the patient remains conscious. General anesthetics block pain sensation by depressing the CNS, causing unconsciousness.

Some Common Local Anesthetics

Type	Brand Name	Generic Name
Ester	Novocain	procaine
Ester	n/a	tetracaine
Amide	Xylocaine	lidocaine
Amide	Marcaine	bupivacaine
Other	Sucrets	dyclonine

See Additional Common Drugs by Classification on pp 533-537 for more drugs in this class.

medullary paralysis an overdose of anesthesia that paralyzes the respiratory and heart centers of the medulla, leading to death.

surgical anesthesia the stage of anesthesia in which surgery can be safely conducted.

GENERAL ANESTHESIA

The Four Stages

There are four stages of general anesthesia:

Stage I—Analgesia Euphoria with loss of pain and consciousness.

Stage II—Excitement Increase in sympathetic nervous system effects such as blood pressure, heart and respiratory rate.

Stage III—*Surgical Anesthesia* The stage in which surgery can safely be conducted. There are four levels of surgical anesthesia, with the higher numbered levels producing deeper anesthesia and more serious systemic effects.

Stage IV—*Medullary Paralysis* An overdose of anesthesia can compromise the respiratory and heart centers of the brain's medulla and cause death.

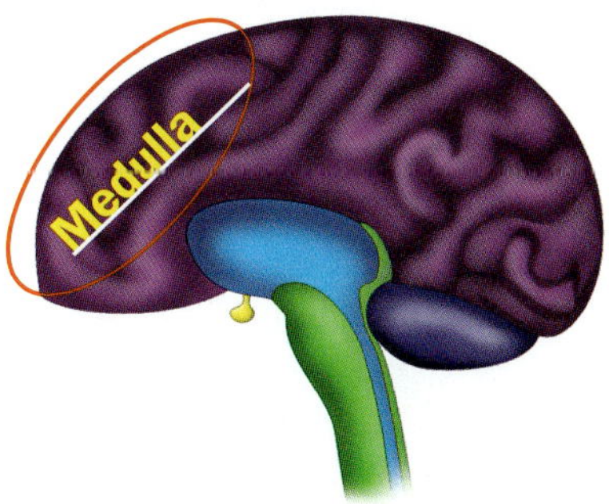

General anesthetics depress the central nervous system to the level of unconsciousness.

The first general anesthetic, nitrous oxide (laughing gas), was developed about 150 years ago. The vapors ethyl ether and chloroform followed soon after. However, these products were found to have many safety concerns and less hazardous agents have been subsequently developed.

General anesthetics are generally classified according to their route of administration: inhalation or intravenous (IV).

IV anesthesia often produces a more pleasant, smoother, and quicker onset than the inhaled anesthetics. A combination of various agents is widely used to avoid undesired side effects and produce the best effects of general anesthesia.

General anesthesia is administered by a medical doctor called an anesthesiologist.

The desired level of general anesthesia can be controlled by balancing the amount of anesthesia the patient receives with the amount their lungs eliminate through exhalation. In ceasing the administration of anesthesia, the process will reverse and the level of anesthesia lighten.

Adjunctive drugs such as analgesics and anti-infectives may be used with anesthetics.

This is to prevent certain negative side effects (those that occur from too much of one anesthetic), potentiate other desired effects (such as pain relief and reduced amount of anesthesia), cause the drying of secretions (preventing aspiration during surgery), or act to prevent infections (post–op). The safety, comfort, and general well-being of the patient are of utmost concern when an anesthesiologist chooses an anesthetic or combination of anesthetics.

Some Common General Anesthetics

Type	Brand Name	Generic Name
Inhalation	Forane	isoflurane
Inhalation	Ultane	sevoflurane
Inhalation	Suprane	desflurane
IV	Diprivan	propofol
IV	Valium	diazepam
IV	Amidate	etomidate

See Additional Common Drugs by Classification on pp 533-537 for more drugs in this class.

ANTI-INFECTIVES

Anti-infectives treat disease produced by microorganisms such as bacteria, viruses, fungi, protozoa, and parasitic worms.

Historically, natural chemicals from the earth such as mercury and molds have been used to treat infections, but it wasn't until Paul Ehrlich synthesized hundreds of chemicals in the 1930s, that a chemotherapeutic approach was widely used. There are now a large number of naturally occurring, semi-synthetic and synthetic drugs and vaccines available for treatments of infectious diseases.

In this section, antibiotics (antimicrobials), antivirals, and antifungals will be discussed and explored.

Other forms of anti-infectives include: antimycobacterials (agents that treat tuberculosis, leprosy, and the MAC complex in AIDS); antiprotozoals (agents that treat malaria, vaginitis, and sleeping sickness); and ***anthelmintics*** (agents that treat parasitic worms in the GI tract).

types of antibiotic action

- **damage bacterial cell wall**
  (e.g., penicillins and cephalosporins)
- **modify protein synthesis**
  (e.g., erythromycin and tetracycline)
- **modify energy metabolism**
  (e.g., sulfonamides)
- **modify DNA synthesis**
  (e.g., ofloxacin and ciprofloxacin)

℞ safety you should know

- Do NOT refrigerate Biaxin® suspension.
- Erythromycins and Biaxin® have many serious drug interactions.
- Many antibiotics can decrease the effectiveness of oral contraceptives.
- Tetracyclines should not be used during pregnancy.
- Tetracyclines should not be used in children under eight years old.
- Tetracyclines and some other antibiotics can cause photosensitivity.
- Avoid dairy products, vitamins, or antacids within two hours of taking tetracyclines.
- Many antibiotics have serious interactions with warfarin (Coumadin®).
- Alcohol should be avoided until one day after therapy with metronidazole.
- Patients taking sulfa drugs should drink plenty of water.

CLASSES

Antibiotics (Antimicrobials)

The term *antibiotic* (or *antimicrobial*) refers to chemicals of bacterial microorganisms that suppress the growth of other microorganisms. Early discovery of antibiotics came from Sir Alexander Fleming and his work isolating the naturally occurring penicillin. Later, a team from Oxford reinvestigated this research and developed potent extracts, which were important in fighting infections during WWII. Since that time, synthetic penicillins such as ampicillin and amoxicillin have been introduced. Other forms of antibiotics include: cephalosporins (cefazolin, cefoxitin, ceftibuten, cefepime, etc.); tetracyclines (tetracycline, doxycycline, etc.); sulfonamides or "sulfa drugs" (sulfamethoxazole, etc.). Some other common antibiotics are azithromycin (Zithromax®) and amoxicillin with potassium clavulanate (Augmentin®).

Antimicrobials can be either ***bacteriostatic*** (inhibiting bacterial growth) or ***bactericidal*** (bacteria killing). Different antibiotics have different types of action such as modifying protein synthesis, modifying energy metabolism, modifying DNA metabolism, or damaging the bacteria's cell wall.

Antivirals

Antivirals inhibit the replication of viruses (and so are virustatic). The viral microorganism will invade the host cell and proliferate using the cell's DNA and RNA. To effectively treat viral infections, the drug needs to stop the viral replication without destroying the patient's healthy cells. Mutations and resistance are common setbacks with this therapy. Antimicrobials are not effective with viral infections, but may be used in cases of accompanying secondary bacterial infection. ***Protease inhibitors*** such as nelfinavir (Viracept®) are a class of medications used to treat HIV and hepatitis C by blocking the enzyme responsible for viral replication. Other common antiviral agents include: valacyclovir (Valtrex®) and acyclovir (Zovirax®).

Antifungals

Antifungals are used to treat fungal infections. Fungi are plant-like microorganisms commonly found in molds and yeast. The drugs chosen to treat these mycosis or mycotic infections are usually fungicidal. The fungal cell is destroyed as the drug prevents cell permeability and nutrition. Common fungal infections include: candidiasis (vaginal yeast infection), ringworm, and athlete's foot. Nystatin and fluconazole (Diflucan®) are popular antifungal drugs.

anthelmintics drugs that destroy worms.
bactericidal bacteria killing.
bacteriostatic bacteria inhibiting.
protease inhibitor an antiviral used for HIV and hepatitis C that blocks the enzyme responsible for viral replication.

ANTI-INFECTIVES (cont'd)

Some Common Anti-infectives		
Type	**Brand Name**	**Generic Name**
Anthelmintic	Albenza	albendazole
Antibiotic/antiprotozoal	Flagyl	metronidazole
Antibiotic/cephalosporin	n/a	cefaclor
Antibiotic/cephalosporin	Ceftin	cefuroxime
Antibiotic/cephalosporin	Cefzil	cefprozil
Antibiotic/cephalosporin	n/a	cefadroxil
Antibiotic/cephalosporin	Fortaz	ceftazidime
Antibiotic/cephalosporin	Keflex	cephalexin
Antibiotic/cephalosporin	Maxipime	cefepime
Antibiotic/cephalosporin	Omnicef	cefdinir
Antibiotic/cephalosporin	Rocephin	ceftriaxone
Antibiotic/cephalosporin	Suprax	cefixime
Antibiotic/penicillin	Bicillin L-A	penicillin G
Antibiotic/penicillin	n/a	dicloxacillin
Antibiotic/penicillin	Timentin	ticarcillin, clavulanate
Antibiotic/penicillin	Unasyn	ampicillin, sulbactam
Antibiotic/penicillin	n/a	penicillin V potassium
Antibiotic/penicillin	Zosyn	piperacillin, tazobactam
Antibiotic/sulfonamide	Bactrim, Septra	trimethoprim/sulfamethoxazole
Antibiotic/synthetic penicillin	Moxatag	amoxicillin
Antibiotic/synthetic penicillin	Augmentin	amoxicillin, clavulanate
Antibiotic/synthetic penicillin	n/a	ampicillin
Antibiotic/tetracycline	Minocin	minocycline
Antibiotic/tetracycline	n/a	tetracycline
Antibiotic/tetracycline	Vibramycin	doxycycline
Antibiotic/other	n/a	amikacin
Antibiotic/other	Avelox	moxifloxacin
Antibiotic/other	Azactam	aztreonam
Antibiotic/other	Bactroban	mupirocin
Antibiotic/other	Biaxin	clarithromycin
Antibiotic/other	Cipro	ciprofloxacin
Antibiotic/other	Cleocin	clindamycin
Antibiotic/other	Cubicin	daptomycin
Antibiotic/other	Erythrocin	erythromycin
Antibiotic/other	n/a	gentamicin
Antibiotic/other	Invanz	ertapenem

Some Common Anti-infectives (cont'd)		
Type	**Brand Name**	**Generic Name**
Antibiotic/other	Levaquin	levofloxacin
Antibiotic/other	Macrodantin, Macrobid	nitrofurantoin
Antibiotic/other	Merrem	meropenem
Antibiotic/other	Primaxin	imipenem, cilastatin
Antibiotic/other	n/a	streptomycin
Antibiotic/other	Tobrex	tobramycin
Antibiotic/other	Vancocin	vancomycin
Antibiotic/other	Zithromax	azithromycin
Antibiotic/other	Zyvox	linezolid
Antifungal	n/a	amphotericin B
Antifungal	Cancidas	caspofungin
Antifungal	Diflucan	fluconazole
Antifungal	Lamisil	terbinafine
Antifungal	Loprox, Penlac	ciclopirox
Antifungal	Mentax	butenafine
Antifungal	Monistat 1, Monistat 3, Monistat 7	miconazole
Antifungal	n/a	nystatin
Antifungal	Nizoral	ketoconazole
Antifungal	Sporanox	itraconazole
Antifungal	Terazol	terconazole
Antimycobacterial	n/a	isoniazid
Antiprotozoal	Flagyl	metronidazole
Antiviral	Atripla	efavirenz, emtricitabine, tenofovir
Antiviral	Isentress	raltegravir
Antiviral	Norvir	ritonavir
Antiviral	Prezista	darunavir
Antiviral	Relenza	zanamivir
Antiviral	Reyataz	atazanavir
Antiviral	n/a	amantadine
Antiviral	Synagis	palivizumab
Antiviral	Tamiflu	oseltamivir
Antiviral	Truvada	emtricitabine, tenofovir
Antiviral	Valtrex	valacyclovir
Antiviral	Zovirax	acyclovir
Antiviral/protease inhibitor	Viracept	nelfinavir

See Additional Common Drugs by Classification on pp 533-537 for more drugs in this class.

ANTINEOPLASTICS

Oncology is the branch of medicine that deals with the study and treatment of cancer.

Antineoplastics inhibit the new growth of cancer cells or ***neoplasms***. Typically, cancer cells are abnormal in structure and growth rate. They offer no useful function, have unusual genetic content, and often reproduce quickly and uncontrollably. Antineoplastics present a chemotherapeutic approach to the treatment of cancer and together with surgery, radiation, and perhaps alternative medicine, comprise an often hopeful and successful treatment protocol.

Malignancy means a life-threatening, cancerous group of cells or tumor is present.

If this original (primary) cell group spreads to other areas, often via the lymphatic or circulatory systems, it is said to have ***metastasized***. Treatment to ***remission*** (state of cancer inactivity) or cure is more successful if little or no metastasis has occurred. However, current chemotherapeutic research and development is offering encouragement for cancers in later stages of growth.

The side effects caused by many of these drugs are often uncomfortable and serious.

They include immunosuppression, anemia (decreased count of red blood cells), alopecia (hair loss), GI ulceration, and dehydration/weight loss from nausea and vomiting.

The Lymphatic System

The lymphatic system is the center of the body's immune system. It collects plasma water from the blood vessels, filters it for impurities through the lymph nodes, and returns the lymph fluid back to the general circulation. Carried in the lymph are ***lymphocytes***, a type of white blood cell that releases antibodies that attack and destroy antigens like bacteria and disease cells (including cancer). This is the body's immune response to antigens. T cells and B cells are the primary lymphocytes. Maintenance of the body's lymphocyte supply is largely performed by the bone marrow.

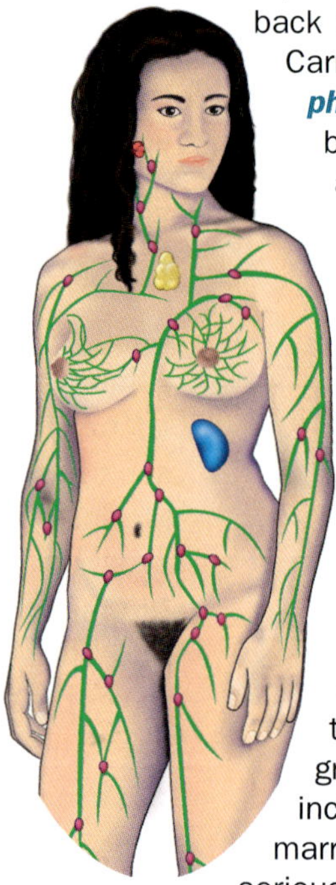

Antineoplastic drugs are targeted at cells with fast growth rates, which not only includes cancer cells but bone marrow as well. As a result, a serious side effect of antineoplastics is that they depress the immune system (immunosuppression), leaving chemotherapy patients prone to infections.

lymphocyte a type of white blood cells that helps the body defend against bacteria and diseased cells.

metastasis when cancer cells spread beyond their original site.

neoplasm a new and abnormal tissue growth, often referring to cancer cells.

remission a state in which cancer cells are inactive.

Controlling Cell Growth

Normal cell growth is highly structured and steady, but cancer cells often reproduce quickly and uncontrollably. Antineoplastic drugs act on various stages of the cell replication process to stop the growth of cancerous cells.

Since cancer cells can mutate in many ways, different chemicals are used to stop their growth. This results in the cocktail approach to chemotherapy, in which a number of drugs are administered to a patient. Because these cocktails also affect normal cells, they are administered in cycles to allow patients to recover from adverse effects before the next round of administration.

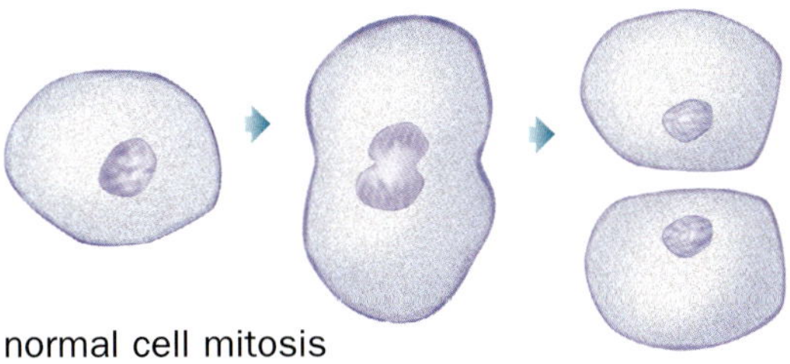

normal cell mitosis

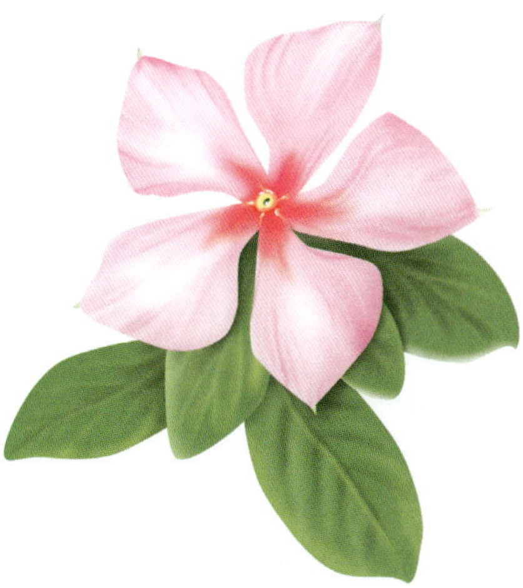

The rosy periwinkle of Madagascar is the source of the antineoplastic vincristine.

Due to the toxicity of many antineoplastics, normal healthy cells are destroyed along with the cancerous cells.

Rapidly replicating cells such as those of the GI tract, bone marrow, and hair follicles are most often affected by selected antineoplastics, causing nausea/vomiting, bone marrow suppression, and hair loss.

Current widely used antineoplastic drugs include alkylating agents (nitrogen mustards), antimetabolites, and plant alkaloids.

They are usually given in cycles (e.g., 3–4 weeks between treatments), allowing rest and recovery periods for the patient. Drug resistance to a particular antineoplastic agent may occur, however, so a combination of these drugs may be given at one time to assure effectiveness. This cocktail, as it is sometimes called, offers drugs of different actions and structure to address whatever type of cancerous cell group is suspected to be present.

Hormones, antitumor antibiotics, and radioactive isotopes are also classified as antineoplastic agents, generally for specific site treatment.

For example, if a tumor is found to be hormone dependent, surgical removal of the affected organ is often indicated (e.g., prostate, breast, or uterus), thus eliminating the chance for hormonal support. In addition, the synthetic antiestrogen agent, tamoxifen, is often used for the treatment of breast cancer in post-menopausal women. Certain antibiotics such as bleomycin and doxorubicin will be ordered to treat skin cancers, lymphomas, and leukemias. The radioactive isotopes, such as gold (AU-198) and iodine (I-131), are also generally organ specific, but are radioactive and special caution is needed during their use.

ANTINEOPLASTICS (cont'd)

CLASSES

Antimetabolites

Classified in accordance with the substances with which they interfere, these antineoplastic drugs inhibit cell growth and replication by mimicking natural metabolites and taking their place within the cells. These fake metabolites inhibit the synthesis of important cellular enzymes, including DNA.

Alkylating Agents

These drugs interfere with mitosis or cell division by binding with DNA and preventing cellular replication. The early alkylating drugs were developed during World War I to introduce chemical warfare. Known as nitrogen mustard gases, these chemicals possessed properties that inhibited cellular growth and sperm counts while depressing bone marrow and damaging intestinal mucosa. Although these agents will adversely affect all cells, those that are growing at a more rapid rate (presumably cancerous) will be more affected. Nitrosureas, a more recent type of alkylating agent, are lipid soluble and pass easily into the brain, where they are effective in treating brain cancers.

Plant Alkaloids

Derived from natural products or semisynthetically produced using natural products, some of these drugs inhibit the enzyme topoisomerase.

Topoisomerase is required for molecular cell growth or mitosis and therefore certain plant alkaloids interfere with cellular DNA replication. Other mechanisms of growth inhibition are not clearly understood.

Some Common Antineoplastics

Type	Brand Name	Generic Name
Antimetabolite	n/a	fluorouracil
Antimetabolite	Rheumatrex	methotrexate
Alkylating agent/nitrogen mustard	Mustargen	mechlorethamine
Alkylating agent/nitrosurea	BiCNU	carmustine
Plant alkaloid	n/a	vincristine
Plant alkaloid	n/a	vinblastine
Hormone agonist	n/a	leuprolide
Hormone/antiestrogen	Soltamox	tamoxifen
Antitumor antibiotic	Blenoxane	bleomycin
Antitumor antibiotic	Adriamycin	doxorubicin
Antitumor antibiotic	Cerubidine	daunorubicin
Radioactive isotope	Bexxar	tositumomab and iodine I-131

See Additional Common Drugs by Classification on pp 533-537 for more drugs in this class.

Note: Drugs highlighted in green in the text and tables are parenteral drugs commonly found in hospitals and other institutional settings.

Hormones

Hormone therapy can be used to treat certain cancers that require hormones to grow. Hormone therapy works by preventing cancer cells from using the hormones they need to grow. Examples include tamoxifen (Soltamox®) and leuprolide.

Antitumor Antibiotics

Antitumor antibiotics are drugs that interact directly with cancer cells to prevent the DNA from functioning normally. This can sometimes result in killing the cancer cells. Examples include bleomycin (Blenoxane®), daunorubicin (Cerubidine®), and doxorubicin (Adriamycin®).

Radioactive Isotopes

Radioactive substances can be used to kill cancer cells in a targeted area. Radiation treatments can be given by a machine that directs radiation at the tumor area. Treatments can otherwise be given internally using needles, seeds, wires, or catheters that contain a radioactive substance and are placed directly in or near the tumor. Radioactive isotopes are sometimes given in combination with other therapeutic approaches. For example, Bexxar® contains tositumomab and iodine I-131 and is used to treat some types of non-Hodgkins lymphoma. It attaches to cancer cells and releases radiation that damages the cancer cells.

Rx safety you should know

- Drugs that are used to treat cancer may cause very serious side effects.
- Pharmacists and pharmacy technicians must be very careful with all calculations associated with drugs that are used to treat cancer.
- Some of the drugs that are used to treat cancer are also used to treat other conditions besides cancer.

CARDIOVASCULAR AGENTS

Some of the most widely used medications available are used to treat diseases and conditions of the cardiovascular system.

Cardiovascular agents include antianginals, antiarrhythmics, antihypertensives, vasopressors, antihyperlipidemics, thrombolytics, and anticoagulants. They are used to treat myocardial infarction (heart attack), angina, cerebral vascular accident (CVA) or stroke, hyper/hypotension (high/low blood pressure), congestive heart failure (CHF), coronary artery disease (CAD), arrhythmias, high cholesterol, unwanted blood clots, and arteriosclerosis.

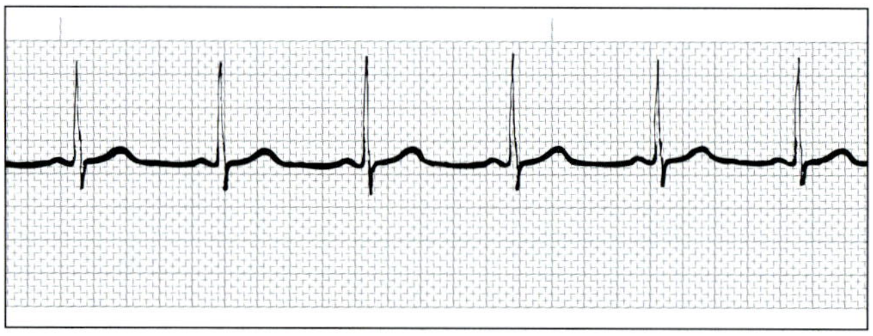

An EKG strip for a normal heart rhythm—variations from this pattern indicate an arrhythmia. The type of arrhythmia can be determined by the nature of the variation.

Arrhythmias

Normally, the electrical system of the heart causes it to contract (or beat) in a regular and organized rhythm that can be graphed by an ***electrocardiogram (EKG or ECG)***. An ***arrhythmia*** is an abnormal heart rhythm that can interfere with the heart's ability to pump in an effective, organized manner. Arrhythmias range from minor to life-threatening. They are classified by degree of seriousness, site of origin (where the electrical impulse causing the rhythm came from), and rate or speed. Familiar arrhythmias include:

- tachycardia;
- bradycardia;
- premature or ectopic beats;
- flutter and fibrillation.

THE HEART

Conduction

The heart is a pump that uses complex chemical and electrical processes to function. Chemically charged particles (ions) stimulate heart muscle to contract and relax systematically, pumping blood through the cardiovascular system. This contraction and relaxation is referred to as the ***cardiac cycle***.

The SA node is the fastest generating electrical impulse area of the heart and it sets the pace. The atria and ventricles follow the conduction signal while the AV node together with the fine fibers (Purkinje fibers) at the base of the heart transmit the impulse.

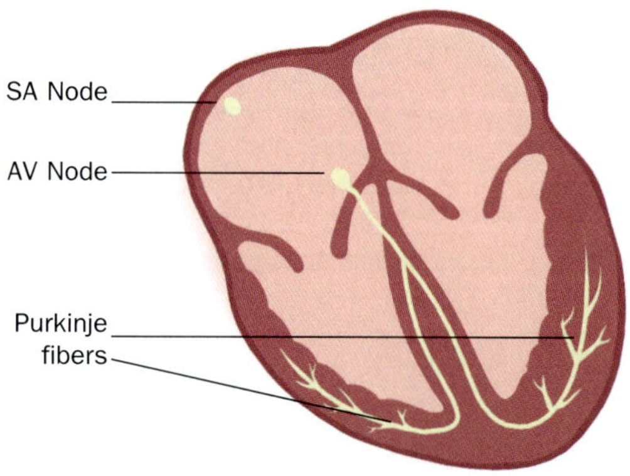

arrhythmia an abnormal heart rhythm.

cardiac cycle the contraction and relaxation of the heart that pumps blood through the cardiovascular system.

diastolic pressure the minimum blood pressure when the heart relaxes; the second number in a blood pressure reading.

The Heart and Circulation

The heart is a muscular organ that powers blood circulation for the entire body. Divided into four chambers, the right and left atria (top chambers) and the right and left ventricles (bottom chambers), the heart receives de-oxygenated blood into the right side (referred to as pulmonary circulation) and oxygenated blood into the left side (referred to as systemic circulation).

The right ventricle pumps blood to the lungs where it mixes with oxygen. The left ventricle pumps oxygenated blood to the body. The ***myocardium*** (heart muscle) is supplied fresh, oxygen-rich blood by the coronary arteries, which branch from the aorta and circle back to the heart.

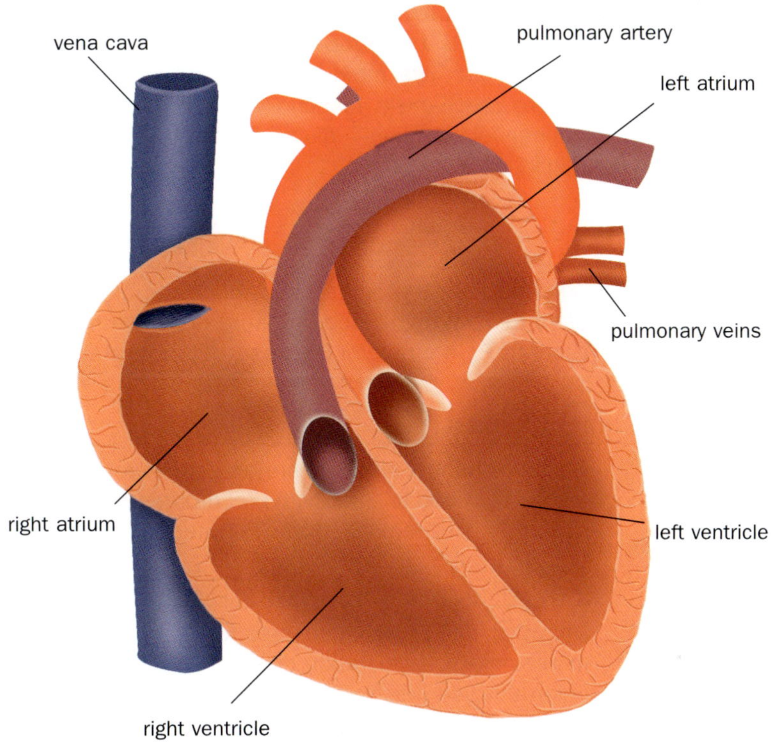

Blood Clotting

Clotting is an essential function of blood that prevents excessive blood loss from injuries. Though clotting factors are the primary influence on clotting, adequate platelets and healthy blood vessel walls are also important. Too much clotting can be dangerous, however. If a clot (***thrombus***) is formed in the bloodstream, it can be carried to a location where it blocks a blood vessel and blood flow. Such blockages are called ***embolisms*** and can cause strokes and death.

Blood Pressure

Blood pressure is the outward pressure of the blood against the arteries as it is pumped through the body by the heart. Current literature recommends a blood pressure no higher than 126/76 for 40% of a normal healthy adult's day. The first number is the ***systolic*** value that represents the maximum pressure as the heart contracts to pump blood out. The second number is the ***diastolic*** value that represents the minimum pressure in the artery as the heart relaxes.

electrocardiogram (EKG or ECG) a graph of the heart's rhythms.

embolism, embolus a clot that has traveled in the bloodstream to a point where it obstructs flow.

myocardium heart muscle.

systolic pressure the maximum blood pressure when the heart contracts; the first number in a blood pressure reading.

thrombus a blood clot.

CARDIOVASCULAR AGENTS (cont'd)

CLASSES BY MECHANISM OF ACTION

In addition to classifying cardiovascular drugs by the conditions they treat, some of these drugs are also grouped by their mechanisms of action or how they work in the body. There are five main groupings of cardiovascular drugs by mechanism of action: beta-blockers, calcium channel blockers, diuretics, ace inhibitors, and vasodilators.

Some beta blockers or calcium channel blockers can be used to treat a variety of conditions including hypertension, arrhythmias, and angina. You will also find different ACE inhibitors have indications for different conditions.

Beta-blockers

Beta-blockers are drugs that reduce the oxygen demands of the heart muscle. They are often used to treat high blood pressure or arrhythmias. Some examples include propranolol, nadolol (Corgard®), metoprolol (Lopressor®), and atenolol (Tenormin®).

Calcium Channel Blockers

Calcium channel blockers are drugs that relax the heart by reducing heart conduction. They are also often used to treat high blood pressure or arrhythmias. Some examples include verapamil (Calan®), diltiazem (Cardizem®), nifedipine (Procardia®), and amlodipine (Norvasc®).

Diuretics

Diuretics decrease blood pressure by decreasing blood volume. They decrease volume by increasing the elimination of salts and water through urination. Some examples include hydrochlorothiazide (Microzide®), furosemide (Lasix®), and bumetanide.

ACE Inhibitors

The "-pril" drugs, ace inhibitors relax the blood vessels. They are often used to treat high blood pressure. Note: the "-sartan" drugs are considered a subgroup of ACE inhibitors. Some examples include captopril (Capoten®), enalapril (Vasotec®), and lisinopril (Zestril®).

Vasodilators

Vasodilators relax and expand the blood vessels. Some examples include hydralazine, and minoxidil.

Rx safety you should know

- Beta-blockers and calcium channel blockers should not be discontinued abruptly without medical supervision.
- Some calcium channel blockers have important drug interactions. Check with your pharmacist when drug interactions are detected by the computer.
- Some diuretics cause sun sensitivity.
- Some cardiovascular drugs have significant interactions with grapefruit juice.
- Most diuretics can cause hypokalemia (low levels of potassium). Exceptions are triamterene and spironolactone, which can cause hyperkalemia (high potassium levels).
- ACE inhibitors have special warnings in pregnancy.
- Some ACE inhibitors may cause hyperkalemia (high levels of potassium).
- Some ACE inhibitors may cause coughing.

Some Common Cardiovascular Drugs by Mechanism of Action		
Type	**Brand Name**	**Generic Name**
Beta-blocker	n/a	propranolol
Beta-blocker	Tenormin	atenolol
Beta-blocker	Corgard	nadolol
Beta-blocker	Lopressor	metoprolol
Calcium channel blocker	Calan	verapamil
Calcium channel blocker	Norvasc	amlodipine
Calcium channel blocker	Procardia	nifedipine
Calcium channel blocker	Cardizem	diltiazem
Diuretics	Lasix	furosemide
Diuretics	Microzide	hydrochlorothiazide
Diuretics	Aldactone	spironolactone
ACE inhibitor	Capoten	captopril
ACE inhibitor	Vasotec	enalapril
ACE inhibitor	Zestril	lisinopril
Vasodilator	n/a	hydralazine

CLASSES BY CONDITION

Antianginals

Antianginals are used to treat cardiac related chest pain (angina) resulting from ischemic heart disease. Patients with this condition suffer a lack of oxygen and blood flow to the myocardium. Nitrates, beta-blockers, and calcium channel blockers such as nitroglycerin (Nitrostat®) and nifedipine (Procardia®), are examples of antianginals.

Antiarrhythmics

Antiarrhythmics are used to treat irregular heart rhythms. They regulate the conduction activity of the heart by inhibiting abnormal pacemaker cells or recurring abnormal impulses and restoring a normal rhythm. Antiarrhythmics such as digoxin (Lanoxin®) and sotalol (Betapace®) include beta-blockers and drugs that block sodium, potassium ion, and calcium channels.

Antihyperlipidemics

Antihyperlipidemics are used to lower high levels of cholesterol that can lead to blocked blood vessels. Cholesterol is a lipid normally present in the body and is essential for healthy cell function. Proteins and carbohydrates, as well as fat, are responsible for natural cholesterol production. Cholesterol levels are measured as total cholesterol, LDL (low-density lipoprotein), and HDL (high-density lipoprotein). Excess amounts of LDL can lead to blocked blood vessels and other cardiovascular problems. HMG-CoA Reductase inhibitors are used to treat high LDL levels. Examples are simvastatin (Zocor®), ezetimibe with simvastatin (Vytorin®), and pravastatin (Pravachol®).

CARDIOVASCULAR AGENTS (cont'd)

CLASSES BY CONDITION (cont'd)

Antihypertensives

Antihypertensives are used to reduce a sustained elevation in blood pressure. Factors affecting blood pressure include stress, blood volume, arterial narrowing, age, gender, and general condition of health. Common antihypertensives include beta-blockers to reduce cardiac output, diuretics to decrease fluid volume, ACE inhibitors to reduce salt and water retention and inhibit vascular constriction, and calcium channel blockers to relax blood vessels. Examples of diuretics are furosemide (Lasix®) and ramipril (Altace®). An example of a potassium sparing diuretic is spironolactone (Aldactone®). (Note that some antihypertensive agents also have other uses such as treating heart conditions and preventing migraine headaches.)

Thrombolytics/Anticoagulants

Thrombolytics dissolve blood clots and anticoagulants prevent their formation. Thrombolytics can be dangerous since blood clotting can be disturbed, resulting in profuse bleeding and even bleeding to death. However, in cases of impending myocardial infarction or stroke, a travelling blood clot (embolus) can be dissolved and the stroke prevented. There has been much success with this group of drugs in recent years. A common thrombolytic agent is alteplase. Common anticoagulants include warfarin (Coumadin®) and heparin.

Vasopressors

Vasopressors act to increase blood pressure. If a patient is in a state of shock due to decreased blood volume, inadequate cardiac output, or severe infection, fluids may be introduced to provide adequate blood volume. In addition to fluid replacement, vasopressors may be used to help supply blood to the brain and kidney. The patient may for example be given an intravenous solution containing dobutamine.

℞ safety you should know

- Many antianginal drugs cause headaches, dizziness, and/or flushing.
- Nitroglycerin products should be kept in the container they came in, tightly closed, and out of reach of children.
- Nitroglycerin tablets that are more than 12 months old should not be used.
- Digoxin (Lanoxin®) is associated with several serious drug interactions.
- Many antihypertensive drugs can cause dizziness and can cause orthostatic hypotension (dizziness associated with standing up quickly).

Note: Drugs highlighted in green in the text and tables are parenteral drugs commonly found in hospitals and other institutional settings.

Some Common Cardiovascular Drugs by Condition

Type	Brand Name	Generic Name
Antianginal	Nitrostat	nitroglycerin
Antianginal	Procardia	nifedipine
Antiarryhthmic	Lanoxin	digoxin
Antiarryhthmic	Betapace	sotalol
Antihyperlipidemic	Vytorin	ezetimibe w/simvastatin
Antihyperlipidemic	Zocor	simvastatin
Antihyperlipidemic	Pravachol	pravastatin
Antihypertensive/diuretic	Lasix	furosemide
Antihypertensive/ACE inhibitor	Altace	ramipril
Antihypertensive/diuretic	Aldactone	spironolactone
Thrombolytic	Cathflo Activase	alteplase
Anticoagulant	Coumadin	warfarin
Anticoagulant	n/a	heparin
Anticoagulant	Pradaxa	dabigatran
Anticoagulant	Xarelto	rivaroxaban
Vasopressor	n/a	dobutamine

See Additional Common Drugs by Classification on pp 533-537 for more drugs in this class.

safety you should know: warfarin (Coumadin®)

- Warfarin (Coumadin®) has many significant drug interactions.
- There is a serious drug interaction with aspirin and warfarin. Patients taking warfarin should carefully check all OTC products to be sure they are not inadvertently taking aspirin.
- Dosing for warfarin is individualized and is carefully adjusted according to blood tests.
- Overdosing with warfarin can cause life-threatening conditions. Special care is needed with the many different strengths that are available.

DERMATOLOGICALS

The skin is the body's protective barrier.

It is the largest of the body's organs and protects the other organs against microorganisms, trauma, extreme temperature, and other harmful elements. It is comprised of several layers: the epidermis (top layer), dermis (middle layer), and subcutaneous tissue (bottom layer). Within these layers, structures such as hair follicles and shafts, sebaceous and sweat glands, veins, arteries, and sensory nerves are found.

Dermatological **refers to a drug used to treat a condition or disease related to the skin.**

Medical conditions and diseases that occur on or in the skin can be caused by inflammation, infection, growth rate changes, trauma, or structural dysfunction. Examples of skin conditions are burns, cuts, rashes, dandruff, eczema, and skin cancer.

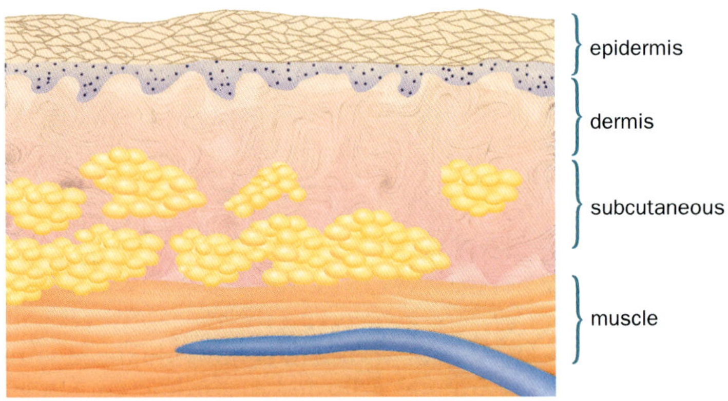

THE SKIN

The skin, also called the ***integumentary system***, is generally 3–5 millimeters thick, though it is thicker in the palms of the hands and soles of the feet and thinner in the eyelids and genitals.

The outer layer of the epidermis (called the stratum corneum) is constantly replenished with new cells from underneath. The turnover time from cell development to shedding (sloughing) is about 21 days.

Contained within the skin are accessory structures: hair follicles, sweat glands, sebaceous glands, and nails.

The subcutaneous layer is not always considered a part of the skin but simply a loose connective tissue separating the skin from the underlying organs. It is, however, so closely interconnected that it is generally described with the integumentary system.

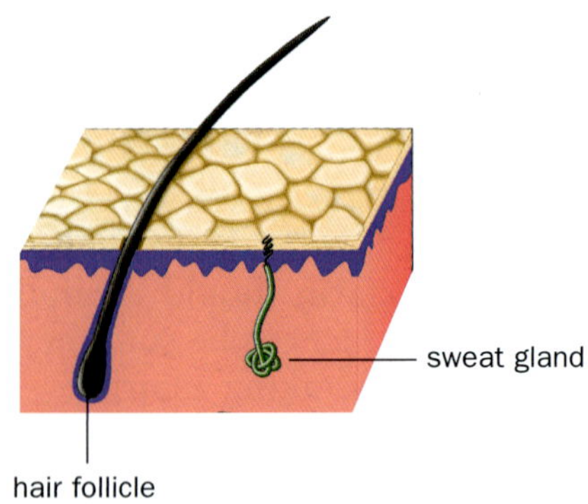

dermatological a product used to treat a skin condition.
integumentary system the body covering, i.e., skin, hair, and nails.

Skin Conditions

The following are examples of skin reactions that selected dermatologicals address:

- trauma (burns, cuts, abrasions, bruises)
- fluid accumulation (edema, cellulitis, blisters)
- discoloration and pigmentation, rashes, freckles, drug or allergy related photosensitivity
- hyper- or hypo-melanin (skin pigment)
- dry skin or scaling (dandruff)
- cancers (basal cell, squamous cell, or melanoma)
- nonmalignant growths (keratoses)

In addition, the following common skin diseases are often treated with both prescription and non-prescription medications:

- eczema
- psoriasis
- acne
- fungal infections (athlete's foot, ringworm)
- viral infections (herpes simplex)
- general dermatitis, hives, or other allergic reactions caused by food, plants, insects, or sunburn

Some Common Dermatologicals

Type	Brand Name	Generic Name
Steroid	Westcort	hydrocortisone cream
Antihistamine	Benadryl	diphenhydramine
Anti-infective	Silvadene	silver sulfadiazine cream
Anti-infective	Vibramycin	doxycycline hyclate
Anti-infective	n/a	ofloxacin
Antimetabolite	Efudex	fluorouracil cream

See Additional Common Drugs by Classification on pp 533-537 for more drugs in this class.

safety you should know

- Do not apply fluorouracil to tender skin areas such as the eyelids or the eyes, nose, or mouth.
- Topical products are for external use.
- Wash hands before and after use of topical products.

tip

The drying agent zinc oxide is often seen in a combination product with the local anesthetic camphor, moisture absorbing agent kaolin, and an anti-infective such as triclosan when treating diaper rash.

ELECTROLYTIC AGENTS

Maintaining the proper balance of body fluids is essential for good health and body function.

Water is the primary element in the body, accounting for more than half of body weight. It is found inside cells (*intracellular fluid*) and outside them (*extracellular fluid*) in plasma and tissue (*interstitial fluid*).

Electrolytes **are water soluble substances that are contained in our body fluids as salts.**

They form electrically charged particles called *ions*, which attract water. They have both positive (*cations*) and negative (*anions*) charges and are responsible for fluid movement into and out of cells. Changes in the body's normal electrolyte count affect fluid movement and balance and consequently various body functions.

Examples of common electrolytes include sodium (Na^+), potassium (K^+), calcium (Ca^{++}), chloride (Cl^-) and bicarbonate (HCO_3^-).

The plus and minus signs indicate their electrical charges. Functions these electrolytes affect include blood pressure, blood coagulation, muscle contractions, myocardial conduction, energy levels, and enzyme production. Electrolytic therapy is aimed at restoring normal sodium, potassium, calcium, and magnesium balances.

COMMON ELECTROLYTES

Sodium

Sodium is the major cation in fluid outside of cells and it regulates the amount of water in the body. Excess sodium is normally excreted in urine.

Potassium

Potassium is the major cation found inside cells. Proper potassium balance is important for normal cell function and is especially important for heart and muscle functions. Hypokalemia is the term for low potassium; hyperkalemia is the term for abnormally high potassium. Extreme hypokalemia can be fatal.

Chloride

Chloride is the major anion in the fluid outside of cells.

Bicarbonate

Bicarbonate is an ion that works as a buffer to maintain a proper acid–base balance.

Opposites Attract

Water molecules (H_2O) are polarized. That is, they have positively and negatively charged sides. For this reason, many compounds ***dissociate*** (come apart) in water to form ions and the ions in turn associate with the water molecules.

The dissociation of sodium chloride (NaCl) into Na+ and Cl^- ions followed by their association with water molecules is depicted at right. H_2O is attracted at its negative pole to the positive sodium ion and at its positive pole to the negative chloride ion.

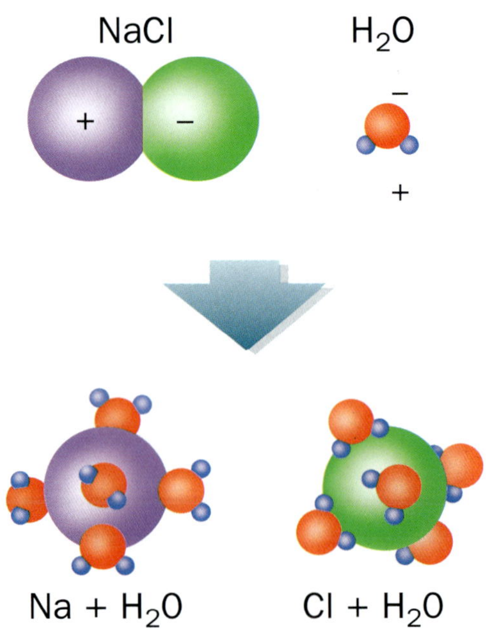

Note: Drugs highlighted in green in the text and tables are parenteral drugs commonly found in hospitals and other institutional settings.

SOME ELECTROLYTE SOLUTIONS

Lactated Ringer's™ Solution is a balanced and isotonic solution. Balanced means the electrolyte concentration is similar to serum and isotonic means the osmolarity is similar to serum. Lactated Ringer's™ Solution contains sodium, potassium calcium, and lactate.

Polyionic R-148 is a balanced and isotonic solution and contains sodium, potassium, magnesium, chloride, acetate, and gluconate.

Polyionic R-148D5 is a balanced and hypertonic solution and contains sodium, potassium, magnesium, chloride, acetate, gluconate, and dextrose.

D5LR is a balanced and hypertonic solution and contains sodium, potassium calcium, lactate, and dextrose.

Normal saline is an isotonic solution of sodium chloride.

Electrolyte balance is important for healthy body function.

Electrolytes are especially important in the regulation of heart function, as well as fluid balance, acid–base balance, and neurological function. The most common cause of electrolyte disturbances is kidney failure. Additionally, dehydration can lead to electrolyte imbalance. Severe diarrhea or vomiting, along with other causes, can also lead to electrolyte disturbances. Serious problems can arise when electrolyte imbalances involve potassium, sodium, and/or calcium.

℞ safety you should know

- Oral potassium supplements may cause gastrointestinal upset.
- Appropriate potassium balance is important for cardiac function.

Some Common Electrolytic Agents

Type	Brand Name	Generic Name
Potassium supplement	Micro-K, Klor-Con	potassium chloride
Electrolyte replacement	Rehydralyte Solution	sodium, potassium, chloride, citrate
Electrolyte replacement	Infalyte Oral Solution	sodium, potassium, chloride, citrate
Electrolyte replacement	Resol Solution	sodium, potassium, chloride, citrate, calcium, magnesium, phosphate
Electrolyte replacement	Naturalyte Solution	sodium, potassium, chloride, citrate
Electrolyte replacement	Pedialyte Solution	sodium, potassium, chloride, citrate

anions negatively charged particles.

cations positively charged particles.

dissociation when a compound breaks down and separates into smaller components.

electrolytes substances that in solution form ions that conduct an electrical current.

extracellular fluid the fluid outside the body's individual cells found in plasma and tissue fluid.

interstitial fluid tissue fluid.

intracellular fluid cell fluid.

ions electrically charged particles.

GASTROINTESTINAL & URINARY TRACT AGENTS

Gastrointestinal agents are used to treat disorders of the stomach and/or the intestines.

The drugs that address and treat various stomach and intestinal disorders include enzymes, antidiarrheals, antiemetics (anti-vomiting), antiulcer agents, laxatives, and stool softeners.

The GI organs are intimately related to the digestive system as a whole.

The other alimentary tract organs (mouth and esophagus), the accessory organs of digestion (salivary, gastric, and intestinal glands, liver, gall bladder, and pancreas), and the organs of elimination (rectum and anus) are often affected by direct GI disorders. For example, it is not uncommon for a colon cancer to metastasize not only to the stomach, but to the pancreas, liver, and rectum as well. As a result, although specific site antineoplastic drugs and treatments are available, agents may be used that treat more than one site and cell type at a time. Gastric reflux is another example. Gastric hyperacidity will often travel toward the chest and throat area via the esophagus. Antacid drugs that inhibit acidity of the stomach will provide for rest and healing of the esophagus when this happens.

THE DIGESTIVE SYSTEM

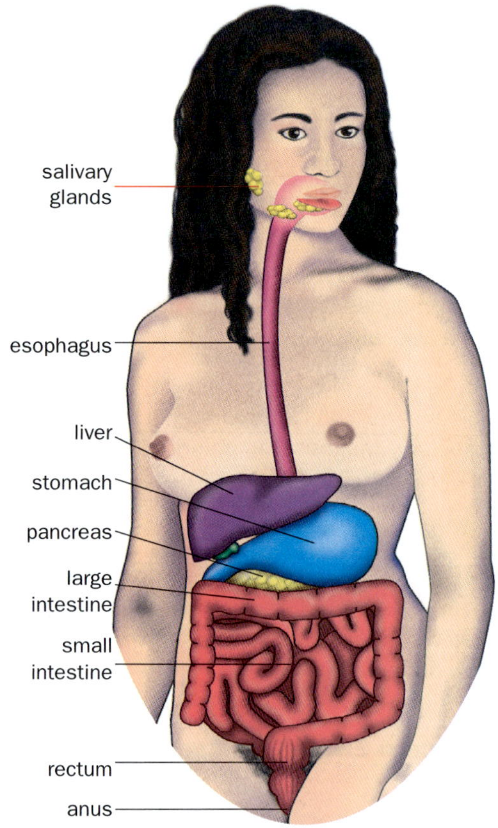

The stomach lies in the upper left quadrant of the abdomen between the lower end of the esophagus and the beginning of the small intestine (duodenum). This organ serves to store and chemically break down food using hydrochloric acid and pepsinogen. ***Chyme*** is the semiliquid form of food as it enters the duodenum. ***Peristalsis*** is the wave-like motion that moves the food products along the intestinal tract.

Together, the small intestine and the large intestine make up about 28 feet of bowel (intestine). Most food absorption takes place in the small intestine. The large intestine absorbs water and connects to the rectum and anus for stool evacuation.

The GI organs are large in mass compared to other systems' organs and play a major role in normal body function. As a result, dysfunction, abnormality, or other pathologic medical conditions of the GI tract may require serious and immediate drug therapy as well as other forms of medical or surgical intervention. Similar to other organ systems, preventive care and early detection of pathology is suggested and encouraged.

The urinary system produces, stores, and eliminates urine and consists of the kidneys, ureters, bladder, urethra, and the penis in males. It is sometimes called the genitourinary system.

chyme the semiliquid form of food as it enters the intestinal tract.

peristalsis the wave-like motion of the intestines that moves food through them.

CLASSES

Enzymes

Pepsin is a normally present gastric enzyme that breaks down proteins. However, in the absence of pepsin, it is still possible for the digestive system to break down protein molecules into amino acids using proteolytic enzymes from the pancreas that are found in the small intestine. These enzymes are capable of attacking starches and fats. If a patient's condition warrants treatment using enzyme therapy (as with cystic fibrosis and chronic pancreatitis), products that contain pancreatin, an agent prepared from hog pancreas, or pancrelipase may be indicated. Malabsorption conditions such as steatorrhea, where fat is inadequately digested and is excreted in large amounts in feces, may be treated with pancrelipase.

Antidiarrheals

Diarrhea is a condition of frequent watery stools that results from microorganism invasion, drug or stress reaction, and/or other circumstances causing a decrease in intestinal absorption of water, an increased secretion of electrolytes into the intestines or an excessive amount of mucus production. Antiperistalsis drugs slow the movement of the intestinal contents to allow for greater water and electrolyte absorption. Loperamide (Imodium®) is a common antiperistalsis agent and diphenoxylate plus atropine (Lomotil®) is another popular antidiarrheal agent. Bismuth subsalicylate (Pepto-Bismol®) is a secretion inhibitor that acts to prevent organisms from attaching to the intestinal mucosa and may deactivate certain toxins as well. In cases of infectious diarrhea, antibiotics such as metronidazole and vancomycin may also be indicated and ordered in conjunction with other therapies. Note: Some antibiotics can kill normal bacterial flora or facilitate regrowth of resistant microorganisms, and so lead to diarrhea.

Antiemetics

This class of drugs treats the condition of nausea and vomiting. There are many causes for this condition, which is usually a symptom or side effect as opposed to being the actual condition itself: food or drug reaction or allergy, pregnancy, anxiety, exhaustion, dehydration, and a large number of diseases or illnesses such as cancer, or a microorganism related infectious process such as a middle ear infection. Often, antiemetics are ordered concurrently with other drug therapies used to treat the underlying condition. Examples are trimethobenzamide (Tigan®) and prochlorperazine. Vomiting is a reflex that occurs from a variety of stimuli. The treatment is to reduce the hyperactivity of stimuli receptors and lower the impulse rate. Also, decreasing the sensitivity to emetic chemicals found in the blood will inhibit the vomiting reflex. Dehydration and electrolyte imbalance are of major concern with prolonged vomiting.

Some Common Gastrointestinal Tract Drugs: Enzymes, Antidiarrheals, and Antiemetics

Type	Brand Name	Generic Name
Enzyme	Creon	pancrelipase
Enzyme	Pancreaze	pancrelipase
Enzyme	Viokace	pancrelipase
Antidiarrheal	Imodium	loperamide
Antidiarrheal	Lomotil	diphenoxylate plus atropine
Antidiarrheal	Pepto-Bismol	bismuth subsalicylate
Antiemetic	Tigan	trimethobenzamide
Antiemetic	n/a	prochlorperazine

See Additional Common Drugs by Classification on pp 533-537 for more drugs in this class.

GASTROINTESTINAL & URINARY TRACT AGENTS

Antacid/Antiulcer Agents

Antacids, generally composed of inorganic salts such as calcium carbonate, aluminum hydroxide, and magnesium hydroxide, are popular antiulcer agents that act to neutralize existing acid, as opposed to inhibiting its production. Antacids are most indicated at the onset of hypergastric activity, are pain relieving yet short acting, and not strong enough for a diagnosed ulcer condition. Caution should be exercised to not rely on antacids alone or for a prolonged time. If ulcer symptoms persist, the physician should be notified. Maalox® Advanced Liquid is an example of a common antacid.

Cimetidine is a histamine receptor antagonist. It inhibits the secretion of gastric acid by blocking the effects of histamine. This type of agent was first approved for use in 1977 and revolutionized standard antacid therapy. Cimetidine has a history of drug interactions, however, and improved histamine antagonists such as ranitidine (Zantac®), famotidine (Pepcid®), and nizatidine (Axid®) have since been developed.

Omeprazole (Prilosec®) is a proton pump inhibitor. It works by decreasing the amount of acid made in the stomach. Omeprazole is available in a delayed-release capsule (Prilosec®), a nonprescription delayed-release tablet (Prilosec OTC®), a powder for suspension (Zegerid®), and a regular capsule (Zegerid®).

Peptic ulcer is caused by hypergastric acidity that erodes tissue in localized areas of the stomach and intestines. While these lesions are normally benign, they may produce symptoms that are mild and of minor discomfort or they may be more serious and extend to underlying layers of connective tissue and smooth muscle. In these cases, blood vessels can be affected and bleeding can occur. A special dietary regime (i.e., frequent, small, bland, nonacid containing meals) together with selected drug therapy is commonly recommended to treat this condition.

Gastric reflux is a more serious gastric acid condition that is often treated with a strong antacid.

Laxatives and Stool Softeners

These agents are commonly prescribed to treat constipation, the condition of dehydrated stool in which bowel movements are infrequent, hard, and often painful and difficult. Aside from changing a patient's diet, fluid intake, and activity level, drug therapy may be suggested. Laxatives promote defecation without stress or pain and are often suggested for use prior to certain medical procedures related to the bowel (e.g., colonoscopy, barium enema), for constipation, and for patients who have hemorrhoids, recent hernia surgery, or a heart attack.

There are several types of laxatives available: bulk forming, that swell as they mix with intestinal contents; stimulant, that irritate the lining and nerves of the intestine; saline, that rapidly promote watery stool by drawing water into the intestine; and osmotic, that increase the stool's water content using osmosis. The osmotic laxative is often used as a retention enema, although it can be powerful and cause cramping. Lactulose (Kristalose®) is an example of a commonly prescribed saline laxative.

Docusate sodium (Colace®) is a commonly ordered stool softener, or emollient laxative. It promotes the mixing of fatty and watery intestinal substances to soften the stool's contents and ease the evacuation of feces.

Enemas may be placed into this category since they are indicated in cases of constipation, premedical treatment, and to ease the stress of bowel movements. Fleets®, sodium biphosphate and sodium phosphate, is a popular saline enema.

℞ **tip**

➥ Phenazopyridine may discolor urine reddish orange and an auxiliary label about urine discoloration may be helpful to the patient.

Urinary Tract Agents

Urinary agents are used to treat conditions affecting the flow of urine. Symptoms can include difficulty urinating, painful urination, urinary frequency, and urgency. One common condition that affects urination in males is benign prostatic hyperplasia (BPH). Examples of drugs that are used include drugs to treat BPH include tamsulosin (Flomax®), alfuzosin (Uroxatral®), finasteride (Proscar®), and dutasteride (Avodart®). Urinary drugs used to treat urinary frequency include tolterodine (Detrol LA®), darifenacin (Enablex®), and solifenacin (Vesicare®).

Some Common Gastrointestinal Tract Drugs: Antacid/Antiulcer and Laxatives & Stool Softeners

Type	Brand Name	Generic Name
Antacid/antiulcer	Maalox Advanced Liquid	magnesium hydroxide, aluminum hydroxide, simethicone
Antacid/antiulcer	Tagamet	cimetidine
Antacid/antiulcer	Zantac	ranitidine
Antacid/antiulcer	Pepcid	famotidine
Antacid/antiulcer	Axid	nizatidine
Antacid/antiulcer; proton pump inhibitor	Prilosec	omeprazole
Laxative	Kristalose	lactulose
Stool softener	Colace	docusate sodium

See Additional Common Drugs by Classification on pp 533-537 for more drugs in this class.

Some Common Urinary Tract Agents

Type	Brand Name	Generic Name
Urinary tract agent	Flomax	tamsulosin
Urinary tract agent	Uroxatral	alfuzosin
Urinary tract agent	Proscar	finasteride
Urinary tract agent	Avodart	dutasteride
Urinary tract agent	Detrol LA	tolterodine
Urinary tract agent	Enablex	darifenacin
Urinary tract agent	Vesicare	solifenacin
Urinary tract agent	n/a	phenazopyridine

℞ **safety you should know**

➥ Cimetidine has several significant drug interactions. Check with the pharmacist when alerted to drug interactions with cimetidine.

➥ Misoprostol is contra-indicated during pregnancy.

➥ Some antacids have significant drug interactions with tetracyclines.

➥ Most antispasmodics can cause dizziness, drowsiness or blurred vision.

➥ Sulfasalazine is contra-indicated in patients who are hypersensitive to sulfasalazine, its metabolites, sulfonamides, or salicylates.

➥ Women who are, could become, or may be pregnant should not touch broken or crushed finasteride tablets. If taken by pregnant women, finasteride can harm the male fetus.

HEMATOLOGICAL AGENTS

Blood coagulation (clotting) is a complex process.

Each stage of clot development can be affected by *clotting factors* as well as drugs. For example, patients with hemophilia A have a genetic deficiency in factor VIII (most clotting factors are denoted by Roman numerals) and can be successfully treated with concentrates of antihemophilic factor (AHF) that are commercially available. Factor VIII concentrate or cryoprecipitate and desmopressin acetate (DDAVP®) are other agents that will act to shorten bleeding time. Von Willebrand disease, a very common congenital coagulation disorder, is also caused by a deficiency in factor VIII. Factor IX concentrates (Christmas factor) are available for patients with hemophilia B, a condition marked by a deficiency in clotting factor IX.

Phytonadione (Mephyton®), or vitamin K1, is a drug that stimulates the liver to produce several clotting factors and mimics the action of vitamin K (a natural clotting promoter).

Patients who may develop vitamin K deficiency and require coagulation enhancer therapy include at risk infants whose liver and intestines are not fully developed, users of antibiotics that "sterilize" the intestines and prevent vitamin K synthesis, and those with malabsorption disorders such as Whipple's disease and obstructive jaundice. In addition, patients with liver disease may suffer with bleeding disorders since the liver is responsible for the synthesizing of many clotting factors.

Clotting

The main stages of natural clot formation and dissolution are:

Thromboplastin is formed from blood and tissue (platelet aggregation at the injury site).

↓

Thrombin is formed from prothrombin and thromboplastin.

↓

The fiber ***fibrin*** is formed from thrombin acting on ***fibrinogen*** (clot formation).

↓

Fibrinolysin breaks down fibrin (clot breakdown).

Some Common Hematological Drugs

Type	Brand Name	Generic Name
Hematopoietic	Feraheme	ferumoxytol
Hematopoietic	Slow Fe	ferrous sulfate
Hematopoietic	n/a	cyanocobalmin
Hemostatic	Amicar	aminocaproic acid
Hemostatic	Cyklokapron	tranexamic acid
Hemostatic/topical	Surgicel	oxidized cellulose

See Additional Common Drugs by Classification on pp 533-537 for more drugs in this class.

℞ safety you should know

- Accidental overdose of products containing iron is a leading cause of fatal poisoning in children under the age of six.
- Although symptoms of iron deficiency usually improve within a few days, patients may have to take ferrous sulfate for several months.

Drugs highlighted in green in the text and tables are parenteral drugs commonly found in hospitals and other institutional settings.

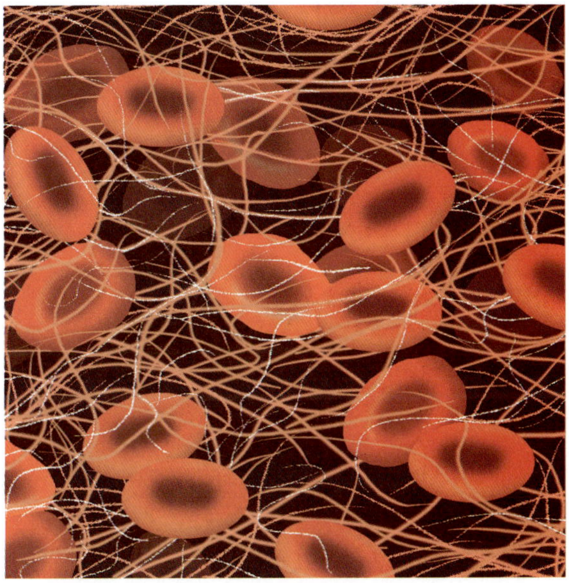

Strands of fibrin interweave and trap red blood cells to form a blood clot.

anemia a decrease in hemoglobin or red blood cells.

clotting factors factors in the blood coagulation process.

fibrin the fiber that serves as the structure for clot formation.

fibrinogen Factor I.

hematopoietics drugs used to treat anemia.

hemostatic drugs drugs that prevent excessive bleeding.

topical hemostatics drugs used for minor bleeding when sutures are not appropriate.

Hematopoietics are drugs that treat various forms of anemias by stimulating or helping to stimulate blood cell growth.

Anemias are generally characterized by a decrease in hemoglobin or red blood cells, which leads to a series of other disorders manifested by oxygen deficiency. The classifications of anemias include cell shape and structure, cause, and the pathophysiology or disease tract the particular anemia will take.

Most commonly, anemias develop in the elderly from iron deficiency, as a result of genetic predisposition (e.g., sickle cell anemia), or due to vitamin B12 deficiency (pernicious anemia).

An additional type of anemia is associated with chronic disease. Correction of the underlying illness will improve this anemia. Anemias may also occur as a result of cancer or other diseases and treatments that cause bone marrow suppression and decrease of erythropoietin (which stimulates red blood cell production). In addition, a decrease in the granulocyte colony stimulating factor (G-CSF) and granulocyte macrophage colony stimulating factor (GM-CSF), excessive blood loss, infections, and inflammatory processes contribute to anemia. Common drug therapies for anemias include ferrous sulfate (Slow Fe®) for iron-deficiency anemia and cyanocobalamin (Crystamine®) for vitamin B12 deficiency anemia.

***Hemostatic drugs* are used to treat or prevent excessive bleeding.**

Patients who have hemophilia or thrombocytic purpura may receive hemostatic medications. They suffer from a lack of platelets and/or blood clotting factors found in the first stage of clotting. Systemic hemostatic agents include aminocaproic acid and tranexamic acid. Their indications range from preventing hemorrhages during dental procedures to prevention of blood loss in cardiopulmonary bypass surgery. Their primary action is to inhibit the activation of plasminogen. *Topical hemostatics* are used for minor bleeding of small blood vessels when sutures are not appropriate. An example of a topical hemostatic is oxidized cellulose.

tip

Aside from drug therapy, patients with excessive bleeding may receive whole blood and blood products such as packed cells, platelets, and plasma to treat this serious situation.

HORMONES & MODIFIERS

H*ormones* are secretions of the *endocrine system's* ductless glands.

These substances control or influence a selected organ or set of organs to produce an effect. If a patient does not naturally produce enough or produces too much of a particular hormone, selected drugs can be prescribed to stimulate or inhibit hormone secretion. These hormones and hormone modifiers can either be extracted from animals or reproduced synthetically.

The pituitary gland is also known as the master gland because it regulates the activities of the entire endocrine system.

This pea-sized organ is located at the base of the skull. In turn, another major system, the nervous system, greatly controls the pituitary gland and together these two systems are responsible for a large number of our body's regulatory processes.

The thyroid gland is located in front of the trachea and secretes hormones that affect metabolism, growth, and central nervous system development.

Thyroxine (T_4) and triiodothyronine (T_3) are thyroid hormones. Their normal secretion is dependent on appropriate amounts of iodine and TSH (thyroid stimulating hormone) in the circulating blood. *Hyperthyroidism* is a disorder of overproduction of thyroid hormones that increases the metabolism. Symptoms include increased nervousness and heart rate. Treatment includes surgery and antithyroid medications. *Hypothyroidism* is a disorder of underproduction of thyroid hormone, resulting in a lower metabolism. Symptoms include tiredness, low blood pressure, slow heart rate, and weight gain. Treatment includes thyroid hormone and increased dietary intake of iodine.

endocrine system a system of glands that secrete hormones into the bloodstream.

hormones chemicals produced by the body that regulate body functions and processes.

hyperthyroidism a condition in which thyroid hormone secretions are above normal, often referred to as an overactive thyroid.

hypothyroidism a condition in which thyroid hormone secretions are below normal, often referred to as an underactive thyroid.

THE ENDOCRINE SYSTEM

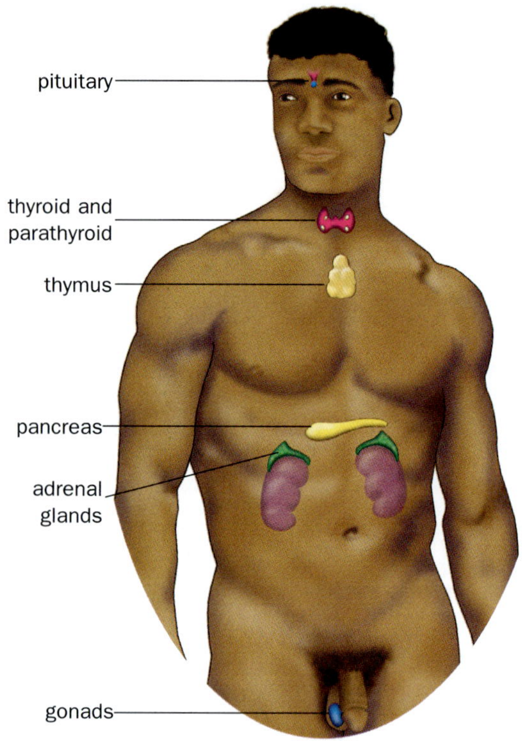

Note: the gonads of males are called testes and of females, ovaries.

Pituitary Gland

- Regulation of endocrine system and growth

Thyroid and Parathyroid

- Metabolic and calcium regulation

Thymus

- Lymphatic regulation

Pancreas

- Blood sugar regulation

Adrenal Glands

- Metabolism and energy regulation

Gonads

- Sexual characteristics

Note: Drugs highlighted in green in the text and tables are parenteral drugs commonly found in hospitals and other institutional settings.

The Parathyroid Glands

PTH (parathyroid hormone) and calcitonin are the hormones secreted by the parathyroid glands.

These hormones regulate the body's serum calcium and phosphorus levels, which are integral to normal muscle contraction, bone formation, blood coagulation, milk production in the lactating mother, and nerve impulse conduction. These four small, round organs are located behind the thyroid gland and reduction of their function can cause low calcium levels, convulsions, and possible death. Calcitonin-salmon is a common parathyroid gland synthetic hormone.

Divided into posterior and anterior lobes, the pituitary gland controls metabolism, growth, water loss and retention, electrolyte balance, and the reproductive cycle.

An example of a hormone secreted by the posterior lobe is ADH or antidiuretic hormone. Also known as vasopressin, this hormone helps the kidneys conserve water and prevent dehydration. Diabetes insipidus is caused by a deficiency in this hormone and marked by excretion of large amounts of urine (polyuria) and excessive thirst (polydipsia).

Oxytocin is another posterior lobe hormone.

It helps stimulate uterine contraction and promote birth or inhibit uterine bleeding post birth.

FSH or follicle stimulating hormone is an anterior lobe hormone called a gonadatropin (stimulator of reproductive organ function).

It acts to stimulate the egg follicle to produce eggs. Clomiphene is a popular synthetic nonsteroidal agent used to induce ovulation and establish fertility in otherwise unfertile women.

Rx safety you should know

- Brands of drugs used for thyroid hormone replacement are not generally interchangeable. Take special care to check with your pharmacist before substituting.

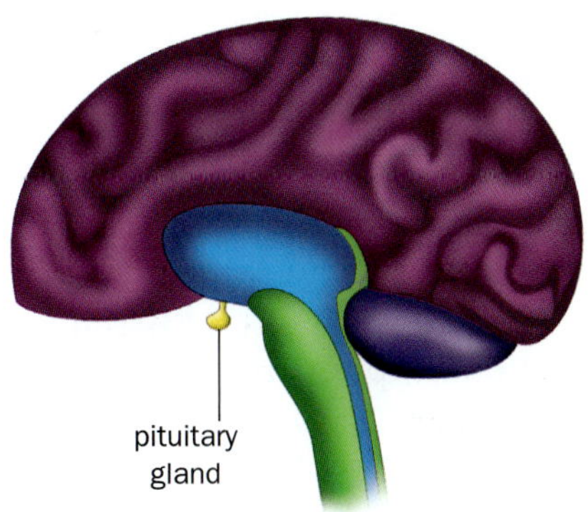

Some Common Hormones & Modifiers: Thyroid, Parathyroid, and Pituitary Drugs

Type	Brand Name	Generic Name
Thyroid	Armour Thyroid	thyroid desiccated
Thyroid	Synthroid	levothyroxine
Parathyroid	Miacalcin	calcitonin-salmon
Pituitary/ovulatory stimulant	Clomid	clomiphene
Pituitary/hypothalamus	Pitocin	oxytocin

See Additional Common Drugs by Classification on pp 533-537 for more drugs in this class.

HORMONES & MODIFIERS

Located above each kidney, the adrenal glands consist of an outer section, the cortex, and an inner section, the medulla.

The cortex secretes ***corticosteroids***, which regulate the body's ability to handle stress; resist infection; affect glucose, fat, protein, and carbohydrate metabolism; and maintain salt and water balance. The adrenal medulla secretes the neurotransmitter ***epinephrine***, which acts as a stimulator to the sympathetic nervous system.

This hormone, referred to as a catecholamine, is generally released during stress or activities of "fight or flight."

Epinephrine will generally cause a rise in blood pressure, strength and rate of heart beat, blood glucose, metabolic rate, a relaxation of bronchi muscles, coronary and uterine muscles, and dilation of the eye's pupil. Epinephrine is commercially available and used often in serious or medical emergency situations.

Adrenal Glands

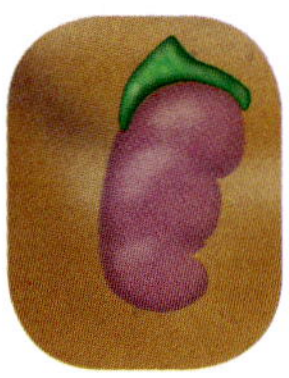

The adrenal glands sit atop the kidneys. They secrete corticosteroids and epinephrine, which influence many aspects of metabolism and energy regulation.

Corticosteroids

Hydrocortisone and methylprednisolone are two adrenal cortex corticosteroids that act to control anti-inflammatory response and the immune response system. In the 1940s cortisone was recognized as having anti-inflammatory properties. Since then, many synthetic corticosteroids such as prednisone (Sterapred®) and triamcinolone (Kenalog®) have been developed and indicated for inflammatory conditions such as arthritis, intestinal disorders, and various respiratory pathologies.

The corticosteroid aldosterone helps maintain an adequate supply of serum sodium, which accommodates sufficient extracellular fluid or blood volume. A severe deficiency in aldosterone could lead to low blood pressure and circulatory collapse.

safety you should know

➥ Corticosteroids should not be abruptly discontinued.

Some Common Hormones & Modifiers: Adrenal Drugs

Type	Brand Name	Generic Name
Adrenal/sympathomimetic	Epipen	epinephrine
Adrenal/corticosteroid	Cortef	hydrocortisone
Adrenal/corticosteroid	Medrol	methylprednisolone
Adrenal/corticosteroid	Sterapred	prednisone
Adrenal/corticosteroid	Kenalog	triamcinolone

See Additional Common Drugs by Classification on pp 533-537 for more drugs in this class.

corticosteroid hormonal steroid substances produced by the cortex of the adrenal gland.

diabetes mellitus a condition in which the body does not produce enough insulin or is unable to use it efficiently.

glucagon a hormone that helps convert amino acids to glucose.

insulin a hormone that controls the body's use of glucose.

Islands (or Islets) of Langerhans specialized cells of the pancreas that secrete insulin.

serum glucose blood sugar.

Note: Drugs highlighted in green in the text and tables are parenteral drugs commonly found in hospitals and other institutional settings.

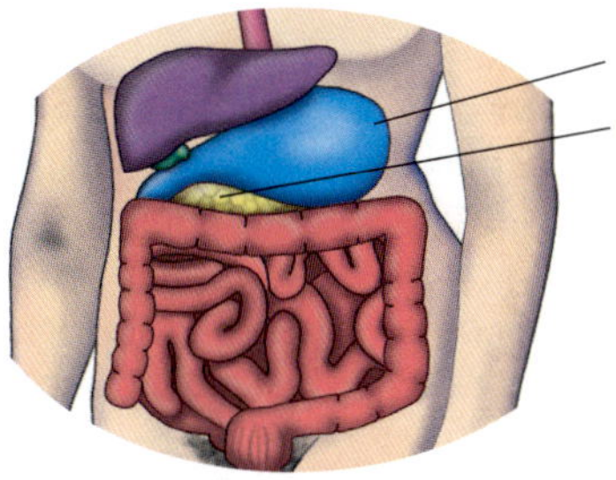

The pancreas is located behind the stomach.

The pancreas secretes the hormones *insulin* and *glucagon*.

The pancreas is an irregularly shaped organ located between the adrenal glands and behind the stomach. A specialized cluster of pancreatic beta cells called the ***Islands (or Islets) of Langerhans*** produce insulin, a hormone that controls the body's use of glucose, its normal source of energy. The alpha cells of the pancreas secrete the hormone glucagon, which helps convert amino acids (by products of protein digestion) to glucose and raise the level of serum glucose (blood sugar). As the serum glucose level increases in a healthy individual, insulin secretion is stimulated. Glucagon and insulin ideally work together to strike a delicate balance and maintain homeostasis. Glucagon is available commercially and given to release glucose into the blood stream for severely hypoglycemic patients.

Without adequate insulin levels, *serum glucose* is not reabsorbed into the intestine, and it spills into the urine for excretion.

Instead of using glucose as it should, the body uses fat and protein as energy sources. This condition, ***diabetes mellitus***, is marked by frequent urination, excessive thirst, elevated blood glucose levels, and positive urine glucose and acetone levels. In the early 1920s, Canadian researchers noted a link between the absence of a pancreas and diabetic symptoms. Insulin (e.g., Humulin® N, Humulin® R, Humulin® 70/30, and Lantus®) is given to treat diabetes mellitus. Several oral diabetic agents are also available (e.g., glyburide and glipizide). Note that insulin does not cure diabetes. It is merely a treatment for it.

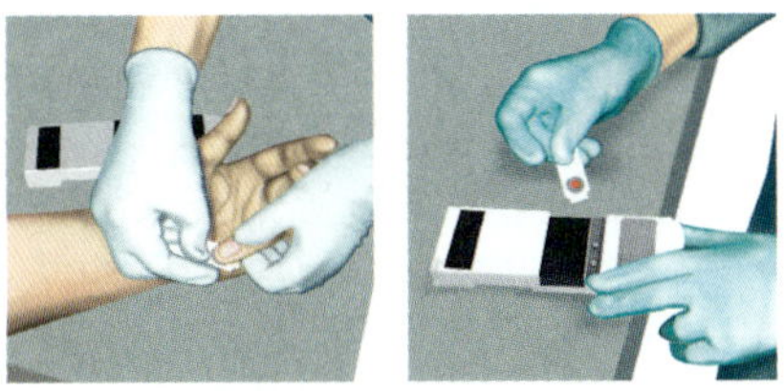

Glucose Monitoring

Patients with diabetes mellitus routinely monitor their blood glucose levels with a glucometer. This involves taking a small blood sample, usually from a fingertip, and inserting the sample into the glucometer for analysis. Newer systems are being developed that read glucose levels through the skin and do not require blood specimens.

℞ safety you should know

- Diabetic patients using insulin should consistently use the same type and brand of syringe.

Some Common Hormones & Modifiers: Insulin and Oral Antidiabetic Drugs

Type	Brand Name	Generic Name
Insulin	Humulin N	NPH
Insulin	Humulin R	regular
Insulin	Lantus	glargine
Oral antidiabetic	Diabeta	glyburide
Oral antidiabetic	Glucotrol	glipizide

See Additional Common Drugs by Classification on pp 533-537 for more drugs in this class.

HORMONES & MODIFIERS

The ovaries are almond shaped organs found on either side of the uterus within the female pelvis.

Under control of the anterior pituitary gland, the ovaries are responsible for the production of ova (eggs) as well as the secretion of the hormones *estrogen* and *progesterone*. These hormones are essential for primary and secondary sex characteristic development, menstruation, healthy pregnancies (gestation), and milk production (lactation).

The testes secretes the male hormone *testosterone*.

Male hormones are called *androgens*. The development and maintenance of the male reproductive tract includes enhancement of secondary sexual characteristics, muscle development, sex organ growth, and body fat distribution. In addition, testosterone also contributes to the building of tissues and prevention of their breakdown. Commercially available testosterone products are often indicated in cases of male hypogonadism or in females for certain breast cancers or engorgement. Methyltestosterone is a common example of this androgen.

Another class of drugs called phosphodiesterase inhibitors is used to treat erectile dysfunction.

Popular erectile dysfunction medications include Cialis® and Viagra®.

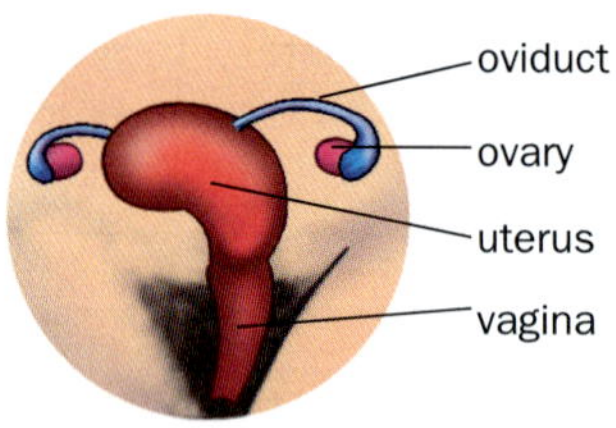

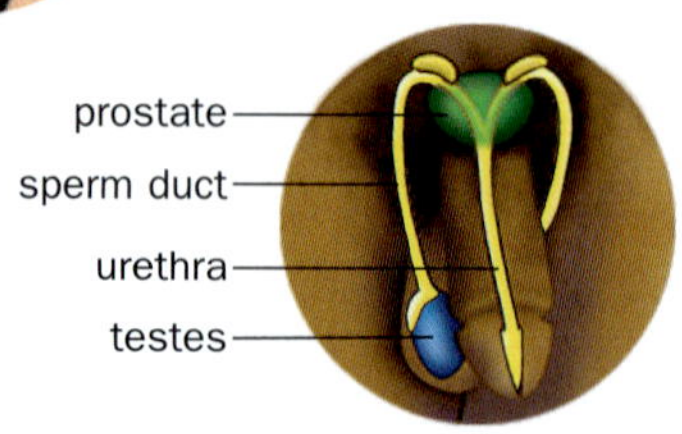

Estrogen

First produced in large quantities at puberty, women secrete estrogens until menopause. Due to their adjunctive role in calcium and phosphorus conservation, many women receive replacement estrogen therapy in their postmenopausal years.

Women who experience a lack of these hormones during their child bearing years and/or postmenopause, may receive them as natural and synthetic products.

Synthetic estrogen may also be indicated in cases of breast engorgement, to stunt female growth in height, and for men with prostate cancer.

Estradiol and Premarin are examples of an estrogen mix/replacement. Estrogens are generally contraindicated in cases of breast and/or genital cancer history or if there has been unexplained uterine bleeding.

Progesterone

Progesterone, which is naturally responsible for placenta development and prevention of ovulation, may be indicated in cases of amenorrhea (absence of menstruation), endometreosis (sloughing off of uterine tissue with subsequent attachment to other pelvic organs), dysfunctional uterine bleeding, and for oral contraceptive use.

androgens male sex characteristic hormones.

estrogens female sex characteristic hormones that are involved in calcium and phosphorus conservation.

progesterone female sex characteristic hormone involved in ovulation prevention.

testosterone the primary androgen.

Oral Contraceptives

There are three types of oral contraceptives:

- monophasic,
- biphasic, and
- triphasic.

Monophasic contraceptives offer a fixed dose of estrogen and progestin (progesterone) while the biphasic and triphasic types deliver the hormones more as they would be naturally secreted by the ovaries.

Ortho Novum®, depending on its estrogen/progestin mix, is an example of an oral contraceptive available as any one of the three above mentioned types.

Other oral contraceptives include Trinessa®, Yasmin 28®, Ortho Tricyclen Lo®, and Ortho Evra®, a contraceptive patch.

Some Common Hormones & Modifiers: Reproductive System Drugs

Type	Brand Name	Generic Name
Androgen	Android	methyltestosterone
Phosphodiesterase inhibitor	Cialis	tadalafil
Phosphodiesterase inhibitor	Viagra	sildenafil
Oral contraceptive	Ortho Novum	norethindrone and ethinyl estradiol
Oral contraceptive	Trinessa	norgestimate and ethinyl estradiol
Oral contraceptive	Yasmin 28	drospirenone and ethinyl estradiol
Oral contraceptive	Ortho Tricyclen Lo	norgestimate and ethinyl estradiol
Contraceptive patch	Ortho Evra Patch	norelgestromin and ethinyl estradiol
Estrogen replacement	Vagifem	estradiol
Estrogen replacement	Premarin	conjugated estrogens
Progestin	Provera	medroxyprogesterone

See Additional Common Drugs by Classification on pp 533-537 for more drugs in this class.

℞ safety you should know

- Antibiotics, especially penicillins, tetracyclines, and griseofulvin, can have significant interactions with oral contraceptives.
- Anticonvulsants (especially Tegretol®, Dilantin®, and Topamax®) can have significant interactions with oral contraceptives.
- St. John's Wort can have a significant interaction with oral contraceptives.
- Cigarette smoking can increase the risk of serious side effects from oral contraceptives; the risk is higher for women over 35 years old and heavy smokers.
- Some oral contraceptives have other uses, including menstrual cycle regularity, dysmenorrhea, and acne vulgaris.

IMMUNOBIOLOGIC AGENTS & VACCINES

Immunity against pathogens is either passive or active.

Passive immunity occurs when a patient is given a preformed antibody from another source, such as with immune globulins. Active immunity occurs when the body is exposed to a pathogen, develops the disease, and manufactures its own antibodies against a future invasion, such as with vaccines.

Immune globulins are specialized proteins that provide passive immunity.

The antibodies used in immune globulins are produced by other humans or animals and are recovered through high tech purification processes. Injections of immune globulins are not as common in contemporary medical practice as they were in the past, but the FDA has approved immune globulins for tetanus, diphtheria, measles, mumps, hepatitis A and B, and chicken pox. Candidates for immune globulin injections include patients who have been exposed to these diseases but have not been previously vaccinated for them, as well as people who have contracted diseases such as botulism and rabies. Immunoglobulins can also address issues associated with blood type and tissue compatibility between kidney donors and recipients.

One negative aspect of passive immunity is that it generally offers a shorter period of protection than does active immunity.

Another concern is the possibility of allergic reaction that may occur in some individuals. Further, hypersensitization may follow the receipt of passive immunity and render the host more prone to allergic response with each subsequent exposure. Severe anaphylactic reactions are possible.

Most vaccines provide an active form of immunity.

Vaccines are suspensions containing infectious agents used to boost the body's own immune system response. Toxoids are sometimes used in some vaccines to cause an immune response. The toxoids of diphtheria and tetanus provide two examples of toxoids that are used in vaccines.

IMMUNE GLOBULINS

Pathogens for which animal antibodies may be used for immune globulins:

- Diphtheria (using Antitoxin, USP)
- Rabies (using Antirabies serum)
- Botulism
- Black Widow Spider Venom

Human antibodies are used in immune globulins in the treatment of:

- Measles (using Measles Immune Globulin, USP)
- Pertussis (using Pertussis Immune Globulin, USP)
- Mumps (using Mumps Immune Globulin, USP)
- Tetanus (using Tetanus Immune Globulin, USP)
- Hepatitis A and B.

Note: Diphtheria, Tetanus, Hepatitis B, Measles, Mumps, and Rabies may also be treated with vaccines.

Common Immune Globulins

Flebogamma®
Octagam®
Gammagard®
Gamunex®
Carimune NF®
Iveegam EN®
Privigen®

Rx safety you should know

In the United States, some versions of the inactivated influenza vaccine use thimerosal, a mercury-based preservative, and other vaccines may still contain trace amounts, as indicated on package inserts.

Source: FDA.gov.

Note: Drugs highlighted in green in the text and tables are parenteral drugs commonly found in hospitals and other institutional settings.

INFLUENZA VACCINES

Because influenza viruses are always changing, the content of the seasonal influenza vaccine changes each year. Protection for three different viruses is included in typical influenza vaccines.

Influenza vaccines are available as an intramuscular injection or nasal spray. The nasal spray contains a live attenuated virus and has been approved only for patients between the ages of 2–49; it is contraindicated for pregnant women and there are restrictions for individuals within the eligible age group who have asthma or wheezing conditions, have experienced Guillain-Barré syndrome, or have a weakened immune system, heart disease, kidney disease, or diabetes.

In the last half of the 20th century many new vaccines were developed.

These include DPT (diphtheria, pertussis, and tetanus), MMR (measles, mumps, and rubella), polio, typhoid, rabies, hepatitis A and B, BCG (an antitubercular agent), Haemophilus influenzae type B (Hib), and chicken pox. Today, state laws require children to have a certification of immunization against most of these diseases, and others, prior to attending school. This has resulted in both a dramatic decrease in the incidence of these diseases and also in the average child receiving 36 doses of 12 different viral and bacterial vaccines by age six.

Vaccine Information Statements (VIS) prepared by the Centers for Disease Control and Prevention (CDC) provide information about the risks and benefits of each vaccine.

The National Childhood Vaccine Injury Act (NCVIA) requires health-care providers to provide a copy of the VIS to either the adult recipient or a child's parent/legal representative before administering the following vaccines: diphtheria, tetanus, pertussis, measles, mumps, rubella, polio, hepatitis A, hepatitis B, Haemophilus influenzae type b (Hib), influenza, and pneumococcal conjugate. The vaccine information statements are available at http://www.immunize.org/vis/. Adverse reactions to vaccines should be reported through the Vaccine Adverse Event Reporting System (VAERS) maintained by the CDC (vaers.hhs.gov/index).

Some Common Vaccines

Brand Name	Vaccine
Daptacel, Infanrix, Tripedia	Diphtheria, Tetanus, Pertussis (DTaP, DT, Tdap, Td)
Liquid Pedvax HIB, ActHIB, HibTITER	Haemophilus influenzae type b (Hib)
Havrix, VAQTA	Hepatitis A (HepA)
Engerix-B, Recombivax HB, Twinrix	Hepatitis B (HepB)
FluMist	Influenza, live attenuated (LAIV)
Afluria, Fluarix, FluLaval, Fluvirin, Fluzone	Influenza, trivalent inactivated (TIV)
Attenuvax, M-M-R II, Mumpsvax, Meruvax II	Measles, mumps, rubella (MMR)
Menomune	Meningococcal, conjugated (MCV4)
Prevnar	Pneumococcal conjugate (PCV)
Pneumovax 23	Pneumococcal polysaccharide (PPV)
Varivax	Varicella (Var)
Comvax	Hib+HepB (combination)
Pediarix	DTaP+HepB+IPV (combination)
ProQuad	MMR+Var (combination)
TriHIBit	DTaP+Hib (combination)

MUSCULOSKELETAL AGENTS

R*heumatoid arthritis* is a chronic and often progressive inflammatory condition linked to the dysfunction of the immune system.

Antibodies called rheumatoid factors contribute to the course of the disease. Inflammation caused by the release of histamine and prostaglandins leads to swelling, feelings of warmth, and pain in joints (especially in the hands, wrists, feet, hips, knees, and ankles). As the disease progresses, a decrease in range of motion and an increase in bony fusion and muscle deformity may occur.

There is no known cure or method of prevention for rheumatoid arthritis.

Treatment may include drug therapy, physical therapy, occupational therapy, weight reduction, rest, and the use of adaptive or assistive devices. Drug therapy primarily consists of NSAIDs that inhibit prostaglandins synthesis and reduce inflammation. They are also the first-line drug of choice due to their analgesic properties. However, as the condition progresses, disease modifying antirheumatic drugs (DMARD's) such as methotrexate (Rheumatrex®) as well as gold preparations, such as aurothioglucose (suspended in oil), are indicated.

***Gout* is an inflammatory condition in which an excess of uric acid and urate crystals accumulate in synovial fluids of the joints.**

This leads to joint swelling, redness, warmth, and pain. Gout may be caused by diet or a metabolism dysfunction. A patient may experience an acute attack of gouty arthritis with severe pain, fever, swelling of joints, and inflammation. A first-line drug used to treat gouty arthritis would be colchicine. *Uricosuric drugs* such as probenecid increase elimination of uric acid and xanthine oxidase inhibitors such as allopurinol (Zyloprim®) interfere with uric acid synthesis.

MUSCULAR SYSTEM

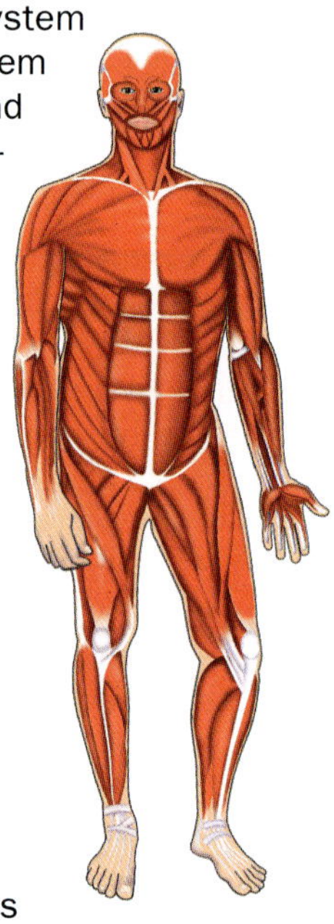

The muscular system is a complex system of connecting and overlapping muscles that completely cover the body. There are cardiac muscles in the heart and smooth muscles in the arteries and digestive tract, but most muscles are skeletal muscles attached to the skeleton by tendons. Skeletal muscles are made up of long fibers that expand and contract to push and pull bones, causing body movement.

gout a painful inflammatory condition in which excess uric acid accumulates in the joints.

osteoarthritis a disorder characterized by weight-bearing bone deterioration, decreasing range of motion, and causing pain and deformity.

Some Common Musculoskeletal Drugs

Type	Brand Name	Generic Name
Disease-modifying antirheumatic	Rheumatrex	methotrexate
Gold preparation	Solganal	aurothioglucose (suspended in oil)
Anti-gout	Colcrys	colchicine
Anti-gout, uricosuric	n/a	probenecid
Anti-gout, xanthine oxidase inhibitor	Zyloprim	allopurinol

See Additional Common Drugs by Classification on pp 533-537 for more drugs in this class.

Note: Drugs highlighted in green in the text and tables are parenteral drugs commonly found in hospitals and other institutional settings.

SKELETAL SYSTEM

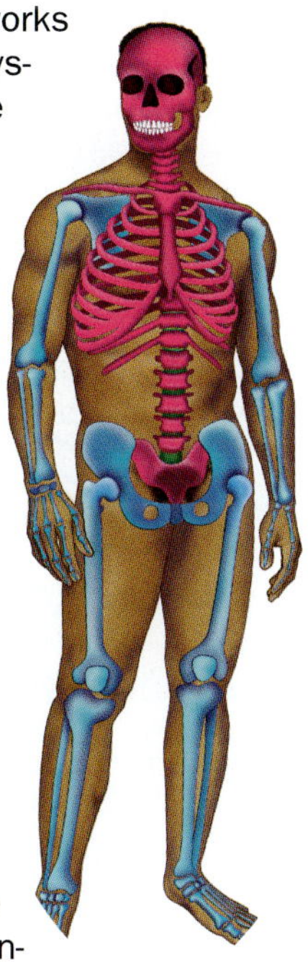

The skeletal system works with the muscular system to provide precise and powerful movement. The system's 206 bones are called axial (brain and spinal column) or appendicular (arms, legs, and connecting bones). They are held together at joints by connective tissue called ligaments and cartilage. Joints range from rigid to those allowing full motion. The hinge joints of the knee, elbow and ankle allow motion along a single axis. The ball-and-socket joints of the hips and shoulders allow a much broader range of movement.

rheumatoid arthritis a disease in which the body's immune system attacks joint tissue.

uricosuric drugs drugs used to treat gout that increase the elimination of uric acid.

O*steoarthritis* and osteoporosis are marked by weight-bearing bone deterioration, decreasing range of motion, and increasing pain, deformity, and disability.

Water content changes in the bone cartilage weakens the bones, causes cartilage damage and prevents repair. Inflammation may occur. Deep aching and local pain is experienced but can initially be relieved by rest. However, as the disease progresses, pain becomes chronic. Deformity also occurs in the later stages and bony enlargements (osteophytes) develop on the fingers and toes. Postmenopausal women, osteoporotic males, and those with Paget disease may suffer from osteoporosis, resulting in bone mass and density loss. Common osteoporotic agents include risedronate (Actonel®) and alendronate (Fosamax®).

Drug therapy, physical therapy, adaptive or assistive devices, patient education, and possibly surgery are part of a comprehensive treatment approach.

Drug therapy primarily consists of analgesics, NSAIDs, and corticosteroids. Since the majority of patients are elderly, drug treatment is directed at pain relief and is traditionally more conservative than aggressive.

Muscle spasms can be infrequent, chronic, or acute, depending on their origin and the patient's underlying medical condition.

Trauma, overwork, or a disorder such as connective tissue irritation can cause painful muscle contractions and involuntary spasms. Severe spasticity is usually linked to central nervous system disorders. Traditionally, treatment of muscle spasms is directed at muscle relaxation, pain relief, ability to exercise the muscle, and preventing loss of motion. Centrally acting antispasmodics such as diazepam (Valium®) eliminate cramps without affecting normal muscle activity. The sedative action of carisoprodol (Soma®) helps relieve acute musculoskeletal pain while cyclobenzaprine (Flexeril®) decreases muscle tone and reduces spasm.

Some Common Musculoskeletal Drugs

Type	Brand Name	Generic Name
Osteoporotic	Actonel	risedronate
Osteoporotic	Fosamax	alendronate
Centrally acting antispasmodics	Valium	diazepam
Muscle relaxant	Soma	carisoprodol
Muscle relaxant	Flexeril	cyclobenzaprine

NEUROLOGICAL AGENTS

Since nerve cells do not contact other neurons or the muscles they affect directly, nerve impulses are communicated by chemical transmission.

These chemical mediators are neurotransmitters or neurohormones. They cross the synapses (the junctions between nerve cells) and allow transmission of impulses from one neuron to another. Two common peripheral nerve neurotransmitters are acetylcholine and norepinephrine.

Several common neurological disorders are affected by abnormalities in neurotransmitter release and/or response.

This includes the following disorders: Parkinson's disease, Alzheimer's disease, epilepsy, migraine headaches, multiple sclerosis, and attention deficit (hyperactivity) disorder.

NERVOUS SYSTEM

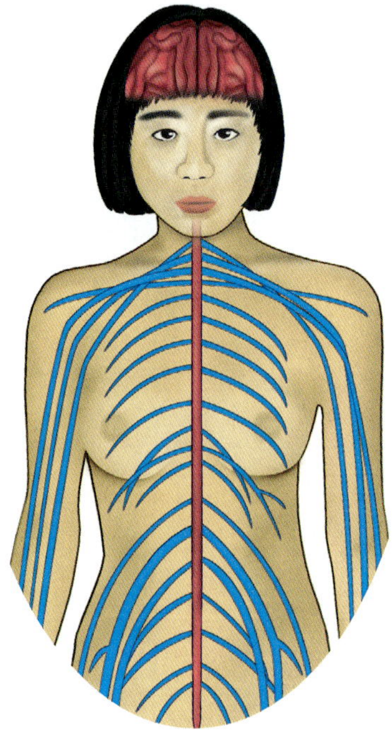

The Nervous System

The nervous system is divided into two main subsystems: the central nervous system (CNS) and the peripheral nervous system (PNS). The central nervous system consists of the brain and spinal cord. The peripheral nervous system carries information throughout the body, linking the body's systems together. It is made up of the somatic and autonomic nervous systems.

The somatic nervous system is associated with voluntary movements of the musculoskeletal system and sensations (heat, cold, pressure, and pain). The autonomic nervous system is responsible for automatic movements (breathing, digestion, etc.).

The autonomic nervous system is divided into the sympathetic and parasympathetic systems. The sympathetic branch works with the adrenal gland's medulla and regulates energy in times of stress such as danger, emotional tensions, and severe illness. The parasympathetic branch influences bodily functions to slow down and conserve energy. The sympathetic and parasympathetic nervous systems effect a delicate balance and maintain homeostasis on a daily basis within the human body. Drugs referred to as mimics act upon these systems to affect this balance and force a reaction.

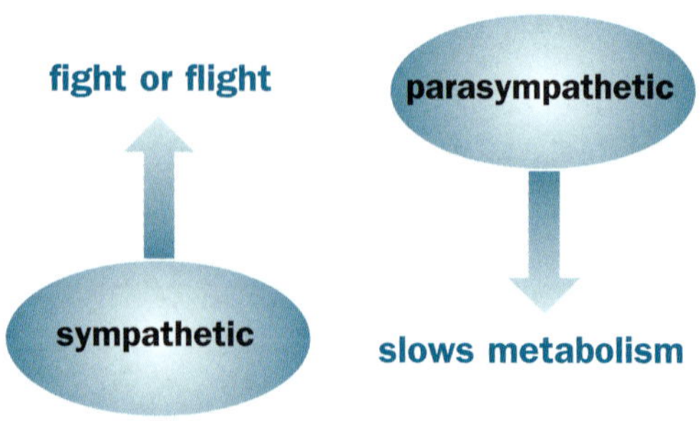

A Delicate Balance

The balance between the sympathetic and parasympathetic systems is illustrated in the "fight or flight" response. In the event of being threatened and frightened, the sympathetic system reacts to increase heart rate, deep breathing, and blood pressure (increases circulation of oxygen), dilate pupils (provides extra light for vision), increase liver glycogen breakdown (supplies glucose and oxygen to muscles for energy), and halt peristalsis. The parasympathetic system will restart digestive and peristaltic actions, constrict the pupils, slow the heart and respiratory rates, and lower blood pressure when the threat is removed.

DISORDERS

Parkinson's Disease

Parkinson's disease is a progressive neuromuscular condition that usually affects patients above 50 years of age and is characterized by flat, emotionless expression, bent posture, shuffling and unsteady gait, fine tremors, and difficulty chewing and swallowing. Early symptoms may include muscle aches, numbness, coldness, and loss of sensation or tingling. It is associated with low levels of the neurotransmitter dopamine in the brain and increased levels of acetylcholine. Brain tumors, arteriosclerosis, severe infectious processes, and excessive use of some antipsychotic drugs may also cause this disease.

THERAPIES

Drug therapy will not stop the progress of this disease. Instead, an increased quality of life, decreased side effects, and minimization of disabilities are the goals of chemical treatment. Levodopa, carbidopa and levodopa together (Sinemet®), amantadine, and selegiline hydrochloride (Eldepryl®) are commonly prescribed antiparkinsonian drugs. In addition, dopamine agonists such as bromocriptine (Parlodel®) are indicated when patients are experiencing a decrease in L-dopa's responsiveness. Anticholinergics are used for the treatment of tremors and decreased muscle tone.

Alzheimer's Disease

Alzheimer's, a progressive dementia often classified as a psychiatric disorder, has been linked to neurotransmitter abnormalities. It primarily affects the elderly. Loss of memory is often one of the first signs of this condition, with speech impairment, frustration, depression, and decreased socialization soon occurring. These symptoms are generally followed by an inability to conduct the activities of daily living as well as a loss of spatial relationships. Ultimately, an inability to recognize familiar people and surroundings, wandering, combative aggression, and incontinence occur.

Drug therapy can be divided into treatment for cognitive symptoms most closely associated with dementias and noncognitive symptoms such as depression. Donepezil (Aricept®) is an example of cognitive symptom agents while secondary amine tricyclic antidepressants such as nortriptyline (Pamelor®) and desipramine (Norpramin®) and SSRI's such as paroxetine (Paxil®) and sertraline (Zoloft®) are indicated for symptoms such as depression in the Alzheimer patient.

Some Common Neurological Drugs: Antiparkinsoniaon and Anti-Alzheimer's

Type	Brand Name	Generic Name
Antiparkinsonian	Sinemet	carbidopa/levodopa
Antiparkinsonian	Eldepryl	selegiline hydrochloride
Antiparkinsonian	n/a	amantadine
Antiparkinsonian/dopamine agonist	Parlodel	bromocriptine
Antiparkinsonian/anticholinergic	Cogentin	benztropine
Cognitive symptom agent	Aricept	donepezil
Antidepressant	Pamelor	nortriptyline
Antidepressant	Norpramin	desipramine
SSRI	Paxil	paroxetine
SSRI	Zoloft	sertraline

See Additional Common Drugs by Classification on pp 533-537 for more drugs in this class.

NEUROLOGICAL AGENTS (cont'd)

DISORDERS

THERAPIES

Epilepsy

Epilepsy is a neurologic disorder associated with neuron transmission instability and characterized by recurrent seizure activity. Though there are other causes for seizures (trauma, fever, stress, etc.), the excess excitability seen in seizures may be linked to an imbalance of dopamine and acetylcholine release coupled with factors such as improper pH balance or an inadequate supply of glucose, oxygen, potassium, calcium, or amino acids.

Common antiepileptic drugs include phenytoin (Dilantin®) and phenobarbital. Other drugs include valproic acid (Depakene®), divalproex sodium (Depakote®), and carbamazepine (Tegretol®). With anticonvulsant agents, the diagnosis needs to be conclusive and the most appropriate drug for the specific seizure type is chosen.

Migraine Headaches

There are two common theories for the causes of migraine headaches: the vascular theory and the nerve theory. The vascular theory is that arterial vasoconstriction causes loss of oxygen and inflammation, which in turn stimulates sensory nerves in the head, resulting in possible auras and pain. An aura is an unusual sensation that can include hallucination. Stress, intense lights, colors, and/or sounds, as well as sleep deprivation are considered stimulants of vasoconstriction. The nerve theory is that the pain is caused by inflammatory neurotransmitters (i.e., prostaglandins) acting on nerve endings in the brain.

Aspirin is considered the drug of choice (using caution when treating children), and NSAIDs are especially useful if the patient is female and menstruating. Other drug therapies include: sumatriptan (Imitrex®), and ibuprofen (Motrin®). Prophylactic treatment may include: beta-blockers, antidepressants, calcium channel blockers, corticosteroids, and anticonvulsants.

Multiple Sclerosis

Multiple sclerosis is a disease in which the body's immune response attacks the person's central nervous system. In multiple sclerosis, nerve cells become demyelinated.

Treatment is aimed at improving function after an attack, preventing new attacks, and preventing disability. Immunomodulators (e.g., interferon beta-1-a and interferon beta-1-b) are used to reduce symptoms and slow the development of disability in patients with some forms of multiple sclerosis.

Attention Deficit Hyperactivity Disorder ADHD

Attention deficit hyperactivity disorder or ADHD is a condition that can affect children and often continues into adulthood. Problems associated with ADHD include inattention, hyperactivity, and impulsive behavior.

Examples of drugs used to treat ADHD include methylphenidate (Concerta®, Methylin®, Ritalin®) and dextroamphetamine/amphetamine (Adderall®).

Some Common Neurological Drugs for Epilepsy, Migraine, Multiple Sclerosis, and ADHD		
Type	**Brand Name**	**Generic Name**
Antiepileptic	Dilantin	phenytoin
Antiepileptic	n/a	phenobarbital
Antiepileptic	Depakene	valproic acid
Antiepileptic	Depakote	divalproex sodium
Antiepileptic	Tegretol	carbamazepine
Antimigraine	Bayer Aspirin	aspirin
Antimigraine	Imitrex	sumatriptan
Antimigraine	Motrin	ibuprofen
Immunomodulator	Avonex	interferon beta-1a
Immunomodulator	Betaseron	interferon beta-1b
Immunomodulator	Copaxone	glatiramer acetate
Immunomodulator	Rebif	interferon beta-1a
ADHD	Concerta	methylphenidate
ADHD	Methylin	methylphenidate
ADHD	Ritalin	methylphenidate
ADHD	Adderall	dextroamphetamine/amphetamine

See Additional Common Drugs by Classification on pp 533-537 for more drugs in this class.

Rx safety you should know

- There are many important drug interactions with some seizure medications such as carbamazepine, phenytoin, and phenobarbital. Some drugs are contraindicated with some seizure medications. Alert your pharmacist when prompted about drug interactions.
- Divalproex sodium and valproic acid have been associated with birth defects if taken by women during pregnancy.
- Anticonvulsants should not be stopped abruptly when used as anticonvulsants.
- Many drugs used to treat ADHD are in DEA Schedule II and have a high potential for abuse. Because they are in DEA Schedule II, they have special requirements for inventory, labeling, and record keeping.
- Some drug interactions for selegiline are dangerous and therefore contraindicated. Alert the pharmacist when drug interactions with selegiline arise.
- Sumatriptan and related drugs have some serious drug interactions and are therefore contraindicated. Alert the pharmacist when drug interactions with sumatriptan or other related drugs for treating migraines arise.

OPHTHALMIC & OTIC AGENTS

Ophthalmic agents are used to treat various conditions or disorders of the eye.

Disorders include *glaucoma*, infection, pain, and inflammation, but agents may also be used for eye examinations and in preparation for surgery. Ophthalmic agents are generally applied topically as drops or ointments.

Due to the special requirements for ophthalmic formulations, there are often many ingredients in a product besides the active ingredient.

Preservatives, antioxidants, buffers, and wetting agents that control such factors as pH, sterility, and proper isotonic percentages are often included.

Glaucoma represents several disorders characterized by abnormally high pressure within the eye that leads to optic nerve damage and progressive loss of vision.

The onset of glaucoma can be a slow process that may not be apparent to the patient and may only be detected during an eye examination. Early detection is essential for successful treatment and prevention of vision loss.

Although infection and inflammation can increase *intraocular* pressure temporarily, the common cause of glaucoma is a structural defect in the eye.

This form is called primary glaucoma and is divided into two types: narrow- or closed-angle and wide- or open-angle. Narrow-angle glaucoma is corrected with surgery. Open-angle glaucoma can be successfully treated with antiglaucoma drugs such as cholinergic receptor agonists, acetylcholinesterase inhibitors, carbonic anhydrase inhibitors, beta-adrenergic receptor antagonists, and adrenergic receptor agonists.

THE EYE

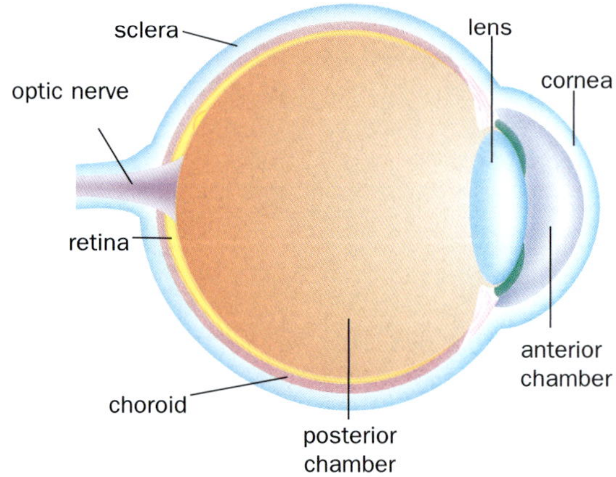

The eyeball has three layers:

- the outer layer contains the sclera (white part) and the cornea (clear);
- the middle vascular layer called the choroid contains the iris and pupil;
- the inner layer contains the retina, responsible for visual reception.

Both the anterior and posterior optic chambers are filled with a liquid called aqueous humor. The lens is located behind the iris. Ocular muscles control the movement of the eyeball and accommodate focusing. The thickness of the lens helps determine the distance at which one can see an object. Behind the lens, a jelly-like substance called the vitreous body helps maintain the shape of the eyeball.

Similar to a camera, the pupil allows light to enter. The lens focuses the light, and the retina receives the image. A complex chemical reaction within the retina processes the picture. The optic nerve then carries the image to the visual area of the brain.

Accessory structures to the eyeball include eyelids, ocular muscles, conjunctiva, eyelashes, and lacrimal glands.

Note: Drugs highlighted in green in the text and tables are parenteral drugs commonly found in hospitals and other institutional settings.

Conjunctivitis ("pink eye") is a common eye infection resulting from conjuctival irritation due to infectious organism or allergy.

Conjunctivitis infections are highly contagious. Symptoms are redness of the conjunctiva and pus-like, crusty exudate that often leads to the eyelid closing. Antibiotics such as gentamicin, sodium sulfacetamide, and norfloxacin are indicated if the infection is bacterial. For viral infections such as herpes simplex and cytomegalovirus retinitis, vidarabine and trifluridine are used. If the conjunctivitis is caused by an allergy, histamine blocking agents such as levocabastine, olopatadine, and emedastine may be ordered.

Inflammation of the eye may be treated with both NSAIDs and corticosteriods.

Agents such as medrysone and prednisolone are common ophthalmic corticosteroids while flurbiprofen and ketorolac are NSAIDs available for ophthalmic application. Note: flurbiprofen and ketorolac are often used following cataract extraction surgery.

Other drugs include *mydriatics*, anesthetics, and lubricating agents.

Mydriatics are drugs that dilate the pupil and are commonly indicated prior to eye exams. When the pupil is dilated, more light is allowed in and visualization into the eye is enhanced. Phenylephrine is a popular example. For optic-related pain, a topical anesthetic such as proparacaine may be prescribed. To provide lubrication to the eyes if abnormal drying is occurring, Lacrisert® is a prescription lubricating drug.

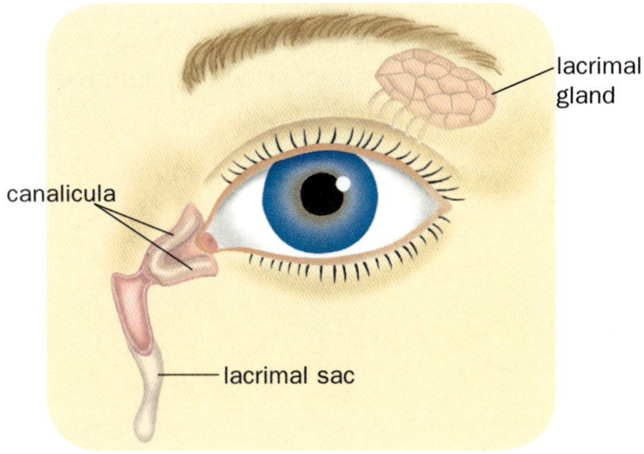

Ophthalmic Administration

- Hands should always be washed prior to drug administration.
- If more than one agent is to be instilled, wait the suggested time (5 minutes between solutions, 10–15 minutes before ointments) between administrations.
- Do not rub eyes. Carefully instill, as per order, onto conjunctiva, one eye at a time.
- Do not touch the applicator to the eye at any time.
- Replace the applicator cap carefully and do not touch the top of the applicator.
- Be aware that temporary vision distortion may occur and encourage the patient accordingly.
- The physician should be notified if symptoms do not alleviate.

Note: The incidence of adverse reactions to ophthalmic agents is small. Systemic absorption may cause allergic response and steroidal side effects in some cases.

conjunctivitis inflammation of the conjunctiva (eyelid lining).

glaucoma abnormally high pressure within the eye leading to optic nerve damage and loss of vision.

intraocular inside the eye.

mydriatics drugs that dilate the pupil.

OPHTHALMIC & OTIC AGENTS (cont'd)

Antiglaucoma Agents

Cholinergic receptor agonists such as pilocarpine and acetylcholine were the first antiglaucoma drugs developed. Beta-adrenergic receptor antagonists are now used more commonly than the cholinergic receptor agonists because they are considered more effective and have fewer side effects. Examples of this type include: betaxolol, carteolol, metipranolol, and timolol.

Adrenergic receptor agonists such as atropine and dipivefrin are used to lower intraocular pressure by increasing outflow of aqueous humor from the eye.

Some Common Ophthalmic Drugs

Type	Brand Name	Generic Name
Antibiotic	Garamycin	gentamicin
Antibiotic	Bleph-10	sulfacetamide
Antibiotic	Ciloxan	ciprofloxacin
Antiviral	Viroptic	trifluridine
Antihistamine	Patanol	olopatadine
Antihistamine	Emadine	emedastine
Ophthalmic corticosteroids	Pred Forte	prednisolone
NSAID	Ocufen	flurbiprofen
NSAID	Acular	ketorolac
Mydriatic	n/a	phenylephrine
Topical anesthetic	Alcaine	proparacaine
Ocular lubricant	Lacrisert	hydroxypropyl cellulose
Antiglaucoma	Betoptic	betaxolol
Antiglaucoma	n/a	carteolol
Antiglaucoma	Optipranolol	metipranolol
Antiglaucoma	Timoptic	timolol
Antiglaucoma	Isopto Atropine	atropine

See Additional Common Drugs by Classification on pp 533-537 for more drugs in this class.

Note: Drugs highlighted in green in the text and tables are parenteral drugs commonly found in hospitals and other institutional settings.

THE EAR

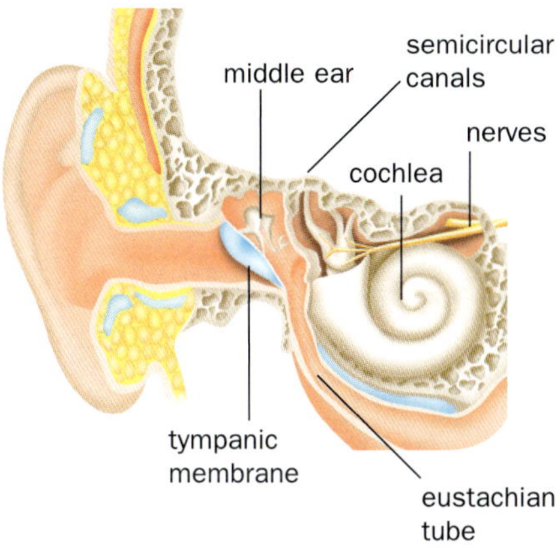

The ear has three main sections: the outer, middle, and inner ear.

The outer ear contains the external part of the ear as well as the part of the ear canal that leads up to the tympanic membrane. Cerumen (earwax) is produced in the skin of the ear canal.

The middle ear contains the three ear bones, or ossicles: the malleus, incus, and stapes. The middle ear also contains the Eustachian tube. The eustachian tube functions to equalize pressure and allow mucus drainage.

The inner ear contains the cochlea, the organ of hearing. The inner ear also contains three semicircular canals and the vestibule, which have function for balance.

Otic agents are used to treat conditions associated with the ear.

The most common conditions treated with otic products are associated with accumulation of earwax and infections of the outer ear. The pH of most otic products is acidic. Otic products can never be used in the eye because the acidity of otic products can damage the eye. However, sometimes ophthalmic products are prescribed to treat infections of the ear.

Otic Administration

- Hands should always be washed prior to drug administration.
- The medicine should be warmed to body temperature by holding the bottle between the hands for a few minutes.
- The head should be placed so the affected ear is on top.
- The ear canal should be straightened
- For children younger than 3 years old: Hold ear lobe and pull down and back.
- For children 3 years and older: Hold upper part of ear and pull up and back.
- The dropper should not touch the ear; the drops should be placed onto the side of the ear canal (not dropped directly down the ear canal).
- The head should remain in place for 5 minutes or insert a cotton plug into the ear.
- The physician should be notified if condition symptoms do not alleviate.

Note: While the incidence of adverse reactions to otic agents is small, systemic absorption may cause allergic response and steroidal side effects.

Some Common Otic Drugs

Type	Brand Name	Generic Name
Anti-infective	Cortisporin Otic Solution	neomycin, polymixin b, hydrocortisone
Earwax softener	Debrox	carbamide peroxide
Anti-infective		acetic acid, hydrocortisone
Anti-infective	Ciprodex	ciprofloxacin/dexamethasone

PSYCHOTROPIC AGENTS

Psychotropic agents are drugs that affect behavior, psychiatric state, and sleep.

They act on specialized areas of the brain to suppress or control symptoms of common psychological disorders such as bipolar disorder, anxiety, depression, schizophrenia, and addiction. The primary types of drugs in this class are antidepressants, antipsychotics, and antianxiety agents. Other related psychotropic agents include sedatives and hypnotics.

THE BRAIN

The brain is an incredibly versatile and complex organ responsible for a vast number of the body's functions. To a great extent, the structures or areas of the brain are specialized by function. These specialized structures are discussed below.

Cerebrum

➥ concerned mostly with learned behavior, thought, memory, sensation, and voluntary motion. It is divided into lobes: frontal, occipital (back), parietal (top), and temporal (side).

Cerebellum

➥ controls balance and muscle coordination.

Medulla Oblongata (brain stem)

➥ controls processes that affect the heart, breathing, temperature control, and circulation.

Pons

➥ bridges from the medulla oblongata to the cerebellum and also works on muscle coordination.

Thalamus

➥ above the pons, receives sensations such as heat, cold, pressure, and pain.

Hypothalamus

➥ below the thalamus, controls blood sugar levels, body temperature, emotions, appetite, and sleep.

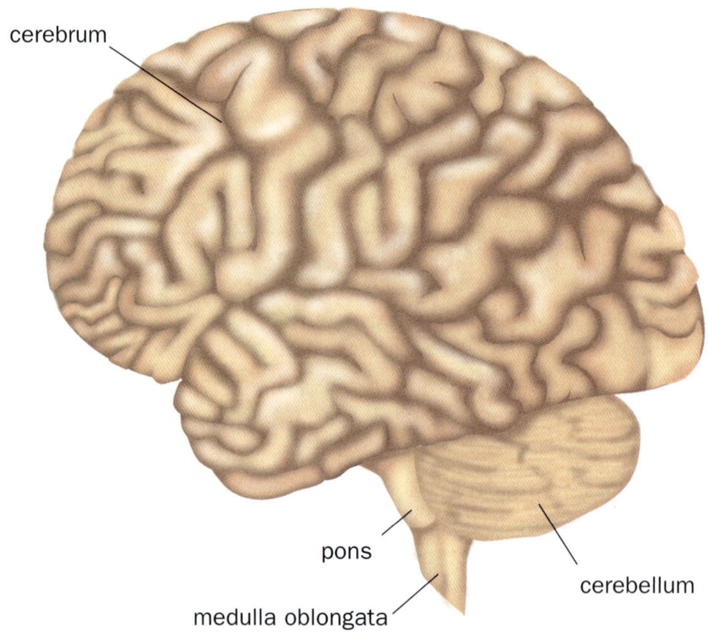

Midbrain

➥ works to control blood pressure and the pineal gland; secretes the hormone melatonin, which affects the body's biological rhythms.

Limbic System

➥ an interconnecting network of brain cells inside the brain that affects behavior, emotions, sociosexual drives, motivation, learning, and memory storage and retrieval.

Sedatives and Hypnotics

Sedatives are drugs that are intended to relax and calm. They reduce restlessness and may produce mild drowsiness. Antianxiety medications that include benzodiazepines (e.g., diazepam and chlordiazepoxide) are included in this group.

Hypnotics are often referred to as sleeping pills and are designed to induce and, in some cases, prolong sleep. This group includes barbiturates such as secobarbital and pentobarbital. Nonbarbiturate sedative-hypnotics include chloral hydrate and meprobamate.

DISORDERS

THERAPIES

Bipolar Disorder

Also known as Manic–Depression, this disorder is characterized by mood, energy, and behavior swings from periods of elation to episodes of depression. These swings are found to occur in a cyclical and recurring pattern. Theories of cause include chemical imbalance and neurotransmitter alterations in the brain. There is a high degree of family history associated with this disorder.

Although psychotherapy is included in the suggested treatment, antipsychotic drugs such as quetiapine (Seroquel®) and risperidon (Risperdal®) are commonly prescribed. Carbamazepine (Tegretol®), valproic acid (Depakene®), and clonazepam (Klonopin®) are often added to this therapy to treat seizure activity secondary to psychotropic agents.

Schizophrenia

This is characterized by extreme and inappropriate behavior and dysfunctional daily routine. Hearing "voices," experiencing delusions, becoming agitated or hostile, and perhaps a lack of response at all (flat affect) are examples of schizophrenic behavior. Theories of cause include: family history and chemical imbalances, especially norepinephrine and serotonin, noted in the limbic system.

Patients experiencing schizophrenia must undergo a complete medical and psychological examination. The drug therapy selected will result from the findings. Antipsychotic agents commonly used may include: chlorpromazine and trifluoperazine.

Some Common Psychotropic Drugs: Antipsychotic and Antiseizure

Type	Brand Name	Generic Name
Antipsychotic/bipolar	Seroquel	quetiapine
Antipsychotic/bipolar	Risperdal	risperidon
Antipsychotic/schizophrenia	n/a	chlorpromazine
Antipsychotic/schizophrenia	n/a	trifluoperazine
Antiseizure	Tegretol	carbamazepine
Antiseizure	Depakene	valproic acid
Antiseizure	Klonopin	clonazepam

Some Common Psychotropic Drugs: Sedatives and Hypnotics

Type	Brand Name	Generic Name
Sedative/antianxiety	Valium	diazepam
Sedative/antianxiety	n/a	chlordiazepoxide
Hypnotic/barbiturate	Seconal	secobarbital
Hypnotic/barbiturate	Nembutal	pentobarbital
Hypnotic/nonbarbiturate	Somnote	chloral hydrate
Hypnotic/nonbarbiturate	n/a	meprobamate

See Additional Common Drugs by Classification on pp 533-537 for more drugs in these classes.

PSYCHOTROPIC AGENTS (cont'd)

DISORDERS

THERAPIES

Anxiety

People experiencing anxiety may appear abnormally tired or energetic, withdrawn, tremorous, tense and restless, and may suffer from insomnia, phobias, and panic attacks. Theories of cause include a hypersensitive sympathetic nervous system, excessive serotonin release, and an inability to chemically receive the body's natural calming agents.

In conjunction with psychotherapy and various relaxation techniques, the commonly prescribed drugs include antianxiety agents such as the benzodiazepines diazepam (Valium®), lorazepam (Ativan®), and alprazolam (Xanax®).

Depression

Depression is characterized by mood disturbances that may be mild (e.g., lack of interest or inability to experience joy) or severe (e.g., physical aggression or suicide attempts). Sleep disturbances, crying episodes, gastrointestinal upset, and heart palpitations may occur. Theories of cause include: experience of trauma (real or perceived), loss, and poor neurotransmitter response of norepinephrine.

While psychotherapy and even shock therapy are often prescribed treatment, antidepressants such as amitriptyline (Elavil®) and sertraline (Zoloft®) are common drug suggestions. Others are escitalopram (Lexapro®), venlafaxine, and fluoxetine (Prozac®).

Some Common Psychotropic Drugs: Antianxiety

Type	Brand Name	Generic Name
Antianxiety	Valium	diazepam
Antianxiety	n/a	chlordiazepoxide
Antianxiety	Ativan	lorazepam
Antianxiety	Xanax	alprazolam

Some Common Psychotropic Drugs: Antidepressant

Type	Brand Name	Generic Name
Antidepressant	n/a	amitriptyline
Antidepressant	Zoloft	sertraline
Antidepressant	Lexapro	escitalopram
Antidepressant	n/a	venlafaxine
Antidepressant	Prozac	fluoxetine

See Additional Common Drugs by Classification on pp 533-537 for more drugs in this class.

DISORDERS

THERAPIES

Drug Dependency

Addiction to drugs and alcohol may occur for various reasons, including chronic usage without adequate physician supervision, chemical intolerance, error in personal judgement, or purposeful abuse. Family history and social situation may be contributing factors.

Treatment for dependency often encompasses an on-site treatment program designed to identify and address the patient holistically. Adjunct drug therapy may or may not be included in this. For example, naltrexone (ReVia®) may be used to dissuade the alcoholic from drinking, desipramine (Norpramin®) curbs cocaine desire, and methadone (Dolophine®) is prescribed for narcotic detoxification.

Some Common Psychotropic Drugs for Treating Alcohol or Drug Dependency

Type	Brand Name	Generic Name
Treatment for alcoholism	Antabuse	disulfiram
Treatment for alcoholism	ReVia	naltrexone
Treatment for cocaine addiction	Norpramin	desipramine
Narcotic detoxification	Dolophine	methadone

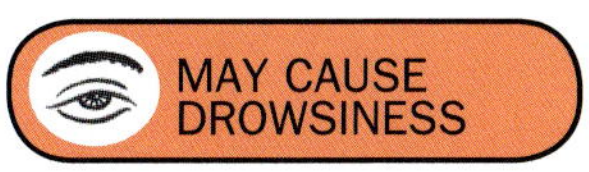

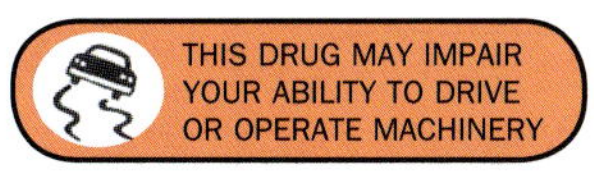

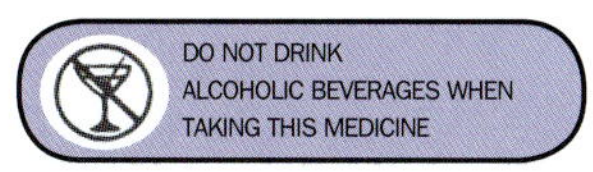

Rx safety you should know

- Psychotropic drugs, by their nature, often impair the central nervous system and can cause drowsiness. Technicians should consult with their pharmacists to see if auxiliary labels should be used to provide a reminder to the patient.

RESPIRATORY AGENTS

Balancing oxygen and carbon dioxide levels correctly is essential to health.

The cells of the body use oxygen for energy and produce carbon dioxide as waste. The respiratory system is responsible for exchanging oxygen from the air with carbon dioxide from the body. High carbon dioxide levels alert the medulla of the brain to signal inspiration (breathing in) to the diaphragm and intercostal muscles of the rib cage. It is their action that drives normal respiration. There are two phases of respiration: the mechanical phase, which involves the diaphragm and the rib cage and allows air to enter the lungs, and the physiologic phase in which oxygen and carbon dioxide are exchanged between the lungs and the blood cells. Dysfunction can occur at any time during either phase.

Emotional stimuli as well as medical disorders may alter gas exchange and breathing patterns.

Abnormal breathing patterns can occur for a variety of reasons and include dyspnea (labored breathing), wheezing, hyperventilation, and apnea (absence of breathing). Common respiratory disorders include: asthma, emphysema, bronchitis, COPD, croup, pneumonia, and allergy (see below).

Drugs commonly indicated in the treatment of respiratory disorders include antihistamines, decongestants, antitussives, and bronchodilators.

These agents act in a variety of ways to clear the airways and restore normal respiration.

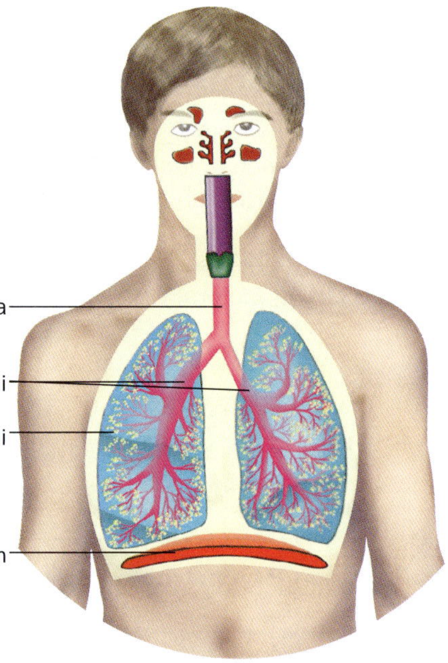

The trachea (windpipe) connects the larynx or voice box and the bronchi, the two airway branches that carry air to the lungs. The smaller bronchial tubes, called bronchioles, carry the air to the alveoli (air sacs) of the lungs where gas exchange takes place.

Common Respiratory Disorders

- **Asthma**: chronic airway inflammation related to stimuli hyperresponsiveness, resulting in airflow obstruction with symptoms such as wheezing and potentially acute spasms and breathlessness.
- **Allergy**: allergic response to food, drugs, animals, insect bites, pollens, or dust.
- **Emphysema:** chronic airway obstruction due to lung hyperinflation and diminished oxygen intake, characterized by breathlessness and flushed color.
- **Croup** (bronchiolitis): an infection of the bronchioles occurring in young children and resulting in airway obstruction and labored breathing.
- **Bronchitis**: infection producing excess mucus in the bronchial tree that makes breathing difficult.
- **COPD** (chronic obstructive pulmonary disease): also termed COLD (lung) or COAD (airway) by some sources. Abnormal lung function that generally encompasses both emphysema and chronic bronchitis that is present at least for 3 months a year for 2 consecutive years.
- **Pneumonia**: infectious process of either bacterial or viral origin whereby fluid accumulates in the lungs causing inadequate, or in severe cases ,impossible air exchange at the alveolar level.

CLASSES

Antihistamines

Antihistamines block the action of histamine from white blood cells or from inflammation-producing substances. Antihistamine agents replace histamine at the inflammation receptor sites to reduce inflammation, swelling, and irritation. Additional properties include: antipruritic (anti-itching), antiemetic, and sedative. Common antihistamines include hydroxyzine (Vistaril®), promethazine (Phenergan®), and loratadine (Claritin®).

Decongestants

Decongestants cause mucous membrane vasoconstriction, reduce nasal passage drainage, and relieve stuffiness. Pseudoephedrine (Sudafed®) is a common decongestant that is restricted by the Combat Methamphetamine Epidemic Act (CMEA) and must be kept behind the pharmacy counter (see Chapter 3 for more information about the CMEA). Phenylephrine (Sudafed PE®) is another common decongestant that is not restricted by the CMEA.

Antitussives

Antitussives treat both productive (with phlegm) and nonproductive (without phlegm) coughs. They are available in both narcotic and non-narcotic preparations. Dextromethorphan is the most widely used antitussive agent. Hydrocodone and chlorpheniramine (Tussionex®) is a common antihistamine/antitussive combination drug. Codeine and hydrocodone are examples of popular narcotic antitussive agents that are used in combination with other respiratory agents to treat coughing.

Some Common Respiratory Drugs: Antihistamines, Decongestants, and Antitussives

Type	Brand Name	Generic Name
Antihistamine	Vistaril	hydroxyzine
Antihistamine	Phenergan	promethazine
Antihistamine	Claritin	loratadine
Decongestant	Sudafed	pseudoephedrine
Decongestant	Sudafed PE	phenylephrine
Antitussive	Delsym	dextromethorphan
Antitussive (narcotic)/antihistamine	Tussionex	hydrocodone and chlorpheniramine

See Additional Common Drugs by Classification on pp 533-537 for more drugs in this class.

℞ safety you should know

➥ Narcotic antitussives and some antihistamines can cause severe drowsiness. Patients should use caution when taking medications that cause drowsiness.

RESPIRATORY AGENTS (cont'd)

CLASSES

Expectorants and Mucolytic Agents

Expectorants are used to treat chest congestion. Expectorants work by thinning the mucus that collects in the breathing passages. As the mucus becomes thinner, it is easier to cough up so the airways become more clear. An example of an expectorant is guaifenesin (Mucinex®). Mucolytic drugs that liquefy thickened bronchial mucus and assist in clearing airways are sometimes included in this category; acetylcysteine is a common mucolytic agent.

Bronchodilators

Bronchodilators relieve bronchospasm (a narrowing of the bronchi, accompanied by wheezing and coughing as seen in disorders such as asthma, emphysema, and bronchitis). Sympathomimetics (e.g., Proventil HFA® and albuterol) dilate the bronchi. Xanthine derivatives such as theopylline (Theo-Dur®) directly relax the smooth muscle of the bronchi. Both categories increase the opening of the bronchi and allow more airflow to occur. Corticosteroids such as beclomethasone (QVAR®) and anticholinergics such as ipratropium (Atrovent®) may be used to decrease respiratory airway inflammation and produce some bronchodilation.

Some Common Respiratory Drugs: Expectorants and Mucolytics

Type	Brand Name	Generic Name
Expectorant	Mucinex	guaifenesin
Expectorant/antitussive (narcotic)	n/a	guaifenesin and codeine
Expectorant/antitussive (non-narcotic)	Mucinex DM	guaifenesin and dextromethorphan
Mucolytic	n/a	acetylcysteine

Some Common Respiratory Drugs: Bronchodilators

Type	Brand Name	Generic Name
Bronchodilator/sympathomimetic	Proventil HFA	albuterol
Bronchodilator/xanthine derivative	Theo-24	theopylline
Bronchial corticosteroid	QVAR	beclomethasone
Anticholinergic	Atrovent HFA	ipratropium

See Additional Common Drugs by Classification on pp 533-537 for more drugs in this class.

℞ safety you should know

➡ Inhalers should be cleaned regularly. If inhalers are not properly cleaned they may become blocked and may not spray medication. Cleaning is also important to prevent germs from growing on the devices. Manufacturers provide instructions for patients to clean their inhalers.

ADDITIONAL COMMON DRUGS BY CLASSIFICATION 18

Following are additional common drugs from Drug Topics' 2010 Top 200 list that are not already included in the tables for each of the classification sections in this chapter. Drug Topics' website is http://drugtopics.modernmedicine.com/Pharmacy+Facts+&+Figures.

Class/Type	Brand Name	Generic Name
Analgesics		
NSAID	Arthrotec	diclofenac and misoprostol
NSAID	Celebrex	celecoxib
NSAID	Voltaren gel	diclofenac topical
Opiate	Opana ER	oxymorphone
Opiate	OxyContin	oxycodone
Anesthetics		
Local	Lidoderm	lidocaine transdermal
Anti-infectives		
Anti-Infective	Doryx	doxycycline
Anti-Infective	Solodyn	minocycline
Antineoplastics		
Hormone	Arimidex	anastrozole
Hormone	Femara	letrozole
Cardiovascular Agents		
Cardiovascular	Aggrenox	aspirin and dipyridamole
Cardiovascular	Aspir-Low	aspirin and dipyridamole
Cardiovascular	Plavix	clopidogrel
Anti-Angina	Ranexa	ranolazine
Anticoagulant	Lovenox	enoxaparin
Antihyperlipidemic	Crestor	rosuvastatin
Antihyperlipidemic	Lipitor	atorvastatin
Antihyperlipidemic	Lovaza	omega-3 fatty acid
Antihyperlipidemic	Niaspan	niacin
Antihyperlipidemic	Simcor	niacin
Antihyperlipidemic	Tricor	fenofibrate
Antihyperlipidemic	Trilipix	fenofibrate
Antihyperlipidemic	Welchol	colesevelam
Antihyperlipidemic	Zetia	ezetimibe
Antihyperlipidemic, Antihypertensive*	Caduet	amlodipine and atorvastatin
Antihypertensive*	Atacand	candesartan

**An asterisk next to a drug's classification indicates there are additional common uses for that drug.*

ADDITIONAL COMMON DRUGS BY CLASSIFICATION

Class/Type	Brand Name	Generic Name
Antihypertensive*	Avalide	irbesartan and hydrochlorothiazide
Antihypertensive*	Avapro	irbesartan
Antihypertensive*	Azor	amlodipine and olmesartan
Antihypertensive*	Benicar	olmesartan
Antihypertensive*	Benicar HCT	olmesartan and hydrochlorothiazide
Antihypertensive*	Bystolic	nebivolol
Antihypertensive*	Coreg CR	carvedilol
Antihypertensive*	Cozaar	losartan
Antihypertensive*	Diovan	valsartan
Antihypertensive*	Diovan HCT	hydrochlorothiazide and valsartan
Antihypertensive*	Exforge	amlodipine and valsartan
Antihypertensive*	Hyzaar	losartan and hydrochlorothiazide
Antihypertensive*	Lotrel	amlodipine and benazepril
Antihypertensive*	Micardis	telmisartan
Antihypertensive*	Micardis HCT	telmisartan and hydrochlorothiazide
Antihypertensive*	Tekturna	aliskiren
Antihypertensive*	Toprol XL	metoprolol
Dental		
Dental	SF 5000 Plus	fluoride
Dermatologicals		
Dermatological	Bactroban	mupirocin
Dermatological	BenzaClin	clindamycin and benzoyl peroxide
Dermatological	Differin	adapalene
Dermatological	Duac Care System	clindamycin and benzoyl peroxide
Dermatological	Epiduo	adapalene and benzoyl peroxide
Dermatological	Zovirax topical	acyclovir
Gastrointestinal Agents		
Gastrointentinal	Moviprep	polyethylene glycol electrolyte
Gastrointestinal	Amitiza	lubiprostone
Gastrointestinal	Asacol	mesalamine
Gastrointestinal	Dexilant/Kapidex	dexlansoprazole
Gastrointestinal	Relpax	for oral solution and bisacodyl
Gastrointestinal	Transderm-Scop	scopolamine
Antacid/antiulcer	Aciphex	rabeprazole
Antacid/antiulcer	Carafate	sucralfate
Antacid/antiulcer	Nexium	esomeprazole
Antacid/Antiulcer	Prevacid	lansoprazole

Class/Type	Brand Name	Generic Name
Antacid/Antiulcer	Prevacid SoluTab	lansoprazole
Antacid/Antiulcer	Protonix	pantoprazole
Laxative	Halflytely Bowel Prep Kit	PEG-3350, sodium chloride, sodium bicarbonate and potassium chloride
Hormones & Modifiers		
Hormones & Modifiers	Byetta	exenatide
Hormones & Modifiers	Prempro	conjugated estrogens and medroxyprogesterone
Hormones & Modifiers	Propecia	finasteride
Androgen	AndroGel	testosterone
Contraceptive	Apri	desogestrel and ethinyl estradiol
Contraceptive	Kariva	desogestrel and ethinyl estradiol
Contraceptive	Loestrin 24 Fe	ethinyl estradiol and norethindrone and iron
Contraceptive	NuvaRing	etonogestrel and ethinyl estradiol
Contraceptive	Ortho Tri-Cyclen	norgestimate and ethinyl estradiol
Contraceptive	Yaz	drosperinone and ethinyl estradiol
Estrogen	Estrace vaginal	estradiol
Estrogen	Vivelle-DOT	estradiol
Insulin	Humalog	insulin lispro
Insulin	Humalog Mix 75/25 Pen	insulin lispro protamine suspension mixed with soluble insulin lispro
Insulin	Humulin 70/30	insulin (human recombinant)
Insulin	Lantus SoloSTAR	insulin glargine [rDNA origin]
Insulin	Levemir	insulin detemir (rDNAorigin)
Insulin	Novolin 70/30	human insulin isophane suspension and regular, human insulin injection (rDNA origin)
Insulin	NovoLog	insulin aspart (rDNA origin)
Insulin	NovoLog Mix 70/30	insulin aspart protamine and insulin aspart (rDNA origin)
Oral antidiabetic	Actoplus Met	metformin and pioglitazone
Oral antidiabetic	Actos	pioglitazone
Oral antidiabetic	Avandia	rosiglitazone
Oral antidiabetic	Glipizide XL	glipizide
Oral antidiabetic	Janumet	metformin and sitagliptin
Oral antidiabetic	Januvia	sitagliptin
Oral antidiabetic	Prandin	repaglinide

ADDITIONAL COMMON DRUGS BY CLASSIFICATION

Class/Type	Brand Name	Generic Name
Phosphodiesterase inhibitor	Levitra	vardenafil
Progestins	Prometrium	progesterone
Thyroid	Levothroid	levothyroxine
Thyroid	Levoxyl	levothyroxine
Musculoskeletal Agents		
Muscle relaxant	Skelaxin	metaxalone
Osteoporitics	Boniva	ibandronate
Osteoporitics	Evista	raloxifene
Neurological Agents		
Neurological	Lyrica	pregabalin
ADHD	Focalin XR	dexmethylphenidate
ADHD	Metadate CD	methylphenidate
ADHD	Vyvanse	lisdexamfetamine
Anti-Alzheimer's	Exelon Patch	rivastigmine
Anti-Alzheimer's	Namenda	memantine
Antiepileptic*	Lamictal	lamotrigine
Antimigraine	Maxalt	rizatriptan
Antimigraine	Maxalt MLT	rizatriptan
Ophthalmic Agents		
Ophthalmic	Lotemax	loteprednol
Ophthalmic	Nevanac	nepafenac
Ophthalmic	Pataday	olopatadine
Ophthalmic	Restasis	cyclosporine
Ophthalmic	Vigamox	moxifloxacin ophthalmic
Ophthalmic	Zymar	gatifloxacin
Antiglaucoma	Alphagan P	brimonidine
Antiglaucoma	Combigan	brimonidine and timolol
Antiglaucoma	Lumigan	bimatoprost
Antiglaucoma	Travatan Z	travoprost
Antiglaucoma	Xalatan	latanoprost
Psychotropic Agents		
Psychotropic	Cymbalta	duloxetine
Psychotropic	Intuniv	guanfacine extended-release
Psychotropic	Nuvigil	armodafinil
Psychotropic	Provigil	modafinil
Psychotropic	Strattera	atomoxetine

Class/Type	Brand Name	Generic Name
Antidepressant	Pristiq	desvenlafaxine
Antidepressant	Wellbutrin XL	bupropion
Antipsychotic	Abilify	aripiprazole
Antipsychotic	Geodon oral	ziprasidone
Antipsychotic	Zyprexa	olanzapine
Drug dependency	Chantix	varenicline
Drug dependency	Suboxone	buprenorphine and naloxone
Hypnotic	Ambien CR	zolpidem
Hypnotic	Lunesta	eszopiclone
Respiratory Agents		
Respiratory	Advair Diskus	fluticasone and salmeterol
Respiratory	Advair HFA	fluticasone and salmeterol
Respiratory	Allegra-D 24 Hour	fexofenadine and pseudoephedrine
Respiratory	Asmanex	mometasone
Respiratory	Combivent	ipratropium and albuterol
Respiratory	Epipen	epinephrine
Respiratory	Flovent HFA	fluticasone
Respiratory	Nasacort AQ	triamcinolone
Respiratory	Nasonex	mometasone
Respiratory	Omnaris	ciclesonide
Respiratory	Pulmicort Flexhaler	budesonide
Respiratory	Rhinocort Aqua	budesonide
Respiratory	Singulair	montelukast
Respiratory	Spiriva	tiotropium
Respiratory	Symbicort	formoterol and budesonide
Respiratory	Tussionex	hydrocodone and chlorpheniramine
Respiratory	Veramyst	fluticasone
Antihistamine	Astelin	azelastine
Antihistamine	Astepro 0.15%	azelastine
Antihistamine	Clarinex	desloratadine
Antihistamine	Xyzal	levocetirizine
Bronchodilator	ProAir HFA	albuterol
Bronchodilator	Ventolin HFA	albuterol
Bronchodilator	Xopenex	levalbuterol
Bronchodilator	Xopenex HFA	levalbuterol

REVIEW

KEY CONCEPTS

DRUG NAMES AND CLASSES

- ✔ A drug's name begins with a chemical name.
- ✔ Marketed drugs under patent protection have one nonproprietary or generic name and one proprietary or brand name.
- ✔ The United States Adopted Names Council (USAN) designates the official nonproprietary names for drugs.

CLASSIFICATION SCHEMES

- ✔ There are various systems for classifying drugs: by disorder, body system affected, type of receptor acted on, type of action, etc.

ANALGESIC

- ✔ Analgesic drugs create a state in which the pain from a painful medical condition is reduced or not felt.
- ✔ Common types of analgesics include salicylates, acetaminophen, nonsteroidal anti-inflammatory, and opiate-type.

ANESTHETIC AGENTS

- ✔ Anesthetics cause an absence of sensation or pain.
- ✔ Anesthetics are classified as local or general.
- ✔ Local anesthetics block pain conduction without causing a loss of consciousness.
- ✔ General anesthetics are administered by inhalation or intravenously by an anesthesiologist and depress the central nervous system to the level of unconsciousness.

ANTI-INFECTIVES

- ✔ Anti-infectives treat diseases produced by microorganisms such as bacteria, viruses, fungi, protozoa, and parasitic worms.

ANTINEOPLASTICS

- ✔ Antineoplastics inhibit new growth of cancer cells.
- ✔ Side effects caused by many antineoplastic agents are often uncomfortable and serious.
- ✔ Pharmacists and pharmacy technicians must be very careful with all calculations associated with drugs that are used to treat cancer.

CARDIOVASCULAR AGENTS

- ✔ Cardiovascular agents include antianginals, antiarrhythmics, antihypertensives, vasopressors, antihyperlipidemics, thrombolytics, and anticoagulants.

DERMATOLOGICALS

- ✔ The skin is the body's protective barrier and is the largest organ of the body.
- ✔ Dermatologicals are drugs used to treat diseases or conditions related to the skin.

ELECTROLYTIC AGENTS

- ✔ Electrolytes are water-soluble substances that are contained in our body fluids as salts.
- ✔ Electrolyte balance is important for healthy body function.

GASTROINTESTINAL & URINARY TRACT AGENTS

- ✔ Gastrointestinal agents are used to treat disorders of the stomach and/or intestines.
- ✔ Urinary agents are used to treat conditions affecting the flow of urine.

HEMATOLOGICAL AGENTS

- ✔ Each stage in the formation of blood clots can be affected by intrinsic clotting factors and drugs.
- ✔ Hematopoietics are drugs that treat various forms of anemias.
- ✔ Hemostatic drugs are used to treat or prevent excessive bleeding.

HORMONES & MODIFIERS

- ✔ Hormones are secreted by glands of the endocrine system.
- ✔ The pancreas secretes the hormones insulin and glucagon. Insulin and glucagon are involved in regulating serum glucose.

IMMUNOBIOLOGIC AGENTS & VACCINES

- ✔ Immune globulins provide passive immunity.
- ✔ Vaccines provide active immunity.
- ✔ Immune globulins provide a shorter period of protection than vaccines.

MUSCULOSKELETAL AGENTS

- ✔ Musculoskeletal agents are used to treat rheumatoid arthritis, osteoarthritis, gout, osteoporosis, and muscle spasms.

NEUROLOGICAL AGENTS

- ✔ Several common disorders are affected by abnormalities in neurotransmitter release and/or response and include Parkinson's disease, Alzheimer's disease, epilepsy, migraine headaches, multiple sclerosis, and attention deficit hyperactivity disorder.

OPHTHALMIC & OTIC AGENTS

- ✔ Ophthalmic agents are used to treat conditions such as glaucoma, eye infection, eye pain, and inflammation. They are also used for eye examinations and in preparation for surgery.
- ✔ Otic agents are used to treat conditions including accumulation of earwax and infections of the outer ear.

PSYCHOTROPIC AGENTS

- ✔ Psychotropic agents are used to treat conditions such as bipolar disorder, anxiety, depression, schizophrenia, and drug abuse.

RESPIRATORY AGENTS

- ✔ Common respiratory disorders include asthma, allergy, emphysema, croup, bronchitis, chronic obstructive pulmonary disease, and pneumonia.

REVIEW

SELF TEST

the answer key begins on page 569

MATCH THE TERMS: I

1. analgesia ____
2. androgens ____
3. anemia ____
4. anion ____
5. anthelmintic ____
6. antipyretic ____
7. bactericidal ____
8. bacteriostatic ____
9. blocker ____
10. cation ____
11. chyme ____
12. clotting factors ____
13. conjunctivitis ____
14. corticosteroid ____
15. dermatological ____
16. diabetes mellitus ____
17. dissociation ____
18. electrolytes ____
19. endocrine system ____
20. estrogens ____
21. extracellular fluids ____
22. fibrin ____
23. fibrinogen ____

a. inflammation of the conjunctiva (eyelid lining).

b. another term for an antagonist drug, because antagonists block the action of neurotransmitters.

c. a state in which pain is not felt even though a painful condition exists.

d. reduces fever.

e. drug that destroys worms.

f. bacteria killing.

g. bacteria inhibiting.

h. a product used to treat a skin condition.

i. when a compound breaks down and separates into smaller components.

j. a substance that in solution forms ions that conduct an electrical current.

k. the fluid outside the body's individual cells found in plasma and tissue fluid.

l. the semiliquid form of food as it enters the intestinal tract.

m. factors in the blood coagulation process.

n. Factor I.

o. the fiber that serves as the structure for clot formation.

p. a decrease in hemoglobin or red blood cells.

q. a system of glands that secrete hormones into the bloodstream.

r. male sex characteristic hormones.

s. female sex characteristic hormone that are involved in calcium and phosphorus conservation.

t. hormonal steroid substances produced by the cortex of the adrenal gland.

u. a condition in which the body does not produce enough insulin or is unable to use it efficiently.

v. a negatively charged ion.

w. a positively charged ion.

MATCH THE TERMS: II

1. glaucoma ____
2. glucagon ____
3. gout ____
4. hematopoietics ____
5. hemostatic drugs ____
6. homeostasis ____
7. hormone ____
8. hyperthyroidism ____
9. hypothyroidism ____
10. insulin ____
11. ions ____
12. integumentary system ____
13. interstitial fluid ____
14. intracellular fluid ____
15. intraocular ____
16. Islands (or islets) of Langerhans ____
17. lymphocyte ____
18. medullary paralysis ____
19. metastasis ____
20. mimetic ____
21. mydriatics ____
22. neoplasm ____
23. neurotransmitter ____
24. osteoarthritis ____

a. chemicals produced by the body that regulate body functions and processes.
b. a type of white blood cell that helps the body defend itself against bacteria an diseased cells.
c. a hormone that helps convert amino acids to glucose.
d. electrically charged particles.
e. abnormally high pressure within the eye leading to optic nerve damage and loss of vision.
f. the body covering, i.e., skin, hair, and nails.
g. a painful inflammatory condition in which excess uric acid accumulates in the joints.
h. a hormone that controls the body's use of glucose.
i. specialized cells of the pancreas that secrete insulin.
j. the state of equilibrium of the body.
k. drugs that dilate the pupil.
l. inside the eye.
m. drugs used to treat anemia.
n. cell fluid.
o. drugs that prevent excessive bleeding.
p. tissue fluid.
q. underproduction of thyroid hormone.
r. when cancer cells spread beyond their original site.
s. overproduction of thyroid hormone.
t. another term for an agonist, because agonists imitate or mimic the action of the neurotransmitter.
u. a new and abnormal tissue growth, often referring to cancer cells.
v. chemicals released by nerves that interact with receptors to cause an effect.
w. an overdose of anesthesia that paralyzes the respiratory and heart centers of the medulla, leading to death.
x. a disorder characterized by weight-bearing bone deterioration, decreasing range of motion, pain, and deformity.

REVIEW

MATCH THE TERMS: III

1. peristalsis ____
2. progesterone ____
3. protease inhibitor ____
4. remission ____
5. rheumatoid arthritis ____
6. serum glucose ____
7. surgical anesthesia ____
8. testosterone ____
9. topical hemostatics ____
10. uricosuric drugs ____

a. a chronic and often progressive inflammatory condition with symptoms that include swelling, feelings of warmth, and joint pain.
b. drugs used to treat gout that increase the elimination of uric acid.
c. the stage of anesthesia in which surgery can be safely conducted.
d. an antiviral used for HIV and hepatitis C that blocks the enzyme responsible for viral replication.
e. a state in which cancer cells are inactive.
f. the wave-like motion of the intestines that moves food through them.
g. drugs used for minor bleeding when sutures are not appropriate.
h. blood sugar.
i. a female sex characteristic hormone involved in ovulation prevention.
j. the primary androgen.

MATCH THE BRAND AND GENERIC DRUG NAMES: I

Brand	Generic	Brand	Generic
1. Ceclor ____	a. ceftazidime	6. Keflex ____	f. ceftriaxone
2. Ceftin ____	b. cefprozil	7. Maxipime ____	g. cefepime
3. Cefzil ____	c. cefuroxime	8. Omnicef ____	h. cefdinir
4. Duricef ____	d. cefaclor	9. Rocephin ____	i. cefadroxil
5. Fortaz ____	e. cephalexin		

MATCH THE BRAND AND GENERIC DRUG NAMES: II

Brand	Generic	Brand	Generic
1. Amikin ____	a. clindamycin	6. Cipro ____	f. mupirocin
2. Avelox ____	b. aztreonam	7. Cleocin ____	g. clarithromycin
3. Azactam ____	c. amikacin	8. Cubicin ____	h. moxifloxacin
4. Bactroban ____	d. gentamicin	9. Erythrocin ____	i. daptomycin
5. Biaxin ____	e. erythromycin	10. Gentak ____	j. ciprofloxacin

MATCH THE BRAND AND GENERIC DRUG NAMES: III

Brand		Generic		Brand		Generic	
1.	Solodyn _____	a.	ertapenem	6.	Primaxin _____	f.	azithromycin
2.	Invanz _____	b.	minocycline	7.	Streptomycin _____	g.	nitrofurantoin
3.	Levaquin _____	c.	levofloxacin	8.	Tobrex _____	h.	meropenem
4.	Macrodantin _____	d.	tobramycin	9.	Vancocin _____	i.	imipenem, cilastatin
5.	Merrem _____	e.	streptomycin	10.	Zithromax _____	j.	vancomycin

MATCH THE BRAND AND GENERIC DRUG NAMES: IV

Brand		Generic		Brand		Generic	
1.	Zyvox _____	a.	ticarcillin, clavulanate	5.	Timentin _____	e.	penicillin G
2.	Albenza _____	b.	linezolid	6.	Unasyn _____	f.	piperacillin, tazobactam
3.	Flagyl _____	c.	albendazole	7.	Veetids _____	g.	penicillin V potassium
4.	Bicillin L-A _____	d.	metronidazole	8.	Zosyn _____	h.	ampicillin, sulbactam

MATCH THE BRAND AND GENERIC DRUG NAMES: V

Brand		Generic		Brand		Generic	
1.	Bactrim _____	a.	amoxicillin, clavulanate	4.	Minocin _____	d.	tetracycline
2.	Moxatag _____	b.	trimethoprim, sulfamethoxazole	5.	Sumycin _____	e.	minocycline
3.	Augmentin _____	c.	doxycycline	6.	Vibramycin _____	f.	amoxicillin

MATCH THE BRAND AND GENERIC DRUG NAMES: VI

Brand		Generic		Brand		Generic	
1.	Atripla _____	a.	efavirenz, emtricitabine, tenofovir	5.	Relenza _____	e.	ritonavir
2.	Isentress _____	b.	zanamivir	6.	Reyataz _____	f.	darunavir
3.	Norvir _____	c.	oseltamivir	7.	Tamiflu _____	g.	raltegravir
4.	Prezista _____	d.	atazanavir				

REVIEW

MATCH THE BRAND AND GENERIC DRUG NAMES: VII

Brand		Generic		Brand		Generic	
1.	Cardizem _____	a.	metoprolol	7.	Procardia _____	g.	atenolol
2.	Tenormin _____	b.	diltiazem	8.	Lasix _____	h.	nadolol
3.	Corgard _____	c.	nifedipine	9.	Microzide _____	i.	hydrochlorothiazide
4.	Lopressor _____	d.	amlodipine	10.	Capoten _____	j.	furosemide
5.	Calan _____	e.	enalapril	11.	Vasotec _____	k.	verapamil
6.	Norvasc _____	f.	captopril				

MATCH THE BRAND AND GENERIC DRUG NAMES: VIII

Brand		Generic		Brand		Generic	
1.	Nitrostat _____	a.	warfarin	6.	Altace _____	f.	sotalol
2.	Lanoxin _____	b.	digoxin	7.	Coumadin ____	g.	exetimibe, simvastatin
3.	Betapace _____	c.	nitroglycerin	8.	Aldactone ____	h.	spironolactone
4.	Zocor _____	d.	ramipril	9.	Vytorin _____	i.	simvastatin
5.	Pravachol _____	e.	pravastatin				

MATCH THE BRAND AND GENERIC DRUG NAMES: IX

Brand		Generic		Brand		Generic	
1.	Actonel _____	a.	cyclobenzaprine	4.	Soma _____	d.	carisoprodol
2.	Fosamax _____	b.	risedronate	5.	Flexeril _____	e.	diazepam
3.	Valium _____	c.	alendronate				

MATCH THE BRAND AND GENERIC DRUG NAMES: X

Brand		Generic		Brand		Generic	
1.	Sinemet _____	a.	carbidopa/levodopa	6.	Zoloft _____	f.	phenytoin
2.	Eldepryl _____	b.	ibuprofen	7.	Dilantin _____	g.	selegiline
3.	Cogentin _____	c.	methylphenidate	8.	Tegretol _____	h.	carbamazepine
4.	Aricept _____	d.	benztropine	9.	Motrin _____	i.	paroxetine
5.	Paxil _____	e.	sertraline	10.	Ritalin _____	j.	donepezil

CHOOSE THE BEST ANSWER

1. A drug's name that describes its structure and compounds:
   a. proprietary.
   b. nonproprietary.
   c. chemical.
   d. brand.

2. The ________________ designates nonproprietary names for drugs.
   a. APhA
   b. ASH
   c. USAN
   d. pharmaceutical company

3. An example of a naturally occurring opiate drug is
   a. morphine.
   b. meperidine.
   c. ibuprofen.
   d. naproxen.

4. All of the following are antipyretic EXCEPT
   a. opiate-type analgesics.
   b. NSAIDs.
   c. acetaminophen.
   d. salicylates.

5. Which anesthetic is administered through an IV?
   a. propofol
   b. isoflurane
   c. sevoflurane
   d. desflurane

6. Which antibiotic contains sulfa?
   a. Sumycin®
   b. Bactrim DS®
   c. Ceclor®
   d. Geocillin®

7. ____________________ is an example of an antiviral drug.
   a. Zithromax®
   b. Flagyl®
   c. Valtrex®
   d. Vermox®

8. An example of an anthelmintic drug is
   a. Albenza®.
   b. Valtrex®.
   c. Zithromax®.
   d. Augmentin®.

9. A term for a state in which cancer cells are inactive is
   a. neoplasm.
   b. metastasis.
   c. lymphocyte.
   d. remission.

10. ________________ is an example of an ACE inhibitor.
    a. Lasix®
    b. Vasotec®
    c. Cardizem®
    d. Norvasc®

11. ___________________ is an example of an antianginal drug.
    a. Heparin
    b. Pravastatin
    c. Warfarin
    d. Nitroglycerin

12. ________________ is an example of an antihyperlipidemic drug.
    a. simvastatin.
    b. dobutamine.
    c. ramipril.
    d. digoxin.

REVIEW

13. An isotonic solution of sodium chloride:
    a. Lactated Ringer's Solution™.
    b. D5LR.
    c. normal saline.
    d. Klor Con®.

14. An example of an antiemetic is
    a. trimethebenzomide.
    b. loperamide.
    c. pancrilipase.
    d. atropine.

15. An example of a stool softener is
    a. docusate sodium.
    b. loperamide.
    c. diphenoxylate plus atropine.
    d. pancrelipase.

16. Accidental overdose from ___________ is a leading cause of fatal poisoning in children under the age of six.
    a. cyanocobalmin
    b. aprotinin
    c. iron
    d. vitamin K

17. ______________ is the main hormone that controls the body's use of glucose.
    a. Glucagon
    b. Insulin
    c. Epinephrine
    d. Cortisone

18. The generic name for Lantus® is
    a. lente.
    b. glyburide.
    c. glipizide.
    d. glargine.

19. Female sex characteristic hormone involved in ovulation prevention:
    a. progesterone.
    b. estrogens.
    c. androgens.
    d. methylprednisolone.

20. A live attenuated influenza vaccine is
    a. Fluarix®.
    b. Fluvirin®.
    c. Flumist®.
    d. Fluzone®.

21. A disorder characterized by weight-bearing bone deterioration, decreasing range of motion, pain, and deformity is
    a. rheumatoid arthritis.
    b. osteoarthritis.
    c. gout.
    d. osteoporosis.

22. All of the following drugs are used to treat muscle spasms except
    a. cyclobenzaprine.
    b. carisoprodol.
    c. diazepam.
    d. alendronate.

23. A progressive dementia is
    a. Alzheimer's disease.
    b. Parkinson's disease.
    c. rheumatoid arthritis.
    d. osteoarthritis.

24. The following drugs are associated with migraine prophylactic treatment EXCEPT ______________.
    a. beta-blockers
    b. calcium channel blockers
    c. antidepressants
    d. diuretics

25. Which of these statements is false?
    a. Otic products must never be used in the eye.
    b. Ophthalmic products can never be used in the ear.
    c. The most common conditions treated with otic products are associated with accumulation of earwax and infections of the outer ear.
    d. The technique for administering ear drops is different for children under three years than for children older than three years.

26. A disorder also known as manic depression:
    a. schizophrenia.
    b. bipolar disorder.
    c. anxiety.
    d. ADHD.

27. A drug used to treat depression is
    a. Zoloft®.
    b. alprazolam.
    c. Ativan®.
    d. Seconal®.

28. An example of a decongestant is
    a. pseudoephedrine.
    b. dextromethorphan.
    c. guaifenesin.
    d. albuterol.

29. An example of a sympathomimetic agent used to dilate the bronchi in asthma:
    a. albuterol.
    b. prednisone.
    c. Benadryl®.
    d. Claritin®.

30. An infection of the bronchioles that occurs in young children is
    a. COPD.
    b. asthma.
    c. emphysema.
    d. croup.

CRITICAL THINKING QUESTIONS

1. What are some reasons proprietary drug names are easier to remember than non-proprietary drug names?
2. What are some reasons for different classifications of drugs?

THINKING IT THROUGH WRAP-UP

1. A root canal is a major dental procedure that could be associated with infection and pain. Amoxicillin would treat possible infection and ibuprofen would help with pain.
2. An anesthetic could have been used during the procedure to block pain.
3. Taking antibiotics correctly is important to treat and prevent infections. The amount of pain and discomfort would be worse with an infection.

LOOK-ALIKE / SOUNDALIKE

It is important to recognize that a number of drugs have similar sounding or looking names, but very different properties.

Besides similarity, one of the primary problems with accuracy in drug name identification is that prescriptions are still largely written by hand. However, it is also true that there are many ways drug names are miscommunicated (by mispronunciation, typos, etc.). Therefore, the identification of a drug should be verified as many ways as possible.

Accuracy in handling and using drugs is essential.

Confusing one drug with another can lead to terrible and sometimes fatal consequences. It is critical to make certain that you have the name correct when involved in any aspect of the prescription process. At right is a list of drugs that can be mistaken for one another either by their sound or how they appear when written. There are many others, but this should illustrate the need for accuracy in drug names.

Identifying Forms

Frequent handling of a drug will help you remember its physical characteristics (size, shape, color, markings, etc.), and this can be a valuable skill in the safe handling of drugs. It should be noted, however, that the most important step in identifying drugs is identifying the correct name. All drug information from the manufacturer to the prescriber, pharmacist, and ultimately the user is based upon communicating the correct name of the drug.

IDENTIFYING DRUG NAMES

At right is a list of drug names that might be easily misread, mispronounced, or otherwise mistaken for each other. Note that this is only a sample and that there are many other drugs with similar looking or sounding names.

Acetazolamide	Acetohexamide
Alfentanil	Fentanyl, Sufentanil
Amitriptyline	Aminophylline
Atenolol	Albuterol
Azathioprine	Azatadine
Baclofen	Bactroban®, Beclovent®
Bupropion	Buspirone
Calcitonin	Calcitriol
Captopril	Capitrol
Cefamandole	Cefmetazole
Cefonicid	Cefobid®
Cefotaxime	Ceftizoxime
Cefoxitin	Cefotaxime
Ceftizoxime	Ceftazidime
Cephalexin	Cephalothin
Chlorpropamide	Chlorpromazine
Clomiphene	Clomipramine
Clonazepam	Clofazimine
Clorazepate	Clofibrate
Clotrimazole	Co-trimoxazole
Cyclosporine	Cycloserine
Dapsone	Daypro®
Dexamethasone	Desoximetasone
Digoxin	Digitoxin
Diphenhydramine	Dimenhydrinate
Dopamine	Dobutamine
Doxazosin	Doxorubicin
Doxepin	Doxapram, Doxidan®
Dronabinol	Droperidol
Dyclonine	Dicyclomine
Encainide	Flecainide
Enflurane	Isoflurane
Etidronate	Etretinate
Flunisolide	Fluocinonide
Glyburide	Glipizide
Guanadrel	Gonadorelin
Guanethidine	Guanidine
Guanfacine	Guaifenesin, Guanidine
Halcinonide	Halcion®
Hydralazine	Hydroxyzine
Hydrochlorothiazide	Hydroflumethiazide
Hydrocortisone	Hydrocodone
Kanamycin	Garamycin®, Gentamicin
Lisinopril	Fosinopril
Magnesium Sulfate	Manganese Sulfate
Methicillin	Mezlocillin
Metolazone	Metaxalone
Metoprolol	Metaproterenol
Nifedipine	Nicardipine
Oxymorphone	Oxymetholone
Pancuronium	Pipecuronium
Pentobarbital	Phenobarbital
Phenytoin	Mephenytoin
Pramoxine	Pralidoxime
Prazosin	Prednisone
Prednisone	Prednisolone
Primidone	Prednisone
Quazepam	Oxazepam
Reserpine	Risperidone
Ribavirin	Riboflavin
Ritodrine	Ranitidine
Sucralfate	Salsalate
Sulfadiazine	Sulfasalazine
Sulfamethizole	Sulfamethoxazole
Terbutaline	Tolbutamide
Terconazole	Tioconazole
Testoderm®	Estraderm®
Thyrar®	Thyrolar®
Thyrolar®	Theolair®
Timolol	Atenolol
Tolazamide	Tolbutamide
Torsemide	Furosemide
Tretinoin	Trientine
Triamterene	Trimipramine
Vincristine	Vinblastine
Zofran®	Zoloft®

TOP 200 BRAND NAME DRUGS

Following is a list of the Top 200 Brand Name Drugs cross-referenced with corresponding generic drug names and the classifications used in this text. Rankings are based on Drug Topics' 2010 Top 200 list (available at http://drugtopics.modernmedicine.com/Pharmacy+Facts+&+Figures).

Brand Name		Generic Name	Classification
1.	Lipitor	atorvastatin	Cardiovascular, Antihyperlipidemic
2.	Nexium	esomeprazole	Gastrointestinal, Antacid/Antiulcer
3.	Plavix	clopidogrel	Cardiovascular
4.	Singulair	montelukast	Respiratory
5.	Lexapro	escitalopram	Psychotropic, Antidepressant
6.	Crestor	rosuvastatin	Cardiovascular, Antihyperlipidemic
7.	Synthroid	levothyroxine	Hormones & Modifiers, Thyroid
8.	ProAir HFA	albuterol	Respiratory, Bronchodilator
9.	Advair Diskus	fluticasone and salmeterol	Respiratory
10.	Cymbalta	duloxetine	Psychotropic
11.	Diovan	valsartan	Cardiovascular, Antihypertensive*
12.	Ventolin HFA	albuterol	Respiratory, Bronchodilator
13.	Diovan HCT	hydrochlorothiazide and valsartan	Cardiovascular, Antihypertensive*
14.	Actos	pioglitazone	Hormones & Modifiers, Oral antidiabetic
15.	Seroquel	quetiapine	Psychotropic, Antipsychotic
16.	Levaquin	levofloxacin	Anti-infective
17.	Lantus	Insulin glargine	Hormones & Modifiers, Insulin
18.	Nasonex	mometasone	Respiratory
19.	Viagra	sildenafil	Hormones & Modifiers, Phosphodiesterase inhibitor
20.	Lyrica	pregabalin	Neurological
21.	Celebrex	celecoxib	Analgesic, NSAID
22.	Concerta	methylphenidate	Psychotropic/Neurologic/ADHD
23.	Spiriva	tiotropium	Respiratory
24.	Premarin tablets	conjugated estrogens	Hormones & Modifiers, Estrogen
25.	Effexor XR	venlafaxine	Psychotropic, Antidepressant
26.	Tricor	fenofibrate	Cardiovascular, Antihyperlipidemic
27.	Zetia	ezetimibe	Cardiovascular, Antihyperlipidemic
28.	Vytorin	ezetimibe and simvastatin	Cardiovascular, Antihyperlipidemic
29.	OxyContin	oxycodone	Analgesic, Opiate
30.	Abilify	aripiprazole	Psychotropic, Antipsychotic
31.	Loestrin 24 Fe	ethinyl estradiol and norethindrone and iron	Hormones & Modifiers, Contraceptive

**An asterisk next to a drug's classification indicates there are additional common uses for that drug.*

Brand Name	Generic Name	Classification
32. Vyvanse	lisdexamfetamine	Psychotropic
33. Cialis	tadalafil	Hormones & Modifiers, Phosphodiesterase inhibitor
34. Suboxone	buprenorphine and naloxone	Psychotropic, Drug dependency
35. Aricept	donepezil	Neurological, Anti-Alzheimer's
36. Benicar	olmesartan	Cardiovascular, Antihypertensive*
37. Januvia	sitagliptin	Hormones & Modifiers, Oral antidiabetic
38. Lunesta	eszopiclone	Psychotropic, Hypnotic
39. Ambien CR	zolpidem	Psychotropic, Hypnotic
40. Niaspan	niacin	Cardiovascular, Antihyperlipidemic
41. Xalatan	latanoprost	Ophthalmic, Antiglaucoma
42. Levoxyl	levothyroxine	Hormones & Modifiers, Thyroid
43. Benicar HCT	olmesartan and hydrochlorothiazide	Cardiovascular, Antihypertensive*
44. Flovent HFA	fluticasone	Respiratory
45. NuvaRing	etonogestrel and ethinyl estradiol	Hormones & Modifiers, Contraceptive
46. Lovaza	omega-3 fatty acid	Cardiovascular, Antihyperlipidemic
47. Yaz	drosperinone and ethinyl estradiol	Hormones & Modifiers, Contraceptive
48. NovoLog	insulin aspart (rDNA origin)	Hormones & Modifiers, Insulin
49. Combivent	ipratropium and albuterol	Respiratory
50. Namenda	memantine	Neurological, Anti-Alzheimer's
51. Detrol LA	tolterodine	Urinary
52. Ortho Tri Cyclen	norgestimate and ethinyl estradiol	Hormones & Modifiers, Contraceptive
53. Lantus SoloSTAR	insulin glargine (rDNA origin)	Hormones & Modifiers, Insulin
54. Proventil HFA	albuterol	Respiratory, Bronchodilator
55. Aciphex	rabeprazole	Gastrointestinal, Antacid/Antiulcer
56. Avapro	irbesartan	Cardiovascular, Antihypertensive*
57. Bystolic	nebivolol	Cardiovascular, Antihypertensive*
58. Adderall XR	dextroamphetamine and amphetamine	Psychotropic/Neurologic/ADHD
59. Symbicort	formoterol and budesonide	Respiratory
60. Zyprexa	olanzapine	Psychotropic, Antipsychotic
61. Trilipix	fenofibrate	Cardiovascular, Antihyperlipidemic
62. Boniva	ibandronate	Musculoskeletal, Osteoporitic
63. Avodart	dutasteride	Urinary
64. Glipizide XL	glipizide	Hormones & Modifiers, Oral antidiabetic
65. Pristiq	desvenlafaxine	Psychotropic, Antidepressant

TOP 200 BRAND NAME DRUGS

Brand Name		Generic Name	Classification
66.	Lidoderm	lidocaine transdermal	Anesthetic, Local
67.	Humalog	insulin lispro	Hormones & Modifiers, Insulin
68.	Vigamox	moxifloxacin ophthalmic	Ophthalmic
69.	Evista	raloxifene	Musculoskeletal, Osteoporitic
70.	Flomax	tamsulosin	Urinary
71.	Chantix	varenicline	Psychotropic, Drug dependency
72.	Avalide	irbesartan and hydrochlorothiazide	Cardiovascular, Antihypertensive*
73.	Protonix	pantoprazole	Gastrointestinal, Antacid/Antiulcer
74.	Cozaar	losartan	Cardiovascular, Antihypertensive*
75.	Vivelle-DOT	estradiol	Hormones & Modifiers, Estrogen
76.	Vesicare	solifenacin	Urinary
77.	Prempro	conjugated estrogens and medroxyprogesterone	Hormones & Modifiers
78.	Avelox	moxifloxacin	Anti-infective
79.	Dexilant/Kapidex	dexlansoprazole	Gastrointestinal
80.	Focalin XR	dexmethylphenidate	Psychotropic/Neurologic/ADHD
81.	Strattera	atomoxetine	Psychotropic
82.	Xopenex HFA	levalbuterol	Respiratory, Bronchodilator
83.	Actonel	risedronate	Musculoskeletal, Osteoporitic
84.	Travatan Z	travoprost	Ophthalmic, Antiglaucoma
85.	Levemir	insulin detemir (rDNA origin)	Hormones & Modifiers, Insulin
86.	Lumigan	bimatoprost	Ophthalmic, Antiglaucoma
87.	Apri	desogestrel and ethinyl estradiol	Hormones & Modifiers, Contraceptive
88.	Levitra	vardenafil	Hormones & Modifiers, Phosphodiesterase inhibitor
89.	Geodon oral	ziprasidone	Psychotropic, Antipsychotic
90.	Micardis	telmisartan	Cardiovascular, Antihypertensive*
91.	Exforge	amlodipine and valsartan	Cardiovascular, Antihypertensive*
92.	Coumadin tabs	warfarin	Cardiovascular, Anticoagulant
93.	Janumet	metformin and sitagliptin	Hormones & Modifiers, Oral antidiabetic
94.	Ciprodex otic	ciprofloxacin and dexamethasone	Otic
95.	Valtrex	valacyclovir	Anti-infective, Antiviral
96.	Restasis	cyclosporine	Ophthalmic
97.	Seroquel XR	quetiapine	Psychotropic, Antipsychotic
98.	Micardis HCT	telmisartan and hydrochlorothiazide	Cardiovascular, Antihypertensive*
99.	Actonel 150	risedronate	Musculoskeletal, Osteoporitic

Brand Name	Generic Name	Classification
100. Lotrel	amlodipine and benazepril	Cardiovascular, Antihypertensive*
101. Tussionex	hydrocodone and chlorpheniramine	Respiratory
102. Prometrium	progesterone	Hormones & Modifiers, Progestin
103. AndroGel	testosterone	Hormones & Modifiers, Androgen
104. Kariva	desogestrel and ethinyl estradiol	Hormones & Modifiers, Contraceptive
105. Patanol	olopatadine	Ophthalmic
106. Voltaren gel	diclofenac topical	Analgesic, NSAID
107. Hyzaar	losartan and hydrochlorothiazide	Cardiovascular, Antihypertensive*
108. Thyroid, Armour	desiccated thyroid	Hormones & Modifiers, Thyroid
109. Nasacort AQ	triamcinolone	Respiratory
110. Coreg CR	carvedilol	Cardiovascular, Antihypertensive*
111. QVAR	beclomethasone	Respiratory
112. Pataday	olopatadine	Ophthalmic
113. Xyzal	levocetirizine	Respiratory, Antihistamine
114. Humulin N	insulin (human recombinant)	Hormones & Modifiers, Insulin
115. Vagifem	estrogen	Hormones & Modifiers, Estrogen
116. Toprol XL	metoprolol	Cardiovascular, Antihypertensive*
117. Byetta	exenatide	Hormones & Modifiers
118. NovoLog Mix 70/30	insulin aspart protamine and insulin aspart (rDNA origin)	Hormones & Modifiers, Insulin
119. Veramyst	fluticasone	Respiratory
120. Azor	amlodipine and olmesartan	Cardiovascular, Antihypertensive*
121. Caduet	amlodipine and atorvastatin	Cardiovascular, Antihyperlipidemic, Antihypertensive*
122. Welchol	colesevelam	Cardiovascular, Antihyperlipidemic
123. Actoplus Met	metformin and pioglitazone	Hormones & Modifiers, Oral antidiabetic
124. Provigil	modafinil	Psychotropic
125. Epipen	epinephrine	Respiratory
126. Aggrenox	aspirin and dipyridamole	Cardiovascular
127. Dilantin	phenytoin	Neurological, Antiepileptic
128. Enablex	darifenacin	Urinary
129. Alphagan P	brimonidine	Ophthalmic, Antiglaucoma
130. Premarin vaginal	conjugated estrogens	Hormones & Modifiers, Estrogen
131. Xopenex	levalbuterol	Respiratory, Bronchodilator
132. Uroxatral	alfuzosin	Urinary
133. Asmanex	mometasone	Respiratory

TOP 200 BRAND NAME DRUGS

Brand Name	Generic Name	Classification
134. Prevacid SoluTab	lansoprazole	Gastrointestinal, Antacid/Antiulcer
135. Moviprep	Polyethylene glycol electrolyte	Gastrointentinal
136. Avandia	rosiglitazone	Hormones & Modifiers, Oral antidiabetic
137. Tekturna	aliskiren	Cardiovascular, Antihypertensive*
138. Propecia	finasteride	Hormones & Modifiers
139. Ortho Evra	norelgestromin and ethinyl estradiol	Hormones & Modifiers, Contraceptive
140. Solodyn	minocycline	Anti-infective
141 Humulin 70/30	insulin (human recombinant)	Hormones & Modifiers, Insulin
142 Lanoxin	digoxin	Cardiovascular, Antiarrhythmic
143. Asacol	mesalamine	Gastrointestinal
144. Prevacid	lansoprazole	Gastrointestinal, Antacid/Antiulcer
145. Atacand	candesartan	Cardiovascular, Antihypertensive*
146. Nitrostat	nitroglycerin	Cardiovascular
147. Combigan	brimonidine and timolol	Ophthalmic, Antiglaucoma
148. HalfLytely Bowel Prep Kit	PEG-3350, sodium chloride, sodium bicarbonate and potassium chloride for oral solution and bisacodyl	Gastrointestinal, Laxative
149. Relpax	eletriptan	Neurological, Antimigraine
150. Novolin 70/30	human insulin isophane suspension and regular, human insulin injection (rDNA origin)	Hormones & Modifiers, Insulin
151. Femara	letrozole	Antineoplastic, Hormone
152. Tamiflu	oseltamivir	Anti-infective, Antiviral
153. Zovirax topical	acyclovir	Dermatological
184. Lovenox	enoxaparin	Cardiovascular, Anticoagulant
155. Zymar	gatifloxacin	Ophthalmic
156. Maxalt	rizatriptan	Neurological, Antimigraine
157. Estrace vaginal	estradiol	Hormones & Modifiers, Estrogen
158. Exelon patch	rivastigmine	Neurological, Anti-Alzheimer's
159. Intuniv	guanfacine extended-release	Psychotropic
160. Allegra-D 24	fexofenadine and pseudoephedrine	Respiratory
161. Astrepo 0.15%	azelastine	Respiratory, Antihistamine
162. Maxalt MLT	rizatriptan	Neurological, Antimigraine
163. Arimidex	anastrozole	Antineoplastic, Hormone
164. Amitiza	lubiprostone	Gastrointestinal
165. Doryx	doxycycline	Anti-infective
166. Differin	adapalene	Dermatological

Brand Name	Generic Name	Classification
167. Clarinex	desloratadine	Respiratory, Antihistamine
168. Lotemax	loteprednol	Ophthalmic
169. Astelin	azelastine	Respiratory, Antihistamine
170. Transderm-Scop	scopolamine	Gastrointestinal
171. Humulin R	insulin (human recombinant)	Hormones & Modifiers, Insulin
172. Levothroid	levothyroxine	Hormones & Modifiers, Thyroid
173. Advair HFA	fluticasone and salmeterol	Respiratory
174. Truvada	tenofovir/emtricitabine	Anti-Infective, Antiviral
175. Nuvigil	armodafinil	Psychotropic
176. SF 5000 Plus	fluoride	Dental
177. Yasmin 28	drospirenone and ethinyl estradiol	Hormones & Modifiers, Contraceptive
178. Bactroban	mupirocin	Dermatological
179. Ranexa	ranolazine	Cardiovascular, Antiangina
180. Metadate CD	methylphenidate	Psychotropic
181. Lamictal	lamotrigine	Neurological, Antiepileptic*
182. Atrovent HFA	ipratropium	Respiratory
183. Simcor	niacin	Cardiovascular, Antihyperlipidemic
184. Opana ER	oxymorphone	Analgesic, Opiate
185. Rhinocort Aqua	budesonide	Respiratory
186. Humalog Mix 75/25	insulin lispro protamine suspension mixed with soluble insulin lispro	Hormones & Modifiers, Insulin
187. Carafate	sucralfate	Gastrointestinal, Antacid/Antiulcer
188. Norvir	ritonavir	Anti-infective, Antiviral
189. Aspir-Low	aspirin and dipyridamole	Cardiovascular
190. BenzaClin	clindamycin and benzoyl peroxide	Dermatological
191. Skelaxin	metaxalone	Musculoskeletal, Muscle relaxant
192. Duac Care System	clindamycin and benzoyl peroxide	Dermatological
193. Wellbutrin XL	bupropion	Psychotropic, Antidepressant
194. Arthrotec	diclofenac and misoprostol	Analgesic, NSAID
195. Epiduo	adapalene and benzoyl peroxide	Dermatological
196. Pulmicort Flexhaler	budesonide	Respiratory
197. Omnaris	ciclesonide	Respiratory
198. Ortho Tri-Cyclen	norgestimate and ethinyl estradiol	Hormones & Modifiers, Contraceptive
199. Prandin	repaglinide	Hormones & Modifiers, Oral antidiabetic
200. Nevanac	nepafenac	Ophthalmic

TOP 50 CANADIAN DRUGS

Following is a list of the top 50 dispensed medication products in Canada cross-referenced with corresponding generic drug names and the classifications used in this text. Rankings are based on IMS Brograns' Top 50 Dispensed Medications in Canada, 2010 (available at http://www.imshealth.com/deployedfiles/ims/Global/North%20America/Canada/Home%20Page%20Content/Pharma%20Trends/Top50Dispensed_En_11.pdf).

Rank	Product	Generic Name	Classification
1.	Synthroid	levothyroxine sodium	Hormones & Modifiers, Thyroid
2.	Crestor	rosuvastatin	Cardiovascular, Antihyperlipidemic
3.	Lipitor	atorvastatin	Cardiovascular, Antihyperlipidemic
4.	Apo-Furosemide	furosemide	Cardiovascular, Antihypertensive*
5.	Teva-Amoxicillin	amoxicillin	Anti-infective
6.	Nexium	esomeprazole magnesium	Gastrointestinal, Antacid/Antiulcer
7.	Teva-Venlafaxine XR	venlafaxine	Psychotropic, Antidepressant
8.	Apo-Ramipril	ramipril	Cardiovascular, Antihypertensive*
9.	Apo-Hydro	hydrochlorothiazide	Cardiovascular, Antihypertensive*
10.	Plavix	clopidogrel	Cardiovascular
11.	Apo-Atorvastatin	atorvastatin	Cardiovascular, Antihyperlipidemic
12.	Teva-Rabeprazole	rabeprazole	Gastrointestinal, Antacid/Antiulcer
13.	Ativan	lorazepam	Psychotropic
14.	Coversyl	perindopril	Cardiovascular, Antihypertensive*
15.	Celebrex	celecoxib	Analgesic, NSAID
16.	Apo-Salvent CFC FR	salbutamol (albuterol)	Respiratory, Bronchodilator
17.	Sandoz-Bisoprolol	bisoprolol	Cardiovascular, Antihypertensive*
18.	Apo-Lorazepam	lorazepam	Psychotropic
19.	Avapro	irbesartan	Cardiovascular, Antihypertensive*
20.	Diovan	valsartan/hydrochlorothiazide	Cardiovascular, Antihypertensive*
21.	Eltroxin	levothyroxine sodium	Hormones & Modifiers, Thyroid
22.	Ratio-Lenoltec #3	codeine/acetaminophen/caffeine	Analgesic, Opiate
23.	Adalat XL	nifedipine	Cardiovascular, Antihypertensive*
24.	Nasonex	mometasone	Respiratory
25.	Ventolin HFA	salbutamol (albuterol)	Respiratory, Bronchodilator
26.	Ratio-Oxycocet	oxycodone/acetaminophen	Analgesic, Opiate
27.	Tylenol with Codeine #3	codeine/acetaminophen	Analgesic, Opiate

**An asterisk next to a drug's classification indicates there are additional common uses for that drug.*

Rank	Product	Generic Name	Classification
28.	Flovent HFA	fluticasone propionate	Respiratory
29.	Actonel	risedronate	Musculoskeletal, Osteoporotic
30.	Lyrica	pregabalin	Neurological
31.	Atacand	candesartan cilexitil	Cardiovascular, Antihypertensive*
32.	Ratio-Metformin	metformin HCl	Hormones & Modifiers, Oral antidiabetic
33.	Taro-Warfarin	warfarin sodium	Cardiovascular, Anticoagulant
34.	Pro-AAS EC-80	aspirin, delayed release	Analgesic, Salicylate*
35.	Ran-Pantoprazole	pantoprazole	Gastrointestinal, Antacid/Antiulcer
36.	Teva-Metoprolol	metoprolol tartrate	Cardiovascular, Antihypertensive*
37.	Cipralex	escitalopram	Psychotropic, Antidepressant
38.	Ezetrol	ezetimibe	Cardiovascular, Antihyperlipidemic
39.	Flomax CR	tamsulosin	Urinary
40.	Apo-Naproxen	naproxen	Analgesic, NSAID
41.	Apo-Prednisone	prednisone	Hormones & Modifiers, Adrenal corticosteroid
42.	Apo-Metformin	metformin HCl	Hormones & Modifiers, Oral antidiabetic
43.	Teva-Hydrochlorothiazide	hydrochlorothiazide	Cardiovascular, Antihypertensive*
44.	Coumadin	warfarin sodium	Cardiovascular, Anticoagulant
45.	Apo-Oxazepam	oxazepam	Psychotropic
46.	Alesse	levonorgestrel/ethinyl estradiol	Hormones & Modifiers, Oral contraceptive
47.	Diovan HCT	valsartan/hydrochlorothiazide	Cardiovascular, Antihypertensive*
48.	Apo-Metoprolol	metoprolol tartrate	Cardiovascular, Antihypertensive*
49.	Spiriva	tiotropium bromide	Respiratory
50.	Yasmin	drospirenone/ethinyl estradiol	Hormones & Modifiers, Oral contraceptive

COMMONLY REFRIGERATED DRUGS

Many products must be stored at refrigerated temperatures to ensure stability. Following is a list of commonly refrigerated drugs. As per the manufacturer's product information, some products need to be refrigerated immediately upon receipt from the manufacturer. Others may be stored at room temperature but will require refrigeration once reconstituted or when a diluent is added. A few drugs are stored in the refrigerator at the pharmacy but can be kept at room temperature when in use by the patient. For reconstituted products, the manufacturer will provide information as to how long the product is stable once reconstituted.

Brand Name & Dosage Form	Generic Name
ActHib vials	haemophilus b conjugate vaccine (tetanus toxoid conjugate)
Actimmune vials	interferon gamma-1b
Adacel vials	tetanus toxoid, reduced diphtheria toxoid, acellular pertussis vaccine adsorbed (Tdap) vaccine
Alcaine ophthalmic solution	proparacaine
Amoxil suspension	amoxicillin
Anectine vials	succinylcholine chloride
Aspirin Uniserts suppositories	aspirin
Atgam vials	lymphocyte immune globulin
Augmentin suspension	amoxicillin/clavulanic acid
Avonex syringes	interferon beta-1a
Azasite ophthalmic solution	azithromycin
BACiiM vials	bacitracin
Benzamycin gel	erythromycin/benzoyl peroxide
Bicillin syringes	penicillin G benzathine
Cardizem vials	diltiazem hydrochloride
Caverject vials	alprostadil
Ceftin suspension	cefuroxime axetil
Cefzil suspension	cefprozil
Cerebyx vials	fosphenytoin sodium
Cipro suspension	ciprofloxacin
Combipatch transdermal patch	estradiol/norethindrone
Copaxone	glatiramer acetate
DDAVP vials	desmopressin
Digibind vials	digoxin immune Fab
Enbrel syringes	etanercept
Engerix-B vials	hepatitis B vaccine
Epogen vials	epoetin alfa
Genotropin cartridges	somatropin
Havrix vials, syringes	hepatitis A vaccine
Hemabate vial	carboprost tromethamine
Humalog vials, pens	insulin lispro

Brand Name & Dosage Form	Generic Name
Humira syringes	adalimumab
Humulin R vials	regular insulin
Infergen vials	interferon alfacon-1
Kaletra solution, capsules	lopinavir/ritonavir
Lactinex tablets	lactobacillus acidophilus/bulgaricus
Lantus vials, pens	insulin glargine
Leukeran tablets	chlorambucil
Meruvax vials	rubella virus vaccine live
Methergine vials	methylergonovine maleate
Miacalcin nasal spray	calcitonin salmon
MMR II vials	measles, mumps, rubella virus vaccine live
Mycostatin pastilles	nystatin
Neupogen vials, syringes	filgrastim
Nimbex vials	cisatracurium besylate
Norditropin cartridges	somatropin
Norvir soft gels	ritonavir
Neulasta syringe	pegfilgrastim
Neurontin suspension	gabapentin
Pavulon	pancuronium bromide
Phenergan suppositories	promethazine
Pneumovax 23 vaccine	pneumococcal vaccine polyvalent
Premarin Secule® vials	conjugated estrogens
RabAvert vial	rabies vaccine
Rapamune solution	sirolimus
Rebetron	ribavirin/interferon alfa-2b
Regranex gel	becaplermin
Risperdal Consta kits	risperidone
Sandostatin vials	octreotide acetate
Survanta vials	beractant
Tamiflu suspension	oseltamivir phosphate
Thyrolar tablets	liotrix
Tracrium vials	atracurium besylate
Veetids suspension	penicillin V
VePesid capsules	etoposide
Vibramycin suspension	doxycycline
Viroptic ophthalmic solution	trifluridine
Xalatan ophthalmic solution	latanoprost
Zemuron vials	rocuronium bromide
Zithromax suspension	azithromycin

GLOSSARY

absolute bioavailability the bioavailability of a drug product compared to the same drug in the form of a rapidly administered IV solution.

absorption the movement of the drug from the dosage formulation to the blood.

abstracting services services that summarize information from various primary sources for quick reference.

active transport the movement of drugs from an area of lower concentration to an area of higher concentration; cellular energy is required.

acute condition a sudden condition requiring immediate treatment.

acute viral hepatitis an inflammatory condition of the liver caused by viruses.

additive a drug that is added to a parenteral solution.

additive effects the summation in effect when two drugs with similar pharmacological actions are taken.

admixture the resulting solution when a drug is added to a parenteral solution.

adverse drug effect/reaction an unintended side effect of a medication that is negative or in some way injurious to a patient's health.

agonists drugs that activate receptors to accelerate or slow normal cell function.

alimentary tract the organs from the mouth to the anus. The GI tract is a portion of the alimentary tract.

aliquot a portion of a mixture.

alveolar sacs (alveoli) the small sacs of specialized tissue that transfer oxygen out of inspired air into the blood and carbon dioxide out of the blood and into the air for expiration.

ampules sealed glass containers with an elongated neck that must be snapped off.

analgesia a state in which pain is not felt even though a painful condition exists.

anaphylactic shock a potentially fatal hypersensitivity reaction producing severe respiratory distress and cardiovascular collapse.

androgens male sex hormones.

anemia a decrease in hemoglobin or red blood cells.

anhydrous without water molecules.

anions negatively charged particles.

antagonists drugs that bind with receptors but do not activate them. They block receptor action by preventing other drugs or substances from activating them.

anthelmintics drugs that destroys worms.

antibiotic a substance that harms or kills microorganisms like bacteria and fungi.

antibiotic therapy a common home infusion service used for treating AIDS-related and other infections.

antidote a drug that antagonizes the toxic effect of another drug.

antihyperlipidemics drugs that lower cholesterol and triglyceride levels.

antipyretic reduces fever.

antitoxin a substance that acts against a toxin in the body; also, a vaccine containing antitoxins, used to fight disease.

antitussive a drug that acts against a cough.

aqueous water based.

arrest knob the knob on a balance that prevents any movement of the balance pans.

arrhythmia an abnormal heart rhythm.

aseptic techniques methods that maintain the sterile condition of products.

automated dispensing machine a device that dispenses medications at the point-of-use upon confirmation of an order that has been communicated from a centralized computer system.

automated filling machines automated machines that fill and label pill bottles with correct quantities of ordered drugs.

auxiliary labels labels regarding specific warnings, foods or medications to avoid, potential side effects, and other cautionary interactions.

bactericidal kills bacteria.

bacteriostatic retards bacteria growth.

batching preparation of large quantities of unit dose oral solutions/suspensions or small volume parenterals for future use.

bevel an angled surface at the tip of a needle.

bioavailability the amount of an administered dose that reaches the general circulation and the rate at which this occurs.

biocompatibility not irritating; does not promote infection or abscess.

bioequivalency the comparison of bioavailability between two dosage forms.

biopharmaceutics the study of the factors associated with drug products and physiological processes, and the resulting systemic concentrations of the drugs.

blocker another term for an antagonist drug, because antagonists block the action of neurotransmitters.

body surface area a measure used for dosage that is calculated from the height and weight of a person and measured in square meters.

bronchodilators a medication that decongests the bronchial tubes.

browser a software program that allows users to view websites on the World Wide Web.

buccal pouch between the cheek and teeth in the mouth.

buffer system ingredients in a formulation designed to control the pH.

bulk compounding log a record of medications that are compounded in the pharmacy for nonspecific patients. Information must include a list of all the ingredients, amounts used, manufacturer, lot numbers, and expiration dates of each specific ingredient.

calcium channel blockers drugs that lower blood pressure by relaxing blood vessels.

calibrate to set, mark, or check the graduations of a measuring device.

carcinogenicity the ability of a substance to cause cancer.

cardiac cycle the contraction and relaxation of the heart that pumps blood through the cardiovascular system.

cations positively charged particles.

central pharmacy the main in-patient pharmacy in a hospital that has pharmacy satellites. It is the place where most of the hospital's medications are prepared and stored.

certification a legal document certifying that an individual meets certain objective standards, usually provided by a neutral professional organization.

Chapter <795> regulations from USP–NF pertaining to compounding nonsterile formulations.

Chapter <797> regulations from USP–NF pertaining to compounding sterile formulations.

chronic condition a continuing condition that requires ongoing treatment for a prolonged period.

chyme the semiliquid form of food as it enters the intestinal tract.

cirrhosis a chronic liver disease causing loss of function.

clean room area designed for the preparation of sterile products.

closed formulary a limited list of approved medications.

clotting factors factors in the blood coagulation process.

CMS-1500 form the standard form used by health-care providers to bill for services, including disease state management services.

CMS-10114 form the standard form used by health-care providers to apply for a National Provider Identifier (NPI).

co-insurance an agreement for cost-sharing between the insurer and the insured.

co-pay the portion of the price of medication that the patient is required to pay.

code cart a locked cart of medications and other medical equipment designed for emergency use.

colloids particles up to a hundred times smaller than those in suspensions that are, however, likewise suspended in a solution.

Combat Methamphetamine Epidemic Act (CMEA) federal law that sets daily and monthly limits on OTC sale of pseudoephedrine and ephedrine.

combining vowel a vowel used to connect the prefix, root word, or suffix parts of a term.

competent being qualified and capable.

complexation when two different molecules associate or attach to each other.

compliance doing what is required.

compounded sterile preparation (CSP) a compounded sterile parenteral dosage form that will be parenterally administered.

compounding record a record of what actually happened when the formulation was compounded.

compression molding a method of making suppositories in which the ingredients are compressed in a mold.

concentration the strength of a solution as measured by the weight-to-volume or volume-to-volume of the substance being measured.

confidential the requirement of health-care providers to keep all patient information private along the patient, the patient's insurer, and the providers directly involved in the patient's care.

conjunctiva the eyelid lining.

conjunctivitis inflammation of the conjunctiva (eyelid lining).

consultant pharmacist develops and maintains an individual pharmaceutical plan for each long-term care patient.

controlled substance mark the mark (CII-CV) that indicates the control category of a drug with a potential for abuse.

controlled substances five groups of drugs identified by the 1970 Controlled Substances Act (CSA) as having the potential for abuse and whose distribution is therefore strictly controlled by five control schedules set forth in the CSA.

conversions changing one unit of measure into another so that both amounts are equal.

coring when a needle damages the rubber closure of a parenteral container causing fragments of the closure to fall into the container and contaminate its contents.

cornea the transparent outer part of the eye.

corticosteroid hormonal steroid substances produced by the cortex of the adrenal gland.

counting tray a tray designed for counting pills.

CPOE a system in which the physician or agent of the physician enters orders directly into the hospital computer system.

Current Procedural Terminology codes (CPT codes) identifiers used for billing pharmacist-provided MTM services.

GLOSSARY

DAW (dispense as written) mechanism by which a prescriber may indicate that the brand product, not the equivalent generic, must be dispensed.

data information that is entered into and stored in a computer system.

database a collection of information structured so that specific information within it can easily be retrieved and used.

DEA number required on all controlled drug prescriptions; identifies the prescriber.

deductible a set amount that must be paid by the patient for each benefit period before the insurer will cover additional expenses.

denominator the bottom or right number in a fraction.

depot the area in the muscle where a formulation is injected during an intramuscular injection.

depth filter a filter that can filter solutions being drawn into or expelled from a syringe, but not both ways in the same procedure.

dermatological a product used to treat a skin condition.

diabetes mellitus a condition in which the body does not produce enough insulin or is unable to use it efficiently.

dialysis movement of particles in a solution through permeable membranes.

diastolic phase the blood pressure after the heart has completed a pumping stroke.

diastolic pressure the minimum blood pressure when the heart relaxes; the second number in a blood pressure reading.

diluent a solvent that dissolves a freeze-dried powder or dilutes a solution.

disintegration the breaking apart of a tablet into smaller pieces.

displacement a drug that is bound to a plasma protein is removed when another drug of greater binding potential binds to the same protein.

disposition a term sometimes used to refer to all of the ADME processes together.

dissociation when a compound breaks down and separates into smaller components.

dissolution when the smaller pieces of a disintegrated tablet dissolve in solution.

distributive pharmacist makes sure long-term care patients receive the correct medications ordered.

diuretics drugs that increase the elimination of salts and water through urination.

drip rounds a process in which the pharmacy technician goes to specific nursing units to find out what IV drips will be needed later that day.

drug-diet interactions when elements of ingested nutrients interact with a drug and this affects the disposition of the drug.

drug recall voluntary or involuntary removal of a drug product by the manufacturer; usually pertaining to a particular shipment or lot number.

DSL a digital subscriber line that provides digital data transmission over the wires of a local phone network.

dual co-pay co-pays that have two prices: one for generic and one for brand medications.

dual marketing status of medications like Plan B® that are classified as both prescription and OTC drugs.

duration of action the time drug concentration is above the minimum effective concentration (MEC).

edema swelling from abnormal retention of fluid.

electrocardiogram (EKG or ECG) a graph of the heart's rhythms.

electrolytes a substance that in solution forms ions that conduct an electrical current.

electronic medical record (EMR) or electronic health record (EHR) a computerized patient medical record.

elimination the processes of metabolism and excretion.

embolism, embolus a clot that has traveled in the bloodstream to a point where it obstructs flow.

emergency drug procurement to quickly obtain a medication not currently in stock in the pharmacy in situations where the drug is urgently needed.

emulsifier a stabilizing agent in emulsions.

emulsions mixture of two liquids that do not mix with each other; one liquid is spread through the other by mixing and using an emulsifier for stability.

endocrine system a system of glands that secrete hormones into the bloodstream.

enteral a route of administration to any organ in the alimentary tract (i.e., from the mouth to the anus).

enterohepatic cycling the transfer of drugs and their metabolites from the liver to the bile in the gall bladder, and then into the intestine, and then back into circulation.

enzyme a complex protein that catalyzes chemical reactions.

enzyme induction the increase in hepatic enzyme activity that results in greater metabolism of drugs.

enzyme inhibition the decrease in hepatic enzyme activity that results in reduced metabolism of drugs.

epidural a sterile, preservative-free medication administered into a patient's epidural space (located near the spinal cord and backbone).

equivalent weight a drug's molecular weight divided by its valence; a common measure of electrolyte concentration.

estrogens female sex characteristic hormones that are involved in calcium and phosphorus conservation.

ethics a branch of philosophy that helps determine what should be done in a principled sense.

eustachian tube the tube that connects the middle ear to the throat.

exempt narcotics medications with habit-forming ingredients that can be dispensed by a pharmacist without a prescription to persons at least 18 years of age.

extemporaneous compounding the on-demand preparation of a drug product according to a physician's prescription, formula, or recipe, usually because the drug product is not available commercially.

extracellular fluid the fluid outside the body's individual cells found in plasma and tissue fluid.

fibrin the fiber that serves as the structure for clot formation.

fibrinogen Factor I.

final filter a filter that filters solution immediately before it enters a patient's vein.

finger cots protective coverings for fingers.

first-pass metabolism the substantial degradation of an orally administered drug caused by enzyme metabolism in the liver before the drug reaches the systemic circulation.

Flashball flexible rubber bulb near the needle adapter on an administration set; used to determine if the needle is properly placed in the veins.

flexor movement an expansion or outward movement by muscles.

flocculating agent electrolytes used in the preparation of suspensions to form particles that can be easily dispersed.

flow rate the rate (in ml/hour or ml/minute) at which solution is administered to the patient; also known as rate of administration.

Food and Drug Administration (FDA) a national regulatory body in the United States that oversees the approval, manufacture, and distribution of drugs for the safety of the public.

formulary a list of stocked drugs that have been selected based on therapeutic factors as well as cost; a list of medications approved for use.

formulation record formulas and procedures (i.e., recipes) for what should happen when a formulation is compounded.

fusion molding a suppository preparation method in which the active ingredients are dispersed or dissolved in a melted suppository base.

gastric emptying time the time a drug will stay in the stomach before it is emptied into the small intestine.

gauge a measurement with needles: the higher the gauge, the smaller the lumen.

geometric dilution a technique for mixing two powders of unequal quantity.

glaucoma abnormally high pressure within the eye leading to optic nerve damage and loss of vision.

glomerular filtration the blood filtering process of the nephron.

glucagon a hormone that helps convert amino acids to glucose.

gout a painful inflammatory condition in which excess uric acid accumulates in the joints.

Health Insurance Portability and Accountability Act (HIPAA) a federal act that, among other things, protects the privacy of individuals and the sharing of protected health information.

hematopoietics drugs used to treat anemia.

hemorrhoid painful swollen veins in the anal/rectal area, generally caused by strained bowel movements from hard stools.

hemostatic drugs drugs that prevent excessive bleeding.

HEPA filter a high-efficiency particulate air filter.

heparin lock an injection device used when a primary solution is not available.

HMOs a network of providers for which costs are covered inside but not outside of the network.

home care agencies home nursing care businesses that provide a range of health-care services, including infusion.

homeostasis the state of equilibrium of the body.

horizontal flow hood a laminar flow hood with horizontal air flow across the work area.

hormones chemicals produced by the body that regulate body functions and processes.

hub the part of the needle that attaches to the syringe.

human genome the complete set of genetic material contained in a human cell.

hydrates absorbs water.

hydrophilic capable of associating with or absorbing water.

hydrophilic emulsifier a stabilizing agent for water-based dispersion mediums.

hydrophobic water repelling; cannot associate with water.

hypersensitivity an abnormal sensitivity generally resulting in an allergic reaction.

hyperthyroidism a condition in which thyroid hormone secretions are above normal, often referred to as an overactive thyroid.

hypertonic when a solution has a greater osmolarity than that of blood.

hypothyroidism a condition in which thyroid hormone secretions are below normal, often referred to as an underactive thyroid.

hypotonic when a solution has a lesser osmolarity than that of blood.

idiosyncrasy an unexpected reaction the first time a drug is taken, generally due to genetic causes.

GLOSSARY

immiscible cannot be mixed.

infusion the gradual intravenous injection of a volume of fluid into a patient.

injectability the ease of flow when a suspension is injected into a patient.

injunction a court order preventing a specific action, such as the distribution of a potentially dangerous drug.

in-patient pharmacy a pharmacy located in a hospital that services only those patients in the hospital and its ancillary areas.

inspiration breathing in.

insulin a hormone that controls the body's use of glucose.

integumentary system the body covering, i.e., skin, hair, and nails.

Internet service provider (ISP) a company that provides access to the Internet.

interpersonal skills skills involving relationships between people.

interstitial fluid tissue fluid.

intracellular fluid cell fluid.

intraocular inside the eye.

intravenous piggyback (IVPB) a small volume parenteral that will be added into or "piggybacked" into a large volume parenteral (LVP).

inventory a list of goods or items a business uses in its normal operations.

ions molecular particles that carry electric charges.

irrigation solution large volume splash solutions used during surgical or urologic procedures to bathe and moisten body tissues.

Islands (or Islets) of Langerhans specialized cells of the pancreas that secrete insulin.

isotonic when a solution has an osmolarity equivalent to that of blood.

lacrimal canalicula the tear ducts.

lacrimal gland the gland that produces tears for the eye.

laminar flow continuous movement at a uniform rate in one direction.

least common denominator smallest possible denominator for an equivalent fraction so that two fractions can be added or subtracted and have the same denominator.

legend drug any drug that requires a prescription and either of these "legends" on the label: "Caution: Federal law prohibits dispensing without a prescription," or "Rx only."

levigation triturating a powder drug with a solvent in which it is insoluble to reduce its particle size.

liability legal responsibility for costs or damages arising from misconduct or negligence.

lipoidal fat like substance.

lipophilic emulsifier a stabilizing agent for oil-based dispersion mediums.

local effect when drug activity is at the site of administration.

look-alikes drug names that have similar appearance, particularly when written.

lumen the hollow center of a needle.

lymphocyte a type of white blood cell that helps the body defend itself against bacteria and diseased cells.

lyophilized freeze-dried.

maintenance medication a medication that is required on a continuing basis for the treatment of a chronic condition.

markup the difference between the retailer's sale price and their purchase price.

materia medica generally pharmacology, but also refers to the drugs in use (from the Latin *materia*, matter, and *medica*, medical).

Material Safety Data Sheets (MSDS) OSHA required notices for hazardous substances that provide hazard, handling, clean-up, and first aid information.

maximum allowable cost (MAC) the maximum price per tablet (or other dispensing unit) an insurer or PBM will pay for a given product.

Medicaid a federal-state program, administered by the states, providing health care for the needy.

Medicare a federal program providing health care to people with certain disabilities or who are age 65 and over; it includes basic hospital insurance, voluntary medical insurance, and voluntary prescription drug insurance.

Medicare Prescription Drug Improvement and Modernization Act federal legislation that created Medicare Part D and made allowance for Medicare recipients to receive Medicare medical coverage through private health insurance plans.

medication administration record (MAR) a form that tracks the medications administered to a patient.

medication order the form used to prescribe medications for patients in institutional settings.

Medication Therapy Management (MTM) services services provided to some Medicare beneficiaries who are enrolled in Medicare Part D and who are taking multiple medications or have certain diseases.

medullary paralysis an overdose of anesthesia that paralyzes the respiratory and heart centers of the medulla, leading to death.

membrane filter a filter that filters solution as the solution is expelled from the syringe.

meniscus the curved surface of a column of liquid.

metabolite the substance resulting from the body's transformation of an administered drug.

metastasis when cancer cells spread beyond their original site.

milliequivalent (**mEq**) the unit of measure for electrolytes in a solution.

mimetic another term for an agonist, because agonists imitate, or "mimic," the action of the neurotransmitter.

minimum effective concentration (**MEC**) the blood concentration needed for a drug to produce a response.

minimum toxic concentration (**MTC**) the upper limit of the therapeutic window. Drug concentrations above the MTC increase the risk of undesired effects.

miscible capable of being mixed together.

modem computer hardware that enables a computer to communicate through telephone lines.

molecular weight the sum of the atomic weights of a molecule.

mucilage a wet, slimy liquid formed as an initial step in the wet gum method.

mydriatics drugs that dilate the pupil.

myocardium heart muscle.

nasal cavity the cavity behind the nose and above the roof of the mouth that filters air and moves mucous and inhaled contaminants outward and away from the lungs.

nasal inhaler a device that aerosolizes a drug for nasal inhalation.

nasal mucosa the cellular lining of the nose.

National Drug Code (**NDC**) **number** the number assigned by the manufacturer of a drug to the specific strength, form, and packaging of a drug product.

national provider identifier (**NPI**) a code assigned to recognized health-care providers; needed to bill MTM services.

necrosis increase in cell death.

negligence failing to do something that should or must be done.

neoplasm a new and abnormal tissue growth, often referring to cancer cells.

nephron the functional unit of the kidneys.

nephrotoxicity the ability of a substance to harm the kidneys.

neuron the functional unit of the nervous system.

neurotransmitter chemicals released by nerves that interact with receptors to cause an effect.

nomogram a chart showing relationships between measurements.

non-formulary drugs not on the formulary which the physician can order; a physician may have to fill out a form stating why that particular drug is needed.

numerator the top or left number in a fraction.

nurses' station work station for medical personnel located on a nursing unit.

obstructive jaundice an obstruction of the bile duct that causes hepatic waste products and bile to accumulate in the liver.

off-label indication a use of a medication for an indication not approved by the FDA.

oil-in-water emulsion an emulsion in which oil is dispersed through a water base.

Omnibus Budget Reconciliation Act of 1990 (**OBRA '90**) federal legislation requiring pharmacists to provide counseling to Medicaid patients on all new prescriptions.

online adjudication the resolution of prescription coverage through the communication of the pharmacy computer with the third-party computer.

onset of action the time MEC is reached and the response occurs.

open formulary a system that allows the pharmacy to purchase any prescribed medication.

ophthalmic related to the eye.

"Orange Book" the common name for the FDA's *Approved Drug Products with Therapeutic Equivalence.*

osmosis the action in which a drug in a higher concentration solution passes through a permeable membrane to a lower concentration solution.

osmotic pressure a characteristic of a solution determined by the number of dissolved particles in it.

osseous tissue the rigid portion of the bone tissue.

osteoarthritis a disorder characterized by weight-bearing bone deterioration, decreasing range of motion, and causing pain and deformity.

outpatient pharmacy a pharmacy attached to a hospital that services patients who have left the hospital or who are visiting doctors in a hospital outpatient clinic.

over-the-counter (**OTC**) **drugs** medications that do not require a prescription but may be filled with a prescription.

panacea a cure-all (from the Greek *panakeia*, same meaning).

par amount of drug product that should be kept on the pharmacy shelf. Each drug product may have a different par value. Par levels may also be assigned to drug products in automated dispensing cabinets.

parenteral a route of administration to any organ outside of the alimentary tract (e.g., ophthalmic, dermal).

passive diffusion the movement of drugs from an area of higher concentration to lower concentration.

patient assistance programs manufacturer sponsored prescription drug programs for the needy.

GLOSSARY

pediatric having to do with the treatment of children.

percutaneous absorption the absorption of drugs through the skin, often for a systemic effect.

peristalsis the wavelike motion of the intestines that moves food through them.

peritoneal dialysis solution a solution placed in and emptied from the peritoneal cavity to remove toxic substances.

perpetual inventory a system that maintains a continuous record of every item in inventory so that it always shows the stock on hand.

personal inventory an assessment of one's personal characteristics, skills, qualities, etc.

pH the pH scale measures the acidity or the opposite (alkalinity) of a substance. 7 is the neutral midpoint of the scale, values below which represent increasing acidity, and above which represent increasing alkalinity.

pharmaceutical of or about drugs; also, a drug product.

pharmaceutical alternative drug products that contain the same active ingredient, but not necessarily in the same salt form, amount, or dosage form.

pharmaceutical equivalent drug products that contain identical amounts of the same active ingredient in the same dosage form.

pharmacogenomics a field of study that defines the hereditary basis of individual differences in absorption, distribution, metabolism, and excretion (the ADME processes).

pharmacognosy derived from the Greek words *pharmakon,* or drug, and *gnosis,* or knowledge; the study of physical, chemical, biochemical, and biological properties of drugs as well as the search for new drugs from natural sources.

pharmacology the study of drugs—their properties, uses, application, and effects (from the Greek *pharmakon*: drug, and *logos*: word or thought).

pharmacopeia an authoritative listing of drugs and issues related to their use.

pharmacy benefit managers companies that administer drug benefit programs.

pharmacy satellite a branch of the inpatient pharmacy responsible for preparing, dispensing, and monitoring medication for specific patient areas.

piggybacks small volume solutions connected to an LVP.

placebo an inactive substance given in place of a medication.

pneumatic tube a system that shuttles objects through a tube using compressed air as the force; commonly used in hospitals for delivery of medication.

point of sale system (POS) an inventory system in which the item is deducted from inventory as it is sold or dispensed.

positional notation a system used in Roman numerals whereby the position of the number signifies its mathematical value.

POS a network of providers where the patient's primary care physician must be a member and costs outside the network may be partially reimbursed.

potentiation when one drug with no inherent activity of its own increases the activity of another drug that produces an effect.

PPO a network of providers where costs outside the network may be partially reimbursed and the patient's primary care physician need not be a member.

prefix a modifying component of a term located before the other components of the term.

prescription an instruction from a medical practitioner that authorizes a patient to be issued a drug or device.

prescription drug benefit cards cards that contain third-party billing information for prescription drug purchases.

Prescription Drug Plans (PDPs) third-party programs for Medicare Part D.

primary emulsion the initial emulsion to which ingredients are added to create the final product.

primary literature original reports of clinical trials, research, and case studies; used for the most up-to-date information.

PRN order an order for medication to be administered only on an as needed basis (e.g., 1 tablet every 4-6 hours as needed for pain).

product labeling important associated information that is not on the the label of a drug product itself but is provided in the form of an insert, brochure, or other document.

professionals individuals who receive extensive and advanced levels of education before being allowed to practice, such as physicians and pharmacists.

progesterone a female sex characteristic hormone involved in ovulation prevention.

protease inhibitor an antiviral used for HIV and hepatitis C that blocks the enzyme responsible for viral replication.

protected health information (PHI) any personal information that could be used to identify an individual to their health history.

protein binding the attachment of a drug molecule to a plasma or tissue protein, effectively making the drug inactive, but also keeping it within the body.

protocol specific guidelines for practice.

punch method a method for filling capsules by repeatedly pushing or, "punching," the capsule into an amount of drug powder.

purchase order number the number assigned to each order for identification.

pyrogens chemicals produced by microorganisms that can cause pyretic (fever) reactions in patients.

qs ad the quantity needed to make a prescribed amount.

ready-to-mix a specially designed minibag where a drug is put into the SVP just prior to administration.

recall the action taken to remove a drug from the market and have it returned to the manufacturer.

receptor the cellular material located at the site of action that interacts with the drug.

reconstitute addition of water or other diluent to commercially made drug bottles or vials in order to make a solution or suspension from a premade powder form of the drug. This may include oral or parenteral products.

Red Flag Rule a set of provisions created by the Federal Trade Commission (FTC) to help prevent identity theft from patient billing accounts maintained by medical and financial institutions.

relative bioavailability the bioavailability of a drug product compared to the same drug in any other dosage form than a rapidly administered IV solution.

remission a state in which cancer cells are inactive.

reorder points minimum and maximum stock levels that determine when a reorder is placed and for how much.

restricted distribution medications having limited availability due to cost, manufacturing problems, or safety concerns. Typically pharmacies must ensure enrollment before obtaining the restricted drug.

retina the inner lining of the eye that translates light into nerve impulses.

rheumatoid arthritis a disease in which the body's immune system attacks joint tissue.

root word the base component of a term that gives a word its meaning and which may be modified by other components.

safety caps a child-resistant cap.

Schedule II drugs drugs that have a high potential for abuse or addiction but that also have safe and accepted medical uses; they require special handling.

scope of practice what individuals may and may not do in their jobs.

search engine software that searches the Web for information related to criteria entered by the user (e.g., Google, Bing, Yahoo!).

secondary literature general reference works based upon primary literature sources; used to find primary literature.

selective (action) the characteristic of a drug that makes its action specific to certain receptors and the tissues they affect.

sensitivity the amount of weight that will move the balance pointer one division mark on the marker plate.

serum glucose blood sugar.

shaft the stem of the needle that provides the overall length of the needle.

sharps needles, jagged glass or metal objects, or any items that might puncture or cut the skin.

shelf stickers stickers with bar codes that can be scanned for inventory identification.

short stability medication that will expire soon after preparation (e.g., within 1-6 hours after preparation).

signa the directions for use on the prescription that must be printed on the prescription label.

signature log a book or electronic signature capture technology that patients sign for the prescriptions they receive for legal and insurance purposes.

site of action the location where an administered drug produces an effect.

Slip-Tip®, Luer-Lok®, eccentric, oral different types of syringe tips.

solution a clear liquid made up of one or more substances dissolved in a solvent.

solvent a liquid that dissolves another substance in it.

sonication exposure to high-frequency sound waves.

spatulation mixing powders with a spatula.

stability the the extent to which a dosage form retains the same properties and characteristics it possessed when it was made.

standing order a standard medication order for patients to receive medication at scheduled intervals.

STAT order an order for medication to be administered immediately.

sterile a sterile condition is one which is free of all microorganisms, both harmful and harmless.

stratum corneum the outermost cell layer of the epidermis.

sublingual under the tongue.

suffix a modifying component of a term located after the other components of the term.

surgical anesthesia the stage of anesthesia in which surgery can be safely conducted.

suspensions formulations in which the drug does not completely dissolve in the liquid.

synergism when two drugs with similar pharmacological actions produce greater effects than the sum of the individual effects.

synthetic combining simpler chemicals into more complex compounds, creating a new chemical not found in nature as a result.

syringeability the ease with which a suspension can be drawn from a container into a syringe.

systemic effect when a drug is introduced into the venous (circulatory) system and carried to the site of activity.

systolic phase the blood pressure as the heart is pumping blood into the cardiovascular system.

systolic pressure the maximum blood pressure when the heart contracts; the first number in a blood pressure reading.

technicians individuals who are given a basic level of training designed to help them perform specific tasks.

teratogenecity the ability of a substance to cause abnormal fetal development when given to a pregnant woman.

tertiary literature condensed works based on primary literature, e.g., textbooks; used to find background information or a summary of information..

testosterone the primary androgen.

therapeutic equivalent pharmaceutical equivalents that produce the same effects in patients.

therapeutic interchange a policy approved by the hospital P&T Committee that allows the pharmacist to change a medication order to a therapeutically equivalent formulary medication.

therapeutic window a drug's blood concentration range between its minimum effective concentration and minimum toxic concentration.

thickening agent an ingredient used in the preparation of suspensions to increase the viscosity of the liquid.

thrombus a blood clot.

tier categories of medications that are covered by third-party plans.

topical hemostatics drugs used for minor bleeding when sutures are not appropriate.

total nutrient admixture (TNA) solution a TPN solution that contains intravenous fat emulsion. Administration of all nutrients intravenously, also known as hyperalimentation.

total parenteral nutrition (TPN) solution complex solutions with two base solutions (amino acids and dextrose) and additional micronutrients.

trade journals journals published commercially for pharmacists but not produced by the profession; they tend to contain large amounts of advertising material.

transaction window counter area designated for taking written prescriptions and dispensing completed prescription products.

transcorneal transport drug transfer into the eye.

trituration the process of grinding powders to reduce particle size.

turnover the rate at which inventory is used, generally expressed in number of days.

tympanic membrane the membrane that transmits sound waves to the inner ear.

uniform resource locator (URL) a Web address.

unit dose packaging a package containing a single dose of medication.

unit inspection a review of a nursing unit to ensure compliance with hospital medication policies.

unit price the price of a unit of medication, such as an ounce of liquid cold remedy.

universal claim form a standard claim form accepted by many insurers.

uricosuric drugs drugs used to treat gout that increase the elimination of uric acid.

usual and customary (U&C or UCR) the maximum amount of payment for a given prescription, determined by the insurer to be a usual and customary (and reasonable) price.

valence the number of positive or negative charges on an ion.

variable an unknown value in a mathematical equation.

vasodilators drugs that relax and expand the blood vessels.

vertical flow hood a laminar flow hood with vertical air flow across the work area.

viscosity the thickness of a liquid. A measure of a liquid's resistance to flow.

volumetric measures volume. Volumetric vessels are either TD (to deliver) or TC (to contain).

water-in-oil emulsion an emulsion in which water is dispersed through an oil base.

water soluble the property of a substance being able to dissolve in water.

waters of hydration water molecules that attach to drug molecules.

wheal a raised, blister-like area on the skin caused by an intradermal injection.

workers' compensation an employer compensation program for employees accidentally injured on the job.

World Wide Web (WWW) a collection of electronic documents at Internet addresses called websites.

zone of turbulence an area of blocked air flow in a laminar flow hood.

ANSWER KEY

Chapter 1

Match the Terms

1. d
2. c
3. h
4. e
5. f
6. i
7. b
8. j
9. g
10. a

Multiple Choice

1. c
2. b
3. b
4. b
5. a
6. b
7. d
8. c
9. c
10. a
11. d
12. c
13. a
14. c
15. a
16. a
17. b
18. c
19. d
20. c
21. d
22. c
23. a
24. c
25. b
26. d
27. d
28. c

Critical Thinking

1. Dolly, as the first cloned mammal, called into questions the ethics of cloning. While her birth showed an adult sheep cell could be used to create an embryo that would develop into another adult sheep, Dolly had many health problems and was put down at a young age due to health problems.
2. Artificial DNA may lead to scientific advances that could help design and create new living things. Some critics worry about safety and about the role of scientists in creating new life.
3. A career as a pharmacy technician in a hospital pharmacy can lead to an abundance of possible working opportunities since hospitals are widely found in different kinds of cities and communities. Pharmacy technicians in hospitals have important duties and roles that are available for inpatient and outpatient pharmacies.

Chapter 2

Match the Terms

1. e
2. d
3. c
4. b
5. g
6. a
7. f

Multiple Choice

1. d
2. b
3. c
4. c
5. d
6. b
7. b
8. d
9. b
10. a
11. c
12. d
13. d
14. a
15. a
16. a
17. a
18. d
19. b
20. b
21. b
22. c
23. d
24. c
25. c
26. d
27. c

Critical Thinking

1. There are many important details associated with the work of pharmacy technicians, especially when filling prescriptions. Any small mistake or oversight could cause a patient to receive the incorrect medication or dose. Everyone working in health care must pay close attention to details, especially in pharmacies.
2. The most commonly used computer skill is data entry for processing prescriptions. Pharmacy technicians also can use skills with billing and reimbursement programs, and other programs used when providing care services to patients.
3. Certification is sometimes required by state law. Certification provides one piece of evidence for job qualifications. To remain certified, technicians must complete continuing education, so certification also provides evidence of efforts to maintain current knowledge.

Chapter 3

Match the Terms

1. o
2. i
3. r
4. h
5. n
6. f
7. s
8. a
9. p
10. b
11. e
12. c
13. k
14. l
15. j
16. d
17. q
18. g
19. m

Multiple Choice

1. b
2. c
3. d
4. b
5. b
6. c
7. b
8. c
9. a
10. d
11. b
12. d
13. a
14. a
15. b
16. c
17. c
18. b
19. b
20. b
21. a
22. a
23. b
24. b
25. a
26. a
27. d

Critical Thinking

1. Phase 1 trials are conducted on a small number of people to mainly test for safety and they last several months. Phase 2 trials test more patients for a longer period of time for short-term safety and effectiveness. Phase 3 trials test even more patients for one to four years to determine dosage in addition to testing safety and effectiveness.
2. Pharmaceutical equivalents are the identical drug in the same dosage form. Therapeutic equivalents are pharmaceutical equivalents that have been

ANSWER KEY

additionally tested for producing the same effects when taken.

3. In pharmacy, we work together toward the best health outcomes for our patients. The first principle reminds us that above all, the health and safety of our patients must come first.

Chapter 4

Match the Terms: I

1. d
2. g
3. p
4. n
5. w
6. a
7. h
8. o
9. y
10. f
11. j
12. v
13. r
14. k
15. q
16. m
17. x
18. b
19. u
20. e
21. l
22. i
23. c
24. s
25. t

Match the Terms: II

1. a
2. c
3. e
4. d
5. h
6. f
7. g
8. i
9. b

Match the Terms: III

1. b
2. e
3. c
4. d
5. j
6. k
7. h
8. a
9. f
10. g
11. i
12. l

Fill in the Meaning

1. abnormally rapid heart action
2. pertaining to the glands that secrete hormones into the bloodstream
3. liver tumor
4. through the skin
5. a disease in which the blood does not clot normally
6. chronic pain in the muscles
7. difficulty in speaking
8. cancerous bone tumor
9. menstrual pain
10. inability to produce sperm
11. chest pain
12. inflammation of the kidney
13. partial hearing loss
14. drooping of upper eyelid

Multiple Choice

1. b
2. b
3. c
4. b
5. d
6. b
7. a
8. b
9. d
10. d
11. d
12. b
13. b
14. d
15. c
16. c
17. c
18. d
19. a
20. a
21. b
22. a
23. b
24. d
25. b
26. b
27. b
28. c
29. c

Critical Thinking

1. A prefix + root word; a root + suffix; a prefix + root word + suffix; a root word + root word; a prefix + suffix

2. If you always spoke or wrote the entire set of words that the abbreviation stood for, you would waste time. Since health care professionals have very little time with each patient, you need to understand abbreviations and know how to use them to be an effective participant.

Chapter 5

Match the Terms: I

1. d
2. f
3. c
4. b
5. a
6. g
7. e
8. h

Match the Terms: II

1. i
2. b
3. d
4. l
5. j
6. a
7. o
8. p
9. f
10. e
11. m
12. n
13. g
14. k
15. c
16. h

Multiple Choice

1. c
2. b
3. a
4. c
5. d
6. a
7. d
8. c
9. b
10. b
11. b
12. a
13. a
14. a
15. d
16. b
17. c
18. a
19. c
20. d

Critical Thinking

1. The HIPAA privacy rule protects privacy by prohibiting the inappropriate disclosure of protected health information (PHI), such as Mr. Hoyt's prescription information, while at the same time allowing the sharing of PHI as needed for patient care and billing purposes. Thus, it would be appropriate for the pharmacy to share Mr. Hoyt's last fill date with the prescriber under certain circumstances. Kyle should refer the call to the pharmacist so he/she can assess whether sharing Mr. Hoyt's blood pressure medication with his prescriber's office is appropriate.

2. Amy has identified what may be an altered prescription. Altered prescriptions are considered forgeries and should be reported to the pharmacist for evaluation and possible action. Under no circumstances should Amy mention the reason for checking with the pharmacist—

discussing any aspect of a potentially forged prescription with a patient is strictly the responsibility of the pharmacist.

3. Marie has noticed a drug utilization review, or edit, message (DUR/DUE) while filling a prescription. DUR messages appear when there is a potential clinical issue, or other issue, with the drug being filled. Typically the concern is between the new drug and an earlier drug or the patient's health conditions. Marie must follow her pharmacy's protocol for managing DUR edits. In some pharmacies she would need to call the pharmacist and not proceed until the pharmacist has reviewed and signed off on the message. In other pharmacies, protocol may allow Marie to print out the message and keep it with the prescription for the pharmacist to review during his/her final check.

Chapter 6

p. 121

1. XVIII
2. LXIV
3. LXXII
4. CXXVI
5. C
6. VII
7. XXVIII
8. 33
9. 110
10. 1,100
11. 1.5
12. 19
13. 24
14. 14 capsules
15. 9 drops
16. 48 tablets
17. 21 tablets

p. 123

1. 0.33
2. 0.5
3. 0.25
4. 0.3
5. 0.1
6. 5/1
7. 3/2
8. 5/2
9. 9/2
10. 15/1

p. 124

1. 2/4 = 1/2
2. 8/8 = 1
3. 1/5
4. 4/8 = 1/2
5. 5/5 = 1
6. 4/8 = 1/2
7. 9/20
8. 7/15
9. 7/16
10. 3/8

p. 125

1. 1/16
2. 3/24 = 1/8
3. 2/9
4. 15/64
5. 2/3
6. 4/12 = 1/3
7. 10/5 = 2
8. 24/24 = 1

p. 126

1. 1.3
2. 7.4
3. 4.34
4. 23.798
5. 72.31
6. 4.6926
7. 276.096
8. 359.3404
9. 230.4465
10. 5288.5529

p. 127

1. -0.16
2. 8.63
3. 14.29
4. 0.9726
5. 71.965
6. 14.592
7. 251.1229
8. 20.6699
9. 459.8842
10. 368.32

p. 128

1. 0.35
2. 0.32
3. 0.09
4. 0.15
5. 22.2
6. 0.159
7. 0.144
8. 0.0264
9. 581.0248
10. 382.6764

p. 133

1. mcg
2. l or L
3. ml or mL
4. g
5. mg
6. kg
7. 1,000
8. 1,000
9. 129.6
10. 1,000
11. 0.001
12. 0.001

p. 133

1. 7,000
2. 3,200
3. 0.0648
4. 30
5. 300
6. 7,000
7. 437.5
8. 1.1
9. 2
10. 1
11. 32
12. 0.25

p. 143

1. 2 ml
2. 8 ml
3. 75 ml
4. 2.08 ml/mn
5. 4.8 ml

p. 145

1. 60%
2. 80%
3. 12%
4. .5
5. .125
6. .99
7. 35 g
8. 52.5 g
9. 14 g
10. 50 ml
11. 70 ml
12. 20 ml
13. 0.12%

p. 150

1. 73.5 ml Amin. 8.5%
2. 37.5 ml dext 50%
3. 2 ml KCl
4. 0.45 ml Ca Gl
5. 5 ml Ped MVI
6. 131.55 mL sterile water is needed

p. 161

1. $45.76
2. $18.40
3. $11.50
4. $328.38
5. $27.05

p. 161

1. $8.54
2. $17.49
3. $37.24
4. $94.90
5. $122.09
6. $8.09
7. $16.64
8. $35.37
9. $8.91
10. $162.50

p. 163

1. gross $24.46
net $18.46
2. gross $17.18
net $11.18
3. gross $19.90
net $13.90
4. gross $29.31
net $23.31
5. gross $23.63
net $17.63
6. gross $31.39
net $25.39
7. gross $54.06
net $48.06
8. gross $6.71
net $0.71
9. gross $25.59
net $19.59
10. gross $22.63
net $16.63

ANSWER KEY

Self-Test

Match the Terms: I

1. g
2. e
3. f
4. a
5. c
6. d
7. b

Match the Terms: II

1. g
2. b
3. a
4. e
5. d
6. f
7. c

Multiple Choice

1. b
2. c
3. b
4. c
5. c
6. b
7. c
8. c
9. a
10. c
11. b
12. a
13. c
14. c
15. a
16. b
17. b
18. b
19. b
20. d
21. a
22. d
23. d
24. b
25. b
26. b
27. c
28. c
29. c

Conversion Exercise

1. 5,000 mg
2. 10,000 g
3. 0.3 l
4. 0.6 g
5. 0.12 mg
6. 224.4 lb
7. 2,200 g
8. 0.473 l
9. 65.9 kg
10. 10,000 mg

Problems

1. 7.8°C
2. 2 ml
3. 2.5 ml
4. 143 ml Dext 70% and 357 ml sterile water

Critical Thinking

1. The metric system is the major system of measurement used in medicine.
2. Electrolytes come in different salt forms and the dosage for different salt forms is not equivalent by weight measures. Examples are KCl and K Acetate for potassium and also NaCl and Na Acetate for sodium. To assure the correct dose for an electrolyte such as potassium or sodium, that could sometimes be administered in different salt forms, mEq are used.
3. The relatively small size of children along with their stage of development makes accurate dosing especially critical. Overdoses of medicine in children can have serious or even fatal consequences, so extreme care is absolutely necessary.

Chapter 7

Match the Terms: I

1. p
2. d
3. l
4. f
5. b
6. k
7. o
8. r
9. j
10. h
11. v
12. w
13. x
14. c
15. g
16. a
17. i
18. q
19. n
20. m
21. e
22. s
23. t
24. u

Match the Terms: II

1. l
2. c
3. b
4. g
5. m
6. a
7. j
8. e
9. h
10. f
11. d
12. k
13. i

Multiple Choice

1. b
2. a
3. d
4. c
5. d
6. c
7. b
8. a
9. c
10. c
11. b
12. b
13. a
14. c
15. a
16. c
17. c
18. d
19. b
20. d
21. b
22. c
23. c
24. a
25. a
26. a
27. c

Critical Thinking

1. Pure drugs are rarely administered by themselves. One reason is that a particular route of administration may allow the drug in only one dosage form, but the pure drug is not in that state. For example, a route may only allow solution dosage forms, but the pure drug is a powder. Also, dosage forms make it possible to make modified release products while the pure drug alone would not be extended release. Finally, pure drugs are used in small amounts, which would be hard for patients to use—dosage forms add bulk so the patient can handle the dosage form easily.
2. Systemic effects involve the total body while local effects involve only the site where the dosage form is administered. With a local effect, you get the desired drug action without causing side effects in the rest of the body.
3. This is the least expensive and most convenient route of administration. The patient does not require skilled assistance to take the dosage forms. The dosage forms are not required to be sterile.

Chapter 8

Match the Terms: I

1. h
2. b
3. c
4. i
5. a
6. d
7. g

8. k
9. j
10. m
11. e
12. f
13. l

Match the Terms: II

1. a
2. r
3. q
4. p
5. s
6. d
7. c
8. b
9. l
10. m
11. o
12. f
13. i
14. h
15. e
16. j
17. n
18. g
19. k

Multiple Choice

1. b
2. b
3. d
4. a
5. d
6. d
7. d
8. a
9. a
10. a
11. c
12. c
13. d
14. b
15. d
16. d
17. c
18. a
19. d
20. c
21. c
22. b
23. c
24. b
25 d
26. d
27. a

Critical Thinking

1. One dosage form or route of administration does not meet all the requirements that individual patients will have.
2. These are the two fundamental operations that are needed to obtain the correct amount of the active drug and other ingredients for the compound. If these operations are not correctly done, then the preparation is not correct.
3. This is the only way to ensure a homogenous blend of the powders.
4. If the product is no longer stable, it may not have the correct amount of the active drug and/or some ingredients may have degraded into an undesirable component.

Chapter 9

Match the Terms: I

1. i
2. g
3. a
4. j
5. f
6. d
7. h
8. m
9. k
10. e
11. c
12. l
13. b

Match the Terms: II

1. p
2. j
3. r
4. d
5. w
6. c
7. q
8. i
9. h
10. f
11. n
12. g
13. o
14. s
15. k
16. t
17. a
18. l
19. u
20. m
21. v
22. e
23. b

Match the Terms: III

1. h
2. d
3. e
4. g
5. f
6. b
7. c
8. a
9. i

Multiple Choice

1. d
2. d
3. b
4. d
5. b
6. b
7. c
8. b
9. d
10. c
11. c
12. c
13. d
14. b
15. a
16. d
17. d
18. a
19. a
20. d

Critical Thinking

1. Air coming out of the hood mixes with the air in the room adjacent to the opening of the hood. If work is done 6 inches inside the hood, then only the laminar air flow reaches the materials.
2. A TNA solution has intravenous fat emulsion as one of its ingredients. If a smaller pore size filter is used (i.e., less than 1.2 micron), the emulsion droplets will be filtered out of the TNA solution, and will not be available to produce a therapeutic benefit.
3. When the ampule is opened, there is the possibility that glass shards will dislodge from the neck of the ampule and fall into the drug solution. A filter needle will trap any such particles as the solution is withdrawn from the ampule.

Chapter 10

Match the Terms: I

1. u
2. q
3. p
4. r
5. s
6. d
7. c
8. o
9. n
10. m
11. l
12. k
13. j
14. b
15. i
16. a
17. h
18. g
19. f
20. e
21. t

Match the Terms: II

1. j
2. f
3. i
4. k
5. g
6. c
7. n
8. l
9. a
10. b
11. o
12. d

ANSWER KEY

13. e
14. m
15. h

Multiple Choice

1. a
2. c
3. d
4. b
5. b
6. a
7. d
8. c
9. c
10. c
11. b
12. a
13. d
14. a
15. a
16. c
17. b
18. c
19. b
20. a
21. b
22. b
23. d
24. c

Critical Thinking

1. The blood concentration-time data for these drugs reflects the drug concentration at the site of action. So if the blood concentrations are within the therapeutic window, you can be sure the response at the site of action is a desired therapeutic response. From a cost standpoint, it is not feasible to monitor every drug. But some drugs are more critical to monitor than others, and these are examples of those drugs.

2. Giving an antagonist for long periods of time causes the body to make more receptors or to increase the sensitivity of the receptors. When an antagonist is stopped abruptly, there is an over abundance of receptors or the receptors are hypersensitive. Therefore, if an agonist is given shortly after abruptly stopping the antagonist, there will be a very strong reaction to the agonist, which can cause a severe rebound reaction.

3. Glomerular filtration and secretion transport drug into the urine. Drug is removed from the urine when it is reabsorbed, and is therefore not excreted from the body, but is returned to the systemic circulation where it can again undergo all three processes. This cycling continues until there is no remaining drug to be excreted.

Chapter 11

Match the Terms

1. j
2. f
3. p
4. c
5. h
6. e
7. i
8. a
9. r
10. k
11. t
12. s
13. b
14. m
15. n
16. d
17. l
18. o
19. q
20. g

Multiple Choice

1. c
2. d
3. b
4. c
5. a
6. c
7. c
8. d
9. b
10. b
11. c
12. d
13. d
14. c
15. d
16. a
17. d
18. c
19. d
20. c
21. a
22. a
23. c
24. d
25. c
26. a
27. b

Critical Thinking

1. Many physiological changes occur at different ages, with different genders, and with family genetics, all of which will influence the disposition of drugs. Also, several disease states influence the disposition of drugs.

2. Adverse drug reactions are the result of taking only one drug. Drug-drug interactions are the result of taking two or more drugs.

3. Some drugs influence through other mechanisms besides direct contact with a second drug. For example, a drug may modify a disease state, which in turn will influence the disposition of a second drug.

Chapter 12

Match the Terms

1. c
2. j
3. d
4. f
5. l
6. i
7. a
8. g
9. h
10. b
11. k
12. e

Multiple Choice

1. b
2. b
3. a
4. d
5. b
6. b
7. b
8. c
9. c
10. c
11. d
12. b
13. b
14. a
15. a
16. b
17. d
18. b
19. a
20. b
21. c
22. a
23. b
24. c
25. a

Critical Thinking

1. You should tell the sales rep that HIPAA prohibits sharing patient specific health information and direct them to the pharmacy supervisor/manager/director.

2. You can determine the therapeutic equivalence of a brand and generic drug by using the "Orange Book." You find that phenytoin is a nonequivalent generic medication. Verify this information with the supervising pharmacist.

3. Refer the new pharmacy technician to the 21 Code of Federal Regulations or the State's Uniform Controlled Substance Act. The federal requirements state narcotic records should be kept by the registrant and available for 2 years.

4. One of the most commonly used references for this type of information is the *Red Book*. In the *Red Book* you will find the manufacturer of gelatin capsules and an approximate price.
5. Suggest that your friend check the *Occupational Outlook Handbook* for pharmacy tech job outlook and PTCB's website for pharmacy tech training and certification information.

Chapter 13

Match the Terms

1. m
2. b
3. f
4. n
5. k
6. g
7. a
8. j
9. d
10. h
11. e
12. l
13. c
14. i

Multiple Choice

1. a
2. b
3. a
4. b
5. b
6. c
7. c
8. c
9. a
10. d
11. b
12. a
13. a
14. a
15. b
16. c
17. b
18. b
19. d
20. b
21. a
22. d
23. c
24. c
25. d
26. d
27. a
28. d
29. b
30. a
31. b

Critical Thinking

1. Ask if another staff member recently put the medication on the shelf. Look at the package insert and review the storage requirements. If stored outside the storage requirements, contact the manufacture and see if they will accept its return. If not, let the pharmacist know and discard the product. Bottom line, you cannot dispense the medication if unsure of storage conditions.
2. Controlled substances, especially C-II's, require specific documentation when ordered and checked in. You should question your coworker or bring it to the attention to the pharmacist on duty.
3. Orders with your suppliers require good understanding of inventory controls and processes for your store or hospital. Make sure you are following the min/max numbers on the shelves or the recommended order points set in the computer. Excessive stock is costly for the pharmacy to carry.

Chapter 14

Match the Terms: I

1. i
2. n
3. e
4. b
5. m
6. g
7. f
8. o
9. h
10. c
11. d
12. j
13. k
14. l
15. a

Match the Terms: II

1. d
2. a
3. f
4. g
5. e
6. i
7. j
8. c
9. b
10. h

Multiple Choice

1. a
2. a
3. c
4. b
5. b
6. a
7. b
8. a
9. b
10. a
11. b
12. a
13. a
14. d
15. d
16. b
17. c
18. a
19. a
20. c
21. c
22. d
23. d

Critical Thinking

1. Pharmacy technicians are trained to handle billing and reimbursement. Billing and reimbursement does not require the expertise of a pharmacist. With experience, technicians can develop valuable knowledge and skills in this area.
2. Pharmacies do not receive payment for rejected claims. Technicians are able to develop expert knowledge and skills for resolving rejected claims.
3. People with Medicare Part D have coverage for prescriptions, which saves them money. Additionally, Medicare Part D allows some patients to receive MTM services provided by pharmacists; these patients can therefore have better outcomes from their prescriptions.

Chapter 15

Match the Terms

1. j
2. f
3. k
4. e
5. l
6. a
7. h
8. o
9. m
10. n
11. c
12. i
13. g
14. b
15. d

Multiple Choice

1. d
2. a
3. d
4. c
5. d
6. b
7. b
8. c
9. d
10. a
11. b
12. d
13. d
14. b
15. d
16. d
17. c
18. a

ANSWER KEY

19. c
20. a
21. a
22. d
23. a
24. d
25. c
26. c
27. d
28. c
29. b

Critical Thinking

1. Because patients may have the same name, the technician should ask for the patient's date of birth and address to confirm they are working with the correct patient profile.
2. The technician should enter the prescription into the computer system and generate a prescription label. Next the technician should retrieve the drug from the stock bottle and pour 150 ml into a 6 ounce amber bottle (holds up to 180 ml). Finally the technician will need to affix the label to the prescription bottle.
3. The technician would start by pouring out tablets from the stock bottle onto the counting tray. Next the technician would use a spatula to count the tablets by three or five at a time into the cylinder at the left of the counting tray. The technician would return any extra pills back to the stock bottle using the slide at the upper right corner of the tray. Finally, the technician would slide the 90tablets in the cylinder into a prescription vial.

Chapter 16

Match the Terms: I

1. c
2. e
3. f
4. d
5. b
6. h
7. o
8. l
9. k
10. n
11. i
12. a
13. m
14. g
15. j

Match the Terms: II

1. s
2. r
3. q
4. a
5. m
6. n
7. g
8. b
9. d
10. e
11. f
12. h
13. i
14. j
15. k
16. p
17. c
18. l
19. o

Multiple Choice

1. b
2. c
3. a
4. b
5. d
6. c
7. d
8. a
9. d
10. b
11. b
12. d
13. a
14. a
15. d
16. c
17. c
18. b
19. c
20. d
21. b
22. b
23. b

Critical Thinking

1. The order for meropenem must be approved by the Infectious Disease Service before the pharmacy can dispense it.
2. The pharmacy technician should: 1) Check if there is a current order for the medication; 2) Ask the nurse if she checked the correct area for the medication (e.g., refrigerator, automated dispensing system); 3) Check when the medication was last dispensed from the pharmacy; 4) Check to see if the patient transferred from another unit recently.
3. According to HIPAA, workers should never look at a patient's chart or computer profile unless specifically required to fulfill an assigned task. Kelly should tell her coworker she cannot look up her brother's labs because that would be a violation of HIPAA and could put her at risk of disciplinary action and even termination of her job.

Chapter 17

Match the Terms: I

1. b
2. c
3. d
4. a

Match the Terms: II

1. a
2. d
3. c
4. b

Multiple Choice

1. a
2. a
3. c
4. a
5. b
6. b
7. c
8. d
9. a
10. a
11. a
12. d
13. a
14. c
15. b
16. b
17. d
18. c
19. a
20. c
21. c
22. c
23. b

Critical Thinking

1. Mail order pharmacies send medications in situations where the need for medication is known in advance, usually for chronic conditions.
2. Pharmacy services for long-term care facilities include providing medications as well as clinical services. Long-term care facilities include nursing homes, psychiatric institutions, chronic disease, and rehabilitation facilities.
3. Home infusion services allow for IV medications to be administered to patients in their homes. A home care team works together to provide care to the patient.

Chapter 18

Match the Terms: I

1. c
2. r
3. p
4. v
5. e
6. d
7. f
8. g
9. b
10. w
11. l

12. m
13. a
14. t
15. h
16. u
17. i
18. j
19. q
20. s
21. k
22. o
23. n

Match the Terms: II

1. e
2. c
3. g
4. m
5. o
6. j
7. a
8. s
9. q
10. h
11. d
12. f
13. p
14. n
15. l
16. i
17. b
18. w
19. r
20. t
21. k
22. u
23. v
24. x

Match the Terms: III

1. f
2. i
3. d
4. e
5. a
6. h
7. c
8. j
9. g
10. b

Matching Drug Names: I

1. d
2. c
3. b.
4. i
5. a
6. e
7. g
8. h
9. f

Matching Drug Names: II

1. c
2. h
3. b
4. f
5. *g*
6. *j*
7. *a*
8. *i*
9. *e*
10. *d*

Matching Drug Names: III

1. *b*
2. *a*
3. *c*
4. *g*
5. *h*
6. *i*
7. *e*
8. *d*
9. *j*
10. *f*

Matching Drug Names: IV

1. *b*
2. *c*
3. *d*
4. *e*
5. *a*
6. *h*
7. *g*
8. *f*

Matching Drug Names: V

1. *b*
2. *f*
3. *a*
4. *e*
5. *d*
6. *c*

Matching Drug Names: VI

1. *a*
2. *g*
3. *e*
4. *f*
5. *b*
6. *d*
7. *c*

Matching Drug Names: VII

1. *b*
2. *g*
3. *h*
4. *a*
5. *k*
6. *d*
7. *c*
8. *j*
9. *i*
10. *f*
11. *e*

Matching Drug Names: VIII

1. *c*
2. *b*
3. *f*
4. *i*
5. *e*
6. *d*
7. *a*
8. *h*
9. *g*

Matching Drug Names: IX

1. *b*
2. *c*
3. *e*
4. *d*
5. *a*

Matching Drug Names: X

1. *a*
2. *g*
3. *d*
4. *j*
5. *i*
6. *e*
7. *f*
8. *h*
9. *b*
10. *c*

Multiple Choice

1. c
2. c
3. a
4. a
5. a
6. b
7. c
8. a
9. d
10. b
11. d
12. a
13. c
14. a
15. a
16. c
17. b
18. d
19. a
20. c
21. b
22. d
23. a
24. d
25. b
26. b
27. a
28. a
29 a
30 d

Critical Thinking

1. Proprietary drug names are designed by the manufacturer and can be useful to help promote the drug. Often the manufacturer will create a proprietary name that is easily associated with the condition or disease it is meant to treat. This sometimes serves as encouragement for prescribers to write prescriptions for the drug.
2. Drugs can be classified by chemical structure, how or where the drugs work in the body, as well as diseases or conditions they are used to treat. Some drugs can be used to treat more than one disease or condition.

INDEX A-ANTI

B

E

N